Br

Quality of Life

To
Tessa and Emma Fayers
and
Christine Machin

Quality of Life

The assessment, analysis and reporting
of patient-reported outcomes

Third Edition

PETER M. FAYERS

*Institute of Applied Health Sciences, University of Aberdeen School of Medicine and
Dentistry, Scotland, UK and
Department of Cancer Research and Molecular Medicine, Norwegian University of
Science and Technology (NTNU), Trondheim, Norway*

and

DAVID MACHIN

*Medical Statistics Group, School of Health and Related Research, University of
Sheffield, Sheffield, UK and
Department of Cancer Studies and Molecular Medicine, University of Leicester,
Leicester, UK*

WILEY Blackwell

This edition first published 2016 © 2016 by John Wiley & Sons, Ltd
Second edition published 2007 © 2007 by John Wiley & Sons, Ltd

Registered office: John Wiley & Sons, Ltd, The Atrium, Southern Gate, Chichester, West Sussex,
PO19 8SQ, UK

Editorial offices: 9600 Garsington Road, Oxford, OX4 2DQ, UK
The Atrium, Southern Gate, Chichester, West Sussex, PO19 8SQ, UK
111 River Street, Hoboken, NJ 07030-5774, USA

For details of our global editorial offices, for customer services and for information about how
to apply for permission to reuse the copyright material in this book please see our website at
www.wiley.com/wiley-blackwell

A catalogue record for this book is available from the Library of Congress and British Library.

ISBN 9781444337952 (cloth)

Wiley also publishes its books in a variety of electronic formats. Some content that appears in print may not be
available in electronic books.

Cover image: © istockphoto/bopp63

Set in 10.5/12.5pt Times LT Std by Aptara Inc., New Delhi, India
Printed and bound in Malaysia by Vivar Printing Sdn Bhd

1   2016

Contents

7   Item response theory and differential item functioning   189

8   Item banks, item linking and computer-adaptive tests   223

Preface to the third edition

When the first edition of this book was published in 2000, the assessment of quality of life (QoL) as an important outcome in clinical trials and other research studies was, at best, controversial. More traditional endpoints were the norm – measures such as disease status, cure and patient's survival time dominated in research publications. How times have changed. Nowadays it is generally accepted that the patients' perspective is paramount, patient representatives are commonly involved in the design of clinical trials, and patient-reported outcomes (PROs) have become recognised as standard outcomes that should be assessed and reported in a substantial proportion of trials, either as secondary outcomes or, in many instances, as a primary outcome from the study. Indeed, in 2000 the term 'patient-reported outcome' hardly existed and the focus at that time was on the ill-defined but all embracing concept of 'quality of life'. Now, we regard QoL as but one PRO, with the latter encompassing anything reported by 'asking the patient' – symptoms such as pain or depression, physical or other functioning, mobility, activities of daily living, satisfaction with treatment or other aspects of management, and so on. Drug regulatory bodies have also embraced PROs and QoL as endpoints, while at the same time demanding higher standards of questionnaire development and validation.

In parallel with this, research into instrument development, validation and application continues to grow apace. There is increasing recognition of the importance of qualitative methods to secure a solid foundation when developing new instruments, and a corresponding rigour in applying and reporting qualitative research. In parallel, a major radical shift towards using item response theory both as a tool for developing and validating new instruments and as the basis of computer-adaptive tests (CATs). Many of the major research groups have been developing new CAT instruments for assessing PROs, and this new generation of questionnaires are becoming widely available for use on computer tablets and smart-phones.

Analysis, too, has benefited in various ways for the increased importance being attached to PROs – two examples being (i) methods for handling missing data and in particular reducing the biases that can arise when data are missing, and (ii) greater rigour demanded for the reporting of PROs.

As a consequence of these and many other developments, we have taken the opportunity to update many chapters. The examples, too, have been refreshed and largely brought up-to-date, although some of the classic citations still stand proud and have been retained. A less convenient aspect of the changes is, perhaps, the resultant increase in page-count.

We continue to be grateful to our many colleagues – their continued encouragement and enthusiasm has fuelled the energy to produce this latest edition; Mogens Groenvold in particular contributed to the improvement of Chapter 3.

Peter M. Fayers and David Machin
September 2015

Preface to the second edition

We have been gratified by the reception of the first edition of this book, and this new edition offers the opportunity to respond to the many suggestions we have received for further improving and clarifying certain sections. In most cases the changes have meant expanding the text, to reflect new developments in research.

Chapters have been reorganised, to follow a more logical sequence for teaching. Thus sample size estimation has been moved to Part C, Clinical Trials, because it is needed for trial design. In the first edition it followed the chapters about analysis where we discussed choice of statistical tests, because the sample size computation depends on the test that will be used.

Health-related quality of life is a rapidly evolving field of research, and this is illustrated by shifting names and identity: quality of life (QoL) outcomes are now also commonly called patient- (or person-) reported outcomes (PROs), to reflect more clearly that symptoms and side effects of treatment are included in the assessments; we have adopted that term as part of the subtitle. Drug regulatory bodies have also endorsed this terminology, with the USA Food and Drug Administration (US FDA) bringing out guidance notes concerning the use of PROs in clinical trials for new drug applications; this new edition reflects the FDA (draft) recommendations.

Since the first edition of this book there have been extensive developments in item response theory and, in particular, computer-adaptive testing; these are addressed in a new chapter. Another area of growth has been in systematic reviews and meta-analysis, as evinced by the formation of a Quality of Life Methods Group by the Cochrane Collaboration. QoL presents some particular challenges for meta-analysis, and this led us to include the final chapter.

We are very grateful to the numerous colleagues who reported finding this book useful, some of whom also offered constructive advice for this second edition.

Peter M. Fayers and David Machin
June 2006

Preface to the first edition

Measurement of quality of life has grown to become a standard endpoint in many randomised controlled trials and other clinical studies. In part, this is a consequence of the realisation that many treatments for chronic diseases frequently fail to cure, and that there may be limited benefits gained at the expense of taking toxic or unpleasant therapy. Sometimes therapeutic benefits may be outweighed by quality of life considerations. In studies of palliative therapy, quality of life may become the principal or only endpoint of consideration. In part, it is also recognition that patients should have a say in the choice of their therapy, and that patients place greater emphasis upon non-clinical aspects of treatment than healthcare professionals did in the past. Nowadays, many patients and patient-support groups demand that they should be given full information about the consequences of their disease and its therapy, including impact upon aspects of quality of life, and that they should be allowed to express their opinions. The term *quality of life* has become a catch-phrase, and patients, investigators, funding bodies and ethical review committees often insist that, where appropriate, quality of life should be assessed as an endpoint for clinical trials.

The assessment, analysis and interpretation of quality of life relies upon a variety of psychometric and statistical methods, many of which may be less familiar than the other techniques used in medical research. Our objective is to explain these techniques in a non-technical way. We have assumed some familiarity with basic statistical ideas, but we have avoided detailed statistical theory. Instead, we have tried to write a practical guide that covers a wide range of methods. We emphasise the use of simple techniques in a variety of situations by using numerous examples, taken both from the literature and from our own experience. A number of these inevitably arise from our own particular field of interest - cancer clinical trials. This is also perhaps justifiable in that much of the pioneering work on quality of life assessment occurred in cancer, and cancer still remains the disease area that is associated with the largest number of quality of life instruments and the most publications. However, the issues that arise are common to quality of life assessment in general.

Acknowledgements

We would like to say a general thank you to all those with whom we have worked on aspects of quality of life over the years; especially, past and present members of the EORTC Quality of Life Study Group, and colleagues from the former MRC Cancer Therapy Committee Working Parties. Particular thanks go to Stein Kaasa of the Norwegian University of Science and Technology at Trondheim who permitted PMF to work on this book whilst on sabbatical and whose ideas greatly influenced our thinking about quality of life, and to Kristin Bjordal of The Radium Hospital, Oslo, who made extensive input and comments on many chapters and provided quality of life data that we used in examples. Finn Wisløff, for the Nordic Myeloma Study Group, very kindly allowed us to make extensive use their QoL data for many examples. We are grateful to the National Medical Research Council of Singapore for providing funds and facilities to enable us to complete this work. We also thank Dr Julian Thumboo, Tan Tock Seng Hospital, Singapore, for valuable comments on several chapters. Several chapters, and Chapter 7 in particular, were strongly influenced by manuals and guidelines published by the EORTC Quality of Life Study Group.

Peter M. Fayers and David Machin
January 2000

List of abbreviations

Note: We have adopted the policy of using *italics* to indicate variables, or things that take values.

α	Alpha, Type I error
$\alpha_{Cronbach}$	Cronbach's reliability coefficient
β	Beta, Power, 1-Type II error
κ	Kappa, Cohen's measure of agreement
θ	Theta, an unobservable or "latent" variable
ρ	Rho, the correlation coefficient
σ	Sigma, the population standard deviation, estimated by *SD*
ADL	Activities of daily living
ANOVA	Analysis of variance
ARR	Absolute risk reduction
AUC	Area under the curve
CAT	Computer-adaptive test
CFA	Confirmatory factor analysis
CI	Confidence interval
CONSORT	Consolidated Standards of Reporting Trials (http://www.consort-statement.org/)
CPMP	Committee for Proprietary Medicinal Products (European regulatory body)
DCE	Discrete choice experiment
df	Degrees of freedom
DIF	Differential item functioning
EF	Emotional functioning
EFA	Exploratory factor analysis
ES	Effect size
F-statistic	The ratio of two variance estimates; also called *F*-ratio
F-test	The statistical test used in ANOVA, based on the *F*-statistic
GEE	Generalised estimating equation
HYE	Healthy-years equivalent

IADL	Instrumental activities of daily living
ICC	Intraclass correlation
ICC	Item characteristic curve
IRT	Item response theory
LASA	Linear analogue self-assessment (scale)
MANOVA	Multivariate analysis of variance
MAR	Missing at random
MCAR	Missing completely at random
MIMIC	Multiple indicator multiple cause (model)
ML	Maximum likelihood (estimation)
MNAR	Missing not at random
MTMM	Multitrait–multimethod
NNT	Number needed to treat
NS	Not statistically significant
OR	Odds ratio
p	Probability, as in *p*-value
PF	Physical functioning
PRO	Patient-reported outcome
QALY	Quality-adjusted life years
QoL	*Quality of life*
Q-TWiST	Quality-adjusted time without symptoms and toxicity
RCT	Randomised controlled trial
RE	Relative efficiency
RR	*Relative risk*
RV	Relative validity
SD	Standard deviation of a sample
SE	Standard error
SEM	Standard error of measurement
SEM	Structured equation model
SG	Standard gamble
SMD	Standardised mean difference
SRM	Standardised response mean
t	Student's *t*-statistic
TTO	Time trade-off
TWiST	Time without symptoms and toxicity
VAS	Visual analogue scale
WMD	Weighted mean difference
WTP	Willingness to pay

QoL instruments

AIMS	Arthritis Impact Measurement Scale
AMPS	Assessment of Motor and Process Skills
AQLQ	Asthma Quality of Life Questionnaire
BDI	Beck Depression Inventory
BI	Barthel Index of disability
BPI	Brief Pain Inventory
BPRS	Brief Psychiatric Rating Scale
EORTC QLQ-C30	European Organisation for Research and Treatment of Cancer, Quality of Life Questionnaire, 30-items
EQ-5D	EuroQoL EQ-5D self report questionnaire
FACT-G	Functional Assessment of Cancer–General Version
FAQ	Functional Activity Questionnaire
FLIC	Functional Living Index–Cancer
GPH	*General Perceived Health*
HADS	Hospital Anxiety and Depression Scale
HDQoL	Huntington's Disease health-related Quality of Life questionnaire
HOPES	HIV Overview of Problems–Evaluation System
HRSD	Hamilton Rating Scale for Depression
HUI	Health Utilities Index
MFI-20	Multidimensional Fatigue Inventory 20
MMSE	Mini-Mental State Examination
MPQ	McGill Pain Questionnaire
NHP	Nottingham Health Profile
PACIS	Perceived Adjustment to Chronic Illness Scale
PAQLQ	Pediatric Asthma Quality of Life Questionnaire
PASS	Pain Anxiety Symptoms Scale
PCQLI	Pediatric Cardiac Quality of Life Inventory
PGI	Patient Generated Index
POMS	Profile of Mood States
QOLIE-89	Quality of Life in Epilepsy
RSCL	Rotterdam Symptom Checklist
SEIQoL	Schedule for Evaluation of Individual Quality of Life
SF-36	Short Form 36
SIP	Sickness Impact Profile
WPSI	Washington Psychosocial Seizure Inventory

PART 1
Developing and Validating Instruments for Assessing Quality of Life and Patient-Reported Outcomes

1

Introduction

Summary

A key methodology for the evaluation of therapies is the randomised controlled trial (RCT). These clinical trials traditionally considered relatively objective clinical outcome measures, such as cure, biological response to treatment, or survival. Later, investigators and patients alike have argued that subjective indicators should also be considered. These subjective patient-reported outcomes are often regarded as indicators of quality of life. They comprise a variety of outcome measures, such as emotional functioning (including anxiety and depression), physical functioning, social functioning, pain, fatigue, other symptoms and toxicity. A large number of questionnaires, or *instruments*, have been developed for assessing patient-reported outcomes and quality of life, and these have been used in a wide variety of circumstances. This book is concerned with the development, analysis and interpretation of data from these quality of life instruments.

1.1 Patient-reported outcomes

This book accepts a broad definition of *quality of life*, and discusses the design, application and use of single- and multi-item, subjective, measurement scales. This encompasses not just 'overall quality of life' but also the symptoms and side effects that may or may not reflect – or affect – quality of life. Some researchers prefer to emphasise that we are only interested in health aspects, as in *health-related quality of life* (HRQoL or HRQL), while others adopt the terms *patient-reported outcomes* (PROs) or *patient-reported outcome measures* (PROMs), because those terms indicate interest in a whole host of outcomes, such as pain, fatigue, depression through to physical symptoms such as nausea and vomiting. But not all subjects are 'patients' who are ill; it is also suggested that PRO could mean *person-reported outcome. Health outcomes assessment* has also been proposed, which emphasises that the focus is on health issues and also avoids specifying the respondent: for young children and for the cognitively impaired we may use *proxy assessment* for cognitive reasons. And for

Quality of Life: The Assessment, Analysis and Reporting of Patient-Reported Outcomes, Third Edition.
Peter M. Fayers and David Machin.
© 2016 John Wiley & Sons, Ltd. Published 2016 by John Wiley & Sons, Ltd.

many years some questionnaires have focused on *health status* or *self-reported health* (SRH), with considerable overlap to *quality of life.*

From a measurement perspective, this book is concerned with all the above. For simplicity we will use the now well-established overall term *quality of life* (QoL) to indicate (a) the set of outcomes that contribute to a patient's well-being or overall health, or (b) a summary measure or scale that purports to describe a patient's overall well-being or health. Examples of summary measures for QoL include general questions such as 'How good is your overall quality of life?' or 'How do you rate your overall health?' that represent global assessments. When referring to outcomes that reflect individual dimensions, we use the acronym PROs. Examples of PROs are pain or fatigue; symptoms such as headaches or skin irritation; function, such as social and role functioning; issues such as body image or existential beliefs; and so on. Mostly, we shall assume the respondent is the patient or person whose experience we are interested in (*self-report*), but it could be a proxy.

The measurement issues for all these outcomes are similar. Should we use single- or multi-item scales? Content and construct validity – are we measuring what we intend? Sensitivity, reliability, responsiveness – is the assessment statistically adequate? How should such assessments be incorporated into clinical studies? And how do we analyse, report and interpret the results?

1.2   What is a patient-reported outcome?

The definition of *patient-reported outcome* is straightforward, and has been described as "any report of the status of a patient's health condition that comes directly from the patient, without interpretation of the patient's response by a clinician or anyone else" (US FDA, 2009). A PRO can be measured by self-report or by interview provided that the interviewer records only the patient's response. The outcome can be measured in absolute terms (e.g. severity of a symptom, sign or state of a disease) or as a change from a previous assessment.

1.3   What is *quality of life*?

In contrast to PRO, the term *Quality of life* is ill defined. The World Health Organization (WHO, 1948) declares health to be 'a state of complete physical, mental and social well-being, and not merely the absence of disease'. Many other definitions of both 'health' and 'quality of life' have been attempted, often linking the two and, for QoL, frequently emphasising components of happiness and satisfaction with life. In the absence of any universally accepted definition, some investigators argue that most people, in the Western world at least, are familiar with the expression 'quality of life' and have an intuitive understanding of what it comprises.

However, it is clear that 'QoL' means different things to different people, and takes on different meanings according to the area of application. To a town planner, for example, it might represent access to green space and other facilities. In the context of clinical trials we are rarely interested in QoL in such a broad sense, and instead are concerned only with evaluating those aspects that are affected by disease or treatment for disease. This may sometimes be extended to include indirect consequences of disease, such as unemployment or financial difficulties. To distinguish between QoL in its more general sense and the requirements of clinical medicine and clinical trials the term *health-related quality of life* (HRQoL) is frequently used in order to remove ambiguity.

Health-related QoL is still a loose definition. What aspects of QoL should be included? It is generally agreed that the relevant aspects may vary from study to study but can include general health, physical functioning, physical symptoms and toxicity, emotional functioning, cognitive functioning, role functioning, social well-being and functioning, sexual functioning and existential issues. In the absence of any agreed formal definition of QoL, most investigators circumvent the issues by describing what *they* mean by QoL, and then letting the items (questions) in their questionnaire speak for themselves. Thus some questionnaires focus upon the relatively objective signs such as patient-reported toxicity, and in effect define the relevant aspects of QoL as being, for their purposes, limited to treatment toxicity. Other investigators argue that what matters most is the impact of toxicity, and therefore their questionnaires place greater emphasis upon psychological aspects, such as anxiety and depression. Yet others try to allow for spiritual issues, ability to cope with illness and satisfaction with life.

Some QoL instruments focus upon a single concept, such as emotional functioning. Other instruments regard these individual concepts as aspects, or *dimensions*, of QoL, and therefore include items relating to several concepts. Although there is disagreement about what components should be evaluated, most investigators agree that a number of the above dimensions should be included in QoL questionnaires, and that QoL is a multidimensional construct. Because there are so many potential dimensions, it is impractical to try to assess all these concepts simultaneously in one instrument. Most instruments intended for health-status assessment include at least some items that focus upon physical, emotional and social functioning. For example, if emotional functioning is accepted as being one aspect of QoL that should be investigated, several questions could evaluate anxiety, tension, irritability, depression and so on. Thus instruments may contain many items. Although a single global question such as 'How would you rate your overall quality of life?' is a useful adjunct to multi-item instruments, global questions are often regarded as too vague and non-specific to be used on their own. Most of the general questionnaires that we describe include one or more global questions alongside a number of other items covering specific issues. Some instruments place greater emphasis upon the concept of global questions, and the EQ-5D questionnaire (Appendix E4) asks a parsimonious five questions before using a single global question that enquires about 'your health'. Even more extreme is the Perceived Adjustment to Chronic Illness Scale (PACIS) described by Hürny *et al.* (1993). This instrument consists of a single, carefully phrased question that is a global indicator of coping and adjustment: 'How much effort does it cost you to cope with your illness?' This takes responses ranging between 'No effort at all' and 'A great deal of effort'.

One unifying and non-controversial theme throughout all the approaches is that the concepts forming these dimensions can be assessed only by *subjective measures*, PROs, and that they should be evaluated by asking the patient. *Proxy* assessments, by a relative or other close observer, are usually employed only if the patient is unable to make a coherent response, for example those who are very young, very old, severely ill or have mental impairment. Furthermore, many of these individual concepts – such as emotional functioning and fatigue – lack a formal, agreed definition that is universally understood by patients. In many cases the problem is compounded by language differences, and some concepts do not readily translate to other tongues. There are also cultural differences regarding the importance of the issues. Single-item questions on these aspects of QoL, as for global questions about overall QoL, are likely to be ambiguous and unreliable. Therefore it is usual to develop questionnaires that consist of multi-item measurement scales for each concept.

1.4 Historical development

One of the earliest references that impinges upon a definition of QoL appears in the *Nichomachean Ethics*, in which Aristotle (384–322 BCE) notes: "Both the multitude and persons of refinement … conceive 'the good life' or 'doing well' to be the same thing as 'being happy'. But what constitutes happiness is a matter of dispute … some say one thing and some another, indeed very often the same man says different things at different times: when he falls sick he thinks health is happiness, when he is poor, wealth." The Greek ευδαιμονια is commonly translated as 'happiness' although Rackham, the translator that we cite, noted that a more accurate rendering would embrace 'well-being', with Aristotle denoting by ευδαιμονια both a state of feeling and a kind of activity. In modern parlance this is assuredly quality of life. Although the term 'quality of life' did not exist in the Greek language of 2000 years ago, Aristotle clearly appreciated that QoL means different things to different people. He also recognised that it varies according to a person's current situation – an example of a phenomenon now termed response shift. QoL was rarely mentioned until the twentieth century, although one early commentator on the subject noted that happiness could be sacrificed for QoL: "Life at its noblest leaves mere happiness far behind; and indeed cannot endure it … Happiness is not the object of life: life has no object: it is an end in itself; and courage consists in the readiness to sacrifice happiness for an intenser quality of life" (Shaw, [1900] 1972). It would appear that by this time 'quality of life' had become a familiar term that did not require further explanation. Specific mention of QoL in relation to patients' health came much later. The influential WHO 1948 definition of health cited above was one of the earliest statements recognising and stressing the importance of the three dimensions – physical, mental and social – in the context of disease. Other definitions have been even more general: "Quality of Life: Encompasses the entire range of human experience, states, perceptions, and spheres of thought concerning the life of an individual or a community. Both objective and subjective, quality-of-life can include cultural, physical, psychological, interpersonal, spiritual, financial, political, temporal, and philosophical dimensions. Quality-of-life implies judgement of value placed on experience of communities, groups such as families, or individuals" (Patrick and Erickson, 1993).

One of the first instruments that broadened the assessment of patients beyond physiological and clinical examination was the Karnofsky Performance Scale proposed in 1947 (Karnofsky and Burchenal, 1947) for use in clinical settings. This is a simple scale ranging from 0 for 'dead' to 100 indicating 'normal, no complaints, no evidence of disease'. Healthcare staff make the assessment. Over the years, it has led to a number of other scales for functional ability, physical functioning and *activities of daily living* (ADL), such as the Barthel Index. Although these questionnaires are still sometimes described as QoL instruments, they capture only one aspect of it and provide an inadequate representation of patients' overall well-being and QoL.

The next generation of questionnaires, in the late 1970s and early 1980s, that quantified health status were used for the general evaluation of health. These instruments focused on physical functioning, physical and psychological symptoms, impact of illness, perceived distress and life satisfaction. Examples of such instruments include the Sickness Impact Profile (SIP) and the Nottingham Health Profile (NHP). Although these instruments are frequently described as QoL questionnaires, their authors neither designed them nor claimed them as QoL instruments.

Meanwhile, Priestman and Baum (1976) were adapting linear analogue self-assessment (LASA) methods to assess QoL in breast cancer patients. The LASA approach, which is also sometimes called a visual analogue scale (VAS), provides a 10 cm line, with the ends labelled with words describing the extremes of a condition. The patient is asked to mark the point along the line that corresponds with their feelings. An example of a LASA scale is contained in the EQ-5D (Appendix E4). Priestman and Baum (1976) measured a variety of subjective effects, including well-being, mood, anxiety, activity, pain, social activities and the patient's opinion as to 'Is the treatment helping?' Others took the view that one need only ask a single question to evaluate the QoL of patients with cancer: "How would you rate your QoL today?" (Gough *et al.*, 1983), and supported their position by demonstrating a relatively strong correlation between answers to this single question and scores derived from a more extensive battery of questionnaires.

Much of the development of QoL instruments has built upon these early attempts, first with increasing emphasis on the more subjective aspects, such as emotional, role, social and cognitive functioning, but subsequently with a counter trend towards greater focus on patient-reported symptoms and other relatively objective outcomes. Frequently, one or more general or global questions concerning overall QoL are included. Implicit in all this is that psychological and social aspects, functional capacity and symptomatology all relate to QoL. Thus, if a patient is unable to achieve full physical, psychological or social functioning, it is assumed that their QoL is poorer. Although this may in general seem a reasonable assumption, it can lead to theoretical problems. In particular, many forms of functioning, especially physical functioning, may be regarded as *causal* variables that can be expected to change or affect a patient's QoL but do not necessarily reflect the true level of their QoL (see Section 2.6). For example, a patient may have a poor QoL irrespective of whether their physical functioning is impaired; this might arise because of other factors, such as pain. Therefore scales measuring functional status assess only whether there are problems that *may* cause distress to the patient or impair their QoL; absence of problems in these specific areas does not indicate that a patient has no problems at all, nor does it necessarily indicate that a patient has good QoL. Despite these reservations, most instruments continue to focus on health status, functional status and checklists of symptoms. For clinical purposes this may be logical since, when comparing treatments, the clinician is most concerned with the differences in the symptoms and side effects due to the various therapies, and the impact of these differences upon QoL.

A number of other theoretical models for QoL have been proposed. The *expectations* model of Calman (1984) suggests that individuals have aims and goals in life and that QoL is a measure of the difference between the hopes and expectations of the individual and the individual's present experience. It is concerned with the difference between perceived goals and actual goals. The gap may be narrowed by improving the function of a patient or by modifying their expectations. Instruments such as the Schedule for Evaluation of Individual Quality of Life (SEIQoL) and the Patient Generated Index (PGI), described in Section 1.8, use Calman's expectations model as a conceptual basis and provide the facility to incorporate personal values.

The *needs* model relates QoL to the ability and capacity of patients to satisfy certain human needs. QoL is at its highest when all needs are fulfilled, and at its lowest when few needs are satisfied. Needs include such aspects as identity, status, self-esteem, affection, love, security, enjoyment, creativity, food, sleep, pain avoidance and activity. Hunt and McKenna (1992) use this model to generate several QoL measures. Somewhat related is the *reintegration to normal living* model that has also been regarded as an approach to assessing QoL. Reintegration means the ability to do what one has to do or wants to do, but it does not mean being free of disease or symptoms.

Other definitions or indicators of QoL that have been suggested are *personal wellbeing* and *satisfaction with life*. The *impact of illness* (or treatment) on social, emotional, occupational and family domains emphasises the illness aspect, or the *interference* of symptoms and side effects. The *existential* approach notes that preferences are not fixed and are both individual and vary over time – as was recognised so long ago by Aristotle. Having a 'positive approach to life' can give life high quality, regardless of the medical condition. Therefore it can be important to assess existential beliefs and also *coping*. A patient's perception of their QoL can be altered by influencing their existential beliefs or by helping them to cope better. The existential model of QoL leads to the inclusion of such items as pleasure in life and positive outlook on life.

Patient preference measures differ from other models of QoL in that they explicitly incorporate *weights* that reflect the importance that patients attach to specific dimensions. Different states and dimensions are compared against each other, to establish a ranking in terms of their value or in terms of patients' preferences of one state over another. These and other *utility measure* approaches to QoL assessment are derived from decision-making theory and are frequently employed in any economic evaluations of treatments.

Finally, some authorities simply circumvent the challenges of defining QoL. The US FDA (2009) notes: "Quality of life — A general concept that implies an evaluation of the effect of all aspects of life on general well-being. Because this term implies the evaluation of nonhealth-related aspects of life, and because the term generally is accepted to mean *what the patient thinks it is*, it is too general and undefined to be considered appropriate for a medical product claim." Further, they also define "Health-related quality of life (HRQL) — HRQL is a multidomain concept that represents the patient's general perception of the effect of illness and treatment on physical, psychological, and social aspects of life", but also add the hard-to-satisfy condition that "Claiming a statistical and meaningful improvement in HRQL implies: (1) that all HRQL domains that are important to interpreting change in how the clinical trial's population feels or functions as a result of the targeted disease and its treatment were measured; (2) that a general improvement was demonstrated; and (3) that no decrement was demonstrated in any domain" (US FDA, 2009).

Thus there is continuing philosophical debate about the meaning of QoL and about what should be measured. Perhaps the simplest and most pragmatic view is that all of these concepts reflect issues that are of fundamental importance to patients' well-being. They are all worth investigating and quantifying.

1.5   Why measure quality of life?

There are several reasons why QoL assessments may be included in RCTs, and it is important to distinguish between them as the nature of the measurements, and the questionnaires that are employed, will depend upon the objectives of the trial. Perhaps the most obvious reason is in order to compare the study treatments, in which case it is important to identify those aspects of QoL that may be affected by the therapy. These include both benefits, as may be sought in palliative trials that are expected to improve QoL, and negative changes, such as toxicity and any side effects of therapy.

Clinical trials of treatment with curative intent

Many clinical trial organisations have now introduced the assessment of QoL as being a standard part of new trials. An obvious reason for the emphasis towards QoL as an important endpoint is that treatment of fatal diseases can, and often does, result in limited gains in cure or prolonged survival. With some notable exceptions, little improvement has been seen in patients with major cancer diagnoses, HIV or AIDS. At the same time therapeutic interventions in these diseases frequently cause serious side effects and functional impairment.

There are numerous examples in which QoL assessments have had an unexpectedly important role in the interpretations and conclusions of RCTs, and it is perhaps surprising that it took so long for the relevance of QoL assessment to be appreciated. For example, one of the earliest randomised trials to include QoL assessment was by Coates *et al.* (1987), who reported that, contrary to their initial expectations, continuous as opposed to intermittent chemotherapy for advanced breast cancer not only prolonged survival but most importantly resulted in a superior QoL.

Similarly, other RCTs recognised that QoL may be the principal outcome of interest. For example, an RCT comparing three anti-hypertensive therapies conducted by Croog *et al.* (1986) demonstrated major differences in QoL, and the results of a cancer chemotherapy trial of Buccheri *et al.* (1989) suggested that small treatment benefits may be more than outweighed by the poorer QoL and cost of therapy. In extreme cases, the cure might be worse than the disease.

Example from the literature

Testa *et al.* (1993) describe an RCT evaluating hypertensive therapy in men. Two angiotensin-converting enzyme inhibitors, captopril and enalapril, were compared. In total, 379 active men with mild to moderate hypertension, aged 55 to 79, were randomised between the treatment arms. QoL was one of the main outcome measures. Several QoL scales were used, including an Overall QoL scale based on a mean score from 11 subscales.

In order to interpret the magnitude of the differences in QoL that were observed, stressful life events that produced an equivalent change in QoL scores were considered, and the responses to the Overall QoL scale were re-calibrated accordingly. Overall QoL scores shifted positively for captopril by 0.11 units, and negatively for enalapril by 0.11. Negative shifts of 0.11 corresponded to those encountered when there was 'major change in work responsibility', 'in-law troubles' or 'mortgage foreclosure'. On the basis of these investigations, a clinically important change was deemed to be one between 0.1 and 0.2.

It was concluded that, although the therapies were indistinguishable in terms of clinical assessments of efficacy and safety, they produced substantial and different changes in QoL.

Clinical trials of treatment with palliative intent

One consequence of ageing societies is the corresponding increased prevalence of chronic diseases. The treatment outcome in such diseases cannot be cure but must relate to the improvement of the well-being of patients thus treated. The aim is to palliate symptoms, or to prolong the time without symptoms. Traditionally, clinical and not QoL outcomes have been the principal endpoints. For example, in an RCT of therapy for advanced oesophageal cancer, absence of dysphagia might have been the main outcome measure indicating success of therapy. Nowadays, in trials of palliative care, QoL is more frequently chosen as the outcome measure of choice. Symptom relief is now recognised as but one aspect of palliative intervention, and a comprehensive assessment of QoL is often as important as an evaluation of symptoms.

Example from the literature

Temel *et al.* (2010) randomly assigned patients with newly diagnosed metastatic non–small-cell lung cancer to receive either early palliative care integrated with standard oncologic care or standard oncologic care alone. Quality of life and mood were assessed at baseline and at 12 weeks with the use of the Functional Assessment of Cancer Therapy–Lung (FACT-L) scale and the Hospital Anxiety and Depression Scale. The primary outcome was the change in the quality of life at 12 weeks.

Of the 151 randomised patients, 27 died by 12 weeks and 107 (86% of the remaining patients) completed assessments. Patients assigned to early palliative care had a better quality of life than did patients assigned to standard care (mean score on the FACT-L scale, 98.0 vs. 91.5; $p = 0.03$). In addition, fewer patients in the palliative care group than in the standard care group had depressive symptoms (16% vs. 38%, $p = 0.01$). Despite the fact that fewer patients in the early palliative care group than in the standard care group received aggressive end-of-life care (33% vs. 54%, $p = 0.05$), median survival was longer among patients receiving early palliative care (11.6 months vs. 8.9 months, $p = 0.02$).

Temel *et al.* conclude that, among patients with metastatic non-small-cell lung cancer, early palliative care led to significant improvements in both quality of life and mood. As compared with patients receiving standard care, patients receiving early palliative care had less aggressive care at the end of life but longer survival.

Example from the literature

Fatigue, lethargy, anorexia, nausea and weakness are common in patients with advanced cancer. It had been widely believed at the time that progestagens, including megestrol acetate (MA), might have a useful function for the palliative treatment of advanced endocrine-insensitive tumours. Beller *et al.* (1997) report a double-blind RCT of 240 patients randomised to 12 weeks of high- or low-dose MA, or to matching placebo. Nutritional status was recorded, and QoL was measured using six LASA scales, at randomisation and after four, eight and 12 weeks.

Patients receiving MA reported substantially better appetite, mood and overall QoL than patients receiving placebo, with a larger benefit being seen for the higher dose. Table 1.1 shows the average change from the baseline at time of randomisation. No statistically significant differences were observed in the nutritional status measurements. Side effects of therapy were minor and did not differ across treatments.

The authors conclude that high-dose MA provides useful palliation for patients with endocrine-insensitive advanced cancer. It improves appetite, mood and overall QoL in these patients, although not through a direct effect on nutritional status.

Table 1.1 Average difference in QoL between baseline and subsequent weeks

LASA scores	Placebo	Low dose MA	High dose MA	p-value (trend)
Physical well-being	5.8	6.5	13.9	0.13
Mood	−4.1	0.4	10.2	0.001
Pain	−5.3	−6.9	1.9	0.13
Nausea/vomiting	−1.4	8.7	7.2	0.08
Appetite	9.7	17.0	31.3	0.0001
Overall QoL	−2.7	2.8	13.1	0.001
Combined QoL measure	−2.1	2.4	12.3	0.001

Source: Beller *et al.*, 1997, Table 3. Reproduced with permission of Oxford University Press.

Improving symptom relief, care or rehabilitation

Traditionally, medicine has tended to concentrate upon symptom relief as an outcome measure. Studies using QoL instruments may reveal other issues that are equally or more important to patients. For example, in advanced oesophageal cancer, it was found that many patients say that fatigue has a far greater impact upon their QoL than dyspnoea. Such a finding is contrary to traditional teaching, but has been replicated in many other cancer sites.

Example from the literature

Smets *et al.* (1998) used the Multidimensional Fatigue Inventory (MFI-20, Appendix E14) to assess fatigue in 250 patients who were receiving radiotherapy with curative intent for various cancers. Patients rated their fatigue at two-weekly intervals during treatment and within two weeks after completion of radiotherapy.

There was a gradual increase in fatigue during radiotherapy and a decrease after completion of treatment. After treatment, 46% of the patients reported fatigue as being among the three symptoms causing most distress, and 40% reported having been tired throughout the treatment period.

Smets *et al.* conclude that there is a need to give preparatory information to new patients who are at risk of fatigue, and interventions including exercise and psychotherapy may be beneficial. They also suggested that their results might be underestimations because the oldest and most tired patients were more inclined to refuse participation.

Rehabilitation programmes, too, have traditionally concentrated upon physical aspects of health, functioning and ability to perform ADLs; these physical aspects were most frequently evaluated by healthcare workers or other observers. Increasingly, patient-completed QoL assessment is now perceived as essential to the evaluation of successful rehabilitation. Problems revealed by questioning patients can lead to modifications and improvement in the programme, or alternatively may show that some methods offer little benefit.

Example from the literature

Results from several small trials had suggested that group therapy, counselling, relaxation therapy and psychoeducation might have a role in the rehabilitation of patients following acute myocardial infarction. Jones and West (1996) report an RCT that examined the impact of psychological rehabilitation after myocardial infarction. In this trial, 2328 patients were randomised between policies of no-intervention and intervention consisting of comprehensive rehabilitation with psychological therapy and opportunities for group and individual counselling. Patients were assessed both by interview and by questionnaires for anxiety and depression, state anxiety, expectations of future life, psychological well-being, sexual activity and functional disability.

At six months, 34% of patients receiving intervention had clinically significant levels of anxiety, compared with 32% of no-intervention patients. In both groups, 19% had clinically significant levels of depression. Differences for other domains were also minimal.

The authors conclude that rehabilitation programmes based upon psychological therapy, counselling, relaxation training and stress management seem to offer little objective benefit to myocardial infarction patients.

Facilitating communication with patients

Another reason for assessing QoL is to establish information about the range of problems that affect patients. In this case, the investigator may be less interested in whether there are treatment differences, and might even anticipate that both study arms will experience similar levels of some aspects of QoL. The aim is to collect information in a form that can be communicated to future patients, enabling them to anticipate and understand the consequences of their illness and its treatment. Patients themselves often express the wish for more emphasis upon research into QoL issues, and seek insight into the concomitants of their disease and its treatment.

Example from the literature

The Dartmouth COOP, a primary care research network, developed nine pictorial Charts to measure patient function and QoL (Nelson *et al.*, 1990). Each Chart has a five-point scale, is illustrated, and can be self- or office-staff administered. The Charts are used to measure patients' overall physical functioning, emotional problems, daily activities, social activities, pain, overall health and QoL. The QoL item is presented as a ladder, and was later used in the QOLIE-89 instrument (Appendix E10, question 49).

Nelson *et al.* report results for over 2000 patients in four diverse clinical settings. Most clinicians and patients reported that the Charts were easy to use and provided a valuable tool. For nearly half of the patients in whom the Charts uncovered new information, changes in clinical management were initiated as a consequence.

It was concluded that the COOP Charts are practicable, reliable, valid, sensitive to the effects of disease and useful for measuring patient function quickly.

Patient preferences

Not only does a patient's self-assessment often differ substantially from the judgement of their doctor or other healthcare staff, but patients' preferences also seem to differ from those of other people. Many patients accept toxic chemotherapy for the prospect of minimal benefit in terms of probability of cure or prolongation of life, contrary to the expectations of medical staff. Therefore QoL should be measured from the patient's perspective, using a patient-completed questionnaire.

Example from the literature

Slevin *et al.* (1990) asked 106 consecutive patients with solid tumours to complete questionnaires about their willingness to receive chemotherapy. They were told that the more-intensive regimen was likely to have considerable side effects and drawbacks, such as severe nausea and vomiting, hair loss, frequent tiredness and weakness, frequent use of drips and needles, admission to hospital, decreased sexual interest and possible infertility. They were given different scenarios, such as (i) small (1%) chance of cure, (ii) no cure, but chance of prolonging life by three months and (iii) 1% chance of symptom relief only. All patients knew they were about to commence chemotherapy, and thus considered the questions seriously. Cancer nurses, general practitioners, radiotherapists, oncologists and sociodemographically matched controls were asked the same questions.

Table 1.2 shows the percentage of respondents that would accept chemotherapy under each scenario. There are major and consistent differences between the opinions of patients and the others, and also between the different healthcare staff.

Slevin *et al.* comment that patients appear to regard a minute chance of possible benefit as worthwhile, whatever the cost. They conclude: "It may be that the only people who can evaluate such life and death decisions are those faced with them."

Table 1.2 Percentage of respondents willing to accept intensive or mild chemotherapy with a minimum chance of effectiveness

	Controls	Cancer nurses	General practitioners	Radiotherapists	Oncologists	Cancer patients
Number	100	303	790	88	60	100
Cure (1%)						
Intensive regimen	19	13	12	4	20	53
Mild regimen	35	39	44	27	52	67
Prolonging life by 3 months						
Intensive regimen	10	6	3	0	10	42
Mild regimen	25	25	27	13	45	53
Relief of symptoms (1%)						
Intensive regimen	10	6	2	0	7	43
Mild regimen	19	26	21	2	11	59

Source: Adapted from Slevin *et al.*, 1990, Table II. Reproduced with permission of BMJ Publishing Group Limited.

These results have been closely replicated by others. For example, Lindley *et al.* (1998) examined QoL in 86 breast cancer patients, using the SF-36 and the Functional Living Index – Cancer (FLIC). They note that 'the majority of patients indicated a willingness to accept six months of chemotherapy for small to modest potential benefit'.

Late problems of psychosocial adaptation

Cured patients and long-term survivors may have continuing problems long after their treatment is completed. These late problems may be overlooked, and QoL reported in such patients often gives results that are contrary to expectations.

Example from the literature

Bjordal *et al.* (1994), in a study of long-term survivors from a trial of radio-therapy for head and neck cancer, unexpectedly found that the hypofractionated patients reported slightly better QoL than those who received conventional therapy. Hypofractionated patients had slightly better EORTC QLQ-C30 mean scores for role, social and emotional function and better overall QoL (Table 1.3), and reported less fatigue. However, both groups reported high levels of symptoms 7–11 years after their radiotherapy, such as dryness in the mouth and mucus production, and high levels of psychological distress (30% being clinical 'cases').

The authors conclude that clinicians need to be aware of these problems and that some patients would benefit from social support or medication. It was proposed that the GHQ-20 (General Health Questionnaire) could facilitate the screening for patients whose psychological distress might be treated.

Table 1.3 Quality of life in head and neck cancer patients 7–11 years after curative treatment

	Conventional radiotherapy ($n = 103$)	Hypofractionated radiotherapy ($n = 101$)	p-value
EORTC QLQ-C30 Function scales (mean scores)			
Physical function	74	79	NS
Role function	72	83	0.03
Social function	73	83	0.02
Emotional function	77	84	0.02
Cognitive function	80	83	NS
Overall QoL	61	69	0.04
EORTC QLQ-C30 Symptom scales (mean scores)			
Pain	19	15	NS
Fatigue	32	25	0.04
Emesis	6	5	NS
GHQ scores			
Mean score	20.8	19.7	NS
% cases	31%	32%	NS

Source: Bjordal *et al.*, 1994. Reproduced with permission of Elsevier.

Medical decision-making

QoL can be a predictor of treatment success, and several studies have found that factors such as overall QoL, physical well-being, mood and pain are of prognostic importance. For example, in cancer patients, pre-treatment assessment of QoL has been shown to be strongly predictive of survival, and a better predictor than performance status (Gotay *et al.*, 2008; Quinten *et al.*, 2009). On this basis, it is possible to argue for the routine assessment of QoL in therapy trials.

It is not clear in these circumstances whether QoL scores reflect an early perception by the patient of disease progression or whether QoL status in some way influences the course of disease. If the former, the level of QoL is merely predictive of outcome. If it affects outcome, there could be potential to use improvement in QoL as an active form of therapy. Whatever the nature of the association, these findings underline the importance of evaluating QoL and using it when making medical decisions. Similar results have been observed in various disease areas. For example, Jenkins (1992) observed that preoperative QoL partially predicts the recovery process in heart surgery patients. Changes in QoL scores during treatment have also been shown to have prognostic value.

Example from the literature

Coates *et al.* (1997) showed that patients' self-assessment of QoL is an important prognostic factor of survival in advanced cancer patients. Adult patients with advanced malignancy from 12 institutions in 10 countries completed the EORTC QLQ-C30 questionnaire. Baseline patient and disease characteristics were recorded.

Follow-up information was obtained on 656 patients, of whom 411 had died. In addition to age and performance status, the QLQ-C30 global QoL scale and the scales of physical, role, emotional, cognitive and social function were each predictive of subsequent survival duration. Table 1.4 shows the association of survival with the scores for overall physical condition (Q29) and overall quality of life (Q30). In this table, items Q29 and Q30 were each divided about their respective medians, and the hazard ratios show that patients with high scores were less likely to die than those below the median. For example, the hazard ratio of 0.89 for Q29 indicates that the rate of death in patients with high scores was only 89% of the death rate in those with low scores.

Coates *et al.* conclude that QoL scores carry prognostic information independent of other recorded factors.

Table 1.4   Prognostic significance for survival of two single-item QoL scores in patients with cancer, after allowing for performance status and age

QoL Variable	Hazard ratio	95% Confidence Interval	*p*-value
Physical condition (Q29)	0.89	0.82 to 0.96	0.003
Overall QoL (Q30)	0.87	0.80 to 0.94	0.001

Source: Coates *et al.*, 1997. Reproduced with permission of Elsevier.

1.6   Which clinical trials should assess QoL?

It would be inappropriate to suggest that *all* RCTs, even in cancer, HIV or chronic diseases, should make a formal assessment of QoL. Clearly, there are situations where such information is not relevant. For example, when evaluating a potentially curative treatment that is not very likely to have adverse side effects, or if the treatments and side effects are similar in the various study arms, it might be unnecessary to make such assessment. However, many trial groups now insist that the investigators should at least consider the QoL implications and should positively justify *not* including the assessment of QoL.

When is QoL assessment a relevant endpoint? Gotay and Moore (1992) propose the following classification of trials for QoL purposes:

1. QoL may be the main endpoint. This is frequently true in palliative care, or when patients are seriously ill with incurable disease.

2. Treatments may be expected to be equivalent in efficacy, and a new treatment would be deemed preferable if it confers QoL benefits.

3. A new treatment may show a small benefit in cure rates or survival advantage, but this might be offset by QoL deterioration.

4. Treatments may differ considerably in their short-term efficacy, but if the overall failure rate is high then QoL issues should be considered.

Furthermore, despite the optimism of those who launch trials that seek a survival break-through, all too often completed trials show a limited survival advantage. Thus in these cases the relevance of QoL assessment has to be considered, since any gain in therapeutic efficacy would have to be weighed against possible negative effects pertaining to QoL.

1.7   How to measure quality of life

Ask the patient

Observers are poor judges of patients' opinions. Many studies have shown that inde-pendent assessments by either healthcare professionals or patients' relatives differ from the responses obtained when patients complete self-reported questionnaires. In some conditions observers appear to consistently overestimate QoL scores, in others, underestimate. There is general agreement that patients' opinions vary considerably from the expectations of both staff and relatives. It has been suggested that observers tend to underestimate the impact of psychological aspects and tend to emphasise the importance of the more obvious symptoms. The impacts of pain, nausea and vomit-ing have all been reported as being underestimated. Expected symptoms and toxicity tend to be accepted and hence ignored by clinical staff. Studies of nausea and vomit-ing in cancer patients receiving chemotherapy have found that doctors assume these symptoms are likely to occur and, as a consequence, often report only the more severe events. However, patients who are reported as having no problems may assert that they suffered quite a lot of vomiting (Fayers *et al.*, 1991).

Observers frequently misjudge the absolute levels of both symptoms and general QoL. In addition, the patients' willingness to trade QoL for possible cure may be misjudged. Many patients are willing to accept unpleasant or toxic therapy for seemingly modest benefits in terms of cure, although a few patients will refuse treatment even when there is a high chance of substantial gain. Physicians and nurses are more likely to say that they would be unwilling to accept the therapy for such small potential benefit. When patients with cancer choose between two treatments, if they believe their disease is likely to be cured they may be willing to accept a treatment that adversely affects their QoL.

Observers, including health professionals, may tend to base their opinions of overall QoL upon physical signs such as symptoms and toxicity. However, in many disease areas, conventional clinical outcomes have been shown to be poorly correlated with patients' assessment of QoL. Thus, for example, in patients with asthma, Juniper *et al.* (1993) observed that correlations between clinical assessments and how patients felt and functioned in day-to-day activities were only modest.

Example from the literature

An early investigation conducted by Jachuk *et al.* (1982) into QoL concerned the effect of hypotensive drugs. Seventy-five patients with controlled hypertension each completed a questionnaire, as did a relative and doctor. A global, summary question was included, about whether there was overall improvement, no change or deterioration.

As Table 1.5 shows, while the physicians assessed all patients as having improved, approximately half the patients thought there was no change or deterioration, and all but one patient was assessed by their relatives as having deteriorated. Patients attributed their deterioration as due to decline in energy, general activity, sexual inactivity and irritability. Physicians, focusing upon control of hypertension, largely ignored these factors. Relatives commonly thought there was moderate or severe impairment of memory, energy and activity, and an increase in hypochondria, irritability and worry.

Nowadays, clinical practice places greater emphasis on patient–physician communication, and it is most unlikely that such extreme results would be observed if this study were to be repeated. The modern physician would be expected to have a far greater awareness of patients' feelings, leading to smaller differences.

Table 1.5 The results of overall assessments of QoL by 75 patients with controlled hypertension, their attending physicians, and the patients' relatives

	Improved	No change	Worse	Total
Physician	75	0	0	75
Patient	36	32	7	75
Relative	1	0	74	75

Source: Jachuk *et al.*, 1982. Reproduced with permission of the Royal College of General Practitioners.

1.8   Instruments

A large number of instruments have been developed for QoL assessment, and we provide a range of examples to illustrate some of the approaches used. Those reproduced (in the Appendix) have been chosen on the grounds of variety, to show particular features, and because these particular instruments are among the most widely used in clinical trials.

The aims and content of each instrument are described, together with an outline of the scoring procedures and any constructed multi-item scales. Most of the instruments use fairly simple forms of scoring, and the following basic procedure is usually used.

First, the successive levels of each categorical item are numbered increasingly. For example, a common scheme with four-category items is to grade responses such as 'not at all', 'a little', 'quite a bit' and 'very much' as being 0 to 3 respectively or, if preferred, 1 to 4, as it makes no difference after standardising the final scores. Second, when a scale contains multiple items, these are usually summed. Thus a four-item scale, with items scored 0 to 3, would yield a working score ranging from 0 to 12. Finally, the working score is usually standardised to a range of 0 to 100, and called the *scale score*. This enables different scales, possibly with different numbers of items and/or where the items have different numbers of categories, to be compared. In our example this would be achieved by multiplying by 100/12. We term this procedure the *standard scoring method*. A number of instruments are now advocating the use of *T*-scores, also called *norm-based scoring*, as described in Chapter 9.

Generic instruments

Some instruments are intended for general use, irrespective of the illness or condition of the patient. These *generic* questionnaires may often be applicable to healthy people, too. Some of the earliest ones were developed initially with population surveys in mind, although they were later applied in clinical trial settings.

There are many instruments that measure physical impairment, disability or handicap. Although commonly described as QoL scales, these instruments are better called *measures of health status* because they focus on physical symptoms. They emphasise the measurement of general health and make the implicit assumption that poorer health indicates poorer QoL. One weakness about this form of assessment is that different patients may react differently to similar levels of impairment. Many of the earlier questionnaires to some degree adopt this approach. We illustrate two of the more influential instruments, the Sickness Impact Profile (SIP) and the Nottingham Health Profile (NIP). Some scales specifically address activities of daily living, and we describe the Barthel questionnaire.

Few of the early instruments had scales that examine the subjective non-physical aspects of QoL, such as emotional, social and existential issues. Newer instruments, however, emphasise these subjective aspects strongly, and also commonly include one or more questions that explicitly enquire about overall QoL. We illustrate this approach by the SF-36. Later, brief instruments that place even less emphasis upon physical functioning have been developed. Two such instruments are the EQ-5D, that is intended to be suitable for use with cost–utility analysis, and the SEIQoL, which allows patients to choose those aspects of QoL that they consider most important to themselves.

Sickness Impact Profile (SIP)

The SIP of Bergner *et al.* (1981) is a measure of perceived health status, as measured by its impact upon behaviour. Appendix E1 shows an extract of SIP – the full question-naire takes 16 pages. It was designed for assessing new treatments and for evaluating health levels in the population, and is applicable across a wide range of types and severities of illness. The SIP consists of 136 items, and takes about 20–30 minutes to complete. The items describe everyday activities, and the respondents have to mark those activities they can accomplish and those statements they agree with. It may be either interviewer- or self-administered. Twelve main areas of dysfunction are covered, but there is no global question about overall health or QoL. It has been shown that the SIP is sensitive even to minor changes in morbidity. However, in line with its original design objectives, it emphasises the impact of health upon activities and behaviour, including social functioning, rather than on feelings and perceptions – although there are some items relating to emotional well-being.

The items are negatively worded, representing dysfunction. Data from a number of field studies were compared against assessments made by healthcare professionals and students, leading to 'scale values'. These scale values are used as weights when summing the individual items to obtain the scale score. The standard scoring method is used for each of the 12 dysfunction scales. Two higher-order dimensions, summarising physical and psychosocial domains respectively, are recognised and these are scored in a similar manner.

Nottingham Health Profile

The NHP of Hunt *et al.* (1981) measures emotional, social and physical distress (Appendix E2). The NHP was influenced by the SIP, but asks about feelings and emo-tions directly rather than by changes in behaviour. Thus, although the authors did not develop or claim it to be a QoL instrument, it does emphasise subjective aspects of health assessment. It was based upon the perceptions and the issues that were men-tioned when patients were interviewed. When it was developed, the idea of asking patients about their feelings was a novel concept.

The version 2 contains 38 items in six sections, covering sleep, pain, emotional reac-tions, social isolation, physical mobility and energy level. Each question takes a yes/ no answer. As with the SIP, each item reflects departures from normal, and items are weighted to reflect their importance. Earlier versions included seven statements about areas of life that may be affected by health, with the respondent indicating whether there has been any impact in those areas. These statements were less applicable to the elderly, unemployed, disabled or those on low income than are the other items, and are usually omitted. The NHP forms a *profile* of six scores corresponding to the different sections of the questionnaire, and there is no single summary index.

The NHP is short compared to the SIP, and is easy to complete. The wording is simple and easily understood. It is often used in population studies of general health evaluation, and has been used in medical and non-medical settings. It is also frequently used in clinical trials, although it was not designed for that purpose. However, it tends to emphasise severe disease states and is perhaps less sensitive to minor – yet important – changes and differences in health state. The NHP assesses whether there are any health problems, but is not sufficiently specific to identify particular problems. Some items do not apply to hospitalised patients, and the developers do not recommend it for these patients. Its simplicity, while being for many purposes an advantage, means that it does not provide suitable coverage for the conditions that apply to patients in many clinical trials.

Medical Outcomes Study 36-Item Short Form (SF-36)

The SF-36 developed by Ware *et al.* (1993) evaluates general health status, and was intended to fill a gap between the much more lengthy questionnaires and other relatively coarse single-item measures (Appendix E3). It is designed to provide assessments involving generic health concepts that are not specific to any age, disease or treatment group. Emphasis is placed upon physical, social and emotional functioning. The SF-36 has become the most widely used of the general health-status measures. It can be either self-assessed or administered by a trained interviewer.

As the name implies, there are 36 questions addressing eight health concepts (simpler 12- and eight-question forms are also available). There are two summary measures: physical health and mental health. Physical health is divided into scales for physical functioning (10 items), role-physical (four), bodily pain (two) and general health (five). Mental health comprises scales for vitality (four items), social functioning (two), role-emotional (three) and mental health (five). In addition, there is a general health transition question, which asks: 'Compared to one year ago, how would you rate your general health now?' There is also a global question about the respondent's perception of their health: 'In general, would you say your health is: (excellent, very good, good, fair, poor)?' Most questions refer to the past four weeks, although some relate to the present. A few questions, such as those for 'role-physical', take yes/no responses, while some, such as the physical functioning items, have three categories (limited a lot, limited a little, not limited at all), and other items have five or six categories for responses.

The designers of the SF-36 selected, standardised and tested the items so that they can be scored using the standard scoring method. More recently, norm-based scoring has been advocated (see Chapter 9).

Most of the items appear broadly sensible. However, the physical functioning scale, in common with many similar scales, poses questions about interpretation. Questions ask whether your health limits you in 'vigorous activities, such as running, lifting heavy objects, participating in strenuous sports' or in 'walking more than a mile'. It is not clear how those who never participate in such activities should respond – for example, suppose someone who never participates in sports has severely impaired health: if they respond 'No, not limited at all' they will receive a score indicating better functioning than might be expected. Some questionnaires therefore restrict physical functioning questions to activities that are expected to be applicable to everyone, while others stress that the questions are hypothetical ('we wish to know whether you *could* participate in sports if you wanted to').

For health economic evaluations, the SF-6D has been derived from the 12-item SF-12 subset of the SF-36 questionnaire (Brazier and Roberts, 2004). The SF-6D provides a preference-based single index measure for health, estimated from values of the SF-12.

EuroQol (EQ-5D)

The EQ-5D of Brooks *et al.* (1996) is another general-purpose instrument, this time emphasising both simplicity and the multi-country aspects (Appendix E4). It takes about two minutes to complete and aims to capture physical, mental and social functioning. It is intended to be applicable over a wide range of health interventions. The EuroQol group, acknowledging its simplicity, recommend using it alongside other instruments.

Most of the questionnaires we describe are *profile* instruments because they provide a descriptive profile of the patient's functional health and symptom experience. For medical decision-making, therapeutic benefits have to be contrasted against changes in QoL: if more efficacious therapy is associated with poorer QoL outcomes, is it worthwhile? Answering this involves weighing QoL against survival and combining them into a single summary score, most commonly by determining patient 'preference ratings' or 'utilities'. Overall benefits of treatment or management policies can then be contrasted. The EQ-5D, like the SF-6D which is based on the SF-36 and described above, is described as a *utility measure* or *preference measure*, in which the scores are weighted on the basis of preferences (or utilities) for discrete health states or combinations of health states derived from a reference sample.

Five dimensions of QoL are recognised: mobility, self-care, usual activities, pain/ discomfort and anxiety/depression. In the first version of the EQ-5D each of these was addressed by a simple three-level response scale; a revised version, the EQ-5D-5L, extended this to five levels per item as shown in Appendix E4 (Herdman *et al.*, 2011). The principal EQ-5D question is represented by a 20 cm vertical VAS, scored from 0 to 100, on which the respondent should mark 'your own health state today', ranging from best imaginable health state to the worst imaginable health state. A single index is generated for all health states. Perhaps because of its extreme simplicity, the EQ-5D has been less frequently used as the outcome measure for clinical trials. It has been used most widely for general healthcare evaluation, including cost–utility evaluation. It is especially used in the UK, where the government-funded National Institute for Health and Care Excellence (NICE) declares: "Health effects should be expressed in QALYs. The EQ-5D is the preferred measure of health-related quality of life in adults" (NICE, 2013).

Schedule for Evaluation of Individual Quality of Life (SEIQoL) and the Patient Generated Index (PGI)

The SEIQoL (Hickey *et al.*, 1996) and the PGI (Ruta *et al.*, 1994) are examples of instruments that were developed to assess QoL from the individual's perspective. For both instruments, the respondents identify areas of life that are particularly important to them, and the current level of functioning in each of these domains is evaluated. The practical procedure is as follows. First, the patient is invited to nominate the five most important aspects of their quality of life. Most patients readily list five domains, but if they find it difficult a standard list of prompts is used. Second, the patient is asked to score each nominated item or aspect, according to its severity. The third and final stage is to provide relative weights for the importance of each domain. Although the first stage is similar for both the PGI and SEIQoL, the two instruments differ in the way they implement the second and third stages. The PGI is somewhat simpler than the SEIQoL, and is described first.

For the second stage, the PGI (Appendix E5) invites the patient to score their chosen items using scales from 0, 'the worst you could imagine', to 10, 'exactly as you would like to be'. Then, for the third stage, the PGI asks patients to 'spend' a total of 10 imaginary points to improve areas of their life. At the second stage of the SEIQoL, the patient is offered a vertical 10 cm VAS for each of their chosen areas and asked to rate themselves on the scale between 'worst possible' and 'best possible'. Each SEIQoL scale generates a score between 0 and 100. For the third stage, obtaining importance weights, there are two approaches. The original SEIQoL then made use of a judgement analysis in which the patients grade a series of presented cases (Joyce *et al.*, 2003). A simpler direct-weighting approach is adopted for the SEIQoL-DW (Browne *et al.*, 1997). In this, patients are provided with a plastic disc that consists of five overlapping segments corresponding to the five domains that the patient has nominated; each segment can be rotated around the central pivot, allowing its exposed size to be adjusted relative to the other segments. The patient is asked: 'How do the five domains compare in importance to each other?' This procedure generates five weights that sum to 100%. For both instruments, the investigator calculates a score by multiplying the individual's self-rating in each of their chosen areas by the relative weight that they assigned to it, and summing the products over the five areas.

Both the SEIQoL and the PGI recognise that sometimes seemingly trivial problems may be of major significance to certain patients, while other issues that are thought by observers to be important may in fact be considered unimportant. Martin *et al.* (2007) review studies using PGI, and Wettergren *et al.* (2009) review use of SEIQoL-DW. Overall, patient-generated outcome measures are cumbersome to implement, make greater cognitive demands than traditional instruments. They appear to be useful primarily in complementing other measures and in guiding management decisions for individual patients, but may be less practical for clinical trial settings or when comparing groups of patients.

Disease-specific instruments

Generic instruments, intended to cover a wide range of conditions, have the advantage that scores from patients with various diseases may be compared against each other and against the general population. On the other hand, these instruments fail to focus on the issues of particular concern to patients with disease, and may often lack the sensitivity to detect differences that arise as a consequence of treatment policies which are compared in clinical trials. This has led to the development of disease-specific questionnaires. We describe three contrasting questionnaires that are used in a single disease area – cancer – and very different questionnaires that are widely used in epilepsy and asthma.

It may be observed that, even in the three cancer-specific instruments, there is substantial variation in content and wording. Although all of these questionnaires assess similar content areas, the relative emphasis placed on any given QoL domain and the specific ways in which questions are posed vary considerably. For example, in comparison to the FACT-G, the RSCL and the EORTC QLQ-C30 include a relatively larger number of questions addressing physical symptoms. There are also semantic and stylistic differences: when assessing depression, the generic SF-36, the FACT-G and the QLQ-C30 use the following item phrasing, respectively: (i) "Have you felt so down in the dumps that nothing could cheer you up?" and "Have you felt downhearted and blue?"; (ii) "I feel sad"; and (iii) "Did you feel depressed?" These items differ in both the degree to which they rely on idiomatic expressions and in the directness with which the questions are posed.

European Organisation for Research and Treatment of Cancer (EORTC) QLQ-C30

The EORTC QLQ-C30 is a cancer-specific 30-item questionnaire (Aaronson *et al.*, 1993); see Appendix E6. The QLQ-C30 questionnaire was designed to be multidimensional in structure, appropriate for self-administration and hence brief and easy to complete, applicable across a range of cultural settings and suitable for use in clinical trials of cancer therapy. It incorporates five functional scales (physical, role, cognitive, emotional and social), three symptom scales (fatigue, pain, and nausea and vomiting), a global health-status/QoL scale, and a number of single items assessing additional symptoms commonly reported by cancer patients (dyspnoea, loss of appetite, insomnia, constipation and diarrhoea) and the perceived financial impact of the disease.

In the QLQ-C30 version 3.0 all items have response categories with four levels, from 'not at all' to 'very much', except the two items for overall physical condition and overall QoL, which use seven-point items ranging from 'very poor' to 'excellent'. The standard scoring method is used. High scale scores represent high response levels, with high functional scale scores representing high/healthy levels of functioning, and high scores for symptom scales/items representing high levels of symptomatology/problems (Fayers *et al.*, 2001).

The QLQ-C30 is available in a range of languages and has been widely used in multinational cancer clinical trials. It has been found to be sensitive to differences between patients, treatment effects and changes over time.

EORTC disease- or treatment-specific modules

The EORTC QLQ-C30 is an example of an instrument that is designed to be modular, with the core questionnaire evaluating those aspects of QoL which are likely to be relevant to a wide range of cancer patients. For each cancer site particular issues are often important, such as specific disease-related symptoms or aspects of morbidity that are consequences of specific forms of therapy. The QLQ-ELD14, described by Wheelwright *et al.* (2013), is one of several modules that address additional issues (Appendix E7). This supplements the core QLQ-C30 with an additional 14 items for elderly patients with cancer.

Functional Assessment of Cancer Therapy – General (FACT-G)

The Functional Assessment of Chronic Illness Therapy (FACIT) Measurement System is a collection of QoL questionnaires targeting chronic illnesses. The core questionnaire, or FACT-G, was developed by Cella *et al.* (1993) and is a widely used cancer-specific instrument (Appendix E8). Similar to the EORTC QLQ-C30, the FACIT questionnaires adopt a modular approach and so a number of supplementary modules specific to a tumour type, treatment or condition are available. Non-cancer-specific FACIT questionnaires are also available for other diseases, such as HIV infection and multiple sclerosis.

The FACT-G version 4 contains 27 items arranged in subscales covering four dimensions of QoL: physical well-being, social/family well-being, emotional well-being and functional well-being. Items are rated from 0 to 4. The items are labelled from 'not at all' to 'very much', which is the same as for the QLQ-C30 but with the addition of a central 'somewhat'. Some items are phrased negatively, and should be reverse-scored. Subscale scores are derived by summing item responses, and a total score is derived by summing the subscale scores. Version 3 included an additional item after each subscale, enabling patients to weight each domain on an 11-point scale from 'not at all' to 'very much so'. These questions were of the form: 'Looking at the above 7 questions, how much would you say your PHYSICAL WELL-BEING affects your quality of life?' A similar set of items is optional for version 4.

Individual questions are phrased in the first person ('I have a lack of energy'), as compared with the QLQ-C30 which asks questions in the second person ('Have you felt weak?'). Both questionnaires relate to the past week, both make similar claims regarding validity and sensitivity and both target similar patients. Yet the FACT-G and the QLQ-C30 are conceptually very different from each other, with the QLQ-C30 emphasising clinical symptoms and ability to function, in contrast to the FACT-G which addresses feelings and concerns (Luckett *et al.*, 2011).

Rotterdam Symptom Checklist (RSCL)

The RSCL (de Haes *et al.*, 1996) is another instrument that is intended for measuring the QoL of cancer patients (Appendix E9). In the past the RSCL was used extensively in European cancer clinical trials, although less so nowadays. It covers broadly similar ground to the EORTC QLQ-C30 and has a similar number of questions. As its name implies, greater emphasis is placed upon the symptoms and side effects that are commonly experienced by cancer patients.

There are two features that are worthy of special note. First, the RSCL has an introductory text explaining 'for all symptoms mentioned, indicate to what extent you have been bothered by it ...' This is in contrast to the QLQ-C30 and most other QoL instruments, which merely inquire about the presence of symptoms. Thus one patient might have 'a little' stomach ache but, when asked if it bothers them, might respond 'not at all'; another might respond that the same ache bothers them 'quite a bit'. What is less clear is whether most patients read the questionnaire with sufficient care to appreciate the subtle significance of the instructions. The second feature relates to the ADL scale. Here, too, there are explicit instructions, stating: 'We do not want to know whether you actually do these, but only whether you are able to perform them presently.' Thus a patient might not 'go shopping' but is requested to indicate whether they could if they wanted to. This is in marked contrast with the equivalent scale on the SF-36 that not only asks about actual functioning but also includes some strenuous tasks which are perhaps less likely to be applicable to the chronically ill.

The RSCL consists of 30 questions on four-point scales ('not at all', 'a little', 'quite a bit', 'very much'), a question about activity level, and a global question about 'your quality of life during the past week' with seven categories. There are two main scales – physical symptom distress and psychological distress – in addition to the scales for activity level and overall valuation. The standard scoring method is used.

Quality of Life in Epilepsy (QOLIE-89)

In contrast with the previous examples, the QOLIE-89 is a 13-page, 89-item questionnaire aimed at patients with epilepsy (Devinsky *et al.*, 1995); Appendix E10 shows extracts. It is based upon a number of other instruments, in particular the SF-36, with additional items from other sources. It contains five questions concerning worry about seizures, and questions about specific 'bothersome' epilepsy-related limitations such as driving restrictions. Shorter versions with 31 and 10 items are available. The QOLIE-89 contains 17 multi-item scales that tap into a number of health concepts, including overall QoL, emotional well-being, role limitations owing to emotional support, social support, social isolation, energy/fatigue, seizure worry, health discouragement, attention/concentration, language, memory, physical function and health perceptions. An overall score is derived by weighting and summing the scale scores. There are also four composite scores representing issues related to epilepsy, cognition, mental health and physical health.

The QOLIE-89 has been developed and tested upon adults. Epilepsy is a serious problem for younger patients too, but children and adolescents experience very different problems from adults. Adolescents may be particularly concerned about problems of forming relationships with friends of the opposite sex, and anxious about possibilities of marriage and their dependence upon parents. Children may feel excluded from school or other activities, and may be teased by other children. Very young children may be unable to complete the questionnaire alone, and parents or others will have to assist. Thus QoL questionnaires intended for adults are unlikely to be satisfactory for younger age groups. One example of a generic QoL questionnaire that has been used for children with epilepsy is the 16-dimensional 16D, which Apajasalo *et al.* (1996) used in young adolescents aged 12–15, comparing normal children against patients with epilepsy. One interesting feature of the QOLIE-89 is that there are five questions about general QoL issues. Questions 1, 2, 3, 49 and 89 use various formats to enquire about health perceptions, overall QoL, overall health and change in health.

Paediatric Asthma Quality of Life Questionnaire (PAQLQ)

The PAQLQ developed by Juniper *et al.* (1996) has been designed to measure the problems that children between the ages of seven and 17 experience as a result of asthma; extracts from the self-administered version are shown in Appendix E11. The PAQLQ has 23 items relating to three dimensions, namely symptoms, activity limitations and emotional function. Items are scored from 1 to 7. Three of the activity questions are 'individualised', with the children identifying important activities at the beginning of the study. There is a global question, in which children are asked to think about all the activities they did in the past week, and to indicate how much they were bothered by their asthma during these activities. The items reflecting each dimension are averaged, forming three summary scales that take values between 1 and 7.

Parents often have a poor perception of their child's health-related QoL, and so it is important to ask the children themselves about their experiences. Since children may have difficulty in completing the self-administered questionnaire, Juniper *et al.* (1996) suggest using the interviewer-administered version, administered by a trained interviewer who has experience of working with children. Children may be strongly influenced by adults and by their surroundings, and so detailed guidelines and interviewing tips are provided. The PAQLQ has been tested in children aged between seven and 17 years, and has demonstrated good measurement properties in this age group.

Instruments for specific aspects of QoL

The instruments described above purport to measure general QoL, and include at least one general question about overall QoL or health. In many clinical trials this may be adequate for treatment comparison, but sometimes the investigators will wish to explore particular issues in greater depth. We describe four instruments that are widely used in clinical trials to explore anxiety and depression, physical functioning, pain and fatigue. These domains of QoL are particularly important to patients with chronic or advanced diseases. Many other instruments are available, both for these areas and others. Additional examples are *coping* (Hürny *et al.*, 1993), *satisfaction* (Baker and Intagliata, 1982), *existential beliefs* (Salmon *et al.*, 1996) and *self-esteem* (Rosenberg, 1965). Since these questionnaires evaluate specific aspects of QoL, in order for a patient assessment to be called 'quality of life' these instruments would normally be used in conjunction with more general questionnaires.

Hospital Anxiety and Depression Scale (HADS)

The HADS was developed by Zigmond and Snaith (1983) and was initially intended as a clinical screening tool to detect anxiety and depression (Appendix E12). It has become widely used in clinical trials for a wide range of conditions, including arthritis, bowel dysfunction, cancer, dental phobia, osteoporosis and stroke. The HADS consists of 14 questions that are completed by the patients. Each question uses a four-point scale. Seven of these questions were designed to address anxiety, and the other seven depression. The HADS deliberately excludes items that may be associated with emotional or physical impairment, such as dizziness and headaches; it emphasises the psychological signs or consequences of anxiety and depression.

Two particular features of the HADS are interesting from the point of view of scale design. The questions addressing anxiety and depression alternate (odd and even items, respectively), and half of the questions are worded positively and half negatively (e.g. 'I feel cheerful' and 'I get sudden feelings of panic').

Each item is scored 0 to 3, where 3 represents the state associated with the most anxiety or depression. The items are summed after suitable ordering, yielding two subscales ranging from 0 to 21. Based upon psychiatric diagnosis, HADS ratings of 11 or more are regarded as definite cases that would normally require therapy; ratings of 7 or less are non-cases; those scoring 8–10 are doubtful or borderline cases that are usually referred for further psychiatric assessment.

Another widely used instrument is the Beck Depression Inventory (BDI) (Beck *et al.*, 1961), which measures existence and severity of depression. It can be either self-rated or administered orally and emphasises cognitive rather than affective symptoms. The PHQ-9 is another popular depression questionnaire, and is briefer than the BDI (Spitzer *et al.*, 1999).

McGill Pain Questionnaire (MPQ)

Pain is a frequent symptom in many disease areas, and can be distressing. Not surprisingly, many instruments have been developed to assess pain. One such instrument, used extensively in clinical trials, is the Brief Pain Inventory (BPI) short form (Cleeland and Ryan, 1994). Further, many QoL instruments contain one or more items assessing pain. Examples include simple numerical rating scales, in which the respondents rate themselves in the range from 0 for no pain up to 10 for worst imaginable pain, and the more descriptive items as seen in the EORTC QLQ-C30 and the FACT-G.

The MPQ is one of the most widely used tests for the measurement of pain (Melzack, 1975). The MPQ full version has 20 main groups of items, each with between two and six adjectives as response categories, such as flickering, quivering, pulsing, throbbing, beating, pounding. It takes five to 15 minutes to complete. Based upon a literature search of terms used to describe pain, the MPQ uses a list of descriptive words that the subject ticks. The words are chosen from three classes of descriptors – sensory (such as temporal, spatial, pressure, thermal), affective (such as tension, fear) and evaluative (such as intensity, experience of pain). There is a six-point intensity scale for present pain, from no pain through to excruciating pain. Three major measures are derived: a pain rating index using numerical scoring, the number of descriptive words chosen, and the value from the pain intensity scale. Pain-rating index scores can be calculated either across all items or for three major psychological dimensions, called sensory–discriminative, motivational–affective and cognitive–evaluative.

The short version, termed the SF-MPQ (Melzack, 1987), is shown in Appendix E13. It has 15 items that are graded by the respondent from none (0) through to severe (3). There is also a 10 cm VAS, ranging from 'no pain' through to 'worst possible pain', and the same six-point intensity scale as in the full version. It takes two to five minutes to complete. Each description carries a weight that corresponds to severity of pain. This leads to a summary score that ranges from 0 ('no pain') to 5 ('excruciating pain'). The SF-MPQ has subscales for affective and sensory components of pain, as well as a total score. In 2009 the SF-MPQ was revised to include an additional 7 items for neuropathic pain, and all 22 items are now rated from 0 to 10.

Pain is a complicated and controversial area for assessment, although some of the problems serve to illustrate general issues in QoL assessment. For example, the Zung (1983) self-rating Pain and Distress Scale measures physical and emotional distress caused by pain, rather than severity of pain itself. This recognises that severity of pain, either as indicated by pain stimuli or by the subject's verbal description, may result in different levels of distress in different patients. One level of pain stimulus may produce varying levels of suffering, as determined by reactions and emotions, in different patients. Also, pain thresholds can vary. Another issue to be considered when assessing pain is that analgesics can often control pain very effectively. Should one be making an allowance for increasing dosages of, say, opiates when evaluating levels of pain? In some studies it may be appropriate to measure 'uncontrolled pain', in which case one might argue that it is irrelevant to enquire about analgesics. On the other hand, high doses of analgesics can be accompanied by disadvantages.

Multidimensional Fatigue Inventory (MFI)

The MFI of Smets *et al.* (1995) is a 20-item self-report instrument designed to measure fatigue (Appendix E14). It covers five dimensions, each of four items: general fatigue, physical fatigue, mental fatigue, reduced motivation and reduced activity. There are equal numbers of positively and negatively worded statements, to counter possible response bias, and the respondent must indicate to what extent the particular statement applies to him or her. The five-point items take responses between 'yes, that is true' and 'no, that is not true', and are scored 1 to 5, where 5 corresponds to highest fatigue. The five scale scores are calculated by simple summation.

Four of the scales appear to be highly correlated, with mental fatigue behaving differently from the others. This suggests that there may be one or two underlying dimensions for fatigue. However, for descriptive purposes, and for a better understanding of what fatigue entails in different populations, the authors suggest that the separate dimensions be retained and that the five scales should not be combined. If a global score is required, the general fatigue scale should be used.

Many other fatigue questionnaires exist. Some are designed to be disease specific, targeting for example patients with arthritis or with cancer; some assume fatigue is unidimensional, while others use for example a three-dimensional model. Fatigue modules have been developed to complement the EORTC-Q30 and the FACT-G.

Barthel Index of Disability (BI)

Disability scales were among the earliest attempts to evaluate issues that may be regarded as related to QoL. They are still commonly employed, but mainly as a simple indication of one aspect of the patient's overall QoL. The BI (Mahoney and Barthel, 1965) was developed to measure disability, and is one of the most commonly used of the class of scales known as ADL scales. ADL scales focus upon a range of mobility, domestic and self-care tasks, and ignore issues such as pain, emotions and social functioning. The assumption is that a lower ADL score implies a lower QoL.

The BI is used to assess functional dependency before and after treatment, and to indicate the amount of nursing care that is required. It has been used widely for assessing rehabilitation outcome and stroke disability, and has been included in clinical trials. Unlike any of the other scales that we have described, it need not be completed by the patient personally but is more intended for administration by a nurse, physiotherapist or doctor concerned with the patient's care. It therefore provides an interesting contrast against the subjective self-assessment that has been adopted by many of the more recent measures. The BI examines the ability to perform normal or expected activities. Ten activities are assessed, each with two or three response categories, scored 5, 10 or 15; items are left blank and scored 0 when patients fail to meet the defined criteria. Overall scores range for 0 (highest dependency) to 100 (least dependency). It takes about one minute to assess a patient.

The original BI uses a crude scoring system, since changes in points do not appear to correspond to equivalent changes in all the scales. Also, patients can be at the highest (0) point on the scale and still become more dependent, and can similarly exceed the lowest (100) value. Modified versions of the BI largely overcome these deficiencies. For example, Shah et al. (1989) expanded the number of categories and propose changes to the scoring procedures (Appendix El5). The BI and its modified versions continue to be used widely as a simple method of assessing the effectiveness of rehabilitation outcome.

Many ADL scales exist, and the Katz et al. (1963) index is another widely used example. The concept here is that loss of skills occurs in a particular sequence, with complex functions suffering before others. Therefore six items were chosen so as to represent a hierarchical ordering of difficulty. A simplified scoring system is provided, in which the number of activities that require assistance are summed to provide a single score. Thus while '0' indicates that no help is required, '6' means that there is dependency for all the listed activities. The Katz index has been used with both children and adults, and for a wide range of conditions. In contrast to the BI, which measures ability, the Katz index measures independence.

Instrumental activities of daily living (IADL) scales include items that reflect ability to live and adapt to the environment. This includes activities such as shopping and travelling, and thus these scales evaluate one's ability to live independently within the community, as opposed to needing help with basic functions such as dressing and washing oneself. One example is the Functional Activity Questionnaire (FAQ), which was designed for use in community studies of normal ageing and mild senile dementia (Pfeffer *et al.*, 1982).

1.9   Computer-adaptive instruments

Instruments developed in the twentieth century were mainly fixed format and paper based. Most are intended for self-completion by patients or other respondents, although some are designed with other modes of administration in mind such as by interviewer or over telephone. More recently, advances in computer technology have led to a new generation of instruments designed specifically for computer administration. These instruments are typically 'adaptive', in the sense that there is a large pool of potential items and each respondent is presented with a different set of items that are dynamically selected according to the respondent's previous answers. To some extent this mirrors the usual dialogue between a physician and patient: if a patient has said that they have no trouble walking long distances, why ask if they are housebound? It is more informative and efficient to tailor the interview as it progresses. However, computer-adaptive instruments use statistical algorithms to identify dynamically the optimal choice of items. They also calculate scores that are calibrated using a consistent metric across patients, enabling comparisons of PROs both between individual patients and in groups of patients.

Many of the instruments described above are available in their full original paper-based form, as short-form versions and, more recently, teams such as the EORTC group are generating in computer-adaptive versions (Petersen *et al.*, 2010). Other instruments are designed mainly for computer adaptive use; a prominent example is PROMIS (Cella *et al.*, 2010; Reeve *et al.*, 2007), which is developing a wide range of instruments that measure concepts such as pain, fatigue, physical function, depression, anxiety and social function (www.nihpromis.org); PROMIS instruments are available as computer adaptive tests that require three to seven items for precise scores, or four- to 10-item short form versions. Computer-adaptive instruments are described in Chapter 8.

1.10   Conclusions

Definitions of QoL are controversial. Different instruments use different definitions, and frequently no specific model for QoL is stated formally. There is a wide range of QoL instruments available, although this range is likely to be reduced once the purpose of evaluating QoL is considered. In a clinical trial setting, the disease area and therapies being evaluated will usually limit the choice. Common features of the instruments are that the patients themselves are asked, there are frequently several subscales, the scales are often based upon multiple items, and the scales represent constructs that cannot be measured directly. In Chapters 3–7 we shall explain methods for constructing such scales. Most importantly, we describe the desirable measurement properties of scales. We show how to 'validate' scales, and how to confirm whether an instrument appears to be consistent with the hypothetical model that the designers intended.

2

Principles of measurement scales

Summary

The main methods for developing and validating new questionnaires are introduced, and the different approaches are described. These range from simple global questions to detailed psychometric and clinimetric methods. We review traditional psychometric techniques, including summated scales and factor analysis models, as well as psychometric methods that place emphasis upon probabilistic item response models. Whereas psychometric methods lead to scales for QoL that are based upon items reflecting patients' levels of QoL, the clinimetric approach makes use of composite scales that may include symptoms and side effects of treatment. This chapter contrasts the different methods, which are then explained in detail in subsequent chapters.

2.1   Introduction

Questionnaires for assessing QoL usually contain multiple questions, although a few may attempt to rely upon a single global question such as 'Overall, what has your quality of life been like over the last week? (very good, better than average, about average, worse than average, very bad)'. Some QoL questionnaires are designed such that all items are combined together; for example items might be averaged to produce an overall score for QoL. Most instruments, however, recognise that QoL has many dimensions and will attempt to group the items into separate scales corresponding to the different dimensions. Thus we explore the relationship between items and scales, and introduce the concepts underlying scales and their measurement.

2.2   Scales and items

Each question on the QoL questionnaire is an expression in words for an item. Most QoL instruments consist of many questions, representing many items. Some of these items may aim to measure a simple aspect of QoL, such as a physical symptom. In

---

Quality of Life: The Assessment, Analysis and Reporting of Patient-Reported Outcomes, Third Edition.
Peter M. Fayers and David Machin.

such cases, sometimes a single item will suffice to encapsulate all that is required. Other QoL concepts may be more complex, and the developers of an instrument might decide that it is preferable to use several questions that can be combined to form a *multi-item scale*.

For example, some drugs may cause vomiting, and therefore questions for patients receiving potentially emetic drugs might aim to assess the level of vomiting. This is typically true for cytotoxic chemotherapy, which is used as a treatment for cancer. Some cancer-specific instruments contain a single question about vomiting. An example is the question 'Have you vomited? (not at all, a little, quite a bit, very much)' on the EORTC QLQ-C30. However, a single question about vomiting may be considered too imprecise to measure severity, frequency and duration of vomiting, and usage of anti-emetics. The QLQ-C30 already contained 30 questions, and it was felt undesirable to lengthen it. The developers considered it more important to retain questions about other symptoms and functions rather than add extra items about vomiting. Thus a single question about vomiting and one about nausea was thought adequate for general-purpose assessment of QoL. However, vomiting can sometimes be an outcome of particular interest, in which case studies might benefit from the addition of supplementary questions on this topic.

Symptoms are often conceptually simple. For example, vomiting has a clear definition and there is little controversy about its meaning. Multi-item scales are frequently used when assessing more complex issues. For example, the more psychological dimensions may be less well defined in many people's perception. Even when there is a commonly agreed single definition, it may be misunderstood by the patients who complete the questionnaire. For example, terms such as 'anxiety' and 'depression' are rather more abstract in nature than most clinical symptoms, and different investigators may adopt differing definitions. Psychological literature distinguishes these two terms, but patients may be less certain of their distinction and may interpret anxiety and depression in many different ways. They may also have widely differing opinions as to the severity intended by 'very anxious'. Because of the nature of psychological constructs, it is usually impossible to rely upon a single question for the assessment of a patient. Most psychometric tests will contain multiple items addressing each psychological aspect.

QoL instruments commonly contain a mixture of single-item and multi-item scales. A major aspect of scale design is the determination of the number of items that should comprise a particular scale and, if more than one item is appropriate, the assessment of how consistently these items hang together.

2.3   Constructs and latent variables

Some psychological aspects of QoL will have clear, precise and universally agreed definitions. As we have noted, others may be more contentious and may even reflect the opinions of an individual investigator. Many of these psychological aspects are not directly and reliably measurable, and in some cases it may be debatable as to whether the concepts that are being described really do exist as distinct and unique aspects of

QoL. These concepts constitute psychological models that may be regarded as convenient representations of QoL issues in patients. They are commonly described as being postulated *constructs*, *latent traits* or *factors*.

These hypothetical constructs that are believed or postulated to exist are represented or measured by *latent variables*. Examples of latent variables are QoL itself, or its constituent components (such as anxiety). Thus latent variables are the representations of constructs and are used in models. The aims of numerical methods in QoL research may largely be summarised as testing the adequacy and validity of models based upon postulated constructs, and estimation of the values of the latent variables that comprise those models. The term *factor*, apart from its use as a synonym for constructs, is commonly used to denote lower-level constructs such as when one construct, for example overall QoL, is decomposed into a number of components, or *factors*. Thus physical functioning, role functioning, social functioning and emotional functioning are latent variables that are all aspects, or factors, of QoL.

Constructs and latent variables are abstract concepts. Thus Nunnally and Bernstein (1994) describe constructs as 'useful fictions' and 'something that scientists "construct" or put together in their own imaginations'. They also note that the name given to any one specific construct is no more than a word and that, although the name may appear to imply a meaningful set of variables, there is no way to prove that any combination of these variables 'measures' the named construct. Since latent variables cannot be measured directly, they are usually assessed by means of multi-item tests or questionnaires. QoL instruments often contain 20 or more questions. Sometimes a single global question is also used, for example: 'How would you rate your overall quality of life during the past week?'

In contrast to the (unobserved) latent variables that reflect hypothetical constructs, the so-called *manifest variables* are the observed responses made by patients to questionnaire items.

When a single latent trait, or factor, underlies the data, the construct is described as being *unidimensional*. Many models for QoL assume that it can be represented by a number of lower-level factors, such as physical functioning, emotional functioning and cognitive functioning. Therefore QoL is often described as being *multidimensional* in nature. Most QoL instruments recognise the multidimensional nature of QoL and thus aim to evaluate a number of distinct dimensions, with each of these dimensions being addressed either by single items or by multi-item scales. In contrast, some instruments that are designed to target individual PROs may identify only a few dimensions – for example, a pain severity questionnaire might recognise a single dimension for pain severity.

2.4 Single global questions versus multi-item scales

Global questions

As Gill (1995) commented, "The simplest and most overtly sensible approach to measure QoL is to use global rating scales. These ratings, which have been successfully used to assess pain, self-rated health, and a myriad of other complex clinical phenomena,

can allow expression for the disparate values and preferences of individual patients."
Investigators can ask patients to give several global ratings, such as one for overall
QoL and another for health-related QoL or for physical well-being. Global single-
item measures allow the subject to define the concept in a way that is personally
meaningful, providing a measure that can be responsive to individual differences.
Global single-item indicators require that subjects consider all aspects of a phenomenon, ignore aspects that are not relevant to their situations, and differentially weight
the other aspects according to their values and ideals in order to provide a single rating.
A global single-item measure may be a more valid measure of the concept of interest
than a score from a multi-item scale.

Unfortunately, there is considerable disagreement whether it is meaningful to ask
a patient such questions as 'Overall, what would you say your quality of life has been
like during the last week? (excellent, very good, good, fair, poor, very poor, extremely
poor)'. Some authors argue that responses to these global questions are unreliable
and difficult to interpret, and that it is better to ask multiple questions about the
many aspects of QoL. They suggest that responses to the individual questions can be
aggregated to form a summary *global score* that measures overall QoL, using either an
unweighted summation that attaches equal importance to all questions or a weighted
summation that uses patients' opinions of the relative importance of questions. Other
authors dissent, some maintaining that QoL is a multidimensional construct and that it
is meaningless to try to sum the individual items to form a single overall score for QoL.

In practice, as described in the preceding chapter, many instruments include at least
one global question in addition to a number of multi-item scales. Often a global question is used for overall QoL, for overall health, or for similar concepts that are assumed
to be broadly understood by the majority of patients. In a similar way, global single
questions are also used to provide a single rating for individual domains, such as a
global question for overall depression.

Multi-item scales

Multi-item scales are commonly used to assess specific aspects of QoL that are likely
to be unidimensional constructs. Measures from multi-items usually have several
advantages over a score estimated from the responses to a single item.

One of the main objections to the use of single items in global questions is that
latent variables covering constructs such as QoL, role functioning and emotional functioning are complex and ill-defined. Different people may have different ideas as to
their meaning. Multi-item scales are often used when trying to measure latent variables
such as these. Many aspects of scale development have their origins in psychometric
testing. For example, from the earliest days it was accepted that intelligence could
not be defined and measured using a single-question intelligence test. Thus multiple
questions were recognised to be necessary to cover the broad range of aspects of intelligence (such as verbal, spatial and inductive intelligence). An intelligence test is therefore an example of a multi-item test that attempts to measure a postulated construct.
Under the *latent variable model* we assume that the data structure can be divided up

into a number of hypothetical constructs, such that each distinct construct is a latent variable representing a unidimensional concept. Since these constructs may be abstract and therefore not directly measurable, they are commonly assessed using multi-item questionnaires.

Psychometric theory also favours multi-item tests because they are usually more reliable and less prone to random measurement errors than single-item measures for assessing attributes such as intelligence, personality or mood. For example, in educational and intelligence tests, multi-item scales reduce the probability of obtaining a high score through either luck or the correct-guessing of answers.

Another very important reason for using multi-item tests is that a single item with, for example, a seven-category response scale lacks precision and cannot discriminate between fine degrees of an attribute, since for each patient it can assume only one of the specified response levels. By contrast, tests involving large numbers of items are potentially capable of very fine discrimination. Gaining precision is frequently the reason for including more items in a multi-item scale as each item adds more information about the latent variable. As we shall see in Chapter 8, this is also the reason for using computer adaptive tests that at each stage select the most informative successive items until adequate precision is obtained.

Many QoL instruments assess more than one domain. Thus they will contain either single items or multiple items per domain, and may present separate scores for each domain. These scores, and the instruments that produce them, are commonly termed *profile* if they describe related domains, and *battery* if they represent scores of independent concepts (Figure 2.1).

- **Single rating, single-item scale**

  A single question that is used to provide a score, such as a pain rating or a depression rating.

- **Multi-item scale**

  A scale formed by multiple related items. The items should represent a single domain or concept.

- **Scale score**

  A summary score for a single- or multi-item scale.

- **Index**

  A summary score for related items or independent concepts.

- **Profile**

  Multiple scores of multiple related domains.

- **Battery**

  Multiple scores of independent domains or concepts.

Figure 2.1   Scales, indexes, profiles and batteries.

2.5   Single-item versus multi-item scales

Reliability

A reliable test is one that measures something in a consistent, repeatable and reproducible manner. For example, if a patient's QoL were to remain stable over time, a reliable test would be one that would give very similar scores on each measurement occasion. In Chapter 4 we show that reliability of a measurement can be measured by the squared ratio of the true-score standard deviation (*SD*) over the observed-score *SD*, and in Chapter 5 we extend the discussion to include multi-item scales. It is often stated that multi-item scales are more reliable than single-item tests. This is a reasonable claim – in some circumstances.

Consider a questionnaire such as the HADS. The anxiety subscale comprises questions that include 'I feel tense or "wound up"', 'Worrying thoughts go through my mind' and 'I get sudden feelings of panic'. A patient with a given level of anxiety will tend to answer positively to all these items. However, there will be variability in the responses, with some patients responding more strongly to one question than another. This patient variability would render a single-item test unreliable. However, by averaging the responses from a large number of questions we effectively reduce the impact of the variability. In statistical terms, the reliability of the scale is increased by including and averaging a number of items, where each item is associated with an independent *random error term*. Cronbach's coefficient α is a measure of reliability of multi-item scales (see Chapter 5), and can be used to calculate the potential gain of adding extra items to a scale.

Many psychological concepts, for instance depression, are subjective states and difficult to define precisely. If asked a single question such as 'Are you depressed?', patients may vary in the perception of their state and may also be unsure as to how to classify themselves. Thus a large random error may be associated with global questions. Spector (1992) writes: "Single items do not produce responses by people that are consistent over time. Single items are notoriously unreliable." On the other hand, as we shall show, estimates of gain in reliability for multi-item scales are based upon conditions that are often inapplicable to the items found in QoL scales. Therefore it does not necessarily follow that increasing the number of items in a QoL scale will increase its overall reliability. A review of published empirical studies suggests that global questions regarding QoL can possess high reliability (Youngblut and Casper, 1993). Thus opinions continue to differ as to whether or not single-item global questions are reliable.

Precision

Numerical precision concerns the number of digits to which a measurement is made. If a scale has a range from 0 to 100, a measurement made to the nearest 1 is more precise than one rounded to the nearest 10. Precision is important because it indicates the potential ability of the scale to discriminate amongst the respondents. Precision is related to reliability, inasmuch as an imprecise measurement cannot be reliable.

Single-item global questions are frequently categorical in form, and these offer limited precision. For example, the SF-36 asks: 'In general, would you say your health is: …?' (response categories from 1 = excellent to 5 = poor), while the EORTC QLQ-C30 asks: 'How would you rate your overall quality of life during the past week?' (response categories from 1 = very poor to 7 = excellent). These questions have a precision that is delimited by the number of valid categories from which the respondent must choose, and the QLQ-C30, with seven categories, potentially offers more precision that the SF-36 with five. Although it might seem tempting to allow a larger number of response categories, this can lead to difficulties in distinguishing shades of meaning for adjacent ones. Offering a large number of categories also leads to unreliability in the sense that, in repeated testing, respondents will not consistently choose the same answer from the closely adjacent possibilities. When using labelled response options, *verbal rating scales* (VRS) with a maximum of four or five response categories are often recommended, and it would seem of little value to go beyond seven categories. For symptoms, a common format is to use an 11-point *numerical rating scale* (NRS) in which 0 represents absence of symptoms and 10 indicates the worst possible grading; for many applications this may provide adequate precision, although in other situations a multi-item scale may be preferred.

Multi-item tests, on the other hand, can have greater precision. For example, if four-point categorical questions are used, and five questions are summed into a summary score, the resultant score would have 20 possible categories of response.

Some single-item assessments attempt to overcome this by using visual analogue scales (VAS) in which a line, typically 10 cm long, is labelled at each end by extreme values. Respondents are invited to mark the line at a distance from the two ends according to their level of QoL. In principal such scales can provide fine discrimination, since the investigator may choose to measure the positions of the response very precisely. In practice, however, there must be doubt as to whether patients can really discriminate between fine differences of position along the line. (VRS, NRS and VAS are also described in Section 3.8).

Validity

The items of a multi-item scale can be compared against each other, to check whether they are consistent and whether they appear to be measuring the same postulated underlying construct. Psychometric tests of validity are to a large extent based upon an analysis of the inter-item correlation structure. These validation tests cannot be employed on a scale that contains only a single item. It has been argued that the ability to check the internal structure of multi-item scales is an essential feature, and the inability to do the same for single-item measures is their most fundamental problem. Blalock (1982) points out that with a single measure of each variable one can remain blissfully unaware of the possibility of measurement error, but in no sense will this make the inferences more valid.

This criticism of single-item scales serves merely to indicate the need to adopt suitable methods of validation. Internal validity, as typified by Cronbach's reliability coefficient α (see Chapter 5), can only be calculated for multi-item scales and cannot be explored when there is but a single item. However, insight into properties analogous to internal validity may be obtained by introducing additional, temporary items. During the scale development phase, redundant items could be added to the questionnaire purely for validation purposes; they could be abandoned once the scale is approved for use.

Both single- and multi-item scales can, and should, be investigated for external validity. This places emphasis upon an examination of the relationships and correlations with other items and scales, and with external variables such as response to treatment. Assessment of all scales should include evaluation of test–retest reliability, sensitivity and ability to detect expected differences between groups such as treatment or disease, and responsiveness to changes over time (Chapter 4).

Scope

QoL, like many constructs, is a complex issue and not easily assessed by a single question. Many patients, when asked: 'How would you rate your overall quality of life?' may reply: 'Well, it depends what you mean by "QoL". Of course I've got lots of symptoms, if that's what you mean. But I guess that is to be expected.' In other words, the global question oversimplifies the issues and some patients may have difficulty in answering it. They find it more straightforward to describe individual aspects of QoL. This is often advocated as a reason for multi-item questionnaires and is perhaps the most pertinent argument for caution in the use of global questions. If patients have difficulty understanding or answering a question, their responses must surely be regarded with suspicion.

An investigator who uses multi-item tests can choose items so that the scope and coverage of the questionnaire is made explicit. Areas of interest can be defined by the selective inclusion of items, and the scope of the questionnaire can be widened by including as many questions as are deemed necessary to cover all the topics of interest. Alternatively, the scope can be made more restricted or tightly defined, by excluding unwanted items, either at the questionnaire-design stage or during analysis. Multi-item questionnaires allow the investigator greater freedom for creating his or her own definition of QoL – even though this may not correspond to the patient's view of what is meant by 'quality of life'.

2.6   Effect indicators and causal indicators

Much of psychometric theory is based on the premise that there exist hypothetical 'latent' constructs such as QoL, and that scales can be constructed from items that reflect the respondent's level of the latent construct. Over the years it has become apparent that several types of items can be distinguished, according to their relationship with the latent variable that is being assessed. These are known as reflective (or effect) and formative (subdivided into causal and composite) indicators. Essentially, psychometric theory is based largely on reflective (effect) indicators, which also implies that models for 'parallel items' are applicable (Section 2.7).

It must be emphasised that the reflective model describes the relationship between the observed items ('indicators') and the latent construct; frequently a completely different perspective is obtained by redefining the latent variable, as we describe at the end of this Section. For example, when exploring QoL as the latent variable, pain impacts on QoL but does not necessarily reflect the level of QoL; on the other hand, pain may reflect severity or progression of illness.

Reflective (effect) indicators

The majority of items to be found in personality, intelligence or educational attainment tests and other psychometric assessments are designed to reflect either a level of ability or a state of mind, and this reflective model has dominated the psychometric methods that have been developed for test or questionnaire design. These items are commonly given a variety of descriptive names, including *effect indicator* or, because they indicate or 'reflect' the level of the latent variable, *reflective indicator.* They are also the most common type of item in PRO or QoL instruments and that is why we draw so heavily on methods developed in these other fields. However, as we shall see there are some notable exceptions and in those cases other methods of questionnaire design and scoring should be considered.

Items that are reflective indicators do not alter or influence the latent construct that they measure. (Although learning effects can interfere with the measurement of intelligence or education, appearing to alter the latent construct, they are less important for our discussion of QoL.)

Causal indicators

However, the symptoms assessed in QoL scales may cause a change in QoL. If a patient acquires serious symptoms, their overall QoL is affected by those symptoms. In fact, the reason for including symptoms in QoL instruments is principally because they are believed to affect QoL. Conversely, having a poor QoL does not imply that the patient has specific symptoms. Unlike educational tests, in which a person with the highest ability has the greatest probability of answering all questions successfully, a patient with poor QoL need not necessarily be suffering from all symptoms. Symptoms and similar items are *causal indicators* (Fayers and Hand, 1997a). Side effects are another good example of variables that are causal indicators in relation to overall QoL. Although symptoms are indicators of disease and side effects are consequences that are reflective of treatment, neither treatment nor disease is the focus when assessing QoL and, in relation to the assessment of QoL, symptoms and side effects are purely causal. Typical characteristics of causal items are that one on its own may suffice to change the latent variable; it is unnecessary – and usually rare – that patients must suffer from all items in order to have a poor QoL (Fayers *et al.*, 1997a). For example, few patients will experience all possible symptoms and side effects, but one serious symptom – such as pain – suffices to reduce overall QoL.

Variables may frequently be partly effect and partly causal indicators. They may also exchange roles. For example, a patient may experience symptoms, become distressed, and then perceive – and report – the symptoms as being worse than they are. An initially causal item has acquired additional reflective properties. Another example is the phenomenon of anticipatory nausea and vomiting. Cytotoxic chemotherapy for cancer commonly induces these side effects. Some cancer patients who have experienced these problems after their initial course of treatment may start vomiting prior to the administration of a subsequent course. Again, a variable that might seem to be purely causal has acquired some of the properties of an effect indicator. The reverse may also apply. A distressed patient may become unable to sleep; so insomnia is a reflective indicator of psychological distress. Continued insomnia, however, may then cause additional anxiety and distress. Thus there will often be uncertainty and ambiguity about the precise role of variables in QoL assessment. Disease or treatment-related symptom clusters are likely to be predominantly causal; it may be less clear whether psychological and other items are mainly causal or reflective in nature.

How do causal indicators affect QoL assessment? Many models assume that the observed items depend solely upon the latent variable. That is, if QoL is 'high', high levels of the items should reflect this. Furthermore, if the observed values of the items are correlated, these correlations should arise solely because of the effect of the latent variable. These assumptions are clearly untrue for causal indicators. Here, the correlations between, say, symptoms arise mainly because of the changing disease patterns. The correlations between a variable that is a causal indicator and the latent variable, QoL, are likely to be weak or obscured by the stronger correlations between symptom clusters.

Example

The Hospital Anxiety and Depression Scale (HADS) questionnaire is an instrument with a simple latent structure (Appendix E12). Zigmond and Snaith (1983) designed it such that seven questions should relate to anxiety, and seven to depression. The design assumes that 'anxiety' and 'depression' are meaningful concepts, and that they can be quantified. It is postulated that they are two distinct constructs. It is assumed that anxiety and depression cannot be measured reliably and adequately by single questions such as 'How anxious are you? (not at all, a little, quite a bit, very much)', and that multiple questions must be employed. In common with most questionnaires that assess *psychological* aspects of QoL, the HADS items are predominantly reflective indicators. If anxious, patients are expected to have high scores for the anxiety items; if depressed, they should score highly on the depression items.

The distinction between causal indicators and reflective indicators has become widely recognised in the field of structural equation modelling. However, the implications of this distinction are less frequently recognised in clinical scale development, even though these two types of items behave in fundamentally different ways in measurement scales, and have considerable impact upon the design of scales. As we shall see, the inter-item correlations can be more difficult to interpret with causal indicators, and thus the methods of Chapter 5 become less useful (e.g. Cronbach's α is usually irrelevant for causal indicators), exploratory factor analysis of Chapter 6 can sometimes prove misleading (although more complex structural models that may be helpful can be specified), and item response models of Chapters 7 and 8 become inappropriate.

Composite indicators

Some indicator variables may fit neither the reflective nor the causal models just described. Consider an Activities of Daily Living (ADL) instrument. This instrument may well provide a global score for ADL. Perhaps it contains items such as ability to walk a short distance, or ability to eat food unassisted. These items are neither effects of ADL nor do they 'cause' ADL to change. Instead, they are part of the definition of what we mean by ADL, and by including them in the model we are defining ADL as meaning mobility and ability to eat by oneself. Another example is given by the example in Section 5.7, where pain was evaluated by four items targeting, respectively, pain in abdomen, anus, rectum, or when urinating; these items are but weakly correlated, and are composite indicators that define what the investigators mean by 'pain' in the context of colorectal cancer.

Composite indicators thus serve to define, or 'form', their latent variable. In recognition of this, a score that is yielded from such instruments is commonly described as an *index*. Indexes exist in many forms; financial indexes include the FTSE-100, the Dow Jones Industrial Average, Nasdaq Index and many others – and in every case the index is defined by and labelled according to the items included in the respective basket. These and similarly formed indexes are defined by their *composite indicators* (e.g. Bollen and Bauldry, 2011). Formative indicators as originally defined by Fornell and Bookstein (1982) are the same as composite indicators. Confusingly, however, the modern trend is towards using the label *formative indicator* as an umbrella term that includes *both* causal indicators and composite indicators – that is, everything that does not fit the reflective model.

Formative indicators

The terms *causal indicator* and *effect indicator* are widely used in the field of structural equation modelling (Bollen, 1989). They are unfortunate choices of words, since in ordinary speech 'cause' and 'effect' are commonly regarded as dynamic and opposite. In our context, changes in so-called effect indicators need not be an effect 'caused' by the latent variable; they merely reflect its level. In an educational test, correct answers to questions are neither 'caused' by high ability nor cause high ability. As already noted, an alternative widely used term for effect indicator is the more neutral *reflective indicator*, because it reflects the level of the latent variable but need not in a strict sense be an effect or consequence caused by that latent variable. In statistical terms, a good reflective indicator is one that is highly correlated with the latent variable, and no implication of causality need be present. Thus the flavour of such an indicator is captured by such phrases as 'it reflects the latent variable' or 'it is a manifestation of the latent variable'. Similarly, some authors prefer the term *formative indicator* instead of causal indicator.

Distinguishing causal from reflective indicators

How can one identify causal indicators? Perhaps the easiest method is the *thought test*. For example, if we consider vomiting: think of the question 'Could severe vomiting affect QoL level?' Yes, almost certainly. 'Could QoL level affect vomiting?' Possibly, but it is more likely that vomiting is a consequence of the treatment or the disease. Hence, most would conclude, vomiting is likely to be a causal indicator for QoL. Jarvis *et al.* (2003) propose a seven-item check list for determining whether a particular item is formative or reflective. In this, a construct should be modelled as having formative indicators if the following conditions prevail:

1. the indicators are viewed as defining characteristics of the construct,

2. changes in the indicators are expected to cause changes in the construct,

3. changes in the construct are not expected to cause changes in the indicators,

4. the indicators do not necessarily share a common theme,

5. eliminating an indicator may alter the conceptual domain of the construct,

6. a change in the value of one of the indicators is not necessarily expected to be associated with a change in all of the other indicators, and

7. the indicators are not expected to have the same antecedents and consequences.

Table 2.1 compares reflective and formative models, and many of these features also serve to distinguish between the two models. Coltman *et al.* (2008) provide an expanded discussion contrasting these models.

Impact of formative models

For an index based on formative indicators, both causal or composite, correlation between the items is usually of little relevance (apart from very high correlations that may sometimes be indicative of item redundancy), so the methods of Chapters 5 to 8 are irrelevant. Face and content validity in the form of comprehensive coverage of the

Table 2.1 Comparison of reflective models and formative models

	Reflective model	Formative model
Construct	Construct exists independently of the items chosen.	Construct is formed and defined by the combination of indicators chosen.
Causality – 1	Changes in level of construct are reflected by corresponding changes in the items.	Changes in the level of the construct are not necessarily reflected by changes in the items.
Causality – 2	Changes in the items do not cause changes in the construct.	Changes in the items can cause changes in the construct.
Thought test	'Could change in an item affect the latent construct?' No; 'Could change in the latent construct affect an item?' Yes. 'No' and 'Yes' => Reflective model	'Could change in an item affect the latent construct?' Yes; 'Could change in the latent construct affect an item?' Not necessarily. 'Yes' and 'Not necessarily' => Formative model
Parallel items	Individual items are exchangeable. Adding or dropping an item does not change the concept of the construct – an essential property for computer adaptive tests (CAT).	Items define the construct. Adding or dropping an item may change the definition of the construct.
Coverage	Since items are parallel and exchangeable, there is no requirement for comprehensive coverage.	Essential that items provide comprehensive coverage of all aspects of the construct that is being defined.
Impact of items	Items are exchangeable and thus equally important.	Emphasis on items that patients consider most important and which have greatest impact.
Correlations (All items in any one scale should be scored in a consistent direction – e.g. high score = 'good')	Items should have moderately high positive correlations. Very high correlations may indicate unnecessary items.	No pattern of correlations is necessary. As with reflective indicators, very high correlations may indicate item redundancy.
Internal consistency / reliability	Scales should have high internal reliability; Cronbach's alpha and other correlation-based methods are suitable.	Correlation-based methods such as Cronbach's alpha are irrelevant. A scale may have low alpha yet still be useful.
Exploratory factor analysis (EFA)	EFA may be used to explore the construct, its dimensionality and relation to the items.	EFA is of little relevance in exploring the construct, except to identify clusters of items with a common theme. It may be feasible to fit structural models provided the conceptual model includes at least some reflective items (e.g. 'MIMIC' models).

components in the index is usually paramount. It is particularly important to include items for all of the issues that impact on (causal model) or define (composite model) the latent variable, especially if they occur frequently or are rated important by patients. Irrelevant items must not be included, as they might distort the index that is being created. These issues are addressed most strongly by qualitative methods for face and content validity, rather than the correlation-based or other psychometric approaches to construct validity.

Thus the development of scales based on reflective or formative models should follow different principles. This will affect the initial choice and specification of candidate items, and the subsequent selection, retention or deletion of items. Two studies are reported in the examples of Section 3.15, illustrating the substantial differences that occur when scales are developed using methods for formative items instead of psychometric models with reflective items. The distinction between the two types of indicators is of fundamental importance to the design and validation of new instruments, particularly when they are intended to combine multiple items into summary scales. Effect indicators may lead to homogeneous summary scales with high reliability coefficients, whereas causal indicators should be treated with greater caution (Fayers and Hand, 1997a).

Re-specifying the latent variable

We have discussed how a symptom such as pain might be conceptually regarded as a causal indicator when assessing QoL. In this model, QoL is the latent variable and it is assumed that the aim is to obtain a rating for patients' level of QoL. Instead, suppose we are interested in simply rating the level of pain severity. To do this, we now define pain severity as the latent variable, and we seek items in the pain questionnaire that are indicators of pain level. These items can arguably be viewed as reflective of pain severity, and the aim of scale validation now becomes to evaluate whether a reflective model is reasonable, and to test the performance of the individual items.

In other words, it is essential to recognise that items are not in themselves inherently reflective or formative. They only acquire these attributes when they are regarded as indicators of a specified latent variable, and the same item may change its status according to the perspective from which it is viewed. A set of pain items may be reflective for severity of pain, and then standard psychometric methods will be perfectly applicable; the same items can at the same time be formative indicators for an index score of QoL, and for that purpose a different approach to scaling and scoring will be necessary.

2.7　Psychometrics, factor analysis and item response theory

The theory of multi-item tests is based upon measurement models that make various assumptions about the nature of the items. These form what is often called *traditional psychometrics* and are based largely on either summated scales, in which the scores on multiple items are added together, or linear models such as factor analysis models. In contrast, models that stress the importance of item response models, in which patients with a particular level of ability have a *probability of responding positively* to different questions, are often called *modern psychometrics*.

Historically, the early psychometricians were interested in exploring ill-defined constructs such as intelligence, to see if there is an innate form of general intelligence. It was thought that this might be distinct from specific abilities such as verbal or mathematical intelligence, which might be influenced by education (see Section 6.6). This led to the creation of multi-item tests that enabled correlation-based models to be explored for attempting to separate these postulated constructs. Thus one major reason for using what are known as parallel tests is that it becomes possible to explore dimensionality and factor-structure. The use of multiple items also increases the reliability and precision of the assessment.

Parallel items

One of the most common models is founded upon the theory of *parallel tests*. This posits that each individual measurement item is a test or a question that reflects the level of the underlying construct – that is, all items should be reflective indicators (Section 2.6). For example, when evaluating anxiety, each question should reflect the underlying level of a patient's anxiety. Each item should be distinct from the others, yet will nevertheless be similar and comparable in all important respects. The item responses should differ only as a consequence of random error. Such items are described as being parallel. There are a number of assumptions inherent in this model, of which the most important are:

1. Each of the items (say, x_i for the ith item) is a test that gives an unbiased estimate of the latent variable (θ). That is, on average, the value of each item equals the value of the latent variable plus random variability (the *error term*). Thus $x_i = \theta + e_i$, where e_i is an error term that has, on average, a mean value of zero.

2. The e_i error terms are uncorrelated. That is, any two items (x_i, x_j) should only appear to be correlated because the latent variable varies. If we consider a group of patients with an identical level of QoL (constant θ), their x values should be uncorrelated with each other.

3. Each item is assumed to have the same amount of potential error as any other item. That is, $SD(e_i) = SD(e_j)$. This implies that, for a group of patients corresponding to any one particular value of the latent variable, the items x_i and x_j have equal SDs.

4. The error terms are uncorrelated with the latent variable. That is, the correlation between e_i and θ is zero.

The theory of parallel tests underpins the construction of simple summated scales in which the scale score is computed by simply adding together all of the item scores.

These scales are often called *Likert summated scales*, after the influential papers by Likert (1932, 1952). The Likert method is most successful when the response scale for each item covers a wide range of scale levels.

However, the constraints of strictly parallel tests have been recognised as being unnecessarily restrictive. Most of the psychometric properties are retained even when the SDs of the error terms are allowed to differ, so that $SD(e_i) \neq SD(e_j)$. Such models are known as *randomly parallel tests*, or *tau-equivalent tests* since τ (tau) is the mathematical symbol that is often used to represent the true score for a test. This implies that the items are still parallel with respect to how much they are influenced by the latent variable, but they may have different error SDs arising from extraneous non-specified factors. Thus in tau-equivalent tests, like parallel tests, the mean value x_i of item i is on average equal to θ.

Much of the early development of psychometric questionnaires was centred upon educational testing, in which examination questions can be carefully designed so as to comply with these exacting demands. For QoL instruments, one might anticipate that some items in a scale might take responses that are on average higher (or lower) than other items in the scale. In psychometric terms, these may be *essentially tau-equivalent tests*, in which the items have different constant 'bias', or shift in value, relative to the latent variable. Thus the mean value of item i is $\theta + k_i$ where k_i is the constant bias for item i. One thing in common with all these models is the assumption that the tests consist of reflective indicators that are solely linear functions of the latent variable (with a random error component included). Many of the traditional psychometric methods remain applicable to essentially tau-equivalent tests (Lord and Novick, 1968).

The majority of QoL instruments have been designed upon the principles of parallel tests and Likert summated scales. The related psychometric methods (see Chapter 5) to a large extent assume that the scales contain solely reflective indicators. This is usually a reasonable assumption for educational, intelligence and personality tests, as well as for many other psychological and sociological tests. The inter-item correlations that exist between causal indicators in many clinical fields of application may render many psychometric methods inapplicable.

Factor models

Parallel tests and Likert summated scales are unidimensional models; that is, they assume that all the items are measuring a single construct, or factor. If an instrument is thought to consist of several multi-item scales, each will have to be analysed separately. By comparison, *factor analysis* is a much more general approach that can model a number of factors simultaneously, using the inter-item correlations and SDs to estimate the models and carry out statistical 'goodness-of-fit' tests. The factor structure models are linear combinations of the observed variables, with the latent variables being estimated by weighted summation that reflects the importance of each of these variables. The basic factor analysis models belong to traditional psychometrics, and they assume that all items are reflective indicators such that the inter-item correlations arise through the relationship between these observed variables and the latent variable.

However, when causal items are present, the so-called exploratory factor analysis model breaks down. For example, many symptoms will be correlated because they are related to disease progression or treatment side effects; these correlations indicate nothing about the relationship between the symptoms and QoL. *Structural equation models* (SEMs) provide generalisations of the factor model, and also include *multiple-indicator multiple cause* (MIMIC) models. These models are able to handle causal indicators, but place far greater demands upon the data and do not provide a solution in every circumstance. Variables that are composite indicators, and form indexes, do not fit factor models, SEMs or MIMIC models.

Factor analysis seems to work – even with formative indicators!

Exploratory factor analysis is widely used in publications that purport to validate QoL instruments. Mostly, the results appear to be sensible. Which might appear to contradict the assertions about formative indicators and misleading correlations. However, although factor analysis is promoted as a form of validation for exploring the dimensionality and constructs underlying latent variables such as QoL, we will show in Chapter 6 that all it really aims to do is identify clusters of variables that are highly correlated. Thus if a QoL instrument contains several items about mobility, it would be unsurprising to find that those items are strongly correlated and thus form a 'factor'; but the presence of a such a factor cannot be taken as reassurance that mobility is a dimension of QoL. In Chapter 6 we provide additional examples where factor analysis leads to misleading results when formative items are present. Usually, however, the resultant factors which represent clusters of correlated items *will* appear sensible, but for the wrong reasons.

Item response theory

While most QoL and other clinical scales have been developed and based upon traditional psychometric theory, with summated scales being particularly common, newer instruments make greater use of modern psychometric theory. This largely centres on *item response theory* (IRT). For this model, items may have varying 'difficulty'. It is assumed that patients will have different probabilities of responding positively to each item, according to their level of ability (that is, the level of the latent variable). Whereas traditional methods focus upon measures such as averages, IRT places emphasis upon probabilities of responses.

The design of scales using IRT methods is markedly different from when traditional methods are used. Likert summated scales assume items of broadly similar difficulty, with each item having response categories to reflect severity or degree of response level. In contrast, IRT scales are based upon items of varying difficulty. In educational testing, where IRT was to a large extent pioneered, each item will frequently have only two response categories (gradings), such as yes/no or right/wrong. By using items with a wide range of difficulty, ability can be scored with a high level of precision. We cannot separate the most able students from those only slightly less competent if all the questions are too easy; thus an exam should include some difficult questions that enable discrimination at this level. Similarly, easy questions are needed to distinguish among the weaker students.

Unlike the early psychometricians, who were using parallel tests to explore the number of dimensions that underlie concepts such as intelligence, the proponents of IRT instead assume that the dimensions have to a large extent been agreed upon. The focus becomes assessment, with the highest efficiency and precision. In addition, the items in educational tests have to be changed from year to year to prevent cheating. A means of calibrating questions is required, to ensure a consistency of grades over time. IRT offers this facility.

IRT models, like factor models, assume that the observed variables reflect the value of the latent variable, and that the item correlations arise solely by virtue of this relationship with the latent variable. Thus it is implicit that all items are reflective indicators. This model is inappropriate for symptoms and other causal items. IRT also underpins computer adaptive tests (CATs), and one of the assumptions of CATs is that items are exchangeable so that different respondents may receive different subsets of items; clearly that cannot be true if the items are formative indicators, either causal of composite indicators.

2.8   Psychometric versus clinimetric scales

Feinstein (1987) argues that many clinical scales possess fundamentally different attributes from psychometric scales, and that their development and validation should therefore proceed along separate paths. He proposed the name *clinimetrics* for the domain concerned with the construction of clinical indexes. A 'good' and useful clinimetric scale may consist of items comprising a variety of symptoms and other clinical indexes, and does not necessarily need to satisfy the same requirements that are demanded of other scales. Fayers and Hand (2002) characterise this by noting that psychometricians try to measure *a single attribute with multiple items*. The validation methods described in Chapter 5 are then used to demonstrate that the multiple component items are all measuring (more or less) the same single attribute (latent variable). Clinicians try to measure *multiple attributes with a single index*, and aim their strategies at choosing and suitably emphasising the most important attributes to be included in the index.

Example

The Apgar (1953) score is used to assess the health of newborn babies. This index combines five seemingly disparate symptoms related to heart rate, respiratory rate, reflex responses, skin colour and muscle tone. Despite this, it provides an effective and well-established predictor of neonatal outcome. Each item is scored from 0 to 2, and a sum-score of 7 or more indicates good prognosis.

In many applications of clinimetrics, as with Apgar scores, the primary aim is to develop a diagnostic tool, or a prognostic or predictive index. In those settings causal items are particularly frequent because they will be powerful predictors. Of course, the development of these predictive indexes is likely to be fundamentally different from developing a QoL instrument because an external criterion variable – the outcome being predicted – is available for patients who have been followed up. Thus statistical methods usually centre on regression or similar techniques.

When a single attribute (latent variable) is being assessed using multiple items, the investigators will often have a model for the structural relationships in mind. Thus psychometricians usually think in terms of how the latent variable manifests itself in terms of the observed variables. This leads to the use of factor analysis and other techniques for the extraction of scores. On the other hand, the summary indexes that clinicians often seek to encapsulate the values from a number of measured attributes may sometimes be completely arbitrary, and are defined rather than modelled. Sometimes various target criteria are employed when developing an index, such as its prognostic or predictive ability for some future outcome such as length of subsequent survival or cure.

When measuring QoL, one might define a hypothetical construct for the latent variable 'overall QoL'. Using a psychometric model, one would seek indicators that are postulated to reflect overall QoL, and would then collect experimental data to explore and test the model, and to determine whether the variables fit the model. Using a clinimetric approach, one could identify those items that patients regard important for good QoL (that is, causal items affecting QoL), and use these to define a summary index. Whereas the psychometric approach emphasises constructing, validating and testing models, the clinimetric approach usually involves defining and developing an index that is 'clinically sensible' and has desirable properties for prognosis or prediction.

The distinction between *clinimetric indexes* and *psychometric scales* has far-reaching implications for the assessment of reliability and validity. Fayers and Hand (2002) show that it is also closely related to the distinction between *causal indicators* and *reflective indicators*, and these concepts explain and justify most of the supposed differences between psychometric scales and clinimetric indexes. The greater part of psychometric theory presumes that all of the items in a scale are reflective indicators. Clinimetric indexes behave differently from psychometric scales principally because they can contain both formative indicators and reflective indicators.

2.9 Sufficient causes, necessary causes and scoring items

In epidemiology, the concepts of causal variables have been highly developed. Thus in 1976 Rothman introduced the concept of *necessary and sufficient causes* (Rothman, 1976). An epidemiological example is infection with *Mycobacterium tuberculosis* (TB). Nothing else can cause TB, and so bacterial infection by this mycobacterium is a *necessary* condition. It is also a sufficient cause for TB because no additional factors are needed; this mycobacterium on its own is *sufficient* to cause TB. Although necessary causes are only infrequently applicable to scale development, the presence of sufficient causes can be of considerable importance. For example, symptoms are examples of causal items that may also sometimes be sufficient causes; a single symptom, such as pain, may be sufficient to cause QoL to become low. If a QoL instrument contains a scale consisting of several symptoms, a high level of symptomatology for one symptom may be sufficient to impair QoL, irrespective of the values of the other symptoms.

This concept of causal indicators often being sufficient causes has a number of implications for scale development. The latent variable, QoL, is not equally reflected by all the component items of the scale. There are no grounds to assume that a summated scale will be applicable and, to the contrary, frequently it is unlikely that all the items in a symptom scale will be equally important as determinants of QoL. For example, suppose disease progression can cause severe pain in some patients, but causes severe nutritional problems in others. A high score on either one of these symptoms would suffice to reduce QoL, and the maximum symptom score could be a better predictor of QoL than the mean of the two items. Thus, instead of a simple summated scale that gives equal weight (importance) to each item, other functions, for example maximum scores, may be more appropriate. When items represent causal variables that are also sufficient causes, linear models such as Likert summated scales and weighted sum-scores may be unsatisfactory predictors of QoL.

2.10 Discriminative, evaluative and predictive instruments

Throughout the stages of scale development, validation and evaluation it is important to consider the intended use of the measurement scale. Guyatt *et al.* (1993) draw attention to the need to distinguish between discriminative, evaluative and predictive instruments. Some scales are intended to differentiate between people who have a better QoL and those with a worse QoL; these are *discriminative scales*. Other scales are intended to measure how much QoL changes; these are *evaluative scales*. Scales may also be designed to *predict* future outcomes for patients. If an instrument is intended to be discriminative, it may be less important to include symptoms that are common to all patients and unlikely to differ between the various treatment groups. For example, fatigue is not only common for patients with thyroid disease but is also common among patients without the disease, and hence it might be considered an unimportant item in a purely discriminative instrument. However, fatigue is indeed an important symptom for people with thyroid disease, and a change in fatigue over time could be a key item for evaluating effects of therapy.

In general, an instrument that is primarily intended to be *evaluative* or *predictive* should be *responsive* to within-patient changes over time. However, if an instrument is intended to be mainly discriminative, patient-to-patient differences are more important than responsiveness. A *discriminative* instrument should yield consistent measurements when applied repeatedly to a patient whose condition is stable and has not changed; that is, it should provide repeatable, reproducible results. In particular, it should possess high *test–retest reliability*. It should in addition be *sensitive* to between-patient differences.

Sensitivity, responsiveness and repeatability are important to all instruments (Chapter 4), but when the instrument is intended for specific applications one or the other property may receive greater priority or, alternatively, different standards may be set for acceptability of the instrument. Thus the emphasis will vary according to the primary objectives in developing the instrument.

2.11 Measuring quality of life: reflective, causal and composite indicators?

QoL instruments commonly contain both reflective and causal indicators. Whereas the level of QoL is reflected in the values of reflective indicators, it is affected by causal items. However, psychometric methods, which have formed the basis for development and validation for the majority of QoL instruments, are founded upon the assumption that all of the items are reflective indicators. The concept of causal indicators explains many of the differences between psychometric and clinimetric methods, and why psychometric methods are less appropriate in the context of these variables and why the clinimetric approach is often preferable.

Fayers and Hand (2002) and Fayers (2004) demonstrate that the distinction between causal and reflective indicators affects all stages of instrument development, from selection of items through validation to scoring and hence analysis. Thus, for example, when selecting items for an instrument, the psychometric approach leads to items that are multiple (parallel) reflective indicators for each scale, while for causal indicators such as symptoms and for other items that are formative indicators the most important considerations are content validity and breadth of coverage.

Essentially, QoL instruments serve two very different functions, and should be designed accordingly. On the one hand, they serve to alert the clinician about problems concerning symptoms and side effects, and help in the management of patients. For this purpose, the clinician will often want the results of each symptom reported separately. Where multi-item symptom scales are needed, they are often best constructed on clinimetric principles. However, sometimes scale scores have been formed simply by summing disparate symptoms and other physical aspects, even when these cannot form a coherent clinical scale indicating the level of QoL. Such scores may, however, provide a health-related measure of total symptom burden.

On the other hand, many QoL instruments are intended to assess overall QoL as well as its aspects. For this, reflective indicators may be the most effective, and they should be chosen and validated using psychometric techniques. These reflective indicators might be expressions of patients' perception of their QoL, or how aspects of their QoL status are impaired or reduced. That is, the indicators should reflect the effects of impairment rather than being items that cause impairment.

It might be thought, therefore, that QoL is best assessed by forming scales consisting solely of reflective indicators. However, this is tantamount to arguing that if, for example, a patient who suffers many symptoms can cope with their problems and neither reports nor shows visible outward signs of suffering, then their QoL is fine. This clearly raises philosophical issues regarding perceptions and meaning of 'good QoL'. Thus most investigators intuitively feel the need to include information about symptoms and functional problems in any assessment of QoL. Equally, clinicians would generally try to relieve symptoms even though patients might claim that they can cope with their problems or disabilities.

An alternative approach to the assessment of overall QoL is simply to ask the patient, and many instruments do contain a global question such as 'How would you rate your overall quality of life during the past week?' Gill and Feinstein (1994) advocate that all instruments should contain such questions.

2.12   Further reading

Much of the work on formative models and causal/composite items has been in fields outside of healthcare, with burgeoning interest in management, business, consumer and marketing research. In 2008, the *Journal of Business Research* dedicated a whole issue to formative indicators (Diamantopoulos, 2008). Other useful papers are Coltman *et al.* (2008), and Diamantopoulos and Siguaw (2006), both reviewing differences between reflective and formative models; Turner *et al.* (2009a) considers implications on scoring of scales, while Lee and Cadogan (2013) observe that for formative variables to have utility in theoretical models, the loadings of the formative indicators should be specified as part of the construct definition prior to any analysis. Edwards and Bagozzi (2000) were early enthusiasts of formative models, although more recently Edwards (2011) comments "The shortcomings of formative measurement lead to the inexorable conclusion that formative measurement models should be abandoned", and suggests alternative ways of constructing measurement models.

2.13   Conclusions

The distinction between causal, composite and reflective indicators, although rarely recognised, carries far-reaching implications regarding the methods of scale construction and validation, as does the distinction between psychometric and clinimetric methods. The majority of QoL instruments contain a mixture of causal and reflective items.

Most instruments also contain both single- and multi-item scales, and the majority of the modern QoL instruments include at least one global question assessing overall reported QoL.

The following chapters explore the ways in which such instruments may be validated and examined for evidence of reliability and sensitivity.

3

Developing a questionnaire

Summary

Chapter 1 explained some of the basic principles of assessing patient-reported outcomes and QoL, together with examples of existing instruments. Chapter 2 discussed the principles of single- and multi-item scales. We now provide an overview of the principles that are involved in the initial stages of developing a questionnaire. This chapter focuses in particular on the early and crucial qualitative aspects of questionnaire design.

3.1   Introduction

The development of a new QoL instrument requires a considerable amount of painstakingly detailed work, demanding patience, time and resources. Some evidence of this can be seen from the series of publications that are associated with such instruments as the SF-36, the FACT-G and the EORTC QLQ-C30. These and similar instruments have initial publications detailing aspects of their general design issues, followed by reports of numerous validation and field-testing studies.

Many aspects of psychometric validation are described in the chapters that follow. These depend on collecting and analysing data from samples of patients or others. However, the statistical and psychometric techniques can only confirm that a scale is valid in so far as it performs in the manner that is expected. These quantitative techniques rely upon the assumption that the items and their scales in a questionnaire have been carefully and sensibly designed in the first place, by the rigorous application of formal qualitative methods.

Thus the scale development process should follow a specific sequence of stages, and details of the methods and the results of each stage should be documented thoroughly. Reference to this documentation will, in due course, provide much of the justification for claiming content validity. It will also provide the foundation for the hypothetical models concerning the relationships between the items on the questionnaire and the postulated domains of QoL and other PROs, and this *construct validity* can then be explored using quantitative methods.

Quality of Life: The Assessment, Analysis and Reporting of Patient-Reported Outcomes, Third Edition.
Peter M. Fayers and David Machin.
© 2016 John Wiley & Sons, Ltd. Published 2016 by John Wiley & Sons, Ltd.

The importance of the initial qualitative stages cannot be overemphasised. If an important PRO has been overlooked and therefore omitted from the instrument, later quantitative validation will be unable to detect this. Thus, no amount of subsequent quantitative validation can compensate for a poorly designed questionnaire; unfortunately, many forms of so-called validation will leave the investigator completely unaware that the foundations are unsound. Conversely, if the initial development has been carried out with full rigour, the subsequent validation stages will serve to collect evidence in support of the instrument, and will enable fine-tuning of the final product; it is rare to see major changes needed to an instrument that has been designed using careful application of qualitative methods.

3.2   General issues

Before embarking on developing a questionnaire, the research questions should have been formulated clearly. In the case of QoL, this will include specification of the objectives in measuring QoL, a working definition of what is meant by 'quality of life', the identification of the intended groups of respondents, and proposals as to the aspects or main dimensions of QoL that are to be assessed. When the focus is on specific PROs, such as fatigue or depression, similar levels of detail should be specified. Examples of *objectives* are whether the instrument is intended for comparison of treatment groups in clinical trials (a discriminative instrument), or for individual patient evaluation and management. Possible *definitions* of QoL might place greater or lesser importance upon symptoms, psychological, spiritual or other aspects. According to the specific definition of the target *respondents*, there may be particular emphasis upon disease- and treatment-related issues. All these considerations will affect decisions about the *dimensions* of QoL to be assessed, the number of questions, feasible length of the questionnaire and the scope and content of the questions.

When an instrument is intended for use in clinical trials, there is a choice between aiming at a general assessment of health-related QoL that is applicable to a wide range of patients, or a detailed evaluation of treatment- or disease-specific PROs. The former has the advantage of providing results that can be contrasted across patients from trials in completely different disease groups. This can be important when determining healthcare priorities and allocation of funding. The SF-36 is an example of such an instrument. However, disease-specific instruments can provide information that focuses upon the issues considered to be of particular importance to the patient groups under investigation. Treatment-specific instruments will clearly be the most sensitive ones for detecting differences between the treatment groups.

3.3   Defining the target population

Before considering the issues to be addressed by the instrument, it is essential to establish the specification of the target population. What is the range of diseases to be investigated, and are the symptomatology and QoL issues the same for all disease subgroups? What is the range of treatments for which the questionnaire should be applicable? For example, in cancer there can be a wide range of completely different treatment modalities, from hormonal treatment to surgery. Even within a class of treatments, there may be considerable variability; the drugs used in cancer chemotherapy include many with completely different characteristics and toxic side effects. A QoL instrument that will be used for more than the immediate study should ensure that it is appropriate for the full range of intended treatments. Similarly, patient characteristics should be considered. For example, what is the age range of the patients, and might it include young children who have very different priorities and may also require help in completing the questionnaire? Will the target group include very ill patients, who may have high levels of symptomatology and who may find it difficult or even distressing to answer some questions? Might a high proportion of patients be relatively healthy, with few symptoms? If so, will the questions be sufficiently sensitive to discriminate between patients who report 'no problems' in response to most items?

The detailed specification of the intended patient population and their target disease states is second in importance only to the specification of the scientific question and the definition of QoL or of the PROs that are to be investigated. All of these aspects should be carefully specified and recorded.

3.4 Phases of development

Adapting the structure used in *The EORTC Guidelines for Developing Questionnaire Modules* (Johnson *et al.*, 2011), we recognise four phases of development.

Phase 1: Generation of QoL issues

This phase is aimed at compiling an exhaustive list of relevant QoL issues that cover the domain(s) of interest. In the process of compiling this list, three sources are used: (i) literature (including existing questionnaires); (ii) patients with the relevant condition and all relevant stages of disease and treatment; (iii) healthcare professionals (such as physicians, nurses, psychologists, dieticians) with clinical expertise in the area of the questionnaire.

Phase 2: Construction of the item list

The list of QoL issues from Phase 1 is converted into questions with suitable format and time frame. During this phase a model of the hypothetical constructs will emerge, and the forming of multi-item scales should be anticipated by including, where pertinent, several similar or related items either to broaden the scope of the construct or to increase it precision or reliability.

Phase 3: Pre-testing

The aim of pre-testing the questionnaire is to identify and solve potential problems in its administration (e.g. the phrasing of questions or the sequence of questions) and to identify missing or redundant issues. Furthermore, Phase 3 may also be used to gather initial insights into the scale structure and the scoring of multi-item scales. Pre-testing is also relevant if previously developed items are used in a new setting, because:

1. the meaning of questions can be affected by the context of the neighbouring questions;

2. items may require adaptation when used in different languages and cultural settings than those of the initial development;

3. questions developed originally for a particular target group may perform differently when applied in a new setting;

4. the scale structure and the scoring of multi-item scales should be explored.

   Pre-testing consists of:

• administering the questionnaire to new patients belonging to the target population, to obtain a response score for each item, together with rating of relevance and importance; and

• conducting structured interviews with each patient after completion of the questionnaire to ensure completeness and acceptability of the items in the list.

   The pre-testing may also include so-called cognitive interviewing to investigate the patients' understanding of the items in more detail (Section 3.13).

   By the end of this Phase 3 there should be a near-final provisional instrument, with the aim of using Phase 4 to confirm the validity of the postulated constructs and scaling.

Phase 4: Field-testing

The questionnaire and its scale structure should be field-tested in a large, international group of patients in order to determine its acceptability, reliability, validity, responsiveness and cross-cultural applicability.

   It is necessary to field test the questionnaire because:

1. the sample size needed to carry out the requisite psychometric evaluation is substantially larger than that used typically in Phase 3;

2. completion of the questionnaire in Phase 3 is typically done in the presence of a researcher and the instrument may perform differently when completed without such supervision;

3. items may require adaptation when used in different languages and cultural settings than those of the initial development (that is in Phases 1 and 3).

Field-testing consists of:

- administering the instrument to patients belonging to the target population, but who were not involved in Phases 1 or 3; and

- completion of a debriefing questionnaire by each patient after completion of the instrument.

It is anticipated that Phase 4 will lead to few minor modifications of the instrument and its scoring. At this stage, any changes of substance would raise the question of whether there is a need for further validation studies, to confirm the validity following the proposed changes.

Work in each of the four phases will be elaborated in following sections of this chapter.

3.5   Phase 1: Generation of issues

The first phase of developing a QoL instrument is to generate an exhaustive list of all QoL issues and PROs that are relevant to the domains of interest, using literature searches, interviews with healthcare workers and discussions with patients. It is essential to have exhaustive coverage of all symptoms that the patients rate as being severe or important. After identifying all of the relevant issues, items can be generated to reflect these issues.

Some issues, such as anxiety, are often assessed using several items in order to increase the reliability of the measurement. Therefore, at the next stage (Phase 2) the developer will need to decide whether to cover each issue selected for inclusion in the questionnaire with one or more items.

Literature search

The initial stage in item generation usually involves literature searches of relevant journals and bibliographic databases, to ensure that all issues previously thought to be relevant are included. Any existing instruments that address the same or related areas of QoL assessment should be identified and reviewed. From these sources, a list of potential QoL issues for inclusion in the questionnaire can be identified.

Example from the literature

Testicular cancer (TC) is the most common type of cancer in men aged 15–45 years, and its incidence is increasing. There is a high survival rate, and so pre-serving QoL and minimising adverse effects of cancer therapy are major issues. Holzner *et al.* (2013) describe the development of a TC-specific questionnaire, designed to complement the EORTC QLQ-C30.

An extensive literature search was conducted to establish an initial list of QoL issues potentially relevant to TC patients. This list was evaluated in semi-structured interviews with experts in the field and with patients to clarify whether further issues should be included. The literature search in the databases MEDLINE and PsychINFO covered the years 1996–2006. The authors present the details of their searching strategy.

The literature search revealed 37 articles and 26 questionnaires providing QoL issues relevant to TC patients. Following this literature search and expert discussion, an initial list of 20 QoL areas containing 69 issues of potential relevance to TC patients was assembled. This list was edited to remove overlap and redundancy and was assessed in semi-structured interviews with TC experts from nine countries.

Based on this selection procedure, the number of QoL issues on the list was reduced to 37.

Specialist interviews

The list generated by the initial search should be reviewed by a number of healthcare workers who are experienced in treating or managing patients from the disease area in question. This will usually include physicians and nurses, and may well also involve psychiatrists and social workers.

Example from the literature

Holzner *et al.* (2013) collected expert ratings on relevance, priority and breadth of coverage from 28 experts (11 urologists, six radiation oncologists, three psychologists, two medical oncologists, two physicians, two junior physicians, a nurse and an urologist in training). They were working at centres in Austria (10), the Netherlands (7), Italy (7), Canada (3) and England (1). Their average professional experience was 11.9 years. Items were rated separately for patients receiving treatment and for patients after treatment.

Twenty-six of the 37 items met all inclusion criteria relating to priority, relevance and breadth of coverage. The remaining 11 items failed to meet one criterion, mainly patient-rated relevance. The authors describe revisions made to eight items.

They should address issues of content validity: are the issues that are currently proposed relevant, or should some be deleted? If they are recommended for deletion, why? Some possible reasons for deletion of an issue may be because (i) it overlaps closely with other issues that are included, possibly by being too broad in scope; (ii) it is irrelevant to the target group of patients; (iii) it lacks importance to QoL evaluation;

and (iv) it concerns extremely rare conditions and affects only a small minority of patients. Care should be taken to ensure that issues are not deleted at this stage simply because of any fixed opinions of the development team, or simply because the 'specialists' are unaware of the occurrence of particular symptoms or problems.

Of equal importance is that the questionnaire should be comprehensive. What other issues should be added to the list? If new issues are proposed, details of the reasons should be recorded for subsequent justification in reports or publications.

Following this stage, a revised list of issues will have been generated.

Patient interviews

The revised list of issues should be reviewed by a group of patients who are representative of those in the intended target population. For example, the group should contain patients of different ages and with a range of disease severities. Their brief will be similar to that of the healthcare specialists: to recommend candidate items for deletion, and to identify omissions.

Example from the literature

Holzner *et al.* (2013) also asked a patient group that included 62 TC patients from three countries to evaluate the items. Comments by patients were very rare and neither had a substantial impact on item wording nor on generating new items.

3.6   Qualitative methods

We have outlined an interview process, and a similar approach is also described in Section 3.12 about pre-testing the questionnaire. An alternative is to use *focus groups*, either as well as or instead of individual interviews. Considerable research has been carried out into these qualitative methods. We can only briefly cover a few points here, and recommend further reading for example as cited at the end of this chapter. The methods detailed below are largely, but not exclusively, adapted from the approach described by Johnson *et al.* (2011).

Interviews

Interviews can be structured or unstructured. A *structured interview* uses pre-specified questions, and frequently the answers are also pre-specified as a set of valid response options. Thus in its most extreme form a structured interview can be viewed as an interviewer-administered questionnaire. At the opposite extreme, a completely *unstructured interview* may be almost unscripted and resemble a conversation. Not surprisingly, *semi-structured interviews* are generally agreed to be the most effective.

These will use open-ended questions that accept a free-text answer, such as 'What do you think are the most important issues affecting patients with …?' The responses are normally audio-taped, to allow objective analyses to be made later and to allow the interviewer to concentrate on the interview itself rather than the note-taking.

Semi-structured interviews are built around a number of key questions that have been carefully planned, composed and scripted in advance. If the interviewer considers any opinions unclear or worthy of expansion, additional probing should be used. For example, after the general question mentioned above – 'What do you think are the most important issues …?' – some natural probes might concern how and why the mentioned issues affect the respondent, and the interviewer might attempt to solicit an importance or impact rating. The most obvious of these probes should have been pre-planned and a suitable phrasing pre-scripted whenever possible, although the actual wording, ordering and choice of questions will vary according to the issues raised and the direction of responses that the interviewee makes. As the probing becomes deeper, so the less scripted the questions will inevitably become.

Interviewing is a skill, and there are many books and courses on this topic. The interviewer should be sympathetic and encouraging, be sensitive to the respondent's verbal and non-verbal communication, and must probe without leading the respondent or influencing their choice of response. Open questions should be used throughout: 'How does it affect you?', 'Why do you feel that way?', 'What is most important to you?' and 'When does this happen?' are all examples of open questions that avoid implying particular responses. In contrast, a question such as 'Does xxx affect you?' (yes/no) is a deprecated closed question with restricted response options and with possible bias if it influences some respondents to think that 'xxx' is particularly likely to be affecting them.

Appropriate methods for developing conceptual issues and frameworks for qualitative interview research, developing the interview discussion guide, reaching saturation, analysis of data and developing a theoretical model are available (Brod *et al.*, 2009).

When there is a provisional list of issues from patient interviews and the literature review, this list should be administered to a limited number of patients (usually not more than 10 in total), followed by a debriefing interview to determine what the various issues mean to the patients, the extent to which patients have experienced the problems, limitations or positive experiences during the period of their disease and to check for any significant omissions.

Focus groups

A focus group is formed by inviting a number of respondents to meet and discuss the relevant issues. The investigator or a representative acts as *moderator* or facilitator of the group, and has the key responsibility of guiding the group into discussion, without influencing the opinions being expressed. The moderator should facilitate the discussion, encourage interaction and ensure that all members of the group have an opportunity to voice their views. The discussions should be electronically recorded for subsequent analysis, and it can be helpful to have either a video-recording or an independent person keeping records of who speaks when, and non-verbal reactions and interaction.

Some facilitators prefer to have a single focus group comprising a wide range of respondents; others find it easier and more productive to have a number of focus groups, with each group containing similar individuals who are more likely to understand each other and reach consensus about the issues that affect their specific condition.

It remains controversial whether focus groups offer advantages over individual interview approaches. In both cases the communication skills and open-mindedness of the facilitator/interviewer remain paramount. It is essential that the respondents carefully consider the relevant issues and are encouraged to voice all their opinions – but they should in no way be influenced by the prejudices of the investigators. Compared to individual interviews, focus groups tend to reach less extreme conclusions and the results will usually be less polarised. Individual interviews allow greater expression by idiosyncratic individuals and deviant cases. Resources permitting, there can be advantages in using a combination of both focus groups and interviews.

Example from the literature

McEwan *et al.* (2004) used focus groups to explore the issues concerning adolescents with epilepsy. Six focus groups were conducted, with between two and five participants in each. Participants were stratified into focus groups according to age (12–13, 14–15 and 16+ years) to enable the exploration of changes in factors related to QoL at different age points. Groups lasted two hours with a half-hour refreshment break. Groups were audiotaped for verbatim transcription.

Confidentiality and housekeeping issues were addressed at the beginning of the first sessions, and participants were informed that they could write down any issues that they felt were too personal to discuss. Each focus group discussion was divided into three main parts. First, an icebreaker in which everybody introduced themselves and described their hobbies and interests. Participants were then asked to identify the places and people important in their daily lives, which led naturally into discussion about the impact of epilepsy. Identified items were recorded on a flipchart for continued reference during the group. The remainder of this part involved unstructured discussion about the topics, in which adolescents were encouraged to generate issues of most relevance to them. The moderator's role was to encourage the flow and elaboration of discussion using reflective statements and questions and to check the relevance of items for the whole group.

During the second part of the session, two picture sheets were distributed, reflecting some of the issues identified in previous literature. This was designed to promote discussion, should participants have had difficulty generating spontaneous conversation. This also provided an opportunity for testing out the relevance of previously determined items.

Finally, towards the end of the session, participants were given the opportunity to write down more sensitive issues. At this point, participants were also asked to record the three main ways in which epilepsy affected their daily lives.

Sample selection

The patients chosen, either for interview or as members of a focus group, should represent full coverage of the target population. If an instrument will target the young and the elderly, or those with mild illness and those who are severely ill, then all these groups must be represented. When developing an instrument for use internationally or in a heterogeneous society, patients from the various cultural groups should be represented. A balance must be struck between including extreme cases and emphasising the maximum variability in the sample, as opposed to balancing the representation of the major criterion groups – such as age groups, males and females, and disease groups. Thus the sample selected should represent the range and diversity of the people for whom the instrument will be applicable. This is usually a *purposively selected* sample in which breadth of coverage, as opposed to proportional representation, is emphasised; a sample based on statistically accurate proportions representing the number of people from the total population in the various subgroups would be much larger.

3.7　Sample sizes

It is always difficult to prescribe a sample size for qualitative studies. Focus groups are commonly between three to a dozen individuals (plus the moderator and perhaps a person to take notes), with five to seven being found most effective when studying complex issues. A balance must be struck between keeping the group manageably small while recruiting individuals to represent all the relevant age/gender/cultural/disease/treatment perspectives.

Similarly, six to eight patients are commonly found to be sufficient when exploring issues for which there is a reasonable degree of concordance. Larger numbers are clearly required if the QoL experiences vary substantially from individual to individual, or if there might be important differences between particular subgroups of patients. Qualitative data are usually analysed at intervals during the data collection, and while new issues continue to emerge more respondents are recruited. When it is apparent that no new themes are being discovered, the study is described as having reached *data saturation* and may be terminated.

> ### *Example from the literature*
>
> The EORTC Guidelines for Developing Questionnaire Modules recommend that 5–10 patients should be interviewed from each different treatment group or disease stage, with similar numbers of patients recruited from each participating country (Johnson *et al.*, 2011). The age and gender distribution of recruited patients should reflect that of the target population. Interviews should continue until no new issues arise. A minimum of 20 patients should be interviewed; usually no more than 30 are required.

Johnson *et al.* suggest that having developed a provisional list of issues from patient interviews and the literature review, this list is administered to a limited number of patients (usually not more than 10 in total), followed by a debriefing interview to determine what the various issues mean to the patient, the extent to which patients have experienced the problems, limitations, or positive experiences during the period of their disease and to check for any significant omissions. The provisional list of issues and the core instrument should be presented to healthcare professionals, for feedback on appropriateness of content and breadth of coverage. At least five health professional should be included; it is usually unnecessary to recruit more than 20 individuals, drawn from all countries represented. The healthcare professionals may be of any relevant discipline and should have experience with treating patients belonging to the target population.

These recommendations have been applied successfully by the EORTC Group when developing a number of disease- and dimension-specific modules to accompany the QLQ-C30.

Example from the literature

Johnson *et al.* (2010) report the development of a questionnaire for elderly patients with cancer, intended as another supplementary module for use with the QLQ-C30. Patients were recruited for qualitative data collection (generation of additional issues) until no new issues were emerging. The authors anticipated at least 30 patients in each age group would be required. Recruitment was stopped when the researchers were satisfied that data saturation had been achieved. This occurred when at least 40 patients had been recruited in each age group.

Saturation

In instrument development, saturation refers to the point in the data collection process when no new concept-relevant information is being elicited from individual interviews or focus groups. There is no fixed rule on either the sample size or the number of iterations needed to reach saturation. Francis *et al.* (2010) suggest that if there are two or three main stratification factors, one simple algorithm is to specify at least 10 interviews will be conducted, with a subsequent stopping rule of saturation achieved when three further interviews have been conducted with no new themes emerging. Thus under this scheme the stopping criterion would be tested for interviews 11, 12, 13; then interviews 12, 13, 14; and so on, until three consecutive interviews provide no additional information. Saturation can be evaluated and documented through a saturation table structured to show the elicitation of information by successive focus group or interview (individual or by set), organised by concept code. For practical purposes of budgeting projects, it is not uncommon to set a sample size of 20–30 interviews, even though saturation may occur earlier in the interview process. Saturation is then documented for where it occurs in the process, often during the interviewing process or sometimes at the end of all interviews.

Brod *et al.* (2009) propose that preliminary judgements regarding reaching saturation can be made by the construction of a 'saturation grid' in which major domains (topics or themes) are listed along the vertical, and each group/interview is listed along the horizontal. This preliminary saturation grid can be constructed as the interviews proceed to help assist in the determination that saturation is likely to have (or not) been reached and make a determination as to whether additional groups will be necessary. Saturation is reached when the grid column for the current group is empty, suggesting that no new themes or concepts have emerged.

Experience suggests that a saturation grid based on field notes is highly correlated with the feeling of 'I have heard all this before.' A rule-of-thumb, when combining both individual and focus group interviews, is that approximately three to four focus groups, in combination with four to six individual interviews, are generally sufficient to reach saturation whereby no new information is gained by further interviews. However, heterogeneity of sample, data quality, diffuse or vague areas of enquiry and facilitator skills will influence the exact number of interviews required to reach saturation.

3.8   Phase 2: Developing items

The next phase of development is to translate the nominated issues into questions. A decision must be made regarding the format of these questions. Most of the individual questions to be found on QoL questionnaires either take responses in binary format, such as yes/no, or are ordinal in nature. *Ordinal scales* are those in which the patients rank themselves between 'low' and 'high', 'not at all' and 'very much', or some similar range of grading. The example instruments in the Appendix illustrate a variety of formats for ordinal scales.

Ordered categorical or Likert summated scales

The most common ordinal scale is the *labelled categorical scale* or *verbal rating scale* (VRS). For example, the EORTC QLQ-C30 items have four-point labelled categories of 'Not at all', 'A little', 'Quite a bit' and 'Very much'. These labels have been chosen by defining the two extremes, and then devising two intermediate labels with the intention of obtaining a very roughly even spread. However, there is little evidence that the difference between, say, categories 'Not at all' and 'A little' is emotionally, psycho-physically or in any other sense equal to the difference between 'A little' and 'Quite a bit' or between 'Quite a bit' and 'Very much'. Thus there are no grounds for claiming that these *ordinal scales* have the property of being *interval scales*.

Labelled categorical scales usually have four or five categories, although six or even seven are sometimes used. Fewer than four categories are usually regarded as too few, while studies have shown that many respondents cannot reliably and repeat-edly discriminate between categories if there are more than six or seven. There are divided opinions about the advantages or disadvantages of having an odd number of categories for a symmetrical scale. For example, question 11 of the SF-36 ranges from 'Definitely true' to 'Definitely false', leading to a middle category of 'Don't know'. Some investigators argue that it is better to have an even number of categories so that there is no central 'Don't know' or neutral response and respondents must make a choice.

A scale with more than five categories may be presented with only the two endpoints labelled; this is known as a *numerical rating scale* (NRS). For example, question 30 on the EORTC QLQ-C30, 'How would you rate your overall quality of life during the past week?', takes responses 1–7, with only the two ends labelled: 'Very poor' to 'Excellent'. Although it may seem more likely that this could be an interval scale, there is little scientific evidence to support the intervals between successive score points as being equal. The NRS format is commonly used for assessing symptoms, frequently with 11-point scales from 0 to 10 in which 0 represents absence of the symptom and 10 indicates the worst possible severity of the symptom. The Edmonton Symptom Assess-ment Scale (ESAS) is a PRO instrument for use in palliative care that uses NRS-11 for pain, tiredness, nausea, depression, anxiety, drowsiness, appetite, well-being, short-ness of breath and other problems (Bruera *et al.*, 1991).

Ordered categorical scales, when scored in steps of one, are commonly called *Lik-ert summated scales*. Despite the on-going arguments about the lack of equal-interval properties, these scales have consistently shown themselves to provide useful sum-maries that appear to be meaningful, even when averaged across groups of patients.

Visual analogue scales

Visual analogue scales (VAS) consist of lines, usually horizontal and 10 cm long, the ends of which are marked with the extreme states of the item being measured. Patients are asked to mark the line at a point that represents their position between these two extremes. The responses are coded by measuring their distance from the left-hand end of the line. These scales have been used in the assessment of PROs for many years. Although some patients may take some time to get used to them, most find them easy to complete.

VAS are generally thought to have equal-interval properties, although this is not necessarily true. In particular, McCormack *et al.* (1988), reviewing the distribution of responses to VAS questions, suggest that many respondents cluster their answers as high, middle or low. For analyses of the readings, some investigators use the reading in millimetres of the distance along the scale, resulting in readings between 0 and 100.

VAS can take many forms. An example of an instrument with a scale that is similar to a VAS is the EQ-5D (Appendix E4), which contains a 'thermometer' scale. It is vertical, graduated with 100 tick marks and labelled at every tenth.

It has been claimed that the VAS is more sensitive and easier for patients to complete than ordered categorical scales, although this has been disputed in some reviews (McCormack *et al.*, 1988). However, VAS are used less frequently in QoL instruments than ordered categorical scales, possibly because they take greater space on the page and demand more resources for measuring the responses. It will be interesting to see whether VAS methods become more widely used now that interactive computer data-capture methods are available.

Example from the literature

Selby *et al.* (1984) describe an instrument containing VAS for assessing QoL in cancer patients. They called the scales linear analogue self-assessment (LASA) scales. These included a 'Uniscale' assessing overall QoL, and 30 scales for individual items. Each scale was 10 cm long. Three items are shown in Figure 3.1.

PLEASE SCORE HOW YOU FEEL EACH OF THESE ASPECTS OF YOUR LIFE WAS
AFFECTED BY THE STATE OF YOUR HEALTH DURING TODAY (24H)

Nausea
extremely severe
nausea _____ no nausea

Physical activity
completely unable   normal physical
to move my body _____ activity for me

Depression
extremely   not depressed
depressed _____ at all

Figure 3.1 The Linear Analogue Self Assessment scale (LASA) is an example of a visual analogue scale.
Source: Selby *et al.*, 1984, Figure 2. Reproduced with permission of Macmillan Publishers Ltd on behalf of Cancer Research UK.

Example from the literature

In the area of pain measurement, VAS, VRS and 10- or 11-step NRS are all widely used for self-reported assessment of pain intensity. Hjermstad *et al.* (2011) identified 54 studies that compared two or more methods. All studies reported very high compliance, although a few found slightly lower compliance with VAS, associated with older age and greater trauma or impairment. Two studies found that VRS was preferred by the less educated or the elderly, while in a few other studies NRS was preferred. In all studies there were high correlations between the scales, with eleven studies preferring the NRS approach, seven the VRS, and four the VAS. Two of the statistical modelling papers suggested that psychometric properties of the VRS were better for research purposes and that the numerical appearance of the NRS/VAS provide false impressions of being reliable measures. It was noted that ratings were not mathematically equivalent across the different approaches.

In conclusion, the 0–10 NRS, the (7-step) VRS and the VAS all work quite well. The authors concluded that the most important choice is not the type of scale *per se*, but the conditions related to its use, which include a standardised choice of anchor descriptors, methods of administration, time frames, information related to the use of scales, interpretation of cut-offs and clinical significance, and the use of appropriate outcome measures and statistics in clinical trials. They indicated a slight preference for NRS-11 because it makes slightly less cognitive demand and it may also be easier for very elderly patients.

Guttman scales

A Guttman scale consists of several items of varying difficulty. An example is found in many activities-of-daily-living (ADL) scales. These usually consist of a number of items that represent common functions or tasks, sequenced in order of increasing difficulty. Guttman scales are also sometimes called *hierarchical scales*, since the questions can be ranked as a hierarchy in terms of their difficulty or challenge to the respondents.

A Guttman scale is a rigidly hierarchical scale. If a patient can accomplish a difficult task at the upper end of the scale, they *must* be able to accomplish all of the easier tasks. For the EORTC QLQ-C30, and for most other ADL and physical functioning scales, this is clearly untrue. Although climbing stairs, for example, might be regarded as more difficult than taking a short walk, a few patients might be able to climb stairs yet be unable to take a walk. Thus the EORTC physical function scale is *not* a true Guttman scale, because the ordering of item difficulty is not fixed and constant for all patients. As discussed in Chapter 7, item response theory (IRT) provides a more appropriate model. IRT assumes that items are of varying difficulty with a probability of positive response that varies according to each patient's ability. That is, IRT incorporates a probabilistic element for responses, whereas a Guttman scale is strictly deterministic and depends solely upon the patient's ability. Hence, Guttman scales are rarely used nowadays.

Example

The physical functioning scale of the EORTC QLQ-C30 contains five items of varying difficulty, shown in Figure 3.2. In versions 1.0–2.0, each item was scored 'Yes' or 'No'. Originally developed with the intention of being scored as a Guttman scale, it is hierarchical in concept with items ranging from 'easy' (eating, dressing and washing) to 'difficult' (carrying heavy loads). Subsequent experience showed that the hierarchy was violated and it was therefore not scored as a Guttman scale. In a revision of the instrument (version 3.0), the yes/no responses were replaced with four-point ordinal scales.

	No	Yes
Do you have any trouble doing strenuous activities, like carrying a heavy shopping bag or a suitcase?	1	2
Do you have any trouble taking a <u>long</u> walk?	1	2
Do you have any trouble taking a <u>short</u> walk outside of the house?	1	2
Do you need to stay in bed or a chair during the day?	1	2
Do you need help with eating, dressing, washing yourself or using the toilet?	1	2

Figure 3.2   Physical functioning scale of the EORTC QLQ-C30 versions 1.0 and 2.0.

3.9   Multi-item scales

Instead of using a single question or item, many scales are devised using multiple items. There are several reasons for doing this. Greater precision may be obtained by using several related items instead of a single item. For example, instead of asking: 'Are you depressed?' with, say, a five-point rating scale, it may be better to ask a number of questions about characteristics of depression, with each of these items being scored on a five-point scale; most depression questionnaires are developed on this basis. Another advantage of using multiple items for a concept such as depression is that the items can be chosen to cover the full breadth of a complex construct – providing better content validity. Multi-item scales are also frequently developed as a means of improving the repeatability/reliability of the assessment;

often individual characteristics or items can fluctuate more than a set of items that form a broadly based multi-item scale.

Quite often items are also grouped simply as a convenient way of summarising a number of closely related issues. Methods such as factor analysis can identify groups of items that are highly correlated, and if these items are thought to be measuring a single construct it may be logical to group them together as a multi-item scale. Finally, a clinimetric index (such as the Apgar score, which is used to assess the health status of newborn children) may be formed using clinical judgement to develop a cluster of sometimes-heterogeneous items that are deemed clinically related. Some well-developed clinimetric indexes provide useful summary scores.

The defining characteristic of multi-item scales is that the individual items are intended to be combined in some manner, to form a summary score or index. The most common method of combining or aggregating items is simply to sum them (or, equivalently, to average them). This is often called *summated ratings*, and the scales are also known as *Likert summated scales*. Alternatively, IRT can be used (Chapter 7).

3.10   Wording of questions

Having identified the issues considered relevant and having made some decisions regarding the format of the questions, the next stage is to convert the items into questions. It should go without saying that questions should be brief, clearly worded, easily understood, unambiguous and easy to respond to. However, the experience of many investigators is that seemingly simple, lucid questions may present unanticipated problems to patients. All questions should be extensively tested on patients before being used in a large study or a clinical trial.

The book by Bradburn *et al.* (2004) focuses on wording and designing questionnaires. The following suggestions are merely a sample of the many points to consider.

1. Make questions and instructions brief and simple. Ill patients and the elderly, especially, may be confused by long, complicated sentences.

2. Avoid small, unclear typefaces. Elderly patients may not have good eyesight.

3. Questions that are not applicable to some patients may result in missing or ambiguous answers. For example, 'Do you experience difficulty going up stairs?' is not applicable to someone who is confined to bed. Some patients may leave it blank because it is not applicable, some might mark it 'Yes' because they would have difficulty if they tried, and others might mark it 'No' because they never need to try and therefore experience no difficulty. The responses cannot be interpreted.

4. If potentially embarrassing or offending questions are necessary, consider putting them at the end of the instrument or making them optional. For example, the FACT-G has a question about satisfaction with sex life, but precedes this with 'If you prefer not to answer it, please check this box and go to the next section.'

5. 'Don't use no double negatives.' For example, a question such as 'I don't feel less interest in sex (Yes/No)' is ill advised.

6. If two or more questions are similar in their wording, use underlining, bold or italics to draw patients' attention to the differences. For example, questions 4 and 5 of the SF-36 are very similar apart from the underlined phrases 'as a result of your physical health' and 'as a result of any emotional problems'.

7. Use underlining and similar methods also to draw attention to key words or phrases. For example, many of the instruments underline the time frame of the questions, such as 'during the past 7 days'.

8. Consider including items that are positively phrased as well as negatively phrased items. For example, the HADS includes equal numbers of positive and negative items, such as 'I feel tense or "wound up"' and 'I can sit at ease and feel relaxed.'

3.11   Face and content validity of the proposed questionnaire

The results from interviews of staff and patients, and from focus groups, will all have been transcribed and interpreted by the investigators. Despite care, it is likely that there will be errors of interpretation, ambiguities and omissions. It is common practice in qualitative studies to present the conclusions to the interviewees for *respondent validation*. The interviewees are invited to confirm whether their intended meaning is captured by the instrument, and to identify discrepancies or omissions from the resultant questionnaire. Thus, when developing questionnaires, the proposed questionnaire should be shown to patients and staff, asking them to review it for acceptability, comprehensiveness, relevance of items, clarity of wording and ambiguity of items. It is prudent to do this before the next stage, the pre-testing, which involves a larger number of patients completing the questionnaire and answering structured debriefing questions.

3.12   Phase 3: Pre-testing the questionnaire

It is essential that new QoL questionnaires be extensively tested on groups of patients before being released for general use. This testing is best carried out in two stages.

First, before the main *field-test*, a pilot or *pre-test* study should be conducted (the EORTC group describe the pre-test as *Phase 3* and the field-test as *Phase 4*). The purpose of this initial study is to identify and solve potential problems. These might include ambiguous or difficult phrasing of the questions and responses, or might relate to the layout and flow of the questions.

For the pre-test, patients should first be asked to complete the provisional questionnaire and then debriefed using a pre-structured interview. The EORTC group (Johnson *et al.* 2011) suggest that they could be asked about individual items, for example: 'Was this question difficult to respond to?', 'Was it annoying, confusing or upsetting?', 'How would you have asked this question?' and 'Is this experience related to your disease or treatment?' If resources do not permit an item-by-item scrutiny, the whole instrument could be reviewed instead, for example: 'Were there any questions that you found irrelevant?', 'Were there questions that you found confusing or difficult to answer?' and 'Were any questions upsetting or annoying?'

Whichever approach is used, there should be some general questions about the whole instrument: 'Can you think of other important issues that should be covered?' and 'Do you have other comments about this questionnaire?' There should also be questions about how long the questionnaire took to complete and whether assistance was obtained from anyone.

An important aspect of the pre-testing phase is the identification of items that have ambiguous, difficult or poorly worded questions. These items should be rephrased. Results of the pre-testing should also identify any potentially serious problems with the questionnaire. Before carrying out the field study, the wording of items may need to be changed, items deleted or additional items introduced.

Example from the literature

Johnson *et al.* (2010) report the Phase 3 testing of their questionnaire for elderly (aged over 70) patients with cancer. They reported difficulty with questions about carers (family members or professional), which required clarification for accurate translation. Issues about approaching death were clearly important to some patients but found this issue had to be handled sensitively, to avoid distress to patients. It was decided to keep the issue but to phrase the item in relation to 'approaching the end of life', which was more acceptable to patients.

One item 'Have you felt that your life is meaningful?' was considered by nine patients to be misleading or unclear and was rejected; it was thought likely that this single item lacked an appropriate context in the older-person questionnaire, which could account for the loss of clarity for patients.

Representative sample

The pre-testing will usually involve between 10 and 30 patients, selected as representing the range of patients in the target population. These should not be the same patients as those who were used when identifying the issues to be addressed. If a questionnaire is intended to be applicable to various subgroups of patients for whom the QoL issues might vary, it is important to ensure that there is adequate representation of all these types of patients and the sample size may have to be increased accordingly. Thus if a QoL questionnaire is intended to address issues associated with different modalities of treatment, it should be tested separately with patients receiving each of these forms of therapy. For example, an instrument for cancer patients could be tested in those receiving surgery, chemotherapy or radiotherapy. It is crucial to ensure that patients receiving each form of therapy are able to complete the questionnaire without difficulty, distress or embarrassment, and that all patients feel the relevant issues have been covered.

Example from the literature

Johnson *et al.* (2010) report that the aim of their Phase 3 study was to assess the content, acceptability and relevance of the provisional item list in a large representative group of older cancer patients from different countries and languages. Sampling was monitored to ensure an even distribution of patients across six tumour sites. A sampling frame was constructed to define patients with localised or advanced disease and in three treatment stages (before, during or after treatment). Patients receiving only palliative care were included as a separate category. This created seven potential groups defined by disease stage and treatment. As recommended in the EORTC Quality of Life Group Guidelines (Johnson *et al.*, 2011), they aimed to recruit 15 patients to each of the seven disease/treatment groups, creating a target of 105 patients. (A matched group of patients aged 50–69 years was also recruited, making 210 in total.)

Sampling was monitored to ensure even distribution of patients across six tumour sites. However, the sampling frame was revised when it became apparent that recruitment to some categories was very difficult.

Missing data

Interpretation of results is difficult when there is much missing data, and it is best to take precautions to minimise the problems. For example, questions about sexual interest, ability or activity may cause problems. In some clinical trials these questions might be regarded as of little relevance, and it may be reasonable to anticipate similar low levels of sexual problems in both treatment arms. This raises the question of whether it is advisable to exclude these potentially embarrassing items so as to avoid compromising patient compliance over questionnaire completion. Other strategies are to place embarrassing items at the end of the questionnaire, or to make their completion optional.

> **Example from the literature**
>
> Fayers *et al.* (1997b) report that in a wide range of UK MRC cancer trials, approximately 19% of patients left blank a question about '(have you been bothered by) decreased sexual interest'. Females were twice as likely as males to leave this item blank. Possible interpretations are that some patients found the question embarrassing, or that they did not have an active sexual interest before their illness and therefore regarded the question as not applicable. Perhaps wording should be adapted so that lack of sexual activity before the illness (not applicable) can be distinguished from other reasons for missing data.

3.13   Cognitive interviewing

Cognitive interviewing techniques can be seen as an extension of the pre-testing phase based on a psychological understanding of the process people go through when answering a questionnaire item. Tourangeau (1984) and Tourangeau *et al.* (2000) develop a model describing the response process consisting of four phases:

1. comprehension of the question

2. retrieval from memory of relevant information

3. decision processes

4. response processes.

Based on Tourangeau's work, Willis (2005) developed the 'cognitive interviewing' technique. The principle is to elucidate each element in the process and to target the interview to the potential problems that may be suspected (for example, problems related to comprehension if the item is lengthy and complicated).

There are two main approaches to cognitive interviewing:

1. Think-aloud interviewing: the respondent is instructed to report the response process orally by describing his or her thoughts and considerations. Ideally, the person goes though each of the steps and reveals any doubts and uncertainties through the process. Typically, some respondents will give excellent insights in their thought processes, and these results can be analysed according to the four-step model. However, the task is mentally quite demanding and not all respondents will accept the task or will experience difficulties giving informative responses.

2. Verbal probing: After the respondent has completed the questionnaire (or just a questionnaire item) the interviewer asks a number of probes prepared in advance.

Unspecific and specific probes used can be used. Unspecific probes correspond to what we mentioned as standard probes in pre-testing. An example is 'Could you repeat the question you were just asked with your own words?' (Paraphrasing). Each of the four steps in Tourangeau's model should be addressed. Specific probes will address potential problems suspected from a review of the items or from previous interviews.

Example from the literature

Willis (2005, pp. 8–9) describes results from nine cognitive interviews concerning the item 'How many times did you go to the dentist the past year?' Three main problems were identified. First, it was not clear whether 'the dentist' included oral surgeons, dental hygienists, etc. Second, the interpretation of 'the past year' varied considerably, with one respondent perceiving it as the prior calendar year and one person reporting the visits since 1 January. Finally, respondents experienced a significant degree of uncertainty, and this raised the question of whether the exact number of visits was necessary.

In order to address the concerns, the following solutions were considered:

1. To modify the wording of 'the dentist' to 'your main dentist' or 'any dentist'.

2. To use 'the past 12 months' instead of 'the past year'.

3. Whether categorical responses, including the option 'one to three times' (in contrast to those not going at all, or going very frequently), would be sufficient. Such a modification would simplify the response process for many respondents.

Such cognitive interviews may be critical to refine items and avoid ambiguity or other difficulties in the final questionnaire. These interviews may be conducted individually or in a focus group, and rely on intensive verbal probing of volunteer participants by a specially trained interviewer. Cognitive testing is designed to identify otherwise unobservable problems with item comprehension, recall and other cognitive processes that can be remediated through question rewording, reordering or more extensive instrument revision.

Example from the literature

Fortune-Greeley *et al.* (2009) conducted 39 cognitive interviews to evaluate items for measuring sexual functioning across cancer populations. The study population reflected a range of cancer types and stages. Trained same-gender interviewers were used. Interviews were recorded, as were non-verbal signs such as apprehension. The investigators reported findings about the relevance of the items, recall period, wording changes to improve sensitivity, appropriateness, clarity and item ordering.

Participants identified problems with the wording of some items that prompted important revisions. It is instructive that participants identified these problems despite many rounds of review by investigators and survey methodology specialists. In brief, a few of the findings that led to modifications were as follows:

One of the original items read, "When having sex with a partner, how often have you needed fantasies to help you stay interested?" Two participants thought the word "needed" implied a negative judgement towards the use of sexual fantasies. The item was reworded to read, 'When having sex with a partner, how often have you used fantasies to help you stay interested?'

Participants with low literacy had difficulty with the term distracting thoughts in the item "How often have you lost your arousal (been turned off) because of distracting thoughts?"

Originally, the item "Are you married or in a relationship that could involve sexual activity?" was presented before the item "Over the past 30 days, have you had any type of sexual activity with another person?" Five out of 20 participants thought that the question was asking about sexual activity with someone other than their partner.

In conclusion, cognitive interviews were critical for item refinement in the development of the PROMIS measure of sexual function.

Cognitive interviews may be used in relation to existing instruments or as an integrated part of the development process, as an extension of what was described as pre-testing.

Example from the literature

Watt *et al.* (2008) integrated cognitive interviews in the development of a questionnaire for thyroid patients and interviewed 31 patients. The data from interviews were analysed according to Tourangeau's model. Fifty-four problems involved comprehension, one retrieval, 23 judgement, 28 response, and 20 could not be coded in relation to the four-stage model. The interviews were conducted in six rounds and Watt noted that the number of problems declined from an initial average of six per interview to two, mainly due to a reduction in the number of problems associated with comprehension.

3.14　Translation

If a field study is to be conducted in a number of different countries, the QoL questionnaire will need to be translated into other languages. The translation process should be carried out just as rigorously as the instrument development process, to avoid introducing either errors into the questionnaire or shifts in nuances that might affect the way patients respond to items. The aims of the translation process should be to ensure that all versions of the questionnaire are equally clear, precise and equivalent in all ways to the original.

As a minimum, translation should involve a two-stage process. A native speaker of the target language who is also fluent in the original language should first make a forward translation. Some guidelines recommend two or more independent forward translations followed by the development of a consensus version. Then another translator (or two) who is a native speaker of the original language should take the translated version and make a back-translation into the original language. This second translator must be 'blind' to the original questionnaire. Next, an independent person should formally compare each item from this forward–backward translation against the original, and must prepare a written report of all differences. The whole process may need to be iterated until it is agreed that the forward–backward version corresponds precisely in content and meaning to the original.

Following translation, a patient-based validation study has to be carried out. This will be similar in concept to the pre-testing study that we described, and will examine whether patients find the translated version of any item confusing, difficult to understand, ambiguous, irritating or annoying.

Differential item functioning (Section 7.10) also provides a powerful tool for identifying translation problems, but this requires large datasets of, say, several hundred patients for each translation.

Marquise *et al.* (2005) review translation issues in depth, and Wild *et al.* (2005, 2009) make detailed recommendations for translations.

3.15　Phase 4: Field-testing

The final stage in the development of a new questionnaire is field-testing. The objective of field-testing is to determine and confirm the acceptability, validity, sensitivity, responsiveness, reliability and general applicability of the instrument to the target group, including cultural and clinical subgroups.

The field study should involve a large heterogeneous group of patients, and this should include patients who are representative of the full range of intended responders. We have already emphasised the need to include a wide range of patients when determining the issues to be assessed and developing the wording of the questions. At the field-testing stage, it becomes even more important to ensure that the sample includes patients who are representative of the full range of the target population, and that sample sizes are adequate to test the applicability of the instrument to all types of patient. For example, it may be relevant to include males and females, elderly and young, sick and healthy, highly educated and poorly educated. Societies often include individuals from diverse cultures and ethnic origins, and even an instrument intended for use within a single country should be tested for applicability within the relevant cultural, ethnic or linguistic groups. Questions that are perceived as relevant and unambiguous by one group may be misunderstood, misinterpreted and answered in ways that are unexpected by the investigator. In some cases, questions that are acceptable to the majority of people may prove embarrassing or cause distress to minority groups.

A debriefing questionnaire should be used. This will be similar in style to the questionnaire administered during the pre-test stage: 'How long did the questionnaire take to complete?', 'Did anyone help complete the questionnaire, and what was the nature of that help?', 'Were any questions difficult to answer, confusing or upsetting?', 'Were all questions relevant, and were any important issues missed?' and 'Any other comments?'

The analysis of the field study should make use of the techniques described in Chapters 4 and 5 to examine validity, reliability, sensitivity and responsiveness. In addition, the following basic issues should be considered.

Missing values

The extent of missing data should be determined and reported. This includes not only missing responses in which the answers are left blank, but also invalid or uninterpretable responses that will have to be scored 'missing' for analyses of the data. For example, a patient might mark two answers to a categorical question that permits only a single response. If a question is unclear or ambiguous, there can be a high proportion of invalid responses of this type. If the reason for missing data is known, this too should be reported. For example, patients might indicate on the debriefing form that a question is difficult to complete or upsetting.

In general, it is to be expected that for any one item there will always be a few (1% or 2%) patients with missing data. This figure will obviously be reduced if there are resources for trained staff to check each questionnaire immediately upon completion, asking patients to fill in the omitted or unclear responses. Whenever items have missing values for more than 3–4% of patients, the questions should be re-examined. Possible reasons for missing values include:

- *Problems with the wording of response options to a question.* Patients may feel that none of the categories describes their condition. Alternatively, they may be unable to decide between two options that they feel describe their state equally well.

- *Problems with the text of an individual question.* Patients may find the question difficult to understand or upsetting.

- *Problems specific to particular subgroups of patients.* It might be found that elderly patients have a higher-than-average proportion of missing values for questions that they regard as less applicable to them (such as strenuous activities), or which are cognitively demanding.

- *Problems with translation of a question or culture-related difficulties of interpretation.* Items that have been developed for one cultural group may present problems when translated or used in other groups. For example, the question 'When eating, can you cut food with a knife?' might be used to evaluate the strength of grip of arthritis patients, but would be inappropriate in Chinese as the Chinese do not use knives when eating their meal.

- *Problems understanding the structure of the questionnaire.* If a group of consecutive missing responses occurs, it can indicate that respondents do not understand the flow of the questions. For example, this might happen following *filter* questions of the form: 'If you have not experienced this symptom, please skip to the next section.'

- *Problems with a group of related items.* If responses to a group of items are missing, whether or not consecutive questions on the questionnaire, it might indicate that some respondents regard these questions as either embarrassing or not applicable.

- *Exhaustion.* This can be manifested by incomplete responses towards the questionnaire's end.

Missing forms

The proportion of missing forms (questionnaires that are not returned) should be reported, too. Again, any information from debriefing forms or any reasons recorded by staff should be described. A high proportion of missing forms might indicate poor acceptability for the instrument. For example, it may be too complicated, too lengthy and tedious to complete, or it may ask too many upsetting or irritating questions. Patients may think the layout is unclear. The printing may be too small, or the questionnaire may have been printed with an injudicious choice of paper and ink colours.

Distribution of item responses

The range and distribution of responses to each item should be examined. This might be done graphically, or by tabulating the responses of those questions that have few response categories.

Ceiling effects, in which a high proportion of the total respondents grade themselves as having the maximum score, are commonly observed when evaluating instruments, especially if very ill patients are sampled and frequently occurring symptoms are measured. The presence of ceiling effects (or *floor effects*, with an excess of minimum values) indicates that the items or scales will have poor discrimination. Thus sensitivity and responsiveness will be reduced.

The interpretation of ceiling effects is affected by the distinction between reflective and formative/causal indicators (Section 2.6). For reflective indicators, the response categories should ideally be chosen so that the full range will be used and the distribution of responses should ideally be spread across these response categories. If the respondents rarely or never use one of the responses to a four-category item, the question becomes equivalent to a less sensitive one with only three categories. If all respondents select the same response option, no differences will be detected between the groups in a comparative study and the question becomes uninformative. An example of such an extreme case might arise when there are questions about very severe states or conditions, with most or even all of the respondents answering 'none' or 'not at all' to these items. It is questionable whether it is worth retaining such items as components of a larger summated scale, since they are unlikely to vary substantially across patient groups and will therefore tend to reduce the sensitivity of the summated-scale score. Thus an abundance of ceiling or floor effects in the target population could suggest an item should be reviewed, and possibly even deleted.

For formative variables such as symptoms, there are different considerations. In particular, it is important to maintain comprehensive coverage of formative items. A symptom may be rare, but if it relates to a serious, extreme or life-threatening state it may be crucially important to those patients who experience it. Such symptoms are important and should not be ignored, even though they manifest floor effects. Equally, a symptom that is very frequent may result in ceiling effects and, in an extreme case, if all respondents report their problems as 'very much', the item becomes of limited value for discriminative purposes in a clinical trial. That item may, however, still be extremely important for descriptive or evaluative purposes, alerting clinical staff to the extensive problems and symptoms that patients encounter.

Questionnaires often use the same standardised responses for many questions. For example, all questions might consistently use four or five response categories ranging from 'not at all' through to 'very much'. Although this is generally a desirable approach, it may be difficult to ensure that the same range of response options is appropriate to all items. Ceiling effects can indicate simply that the range of the extreme categories is inadequate. For example, possibly a four-point scale should be extended to seven points.

Item reduction

While items were being generated, there was also the possibility of deleting any that appeared unimportant. However, the number of patients and clinicians included in the initial studies is usually small, and the decision to delete items would be based upon the judgement of the investigator. In the later stages of instrument development, there is greater scope for using psychometric methods to identify redundant or inappropriate items.

Ideally, a questionnaire should be brief, should cover all relevant issues, and should explore in detail those issues that are considered of particular interest to the study. Clearly, compromises must be made: first, between shortening a questionnaire that is thought to be too lengthy, while retaining sufficient items to provide comprehensive coverage of QoL (content validity) and, second, between maintaining this breadth of coverage while aiming for detailed in-depth assessment of specific issues. Sometimes the solution will be to use a broadly based questionnaire covering general issues, and supplement this with additional questionnaires that address specific areas of interest in greater depth (see for example Appendixes E12 and E13). This modular approach is also adopted by the EORTC QLQ-C30 and the FACT-G.

Chapter 5 describes several psychometric methods that may be used to indicate whether items could be superfluous. For multi-item scales, *multitrait analysis* can identify items that are very strongly correlated with other items, and are therefore redundant because they add little information to the other items. It can also detect items that are only weakly correlated with their scale score and are therefore either performing poorly or making little contribution. Cronbach's α can in addition be used to explore the effect of removing one or more items from a multi-item scale. If the α reliability remains unchanged after deleting an item, the item may be unnecessary. Item response theory (Chapter 7) provides another approach for investigating the contribution made by each item to the total test information. However, as the following example illustrates, many of these methods may be inappropriate for *clinimetric scales* that have *formative variables*, as described in Sections 2.6 and 2.8.

Example from the literature

Marx *et al.* (1999) report the application of clinimetric and psychometric methods in the reduction of 70 potential items to a 30-item Disabilities of Arm, Shoulder and Hand health measurement scale. The clinimetric strategy relied upon the ratings of patients to determine which items to include in the final scale. Fifteen items were selected in common by both methods. The clinimetric methods selected a greater number of symptoms and psychological function items. In contrast, the psychometric strategy selected a greater number of physical-disability items, and factor analysis suggested that the items constituted a single factor.

These results can be explained in terms of formative and reflective items. The clinimetric strategy favoured the inclusion of symptoms that are formative items. The psychometric strategy favoured the physical-disability items because they were measuring a single latent variable and were therefore more highly and more consistently correlated with each other.

As well as seeking to reduce the number of items in a scale, there is also scope for reduction at the scale level itself. Correlations between different multi-item scales can be investigated, to check whether any are so highly correlated that it would appear they are measuring virtually the same thing.

At all stages, face validity and clinical sensibility should be considered. The principal role of psychometric analysis is to point at potential areas for change, but one would be ill-advised to delete items solely on the basis of very strong or very weak correlations.

Example from the literature

Juniper *et al.* (1997) describe the development of an asthma QoL question-naire, and demonstrate that different approaches lead to appreciably different instruments. They show that methods based on factor analysis will lead to exclusion of some items that are considered important by patients, and inclu-sion of other items that are considered unimportant. Fayers *et al.* (1998b) noted that the discrepancies in item selection under the two approaches – clinimetric or psychometric – could without exception be fully explained in terms of causal (formative) indicators and reflective indicators. Fayers *et al.* also agreed that clinimetric considerations, including patients' assessment of item importance, should dominate the decisions concerning an item's inclu-sion or exclusion.

This and the previous example show that choice of model – reflective or formative – can have a major impact on the selection of items included in multi-item scales.

Cultural and subgroup differences

There may be subgroups of patients with particular problems. Older patients may have different needs and concerns from younger ones, and may also interpret questions dif-ferently. There may be major cultural differences, and a questionnaire developed in one part of the world may be inappropriate in another. For example, respondents from Mediterranean countries can be less willing to answer questions about sexual activity than those from Northern Europe. Subjects from oriental cultures may respond to some items very differently from Europeans.

The field study should be designed with a sufficiently large sample size to be able to detect major differences in responses according to gender, age group or culture. However, it is difficult to ensure that similar patients have been recruited into each subgroup. For example, in a multi-country field study there might be country-specific differences in the initial health of the recruited patients. Some countries might enter patients with earlier-stage disease, and the treatment or management of patients may differ in subtle ways. Thus observed differences in, for example, group mean scores could be attributable to 'sampling bias' in patient recruitment or management, and it is extremely difficult to ascribe any observed mean differences to cultural variation in the response to questions.

Methods of analysis might include comparison of subgroup means and *SD*s. How-ever, to eliminate the possibility of sampling bias, differential item functioning (DIF) is an attractive approach for multi-item scales. DIF analysis, described in Section 7.10, allows for the underlying level of QoL for each patient, and examines whether the individual item responses are consistent with the patients' QoL.

> **Example**
>
> There may be different semantic interpretation of words by different cultures. Nordic and Northern European countries interpret 'anger' as something that is bad and to be avoided; in Mediterranean countries, 'anger' is not only acceptable, but there is something wrong with a person who avoids expressing it. Thus the interpretation of an answer to the question 'Do you feel angry?' would need to take into account the cultural background of the respondent.

3.16 Conclusions

Designing and developing new instruments constitutes a complex and lengthy process. It involves many interviews with patients and others, studies testing the questionnaires upon patients, the collection of data, and statistical and psychometric analyses of the data to confirm and substantiate the claims for the instrument. The full development of an instrument may take many years. If at any stage inadequacies are found in the instrument, there will be a need for refinement and re-testing. Many instruments undergo iterative development through a number of versions, each version being extensively reappraised. For example, the Appendix shows version 3.0 of the EORTC QLQ-C30 and version 4 of the FACT-G. The instruments described in the appendices to this book, like many other instruments, will have undergone extensive development along the lines that we have described.

In this chapter we have emphasised the qualitative aspects of instrument development. In our experience, this is the most crucial phase in developing a new instrument. As noted in the introduction to this chapter, the subsequent validation using quantitative methods as described in the next chapters of this book will only be of value if it builds on a secure foundation developed by the application of a rigorous qualitative approach.

The contrast between the EORTC QLQ-C30 and the FACT-G is in this respect informative. Both instruments target the same population: cancer patients in general. Yet these are two very different instruments, the one focusing on clinical aspects and the other on patients' feelings and concerns. Both instruments have been exhaustively validated. Thus we can see that the initial conceptual foundations determined the nature of each instrument, and no amount of subsequent validation has narrowed the gap between them. The conceptual basis of the postulated constructs should be considered when choosing instruments for use in studies, as it will affect the interpretation of results.

The role of qualitative methods involving not only experts but, most importantly, patients, is now well recognised (Reeve *et al.*, 2013; US FDA, 2009). Thus when developing a new instrument it is essential to fully document the qualitative procedures and results, and in particular the involvement and role of patients from the earliest stages of instrument specification and development. This has now become standard for all new instruments. However, many legacy instruments either do not have the documentation or even failed to involve patients. The United States Food and Drug Administration (US FDA, 2009) states that documentation provided to the FDA to support content validity should include all item generation techniques used, including any theoretical approach; the populations studied; source of items; selection, editing, and reduction of items; cognitive interview summaries or transcripts; pilot testing; importance ratings; and quantitative techniques for item evaluation. Furthermore, "With existing instruments, it cannot be assumed that the instrument has content validity if patients were not involved in instrument development. New qualitative work similar to that conducted when developing a new instrument can provide documentation of content validity for existing instruments if patient interviews or focus groups are conducted using open-ended methods to elicit patient input". Rothman *et al.* (2009) address the issues for evaluating and documenting content validity for the use of existing instruments and their modification.

Developing new instruments is a lengthy and time-consuming task. In summary, our advice is: don't develop your own instrument – unless you have to. Wherever possible, consider using or building upon existing instruments. If you must develop a new instrument, be prepared for much hard work over a period of years.

3.17 Further reading

One of the first groups to develop and publish comprehensive guidelines for developing QoL instruments was the EORTC Quality of Life Group. These guidelines have been influential in the writing of this chapter, and are recommended to those developing questionnaires. They are: *EORTC Quality of Life Group Module Development Guidelines*, currently in a fourth edition, by Johnson *et al.* (2011), and *EORTC Quality of Life Group Translation Procedure* (3rd edn.) by Dewolf *et al.* (2009). These manuals are downloadable from the website http://groups.eortc.be/qol/manuals. The translation issues are also summarised in Koller *et al.* (2007).

Much of the methodological research into questionnaire development has been carried out in other disciplines, such as survey methodology. In recent years cognitive psychology has had a major impact on the understanding of how respondents react to questions, and how to use cognitive-based methods to identify weaknesses in questionnaires. Useful books on modern approaches include: *Asking Questions: The Definitive Guide to Questionnaire Design*, by Bradburn *et al.* (2004), *Cognitive Interviewing: A Tool for Improving Questionnaire Design*, by Willis (2005) and *Focus Groups: A practical guide for applied research,* by Kreuger and Casey (2000). Brod *et al.* 2009 and Rothman *et al.* (2009) discuss qualitative methods for ensuring content validity, Lehoux *et al.* (2006) explore focus groups and Kerr *et al* (2010) cover data saturation.

In addition to Dewolf *et al.* (2009) mentioned above, translation issues are reviewed in detail by Marquise *et al.* (2005) and Wild *et al.* (2005, 2009), who also provide references to key publications in this area.

The COREQ checklist offers useful guidance for the reporting of qualitative studies (Tong *et al.*, 2007).

4

Scores and measurements: validity, reliability, sensitivity

Summary

In this chapter we explore properties that are common to all forms of measures. This includes both single-item measurements, such as the response to a single global question, and summary scores derived from multi-item scales, such as the scores from the summated scales that are used in many QoL instruments. These properties include validity, reliability, sensitivity and responsiveness. This chapter focuses upon those aspects of the properties that apply to single items and summary scale scores. Chapter 5 discusses related techniques that apply to multi-item scales, when the within-scale between-item relationships can be examined.

4.1 Introduction

All measurements, from blood pressures to PRO measures, should satisfy basic properties if they are to be clinically useful. These are primarily validity, reliability, repeatability, sensitivity and responsiveness.

Validity describes how well a measurement represents the attribute being measured, or how well it captures the concept that is the target of measurement. From a statistical aspect, validity is similar to bias, in that a biased measurement is somehow missing the fundamental target.

Validation of instruments is the process of determining whether there are grounds for believing that the instrument measures what it is intended to measure, and that it is useful for its intended purpose. For example, to what extent is it reasonable to claim that a 'quality-of-life questionnaire' really is assessing QoL? Since we are attempting to measure an ill-defined and unobservable latent variable (QoL), we can only infer that the instrument is valid in so far as it correlates with other observable behaviour. This validation process consists of a number of stages, in which it is hoped to collect convincing evidence that the instrument taps into the intended constructs and that it produces useful measurements reflecting patients' QoL. Validity can be subdivided into three main aspects.

Quality of Life: The Assessment, Analysis and Reporting of Patient-Reported Outcomes, Third Edition.
Peter M. Fayers and David Machin.
© 2016 John Wiley & Sons, Ltd. Published 2016 by John Wiley & Sons, Ltd.

Content validity concerns the extent to which the items are sensible and reflect the intended domain of interest. *Criterion validity* considers whether the scale has empirical association with external criteria, such as other established instruments. *Construct validity* examines the theoretical relationship of the items to each other and to the hypothesised scales. Of these three types of validity, construct validity is the most amenable to exploration by numerical analysis. Two aspects of construct validity are *convergent validity* and *discriminant validity*. Some items or scales, such as anxiety and depression, may be expected to be highly correlated, or convergent. Others may be expected to be relatively unrelated, or divergent, and possessing discriminant validity. If a group of patients with a wide range of diagnoses and treatments is included, a very high scale-to-scale correlation could imply low discriminant validity and might suggest that the two scales measure similar things. On the other hand, if scale-to-scale correlations do not correspond roughly to what is expected, the postulated relationships between the constructs are questionable.

Reliability and *repeatability* concern the random variability associated with measurements. Ideally, patients whose status has not changed should make very similar, or repeatable, responses each time they are assessed. If there is considerable random variability, the measurements are unreliable. It would be difficult to know how to interpret the results from individual patients if the measurements are not reliable. Poor reliability can sometimes be a warning that validity might be suspect, and that the measurement is detecting something different from what we intend it to measure.

Sensitivity is the ability of measurements to detect differences between patients or groups of patients. If we can demonstrate that a measurement is sensitive and detects differences believed to exist between groups of patients, such as differences between poor and good prognosis patients, we will be more confident that it is valid and measuring what we believe it to be measuring. Sensitivity is also important in clinical trials since a measurement is of little use if it cannot detect the differences in patient outcomes that may exist between the randomised groups.

Responsiveness is similar to sensitivity, but relates to the ability to detect changes when a patient improves or deteriorates. A measurement has limited use for patient monitoring unless it reflects changes in the patient's condition. A sensitive measurement is usually, but not necessarily, also responsive to changes.

Validity, reliability, sensitivity and responsiveness are interrelated, yet each is separately important. Assessing validity, in particular, is a complex and never-ending task. Validity is not a dichotomy and, in outcomes research, scales can never be proved to be 'valid'. Instead, the process of validation consists of accruing more and more evidence that the scales are sensible and that they behave in the manner that is anticipated.

For a discussion of statistical significance and *p*-values mentioned in this chapter see Section 5.2.

4.2   Content validity

Content validity relates to the adequacy of the content of an instrument in terms of the number and scope of the individual questions that it contains. It makes use of the conceptual definition of the constructs being assessed, and consists of reviewing the instrument to ensure that it appears to be sensible and covers all of the relevant issues. Thus content validation involves the critical examination of the basic structure of the instrument, a review of the procedures used for the development of the questionnaire, and consideration of the applicability to the intended research question. In order to claim content validity, the design and development of an instrument should follow rigorously defined development procedures. It has been defined as: "Content validity is the extent to which a scale or questionnaire represents the most relevant and important aspects of a concept in the context of a given measurement application" (Magasi *et al.*, 2012).

Item coverage and relevance

Comprehensive coverage is one of the more important aspects of content validity, and the entire range of relevant issues should be covered by the instrument. An instrument aiming to assess symptomatology, for example, should include items relating to all major relevant symptoms. Otherwise there could be undetected differences between groups of patients. In an extreme case, important side effects may remain undetected and unreported. Although these side effects may have a substantial effect upon QoL, a single global question about overall QoL may lack the specificity and sensitivity to detect a group difference. Comprehensive coverage is essential at the domain level, but is also particularly important for multi-item scales that consist of formative (causal or composite) indicators; it should be less important for reflective indicators within a scale, where all items are regarded as being parallel and interchangeable (as is also a fundamental assumption of computer adaptive tests – see Chapter 8).

The extent of item coverage is not amenable to formal statistical testing, and depends largely upon ensuring that the instrument has been developed according to a rigorous pre-defined methodology. The item generation process should include input from specialists in the disease area, a review of published data and literature, and interviews with patients suffering from the illness. Evidence of having followed formal, documented procedures will tend to support claims regarding the content validity of the instrument.

At the same time, all the items that *are* included should be relevant to the concept being assessed, and any irrelevant items should be excluded. Item relevance is commonly approached by using an expert panel to assess whether individual items are appropriate to the construct being assessed, and also by asking patients their opinion as to the relevance of the questions. Methods of construct validation can also indicate those items that appear to be behaving differently from other items in a scale (see Section 5.4). These items can then be critically reviewed, to decide whether they really do or do not relate to the construct that is being evaluated. Items should also be excluded if they are redundant because they overlap with or duplicate the information contained in other items.

Face validity

Face validity involves checking whether items in an instrument appear on the face of it to cover the intended topics clearly and unambiguously. Face validity is closely related to content validity, and is often considered to be an aspect of it. The main distinction is that face validity concerns the critical review of an instrument *after* it has been constructed, while the greater part of content validation consists of ensuring that comprehensive and thorough development procedures were rigorously followed and documented.

Example from the literature

Branski *et al.* (2010) compared the content of nine QoL instruments for patients with voice disorders (Table 4.1). The variation in content was substantial. In part this may be attributable to the different objectives of the instruments: the last four (VHI-10 to pVHI) were developed without using patient interviews and of these three were intended for proxy administration to children. None-the-less, the overall differences are striking: of the first five, some focused on communication and social problems, while the remainder addressed emotional, physical and functional problems.

Table 4.1 Number of items and content of nine instruments that assess voice problems

	Instrument								
	VHI	V-RQOL	VOS	VAPP	VoiSS	VHI-10	PVOS	PV-RQOL	pVHI
Number of items	30	10	5	28	30	10	4	10	23
Domains									
Communication problems			✓	✓	✓		✓		
Social		✓	✓	✓	✓		✓	✓	
Emotional	✓	✓		✓		✓		✓	✓
Physical	✓	✓				✓		✓	✓
Functional	✓	✓				✓		✓	✓
Work/school			✓	✓	✓				
Voice sound and variability					✓				

VHI; Voice Handicap Index; VRQOL; Voice Related Quality of Life; VOS; Voice Outcome Survey; VAPP; Voice activity and participation profile; VoiSS; Voice Symptom Scale; VHI-10; Voice Handicap Index-10; PVOS; Pediatric Voice Outcome Survey; PVRQOL; Pediatric Voice-Related Quality of Life; pVHI; Pediatric Voice Handicap Index.
Source: Branski *et al.*, 2010. Reproduced with permission of Elsevier.

Content validity is optimised by including a wide range of individuals in the development process, and face validity may be maximised in a similar way. Thus when confirming face validity the opinion of experts (such as doctors, nurses and social scientists) should be sought, and patients should be asked whether the instrument seems sensible. Although investigators describing the validation of instruments often state that consensus opinion was sought and that the instrument is believed to have good face validity or content validity, explicit details are often lacking. It is important to describe the composition and functioning of the individuals involved in the development and validation processes.

Example from the literature

Luckett *et al.* (2011) compare the EORTC QLQ-C30 and FACT-G cancer-specific questionnaires with a view to informing choice between them. There is substantial evidence for the reliability and validity of both questionnaires in a range of cancer settings, and both are available in a large number of languages; psychometric data were not decisive in recommending one measure or the other. However, there are major differences in the content, social domains, scale structure and overall character of these two instruments.

A first important difference concerns the way in which 'social HRQoL' is conceptualised and measured in the QLQ-C30 versus FACT-G. Low correlations between the QLQ-C30's social functioning (SF) and FACT-G's social well-being (SWB) reflect differences in their content; items in SF assess impacts on social activities and family life while those in SWB focus on social support and relationships.

In addition to the physical, emotional, social and functional/role scales offered by both measures, the QLQ-C30 provides brief scales for cognitive functioning, financial impact and a range of symptoms either not assessed by the FACT-G or else subsumed within its well-being scales. While the QLQ-C30's approach enables scores to be generated for outcomes that may be of specific interest, it provides 15 scores compared with the FACT-G's five, which complicates analysis and raises issues of multiple hypothesis testing.

An overall score on the QLQ-C30 is generated by averaging responses to just two questions (global health and quality of life), while the FACT-G allows summation of all 27 items. The QLQ-C30 and FACT-G both look and feel different. With the exception of its emotional scale, the QLQ-C30 confines its questions to relatively objective aspects of functioning, whereas the FACT-G encourages respondents to reflect on their thoughts and feelings throughout. Studies asking patients and health professionals about relative face validity, ease of comprehension and overall preference have been inconclusive, although the trend has generally favoured the QLQ-C30.

Thus both instruments claim face and content validity, yet they differ substantially in their content. In part, this reflects the different design teams, with the QLQ-C30 placing greater emphasis on clinical aspects as compared to the FACT-G which is more psycho-social in content.

4.3   Criterion validity

Criterion validity involves assessing an instrument against the true value, or against some other standard that is accepted as providing an indication of the true values for the measurements. It can be divided into *concurrent validity* and *predictive validity*.

Concurrent validity

Concurrent validity means agreement with the true value. Such a 'gold standard' is not available for PROs since they measure postulated constructs that are experimental and subjective. Therefore the most common approach involves comparing new questionnaires against one or more well-established instruments. This may be reasonable if the objective of developing a new instrument is to produce a shorter or simpler questionnaire, in which case the more detailed, established instrument may be believed to set a standard at which to aim. More frequently, the rationale for creating a new instrument is that the investigators believe existing ones to be suboptimal. In this case, the comparison of new against established is of limited value since the latter has, in effect, already been rejected as the gold standard. Another approach is to use indirect methods of comparison. A detailed interview, using staff trained in interviewing techniques, might yield estimates of the constructs that are perhaps believed to be approximations to true values for a patient.

Example

Anxiety and depression are psychological concepts that have traditionally been assessed by using in-depth interviews to rate their severity and to detect patient 'cases' needing psychiatric intervention. If the psychiatric assessment is regarded as an approximation of the true level of these states, it can serve as a criterion against which a patient's self-completed questionnaire is compared. Anxiety and depression are perhaps different from more complex QoL scales, in that there is (arguably) a clearer definition and better consensus among psychiatrists of the meaning of these terms. On that assumption, it would seem reasonable to regard a brief patient-questionnaire, taking a few minutes to complete, as a convenient method for estimating the 'true' values of the detailed interview.

As already mentioned, a new instrument is usually compared against values obtained from other well-established or lengthier instruments, an in-depth interview, or an observer's assessment. If agreement between the two methods is considered to be poor, the concurrent validity is low. It may be difficult to determine with certainty whether one or both of the methods has low validity, but the low level of agreement serves as an indicator that something may be amiss.

Example from the literature

When developing the HADS instrument, Zigmond and Snaith (1983) asked 100 patients from a general medical outpatient clinic to complete the questionnaire. Following this, they used a 20-minute psychiatric interview to assess anxiety and depression; this provided the criterion against which the two scales of the HADS were compared. A summary of the results is shown in Table 4.2, with patients grouped into three categories according to whether they were psychiatric cases, doubtful cases or non-cases of anxiety and depression.

For diagnosing psychiatric cases, the depression scale gave 1% false positives and 1% false negatives, and the anxiety scale 5% false positives and 1% false negatives.

Table 4.2 HADS questionnaire completed by 100 patients from a general medical outpatient clinic

HADS score	Depression			Anxiety		
	Non-cases	Doubtful cases	Cases	Non-cases	Doubtful cases	Cases
0–7	57	11	1^-	41	4	1^-
8–10	8	7	3	10	9	1
11–21	1^+	4	8	5^+	15	14

+ False positives. − False negatives.
Source: Zigmond and Snaith, 1983, Table 1. Reproduced with permission of John Wiley & Sons, Ltd.

Predictive validity

Predictive validity concerns the ability of the instrument to predict future health status, future events or future test results. For example, it has frequently been reported that overall QoL scores are predictive of subsequent survival time in cancer trials, and that QoL assessment is providing additional prognostic information to supplement the more objective measures, such as tumour stage and extent of disease. The implication is that future health status can serve as a criterion against which the instrument is compared. Thus, for purposes of criterion validity, future status is regarded as a better indicator of the current true value of the latent variable than the observed patient responses from the instrument being developed. To make such an assumption, the investigator will have to form a conceptual model of the construct being assessed and its relationship with future outcomes. Therefore predictive validity is more conveniently discussed from the perspective of being an aspect of construct validity.

4.4   Construct validity

Construct validity is one of the most important characteristics of a measurement instrument. It is an assessment of the degree to which an instrument is valid in that it appears to measure the construct that it was designed to measure. The subject of construct validity is a difficult and controversial one. It involves first forming a hypothetical model, describing the constructs being assessed and postulating their relationships. Data are then collected, and an assessment is made as to the degree to which these relationships are confirmed. If the results confirm prior expectations about the constructs, the implication is that the instrument *may* be valid and that we may therefore use it to make inferences about patients.

The '*may* be valid' emphasises the controversial aspect of construct validation. The difficulty is that neither the criterion nor the construct is directly measurable. Hence a formal statistical test cannot be developed. Since assessment of construct validity relies upon expressing opinions about expected relationships amongst the constructs, and confirming that the observed measurements behave as expected, we cannot *prove* that questionnaire items are valid measures for the constructs, or that the constructs are valid representations of behaviour. All we can do is collect increasing amounts of evidence that the measurements appear to be sensible, that the postulated constructs behave as anticipated, and that there are no grounds for rejecting them. The greater the supporting evidence, the more confident we are that our model is an adequate representation of the constructs that we label QoL.

More formally, construct validity embraces a variety of techniques, all aimed at assessing two things: first, whether the theoretical postulated construct appears to be an adequate model; and, second, whether the measurement scale appears to correspond to that postulated construct. In this chapter we describe several approaches that are applicable to single-item scales or summary scores from multi-item scales, but in the next chapter we show more powerful methods that are available for multi-item scales, to explore dimensionality, homogeneity and overlap of the constructs.

Mainly, assessment of construct validity makes use of correlations, changes over time, and differences between groups of patients. It involves building and testing conceptual models that express the postulated relationships between the hypothetical domains of QoL and the scales that are being developed to measure these domains. Construct validation is a lengthy and on-going process of learning more about the construct, making new predictions and then testing them. Each study that supports the theoretical construct serves to strengthen the theory, but a single negative finding may call into question the entire construct.

Known-groups validation

One of the simpler forms of construct validation is *known-groups validation*. This is based on the principle that certain specified groups of patients may be anticipated to score differently from others, and the instrument should be sensitive to these differences. For example, patients with advanced cancer might be expected to have poorer overall QoL than those with early disease. A valid scale should show differences, in the predicted direction, between these groups. Known-groups comparisons are therefore a combination of tests for validity and a form of sensitivity or responsiveness assessment. A scale that cannot successfully distinguish between groups with known differences, either because it lacks sensitivity or because it yields results that are contrary to expectations, is hardly likely to be of value for many purposes.

Investigators frequently select patients in whom one may anticipate that there will be substantial differences between the groups. This implies that even a very small study will provide sufficient evidence to confirm that the observed differences are unlikely to be due to chance; what matters most is the magnitude of the differences, not the p-values. Although statistical significance tests are uninformative and not worthy of reporting in these circumstances, it is common to see publications that describe all differences as statistically highly significant with p-values less than 0.0001.

Closely similar to known-groups validation is *validation by application* (Feinstein 1987, p. 205). When a scale is used in a clinical trial and detects the anticipated effects, one can infer that the scale is sensitive and that it is presumably measuring the outcome of interest. However, cynics may claim that this approach (and, indeed, known-groups validation in general) cannot tell whether the scale being validated is addressing the intended construct, or merely evaluating another outcome that is highly correlated with it. Thus, as with known-groups validation, face validity is an important aspect of drawing conclusions from the observations.

Example from the literature

O'Connell and Skevington (2012) described the validation of a short form of the WHOQOL-HIV instrument, the 31-item WHOQOL-HIV-BREF. Survey data from 1,923 HIV-positive adults (selected for age, gender and disease stage) were collected in eight culturally diverse centres. Known-groups validity, based on 1,884 adults, was explored by contrasting three subgroups with disease of varying severity: HIV-asymptomatic, HIV-symptomatic and AIDS. The authors reported the ANOVA F-statistics for each of the 31 items and the six multi-item domains; in Table 4.3 we show just the two general items and the six domains.

For both of the general items and all of the summary scales there is a clear trend according to severity of illness. Given the large sample size, it is not surprising that all ANOVA F-ratios are highly significant ($p < 0.001$). The authors comment that their results confirm that the new instrument shows very good discriminant validity. They also note that the two domains with the largest effects (largest F-ratios) were physical and level of independence.

Known-groups validity is not the same as sensitivity, which we discuss later in this chapter. For sensitivity, we are interested in whether the instrument can detect small group-differences, in sample sizes as used in clinical trials. Here, for known-groups validity, the authors confirm that the anticipated effects were observed.

Table 4.3   Known-groups validity of the Short Form WHOQOL-HIV instrument, in 1,884 adults who are HIV-positive

	HIV asymptomatic N = 776	HIV symptomatic N = 643	AIDS N = 465	F-ratio*
Overall QoL and Health				
General QoL	3.47	3.15	2.98	45.43
General health	3.27	2.77	2.56	84.97
Domain scores				
1. Physical	14.49	12.39	11.12	186.37
2. Psychological	13.77	12.59	11.81	79.95
3. Independence	15.25	13.14	11.75	197.63
4. Social Relationships	13.30	12.56	12.00	25.41
5. Environment	12.87	12.10	11.83	27.59
6. Spirituality, Religion and Personal Beliefs (SRPB)	13.35	12.53	11.85	26.78

* ANOVA F-statistics; all are significant $p < 0.001$.
Source: Extract from O'Connell and Skevington, 2012, Table 3, which displays discriminant validity for all items. Reproduced with permission of Springer Science+Business Media.

Convergent validity

Convergent validity is another important aspect of construct validity, and consists of showing that a postulated dimension of QoL correlates appreciably with all other dimensions that should in theory be related to it. That is, we may believe that some dimensions of QoL are related, and we therefore expect the observed measurements to be correlated. For example, one might anticipate that patients with severe pain are likely to be depressed, and that there should be a correlation between the pain scores and depression ratings.

Many of the dimensions of QoL are interrelated. Very ill patients tend to suffer from a variety of symptoms and have high scores on a wide range of psychological dimensions. Many, and sometimes nearly all, dimensions of QoL are correlated with each other. Therefore an assessment of convergent validity consists of predicting the strongest and weakest correlations, and confirming that subsequent observed values conform to the predictions. Analysis consists of calculating all pairwise correlation coefficients between scores for different QoL scales.

A very high correlation between two scales invites the question of whether both of the scales are measuring the same factor, and of whether they could be combined into a single scale without any loss of information. The decision regarding the amalgamation of scales should take into account the composition of the separate scales, and whether there are clinical, psychological or other grounds for deciding that face validity could be compromised and that it is better to retain separate scales. Alternatively, a very high correlation might imply that one of the scales is redundant and can be deleted from the instrument. Convergent validity is usually considered together with discriminant validity.

Discriminant validity

Discriminant validity, or divergent validity, recognises that some dimensions of QoL are anticipated to be relatively unrelated and that therefore their correlations should be low. Convergent and discriminant validity represent the two extremes in a continuum of associations between the dimensions of QoL. One problem when assessing discriminant validity (and, to a lesser extent, convergent validity) is that two dimensions may correlate because of some third, possibly unrecognised, construct that links the two together; statisticians term this *spurious correlation*. For example, if two dimensions are both affected by age, an apparent correlation can be introduced solely through the differing ages of the respondents. Another extraneous source of correlations could be 'yea-saying', in which patients may report improving QoL on many dimensions simply to please staff or relatives. When specific independent variables are suspected of introducing spurious correlations, the statistical technique of *partial correlation* should be used; this is a method of estimating the correlation between two variables, or dimensions of QoL, while holding constant other variables that statisticians describe as *nuisance variables*. In practice, there are usually many extraneous variables each contributing a little to the spurious correlations.

Convergent validity and discriminant validity are commonly assessed across instruments rather than within an instrument, in which case those scales from each instrument that are intended to measure similar constructs should have higher correlations with each other than with scales that measure unrelated constructs.

Example from the literature

Schag *et al.* (1992) evaluated the HIV Overview of Problems – Evaluation System (HOPES), and predicted the pattern of associations that they expected to observe between scales from the HOPES questionnaire and the MOS-HIV. Table 4.4 shows some of the corresponding observed correlations.

The authors comment that, as predicted, the three MOS-HIV scales of cognitive function, mental health and health distress correlate most highly with the psychosocial summary scale of the HOPES. Similarly, other MOS-HIV subscales correlate most highly with the HOPES physical summary scale.

The high correlations support the predictions of convergent validity, while the lower correlations between other subscales support discriminant validity.

Table 4.4 Correlations between HOPES physical and psychosocial scales and the MOS-HIV scales, in patients with HIV infection

MOS-HIV	Hopes	
	Physical	Psychosocial
General health	0.74	0.41
Physical function	0.74	0.42
Role function	0.70	0.36
Social function	0.75	0.43
Cognitive function	0.55	0.55
Pain score	0.67	0.39
Mental health	0.55	0.70
Energy/fatigue	0.72	0.47
Health distress	0.65	0.67
QoL	0.52	0.44
Health transition	0.25	0.17

Source: Schag *et al.*, 1992, Table 6. Reproduced with permission of Springer Science+Business Media.

Multitrait–multimethod analysis

The *multitrait–multimethod* (MTMM) correlation matrix is a method for examining convergent and discriminant validity, and was described by Campbell and Fiske in 1959. The general principle of this technique is that two or more 'methods', such as different instruments, are each used to assess the same 'traits', for example QoL aspects, items or subscales. Then we can inspect and compare the correlations arising from the same subscale as estimated by the different methods. Various layouts are used for MTMM matrices, the most common being shown in Table 4.5.

In this template the two instruments are methods, while the functioning scales are traits. Cells marked *C* show the correlations of the scores when different instruments

Table 4.5 Template for the multitrait–multimethod (MTMM) correlation matrix

	Instrument	Emotional function		Social function		Role function	
		1	2	1	2	1	2
Emotional function	1	R					
	2	C	R				
Social function	1	D		R			
	2		D	C	R		
Role function	1	D		D		R	
	2		D		D	C	R

are used to assess the same trait. *Convergent validity* is determined by the C cells. If the correlations in these cells are high, say above 0.7, this suggests that both instruments may be measuring the same thing. If the two instruments were developed independently of each other, this would support the inference that the traits are defined in a consistent and presumably meaningful manner.

Similarly, the D cells show the scale-to-scale correlations for each instrument, and these assess *discriminant validity*. Lower correlations are usually expected in these cells, since otherwise scales purporting to measure different aspects of QoL are in fact more strongly related than supposedly similar scales from different instruments.

The main diagonal cells, marked R, can be used to show reliability coefficients, as described later and in Chapter 5. These can be either Cronbach's α for internal reliability or, if repeated QoL assessments are available on patients whose condition is stable, test–retest correlations. Since repeated values of the same trait measured twice by the same method will usually be more similar than values of the same trait measured by different instruments, the R cells containing test–retest repeatability scores should usually contain the highest correlations.

One common variation on the theme of MTMM matrices is to carry out the patient assessments on two different occasions. The unshaded triangular area to the upper-right of Table 4.5 can be used to display the correlations at time 1, and the time 2 data can be shown in the shaded cells as described above. The diagonal cells dividing the two triangular regions, marked R, can then show the test–retest repeatability correlations.

Example from the literature

The FACT-G and the EORTC QLQ-C30 are two instruments that ostensibly measure many of the same aspects of QoL. Silveira *et al.* (2010) used an MTMM matrix, summarised in Table 4.6, to compare these two instruments in 102 patients with head and neck cancer.

Silveira *et al.* used the layout of Table 4.5, subdividing the instruments into traits (QoL dimensions). The correlation between the QLQ-C30 physical function scale and the FACT-G physical well-being scale is 0.80, while the correlation between the QLQ-C30 social function and the FACT-G social well-being is only 0.21.

Convergent validity is determined by the shaded cells, which represent the correlation of two instruments when assessing the traits that are hypothesised as similar. In this example, the correlation for social function and social well-being is very low, indicating that despite the similar names these two scales are measuring very different constructs. The correlation between the two emotional scales is at best only modest, again suggesting that these scales may differ in concept.

These results are not surprising; as we commented when introducing the instruments in Chapter 1, they are conceptually very different from each other, with the QLQ-C30 emphasising clinical symptoms and the FACT-G addressing feelings and concerns. Other authors have reported similar differences (Luckett *et al.*, 2011).

Table 4.6　Multitrait–multimethod correlation matrix for FACT-G scores and EORTC QLQ-C30 scores, in 102 patients with head-and-neck cancer

	Physical		Social		Emotional		Role	
	PF (QLQ)	Pwb (FACT)	SF (QLQ)	Swb (FACT)	EF (QLQ)	Ewb (FACT)	RF (QLQ)	Fwb (FACT)
Physical								
PF								
Pwb	0.80							
Social								
SF	0.62	0.70						
Swb	0.19	0.19	0.21					
Emotional								
EF	0.42	0.49	0.48	0.18				
Ewb	0.51	0.67	0.54	0.35	0.63			
Role								
RF	0.79	0.75	0.72	0.18	0.44	0.56		
Fwb	0.71	0.70	0.65	0.39	0.43	0.60	0.70	

EORTC QLQ-C30: PF physical function; SF social function; EF emotional function; RF role function.
FACT-G: Pwb physical well-being; Swb social well-being; Ewb emotional well-being; Fwb functional well-being.
Source: Silveira *et al.*, 2010, Table 8. CC BY 2.0 (http://creativecommons.org/licenses/by/2.0).

Silveira *et al.* comment on the marked departures of Swb and SF from a normal distribution, but despite this used Pearson correlation and not that of Spearman which is more applicable in such cases.

Example from the literature

Khanna *et al.* (2012) explored the validity of computerised adaptive tests from Patient-Reported Outcomes Measurement Information System (PROMIS) item banks, using data from 143 patients with systemic sclerosis. Construct validity of the PROMIS items was evaluated by examining correlations with corresponding legacy measures using MTMM analysis. The six PROMIS domains selected for analysis were depression, fatigue, pain behaviour, physical function, sleep disturbance and satisfaction with participation in discretionary social activities. The corresponding legacy scales were the depression from CESD-10, FACIT-Fatigue, SF-36 bodily pain, SF-36 physical functioning, MOS 9-item sleep problem index and SF-36 social functioning, respectively.

The correlations are shown in Table 4.7.

Khanna *et al.* used a summary table for the MTMM analysis, presenting only the correlations between the PROMIS scales and the legacy instruments. It was hypothesised that the correlation coefficients between scales for corresponding dimensions (shown as shaded values on the main diagonal in Table 4.7) would be '≥0.50 (a large effect size) and that these would be significantly larger than off-diagonal correlations'.

Table 4.7 Multitrait–multimethod correlation matrix for PROMIS scores compared against legacy instruments, in 143 patients with systemic sclerosis

PROMIS CAT	CESD-10 Depression	FACIT Fatigue	SF-36 Bodily pain	SF-36 Physical func.	MOS Sleep index	SF-36 Social func.
Depression 1.0	0.67	0.44	0.31	0.20	0.33	0.46
Fatigue 1.0	0.59	0.76	0.59	0.51	0.49	0.59
Pain Behavior 1.0	0.44	0.53	0.66	0.38	0.37	0.47
Phys. Function 1.0	0.46	0.72	0.56	0.82	0.43	0.55
Sleep Disturb 1.0	0.50	0.37	0.23	0.24	0.75	0.28
Social Sat Discretionary	0.56	0.62	0.48	0.54	0.46	0.61

Source: Khanna *et al.*, 2012, Table 4. Reproduced with permission of Elsevier.

Khanna *et al.* reported that 'Validity diagonals (correlations among different methods of measuring the same domain) were the largest correlations across the row and column in every case with one exception: the PROMIS scale (satisfaction with participation in discretionary social activities) had about the same size correlation with the legacy scale FACIT-Fatigue ($r = 0.62$) than with the SF-36 social functioning counterpart. Eighty-three percent of the paired correlation t-tests were statistically significantly larger than relevant off-diagonal correlations in the MTMM matrix, providing substantial support of construct validity of the measures.'

It is often useful to consider confidence intervals (*CI*s) of the correlation coefficients, as shown in Section 5.3. The *CI*s reflect the sample size of the study, and a small study will be associated with wide intervals. The intervals enable a critical inspection of whether differences between correlations may be due to chance, or whether there is reasonable confirmation of the expected correlation structure

4.5   Repeated assessments and change over time

The methods described so far have involved a single cross-sectional assessment of the patients. We turn now to validation in which repeated assessments per patient are used:

- repeatability in stable patients, or consistency over time: test–retest reliability;

- responsiveness or sensitivity to changes in patients whose condition has altered over time.

4.6   Reliability

Assessment of *reliability* consists of determining that a scale or measurement yields reproducible and consistent results. Confusingly, this same word is used for two very different levels of scale validation. First, for scales containing multiple items, all the items should be consistent in the sense that they should all measure the same thing. This form of reliability, which is called *internal reliability*, uses item correlations to assess the homogeneity of multi-item scales and is in many senses a form of validity. Second, reliability is also used as a term to describe aspects of *repeatability* and stability of measurements. Any measurement or summary score, whether based upon a single item or multiple items, should yield reproducible or consistent values if it is used repeatedly on the same patient while the patient's condition has not changed materially. Thus reliability, in this sense of repeatability, describes the differences between multiple measurements. From a statistical perspective, reliability is similar to variance, in the sense that an unreliable measure varies between measurement occasions. This second form of reliability is a desirable property of any quantitative measurement, and is a necessary condition for a PRO to be valid. However, reliability does not in itself imply validity: a measure that is measuring something reliably and consistently may not necessarily be measuring the intended construct.

From a statistical point of view, both forms of reliability are assessed using related techniques. Thus *repeatability reliability* is based upon analysis of correlations between repeated measurements, where the measurements are either repeated over time (*test–retest reliability*), by different observers (*inter-rater reliability*) or by different variants of the instrument (*equivalent-forms reliability*). *Internal reliability*, which is also often called *internal consistency,* is based on item-to-item correlations in multi-item scales, and is discussed in Section 5.5. Since these two concepts are mathematically related, estimates of the internal reliability of multi-item scales can often be used to predict the approximate value of their repeatability reliability.

A number of different measures have been proposed. Since reliability is the extent to which repeated measurements will give the same results when the true scale score remains constant, measurement concerns the level of agreement between two or more scores. We describe those measures that are commonly used when there are two assessments per patient. However, we also note that, from a statistical perspective, the reliability of continuous measurements may be more effectively explored using ANOVA models to evaluate the *SE* of the measurements, and to explore the relationship of this *SE* to the other sources of variance; see also Section 5.5.

Binary data: proportion of agreement

Binary assessments include ratings such as yes/no, present/absent, positive/negative, or patients grouped into those greater/less than some threshold value. The simplest method of assessing repeatability is the *proportion of agreement* when the same instrument is applied on two occasions. When patients are assessed twice, the resulting data can be tabulated, as in Table 4.8. Here x_{11} is the number of patients whose QoL response is positive both times, and x_{22} when it is negative.

The number of agreements, that is the number of patients who respond in the same way in both assessments, is $x_{11} + x_{22}$, and so the proportion of agreements is

$$P_{Agree} = \left(x_{11} + x_{22} \right) / N, \tag{4.1}$$

where N is the total number of patients.

Binary data: κ

However, we would expect some agreement purely by chance, even if patients entered random responses on the questionnaire, and p_{Agree} does not only reflect whether the agreement arises mainly from being positive twice, or negative twice. The kappa coefficient, κ, provides a better method by extending the above concept of proportion agreement to allow for some expected chance agreements. It can be shown that the expected number of chance agreements corresponding to cell x_{11} is $c_1 r_1 / N$ and similarly for x_{22}, $c_2 r_2 / N$. Thus the expected proportion of chance agreements is

$$P_{Chance} = \left(\frac{c_1 r_1}{N} + \frac{c_2 r_2}{N} \right) \bigg/ N = \left(c_1 r_1 + c_2 r_2 \right) N^2. \tag{4.2}$$

Table 4.8 Notation for repeated binary data, with two assessments of the same N subjects

Second assessment	First assessment		
	Positive	Negative	Total
Positive	x_{11}	x_{12}	r_1
Negative	x_{21}	x_{22}	r_2
Total	c_1	c_2	N

Table 4.9 Guideline values of κ to indicate the strength of agreement

Agreement:		Agreement:	
κ	Landis & Koch	κ	Hahn *et al.*
< 0.20	Poor/slight	(< 0.40)	Low (high error)
0.21–0.40	Fair		
0.41–0.60	Moderate	(0.40–0.74)	Moderate or good (acceptable error)
0.61–0.80	Substantial		
0.81–1.00	Almost perfect	(> 0.74)	High or excellent (minimal/no error)

Sources: Landis and Koch, 1977. Reproduced with permission of John Wiley & Sons, Inc; Hahn *et al.*, 2007, Table 1. Reproduced with permission of Elsevier.

The excess proportion of agreement above that expected is then $\left(p_{Agree} - p_{Chance} \right)$ Furthermore, since the maximum proportion of agreements is 1 when $x_{11} + x_{22} = N$, the maximum value of $\left(p_{Agree} - p_{Chance} \right)$ is $\left(1 - p_{Chance} \right)$. Hence we can scale the excess proportion of agreement so that it has a maximum value of 1. This leads to the κ index of agreement:

$$\kappa = \left(p_{Agree} - p_{Chance} \right) / \left(1 - p_{Chance} \right). \tag{4.3}$$

The value of κ is equal to 1 if there is perfect agreement, and equals 0 if the agreement is no better than chance. Negative values indicate an agreement that is even less than what would be expected by chance. Interpretation of κ is subjective, but Table 4.9 shows the frequently cited guideline values of Landis and Koch (1977), although later authors such as Hahn *et al.* (2007) agree higher values are desirable.

Although κ may seem intuitively appealing, it has been criticised. Misleading values are often obtained, mainly because κ is affected by the degree of asymmetry or imbalance in the table. The value of κ is also influenced by the total percentage of positives, and it is possible to obtain very different values of κ even when the proportion of agreement remains constant. Further, high agreement can occur even when κ is very low. Thus κ is no substitute for inspecting the table of frequencies, and examining whether the table appears to be symmetrical or whether there is a tendency for patients to respond differently on the two occasions.

Example from the literature

The EQ-5D-Y was developed from the EQ-5D for measuring HRQOL in children and adolescents from 8 years onwards. In addition to the VAS scale of the EQ-5D, it comprises five items referring to mobility, self-care, usual activities, pain and discomfort, and anxiety and depression. Each item has three levels (no problems, some problems and a lot of problems). From a large international validation study, Ravens-Sieberer *et al.* (2010) report the test–retest reliability for Italy and Spain, where a third of the study sample received the questionnaire again 7–10 days after the first examination.

Percentage of agreement is shown in Table 4.10, with κ coefficients calculated after dichotomising the responses into 'no problem' versus 'any problems' for each profile domain.

The percentage agreement was 69.8–93.8% for Italian youths, and in 86.2–99.7% for Spanish. This reasonably high level of agreement was generally confirmed by the κ coefficients. However, the authors noted that the high ceiling effects caused some apparent non-confirmation of the results. In Italy, no κ coefficient could be computed for the self-care domain since all children reported no problems in the retest. Similarly, the κ coefficients in the mobility dimension are of limited value since nearly all retest responses were in the 'no problems' category.

These results illustrate some of the problems in the interpretation of κ.

Table 4.10 Test–retest κ coefficients and percent agreement for the youth-version EQ-5D-Y

	Italy ($N = 415$)		Spain ($N = 973$)	
	κ coefficient	Agreement (%)	κ coefficient	Agreement (%)
Mobility (walking about)	0.222	91.5	−0.003*	99.4
Looking after myself	0.000[a]	93.8	0.665*	99.7
Doing usual activities	0.352*	82.9	0.557*	97.5
Having pain or discomfort	0.350*	69.8	0.435*	86.2
Feeling worried, sad or unhappy	0.549*	78.3	0.468*	87.4

*Significant at $p \leq 0.01$.
[a]The responses in the retest are identical to the test.
Source: Ravens-Siberer *et al.*, 2010, Table 3. CC-BY-NC (http://creativecommons.org/licenses/by-nc/2.0/uk/). Reproduced commercially with kind permission from Springer Science+Business Media and the authors.

Ordered categorical data: weighted κ

QoL assessments frequently consist of ordered categorical response items that are scored according to the level of response. For example, items from some instruments are scored with $g = 4$ categories from 1 for 'not at all' through to 4 for 'very much'.

If we construct the $g \times g$ two-way table of frequencies analogous to Table 4.8, we obtain

$$P_{Agree} = \left(\sum x_{ii}\right)\Big/N \quad \text{and} \quad P_{Chance} = \left(\sum r_i c_i\right)\Big/N^2, \tag{4.4}$$

where the summation is from $i = 1$ to g. Equation (4.3) is then applied to give κ.

However, these equations give equal importance to any disagreement. Although it is possible to use this directly, it is generally more realistic to use a *weighted* form, κ_{Weight}. This takes into account the degree of disagreement, such that a difference between scores of 1 and 3 on the two occasions would be considered of greater importance than the difference between 1 and 2. In terms of the table of frequencies, values along the diagonal, corresponding to x_{11}, x_{22}, x_{33} to x_{gg}, represent perfect agreement. Values that are off the diagonal in row i and column j are given scores or *weights* according to their distance from the diagonal, which corresponds to their degree of discrepancy. Two frequently used choices of weights are

$$w_{ij} = 1 - \frac{i-j}{g-1}, \quad \text{or} \quad w_{ij} = 1 - \left(\frac{i-j}{g-1}\right)^2, \tag{4.5}$$

where $|i - j|$ is the absolute difference of i and j, which ignores the sign of the difference. In equation (4.5), the first represents linear weighting, and the second is quadratic weighting.

Example

Suppose an item has $g = 4$ possible response categories, with 1 for 'not at all', 2 for 'a little', 3 for 'quite a bit' and 4 for 'very much'. If the result of the first assessment on a patient is 1, then for second assessment values of 1, 2, 3 or 4 respectively, the corresponding linear weights would be 1, 0.67, 0.33 and 0, while the quadratic weights would be 1, 0.89, 0.56 and 0. For both weighting schemes 1 indicates perfect agreement and 0 the maximum disagreement. The quadratic weights place greater emphasis upon measurements that agree closely.

Quadratic weights are generally considered preferable, and lead to:

$$p_{Agree}^{W} = \left(\sum_{i=1}^{g}\sum_{j=1}^{g} w_{ij}x_{ij}\right)\Big/N, \; p_{Chance}^{W} = \left(\sum_{i=1}^{g}\sum_{j=1}^{g} w_{ij}r_i c_j\right) = \left(\sum_{i=1}^{g}\sum_{j=1}^{g} w_{ij}r_i c_j\right)\Big/N^2,$$

and hence

$$\kappa_{Weight} = \left(p_{Agree}^{W} - p_{Chance}^{W}\right)\Big/\left(1 - p_{Chance}^{W}\right). \tag{4.6}$$

Similar reservations apply to weighted κ_{Weight} as to simple κ. The value is highly affected by the symmetry of the table, and by the proportion of patients in each category. Also, the number of categories g affects κ_{Weight}. Thus, for example, κ_{Weight} will usually be greater (and sometimes substantially so) if patients are evenly distributed over the range of values for QoL, and will be smaller if most patients have extreme values, for example if most patients have very poor QoL. Thus it can be difficult to know how to interpret or decide what are acceptable values of κ_{Weight}, as it is greatly affected by the weights, making the guideline values of Table 4.9 inapplicable. One use of κ_{Weight} that does not depend upon guideline values is inference about the *relative* stability of different items: those items with largest κ are the most repeatable.

Despite these reservations, when analysing proportions or items, which have only a few ordered categories, κ_{Weight} is a measure for assessing the agreement between two items or between two repeats of an assessment. However, Fleiss and Cohen (1973) showed that quadratic-weighted κ_{Weight} is also equivalent to the intraclass correlation coefficient described next, and we recommend the latter as being simpler to calculate and interpret.

Example from the literature

Lemmens *et al.* (2013) adapted the Swal-Qol, a questionnaire for evaluating the impact of dysphagia on quality of life, to an interview format suitable for dysphagic patients with communicative and/or cognitive problems. Test–retest reliability was assessed by administrating two identical Swal-Qol interviews with the same interviewer. A two-week time interval was considered enough time for patients not to remember their previous answers. The test–retest reliability for each subscale and overall score was reported, with values of κ_{Weight} between 0.40 and 0.75 interpreted as good and those above 0.75 as excellent. To compare the data with previous published studies, Spearman's correlation coefficients and the intraclass correlation coefficients (*ICC*) were also calculated (Table 4.11).

Lemmens *et al.* reported that weighted kappa was excellent ($\kappa_{Weight} > 0.75$) for the overall score and seven subscales, and good for subscales 'fear' ($\kappa_{Weight} = 0.675$) and 'fatigue' ($\kappa_{Weight} = 0.713$).

It was not specified whether quadratic weighting was used. The interpretation criteria correspond to those of Hahn *et al.* in Table 4.9, and are frequently used for κ_{Weight} although as we have noted this is questionable. Lemmens *et al.* additionally presented κ_{Weight} coefficients for two subgroups, one with only 16 patients; some statistical packages provide confidence intervals, and these can aid the interpretation for small sample sizes.

Table 4.11 Test–retest κ_{Weight} coefficients for the Swal-Qol dysphagia questionnaire, adapted for interviewing patients with communicative and/or cognitive problems; results of testing 56 patients

Subscale	Number of items	Number of patients	κ_{Weight}	Spearman's correlation	ICC
1. Burden	2	56	0.849	0.854	0.850
2. Eating duration and desire	5	54	0.822	0.828	0.817
3. Dysphagia symptoms	14	54	0.940	0.934	0.941
4. Food selection	2	53	0.823	0.834	0.818
5. Communication	2	56	0.786	0.777	0.789
6. Fear	4	53	0.675	0.715	0.678
7. Mental health	5	55	0.898	0.877	0.891
8. Social functioning	5	48	0.908	0.909	0.909
9. Fatigue and sleep	5	55	0.713	0.710	0.714
Overall score	44	48	0.953	0.951	0.952

Source: Lemmens et al., 2013, Table 2. CC BY 3.0 (https://creativecommons.org/licenses/by/3.0/).

Pearson's correlation coefficient

The ordinary correlation coefficient, also called Pearson's correlation, is described in Section 5.3. Although it is often advocated as a measure of repeatability, this is to be deprecated because correlation is a measure of association. Repeated measurements may be highly correlated yet systematically different. For example, if patients consistently score higher by exactly 10 points when a test is reapplied, there would be zero agreement between the first and second assessments. Despite this, the correlation coefficient would be 1, indicating perfect association. When one has continuous variables, a more appropriate approach to the assessment of reliability is the *intraclass correlation coefficient* (*ICC*).

Intraclass correlation coefficient (*ICC*)

For continuous data, the *ICC* measures the strength of agreement between repeated measurements, by assessing the proportion of the total variance, σ^2 (the square of the *SD*), of an observation that is associated with the between-patient variability. Thus,

$$ICC = \frac{\sigma^2_{Patient}}{\sigma^2_{Patient} + \sigma^2_{Error}}. \tag{4.7}$$

If the *ICC* is large (close to 1), then the random error variability is low and a high proportion of the variance in the observations is attributable to variation between patients. The measurements are then described as having high reliability. Conversely, if the *ICC* is low (close to 0), the random error variability dominates and the measurements have low reliability. If the error variability is regarded as 'noise' and the true value of patients' scores as the 'signal', the *ICC* measures the signal/noise ratio.

The *ICC* can be estimated from an ANOVA. In brief, ANOVA partitions the total variance into separate components, according to the source of the variability. A table for ANOVA in which *p* patients repeat the same QoL assessment on *r* occasions can be represented as in Table 4.12. Here, we have shown a two-way (repeats and patients) random effects model, without interaction term; because several alternatives are possible, this has been described as a 'case 2A' model by McGraw and Wong (1996). Equation (4.7) describes the average *consistency* of the assessments when there is a single repeat, and has been termed $ICC(C,1)$ (McGraw and Wong, 1996) or $ICC_{Consistency}$ (de Vet *et al.*, 2006).

The *error* variability corresponding to equation (4.7) has been separated into two components, and is now $\sigma^2_{Repeats} + \sigma^2_{Error}$. This leads to:

$$ICC = \frac{\sigma^2_{Patient}}{\sigma^2_{Patient} + \sigma^2_{Repeats} + \sigma^2_{Error}}, \tag{4.8}$$

which includes a term for a random *Repeats* effect. Equation (4.8) is generally preferred over equation (4.7), and has been described as $ICC_{Agreement}$ (de Vet *et al.*, 2006), and for a single repeat corresponds to $ICC(A,1)$ of McGraw and Wong (1996). Solving

Table 4.12   ANOVA table to estimate the intraclass correlation

Source	Sum of squares	Degrees of freedom	Mean squares	Variances
Between-patients	$S_{Patient}$	$p-1$	$V_{Patient} = \dfrac{S_{Patient}}{p-1}$	$= r\sigma^2_{Patient} + \sigma^2_{Error}$
Repeats (Within patients)	$S_{Repeats}$	$r-1$	$V_{Repeats} = \dfrac{S_{Repeats}}{r-1}$	$= p\sigma^2_{Repeats} + \sigma^2_{Error}$
Error	S_{Error}	$rp-r-p+1$	$V_{Error} = \dfrac{S_{Error}}{rp-r-p+1}$	$= \sigma^2_{Error}$
Total	S_{Total}	$rp-1$		

the equations indicated in Table 4.12 for $\sigma^2_{Patient}$, $\sigma^2_{Repeats}$ and σ^2_{Error} gives the more general form of the ICC for p patients and r repeated assessments:

$$ICC = \frac{p\left(V_{Patient} - V_{Error}\right)}{pV_{patient} + rV_{Repeats} + (p-r)V_{Error}}. \tag{4.9}$$

ICC is a form of correlation, and in Section 5.3 we describe how confidence limits may be calculated. It is the most commonly used method for assessing reliability with continuous data, and is also sometimes used for ordered categorical data. A reliability coefficient of at least 0.90 is often recommended if measurements are to be used for evaluating individual patients (e.g. Nunnally and Bernstein, 1994; Kottner *et al.*, 2011), although most QoL instruments fail to attain such a demanding level. For discriminating between groups of patients, as in a clinical trial, it is usually recommended that the reliability should exceed 0.70. Thus Hahn *et al.* (2007) suggest that values from 0.70 to 0.90 represent 'moderate or good reliability (acceptable error)' and above 0.90 are 'high or excellent (minimal or no error)'. The principal effect of using measurements with a low reliability in a clinical trial is that there will be a dilution of the between-treatments effect, and so the sample size will have to be increased accordingly to compensate.

Example from the literature

Table 4.11 shows both the ICC values and κ_{Weight} coefficients that Lemmens *et al.* (2013) reported. The ICC values are, as is to be expected, very similar to those of κ_{Weight} (Fleiss and Cohen, 1973). Although presented by Lemmens *et al.* purely for comparison with other studies, it should be noted that Spearman's correlation coefficient, like Pearson's, is less appropriate than ICC for measuring agreement.

Study size for reliability studies depends upon both the minimum acceptable reliability and the true reliability. For example, if it is desired to show that the reliability is above 0.70 when the anticipated (true) reliability is 0.90, two measurements on 18 patients could suffice; but 118 patients are needed if the anticipated reliability is only 0.80 (Walter *et al.*, 1998). Zou (2012) reviews the approaches to sample size estimation, and presents equations for estimating the required sample size such that the CI is likely to be within a specified width. We illustrate the results for an ICC based on two assessments per patients, with a 95% CI, in Figure 4.1. From this figure, if the estimated ICC is 0.8, then the anticipated width of the CI would be about $2 \times 0.15 = 0.30$ if $N = 40$ and this width would reduce to about 0.16 if $N = 120$. Unless you are certain that the ICC is high or excellent (> 0.9), we suggest a sample size of *at least* 80 patients is usually desirable.

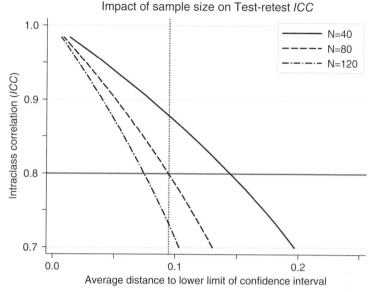

Figure 4.1   Sample size for two-observation *ICC*s, such as test-retest studies. The plot shows the effect of sample size on the average distance to the lower limit of an (asymmetric) two-sided 95% confidence interval. For example, with 80 patients on average the 95% *CI* for an *ICC* of 0.8 will have a lower limit of slightly above 0.7 (distance slightly less than 0.1).

Test–retest reliability

If a patient is in a stable condition, an instrument should yield repeatable and repro-ducible results if it is used repeatedly on that patient. This is usually assessed using a test–retest study, with patients who are thought to have stable disease and who are not expected to experience changes due to treatment effects or toxicity. The patients are asked to complete the same QoL questionnaire on several occasions. The level of agreement between the occasions can be measured by the *ICC*, providing a measure of the reliability of the instrument. It is important to select patients whose condition is stable, and to choose carefully a between-assessment time gap that is neither too short nor too long. Too short a period might allow subjects to recall their earlier responses, and too long a period might allow a true change in the status of the subject. In diseases such as cancer, where one might anticipate that most treatments would cause QoL to vary over time in various ways, the requirement of stability often leads to patients being studied either pre- or post-treatment.

Test–retest reliability is a critical aspect of measurement theory. Examples from biology highlight the issues. Blood pressure has inherently poor test–retest reliabil-ity and as a consequence multiple measurements are required, taken over a period of time. Patients' height has potentially good reliability provided staff are trained to fol-low precise procedures to make the patients stand stretched and fully erect. Patients' weight has, for most applications, adequate reliability provided suitably sensitive, calibrated weighing scales are used so as to avoid measurement error.

Relative comparisons are straightforward. If two instruments address the same construct then, provided all else is equal, the one exhibiting the better test–retest reliability is the one to be preferred. More difficult is the interpretation of absolute values. The range of acceptable values for test–retest reliability will depend upon the use to which the QoL instrument will be put.

Although test–retest reliability is arguably the most important form of reliability for QoL instruments, usually the *ICC* values will follow obvious patterns. Symptoms and physical outcomes are likely to be highly consistent, and it is usually predictable that reliability will be found to be highly satisfactory; rarely do developers of instruments report surprising results. The more subjective items will generally show lower reliability. Another factor is the target population. Instruments being developed for assessing the very young or the very elderly may present particular problems in attaining adequate reliability. The evaluation of patients with cognitive limitations, such as Alzheimer's disease, is especially challenging. Lack of test–retest reliability can be a simple indication of measurement difficulties arising either from the items or scales under investigation, or from the nature of the target population.

In particular situations, poor test–retest reliability may indicate a problem with the construct definition. For example, consider the assessment of *current pain*. If the pain scores exhibit poor reliability it could be indicative of intermittent pain, in which case more appropriate alternatives are 'pain on average', or 'worst pain over a period of time'.

Inter-rater reliability

Inter-rater reliability concerns the agreement between two raters. However, for QoL purposes we are principally interested in the patient's self-assessment. Many studies have shown that observers such as healthcare staff and patients' relatives make very different assessments from the patients themselves. Therefore, for validation of a self-administered QoL instrument, inter-rater reliability is usually of lesser concern than test–retest reliability.

When instruments are to be interviewer-administered, inter-rater reliability becomes critical. Although studies can assess inter-rater reliability using *ICC*s, frequently analysis of variance is used to explore the components of rater-to-rater variability and, for example, the impact of the rater's training and experience.

Since the patients are usually regarded as the best assessor of themselves, there may be interest in determining whether observers are able to predict the patients' scores. This is particularly important when deciding whether to use proxies to assess QoL in patients who are unwilling, too ill, too young or unable to complete questionnaires. In this situation, absolute agreement between patient and proxy is not the issue of interest. Instead, one is usually more interested in prediction or estimation, using techniques such as regression analysis and regarding the patient's self-assessment as the criterion (Section 4.3 discusses other aspects of criterion validity). For these studies it may be necessary to restrict recruitment to patients who have good cognitive functioning, and the implication is that it is hoped that the results so obtained are equally applicable to lower-functioning subjects. If the proxy is a spouse or partner, there is by definition only a single possible assessor. However, when there are multiple potential observers (such as clinical staff), inter-rater reliability is again crucial.

More complex designs are possible. For example, a study of the inter-rater reliability of proxies for patients with Alzheimer's disease might enrol one or more experts to provide a criterion rating, and use analysis of variance to compare the expert ratings against the scores from inexperienced nursing staff.

Example from the literature

Huntington's disease (HD) is a fatal, neurodegenerative disease for which there is no known cure. Proxy evaluation is sometimes necessary as HD can limit the ability of persons to report their HRQoL. Hocaoglu *et al.* (2012) explored patient–proxy ratings of persons at various stages of HD, and examined factors that may affect proxy ratings. A total of 105 patient–proxy pairs completed the Huntington's disease health-related quality of life questionnaire (HDQoL). Table 4.13 shows the patient-proxy *ICC* values and 95% *CI*s for the total sample and divided by HD severity grades.

The authors specified the type of *ICC* that they used: "Intraclass correlation coefficients with a one-way random effects model and their respective confidence intervals were calculated to quantify correlation between self and proxy scores".

Table 4.13 Agreement between proxy assessment and patient self-rating using the HDQoL disease-specific Huntington's disease health-related quality of life questionnaire on 105 patients

HDQoL	Whole sample (N = 105)		Early HD (N = 36)		Moderate HD (N = 18)		Advanced HD (N = 50)	
	ICC	*(95% CI)*	*ICC*	*(95% CI)*	*ICC*	*(95% CI)*	*ICC*	*(95% CI)*
Specific scales								
Cognitive	0.79	(0.71–0.85)	0.78	(0.61–0.88)	−0.03	(−0.47–0.42)	0.61	(0.40–0.76)
Hopes and worries	0.74	(0.63–0.81)	0.83	(0.69–0.91)	0.49	(0.05–0.77)	0.77	(0.63–0.86)
Services	0.71	(0.60–0.79)	0.76	(0.58–0.87)	0.48	(0.04–0.76)	0.74	(0.59–0.85)
Physical and functional	0.88	(0.84–0.92)	0.87	(0.77–0.93)	0.24	(−0.23–0.63)	0.81	(0.69–0.89)
Mood state	0.73	(0.63–0.81)	0.56	(0.29–0.75)	0.46	(0.02–0.76)	0.76	(0.61–0.85)
Self and vitality	0.75	(0.65–0.82)	0.63	(0.39–0.79)	0.65	(−0.28–0.85)	0.59	(0.37–0.74)
Summary scale	0.85	(0.79–0.90)	0.81	(0.65–0.90)	0.37	(−0.09–0.70)	0.81	(0.69–0.89)

HD, Huntington's disease; *ICC*, intraclass correlation coefficient; *CI*, confidence interval; HDQoL, Huntington's disease health-related quality of life questionnaire.
Source: Hocaoglu *et al.*, 2012, Table 3. CC BY 4.0 (http://creativecommons.org/licenses/by/4.0/).

It can be seen in Table 4.13 that for the whole sample the 95% *CI* is reasonably narrow, especially when the *ICC* is high – for example, when *ICC* = 0.88 the *CI* is (0.84–0.92), a width of 0.08; the *CI* is much wider when the *ICC* is 0.71. However, there are only 18 patients classified as having moderate levels of HD, and the *CIs* are then so wide that the results are uninterpretable.

Hocaoglu *et al.* noted that in both the early and advanced groups the objective, observable scale Physical and Functional produced the highest *ICC* values, as previously observed by other investigators. Even the more subjective scales such as Hopes and Worries or Mood State yielded 'substantial' *ICCs*. It was suggested that this may reflect the fact that proxies were long-term companions or close family members who typically show better agreement than unrelated healthcare providers. It was concluded that the HDQoL showed good patient–proxy agreement, not only with early HD patients who could validly assess their own HRQoL, but also with Advanced HD patients who usually have physical or cognitive barriers to self-reporting.

Equivalent-forms reliability

Equivalent-forms reliability concerns the agreement between scores when using two or more instruments that are designed to measure the same attribute. For example, in principle a new QoL instrument could be compared against a well-established one or against a lengthier one. However, as with inter-rater reliability, agreement is often of lesser concern than is prediction; one of the instruments is usually regarded as the standard against which the other is being assessed, and linear regression analysis is more informative than a simple measure of agreement. It is less common to have two

Example from the literature
Gorecki *et al.* (2013) developed the PU-QOL instrument for assessing PROs for patients with pressure ulcers, and as part of the validation carried out an international field test on 229 patients with pressure ulcers. The sample size calculations were based on having sufficient participants to estimate test-retest reliability correlations at levels expected in test-retest situations (e.g. $r \geq 0.80$) with reasonable precision (95% *CI* width of 0.2). Table 4.14 shows the test-retest *ICCs* and the internal consistency.

The authors followed current practice (Kottner *et al.*, 2011) in specifying the types of *ICC* used – both $ICC_{Agreement}$ and $ICC_{Consistency}$. They also provided Pearson's correlations. As is frequently the case, these three measures were closely similar to each other.

Table 4.14 Test–retest intraclass correlations and internal consistency of the PU-QOL instrument for patients with pressure ulcers, tested on 229 patients

Scale (no. of items)	Internal consistency	Test–retest reproducibility		
	Cronbach's alpha	*ICC* consistency	*ICC* absolute	Correlation[a]
Pain (8)	0.89	0.80	0.81	0.80
Exudate (8)	0.91	0.62	0.63	0.62
Odour (6)	0.97	0.68	0.68	0.70
Sleep (6)	0.92	0.82	0.82	0.82
Vitality (6)	0.90	0.74	0.74	0.74
Movement/Mobility (9)	0.93	0.87	0.86	0.88
ADL (8)	0.95	0.87	0.87	0.87
Emotional well-being (15)	0.94	0.83	0.82	0.83
Appearance & self-consciousness (7)	0.89	0.81	0.81	0.81
Participation (9)	0.93	0.63	0.64	0.63

[a]Pearson correlation.
Source: Gorecki *et al.,* 2013, Table 5. CC BY 2.0 (http://creativecommons.org/licenses/by/2.0).

instruments that are believed to be equivalent to each other in QoL research than in areas such as education, where examination questionnaires often aim to use different, but equivalent, test items. When appropriate, the same methods as for test–retest reliability may be used. Ways of analysing method comparison studies are discussed by Bland and Altman (1986).

4.7 Sensitivity and responsiveness

Two closely related properties to repeatability are sensitivity and responsiveness. *Sensitivity* is the ability to detect differences between groups, for example between two treatment groups in a randomised clinical trial or between groups of patients with mild disease and those with more severe disease. *Responsiveness* is the ability of a scale to detect changes. An instrument should not only be reliable, yielding reproducible results when a patient's condition is stable and unchanged, but in addition it should respond to relevant changes in a patient's condition. If disease progression causes deterioration in a patient's overall QoL, we would expect the measurements from a QoL instrument to respond accordingly. In addition, the measurement instrument should be sufficiently responsive to detect relevant changes when the condition of the patient is known to have altered. Similarly, if two groups of patients differ in their QoL, an instrument should be sufficiently sensitive to detect that change.

Both sensitivity and responsiveness are crucially important for any measurement, and a QoL instrument that lacks these properties will be less able to detect important changes in patients. Depending upon the intended application, sometimes one property is more important than the other. An *evaluative* QoL instrument intended for monitoring patients should be responsive to changes. A *discriminative* instrument aimed at diagnosing individual patients will have to be more sensitive than one that is intended for detecting differences between groups of patients in clinical trials. However, if a QoL measurement can be shown to be sensitive to specific changes, it is presumably also responsive to the condition causing those changes.

Sensitivity can be assessed by cross-sectional studies, but responsiveness is evaluated by longitudinal assessment of patients in whom a change is expected to occur. Disease-specific scales, being more focused and tailored towards problems of particular importance to the target group of patients, are generally more responsive than generic health status measures.

The most widely used measures of sensitivity and responsiveness are the standardised response mean (*SRM*) and the effect size (*ES*), which are also used for indicating clinical significance. Briefly, the *SRM* is the ratio of the mean change to the *SD* of that change, and the *ES* is the ratio of the mean change to the *SD* of the initial measurement (Table 4.15). Thus *ES* ignores the variation in the change, while *SRM* is more similar to the paired *t*-test (except that the *t*-test uses the standard error, *SE*, rather than the *SD*). The *SRM* is more frequently used than *ES*.

Table 4.15 Summary of measures of sensitivity and responsiveness, for two measurements x_1 and x_2 with corresponding means $\bar{x}_1, \bar{x}_2$

Measure	Equation	Denominator
Effect size (*ES*)	$\left(\bar{x}_2 - \bar{x}_1\right)/SD(x_1)$	SD of baseline (x_1)
Standardised response mean (*SRM*)	$\left(\bar{x}_2 - \bar{x}_1\right)/SD(x_2 - x_1)$	SD of change
Paired *t*-statistic (t_{Paired})	$\left(\bar{x}_2 - \bar{x}_1\right)/SE(x_2 - x_1)$	SE of change
Responsiveness statistic	$\left(\bar{x}_2 - \bar{x}_1\right)_{Changed}/SD(x_2 - x_1)_{Stable}$	SD of change, in stable patients
Relative change	$\left(\bar{x}_2 - \bar{x}_1\right)/\bar{x}_1$	Mean at baseline
Relative efficiency, *RE* of two scales (Relative validity, *RV*)	Ratio of the squares of the t_{Paired} statistics for the two scales = ratio of the two *SRM* statistics	

Another approach is to argue that the most sensitive scale is the one most likely to result in statistically significant differences between groups of patients, and thus the scale with the largest *t*-statistic is the most sensitive. Therefore, when comparing two scales or items, the ratio of the two *t*-statistics could be a suitable measure. However, in practice, squared *t*-statistics are more often used when calculating the ratios, giving the widely used measure that is called *relative efficiency* (*RE*) or *relative validity* (*RV*). When comparing more than two scales, it is recommended to use the largest of the squared *t*-statistics as the denominator when calculating the ratios, resulting in all coefficients being between 0 (weakest) and 1 (strongest), as illustrated in Table 4.16 (where *RE* is based on the ratio of two *F*-statistics, as described below). This amounts to defining the most sensitive scale as the baseline. Some papers use the smallest value for the denominator, but it should be noted that this value will be unstable if it is small (or if the *t*-statistic used in the denominator is not significant); this uncertainty is readily shown by wide confidence intervals, which will be asymmetric and are most easily calculated using the 'bootstrap' methods that are available in many statistical packages (Deng *et al.*, 2013).

All of the above methods are based upon means and *SD*s, with an implicit assumption that the data follow a Normal distribution. Many QoL scales have a non-Normal distribution, in which case medians and interquartile ranges may replace means and *SD*s. Unfortunately, little work has been carried out into this subject. It should also be noted that some scales are not only non-Normal but may also suffer from *ceiling effects*, in which a large number of patients place responses in the maximum category. This can compromise sensitivity and responsiveness.

Although Table 4.15 summarises the principal measures that may be encountered in the literature, there is controversy as to which is the best measure to use and a number of other alternatives have been proposed. As Wright and Young (1997) conclude when comparing five indices for their ability to rank responsiveness of different instruments: 'Given that the indices provide different rank ordering, the preferred index is unclear.'

When there are more than two groups or more than two measurements only the *RE* can be readily generalised. Just as the *t*-test is replaced by an *F*-test in ANOVA when comparing more than two means, so we can base the *RE* upon the ratio of two *F*-statistics when there are more than two groups. In the case of two groups, the *F*-statistic is identical to the squared *t*-statistic, and so these approaches are consistent with one another.

Sensitivity

Sensitivity is one of the most important attributes of an instrument. The usefulness of a measure is dependent upon its ability to detect clinically relevant differences. In clinical trials, therefore, sensitivity should be sufficient to detect differences of the order of magnitude that might occur between the treatment groups. The level of sensitivity that is adequate depends upon the intended application of the instrument. An instrument should be capable of distinguishing the differences of interest, using real-istically sized study groups. The more sensitive an instrument, the smaller the sample size that is necessary to detect relevant differences.

Usually, but by no means always, sensitive measurements will be reliable. This follows because reliability is usually a prerequisite for sensitivity. An unreliable meas-urement is one that has large background noise, and this will obscure the detection of any group differences that may be present. The converse need not apply: reliable measurements may lack sensitivity. For example, responses to the four-point single item 'Do you have pain? (None, a little, quite a bit, very much)' may be highly reliable in the sense that repeated responses by stable patients are very consistent. However, such a question may be unable to detect small yet clinically important differences in pain levels unless there are large numbers of patients in each treatment group. To take an extreme situation, all patients in both groups could respond 'quite a bit', with 100% reliability, and yet the patients in one group might have more pain than the other group. The pain scale would have zero sensitivity but perfect reliability. This example also serves to illustrate that *floor* and *ceiling* effects may be crucial. If most patients have very poor QoL and respond with the maximum, or 'ceiling' value, or with the minimum, or 'floor' value, the scale will not be sensitive and will not be capable of discriminating between different treatment groups.

Sensitivity is usually assessed by cross-sectional comparison of groups of patients in which there are expected to be QoL differences. Thus it is in practice closely related to *known-groups validity*. The main distinction is that with known-groups validity we are concerned with confirming that anticipated differences are present between groups of patients. Sensitivity analyses, on the other hand, aim to show that a reasonable-sized sample will suffice for the detection of differences of the magnitude that may exist between treatments (or other subdivisions of interest), and which are clinically relevant.

If the anticipated effects can be detected by a statistical significance test on the resulting data, this is often taken to be an indication of adequate sensitivity. However, it should be noted that statistical significance of group differences is also influenced by the selection of the patient sample. For example, a validation study might select a group of very ill patients to compare against patients who are disease-free. Then we know that there are undoubtedly group differences in QoL, and a significance test is of little practical interest. If the differences are large enough, a p-value of less than 0.0001 merely indicates that the sample size is also large enough to reject the possibility that the difference is zero. A sensitive instrument should be able to detect *small* differences, in *modest-sized* studies.

On the one hand, we want to be confident that the groups in the sensitivity study really do differ but, on the other hand, we do not want to select groups that are known to have unusually large differences. For this reason, sensitivity studies that evaluate a new instrument should report a variety of comparisons, covering a range of situations that are typical of the areas of intended future application of the instrument.

It is perhaps easier to interpret the measures of sensitivity (and responsiveness) in terms of relative rather than absolute values. Different scales or instruments can

Example from the literature

Deng *et al.* (2013) compare the SF-12, a generic instrument, against two disease-specific instruments for chronic kidney disease (CKD), the QDIS-CKD quality-of-life disease impact scale for chronic kidney disease and the KDQOL kidney disease quality-of-life questionnaire. Table 4.16 shows the mean scores for 453 patients with chronic kidney disease, divided according to dialysis, pre-dialysis stage 3–5 and transplant. ANOVA was used, obtaining the *F*-ratios and *RE* values that are shown. The QDIS-CKD CAT-5 scale is chosen as the reference measure because it has the largest *F*-statistic, and the *RE* values are calculated using this as the denominator. As might be anticipated, PROs from the disease-specific instruments had the highest *RE* values.

Table 4.16 Sensitivity of PRO measures from two disease-specific instruments and the SF-12, for 453 patients with chronic kidney disease (CKD): mean scores, ANOVA *F*-statistics and *RE*

PRO measure	Dialysis (N=206)	Pre-dialysis, stage 3–5 (N=113)	Transplant (N=134)	F-statistic	RE	95% CI[a]
CKD-specific						
QDIS-CKD						
CAT-5 (Reference group)	39.83	16.19	19.25	57.43**	1	—
Static-6	39.18	16.86	19.60	50.15**	0.87	(0.72–1.03)
Static-34	35.93	14.90	18.71	48.01**	0.84	(0.71–0.97)
KDQOL						
Burden	48.83	76.62	68.21	44.46**	0.77	(0.53–1.09)
Symptoms	71.95	80.58	80.03	15.11**	0.26	(0.13–0.44)
Effects	63.41	84.38	77.86	43.95**	0.77	(0.52–1.10)
Generic						
SF-12						
PF	37.06	45.38	44.88	31.12**	0.54	(0.32–0.85)
RP	38.00	45.12	45.83	34.12**	0.59	(0.38–0.89)
BP	43.19	46.71	47.10	5.84**	0.10	(0.02–0.22)
GH	39.08	41.99	43.71	7.79**	0.14	(0.04–0.28)
VT	45.72	46.40	48.35	3.04*	0.05	(0.00–0.15)
SF	42.75	47.81	47.83	11.02**	0.19	(0.07–0.34)
RE	44.59	48.39	48.39	7.01**	0.12	(0.03–0.25)
PCS	36.60	43.49	44.08	26.61**	0.46	(0.27–0.74)
MCS[b]	49.74	50.42	50.55	0.32	—	—
MH[b]	49.85	50.71	50.31	0.26	—	—

*Significant at the 0.05 level; **Significant at the 0.01 level.

ANOVA, analysis of variance; *RE*, relative efficiency; CKD, chronic kidney disease; QDIS-CKD, quality-of-life disease impact scale for chronic kidney disease; KDQOL, kidney disease quality-of-life; SF-12, Short Form 12; PF, physical functioning; RP, role physical; BP, bodily pain; GH, general health; VT, vitality; SF, social functioning; RE, role emotional; PCS, physical component summary; MCS, mental component summary; MH, mental health.

[a]The 95% confidence interval of the *RE* was derived from the original data using the bootstrap BCa method.

[b]The *F*-statistics for SF-12 MCS and MH are small and non-significant (*p*-values of 0.73 and 0.77 separately), therefore their *RE*s were not computed and are excluded from significance test.

Source: Deng et al., 2013, Table 1. CC BY 2.0 (http://creativecommons.org/licenses/by/2.0).

The authors describe the calculation of confidence intervals from computer-intensive 'bootstrap' simulations, and comment that they "suspect that most studies, without constructing a confidence interval for the *RE* estimate, over-interpreted the observed differences in the *RE*s with small-denominator *F*-statistics".

then be compared to determine which is the most sensitive. The *RE* provides a suitable comparative measure. Another advantage of the comparative approach is that it largely overcomes the criticism that measures of sensitivity are affected by the choice of patient sample and the actual group differences that are present. Thus the magnitude of the specific difference no longer matters; the most sensitive of the concurrently applied instruments is the one with the largest *RE*.

Thus we can compare the different instruments or scales, and identify the ones with the highest sensitivity. The most sensitive ones will usually be the preferred scales for detecting differences between treatments, *provided* they are also thought to be clinically sensible and providing comprehensive coverage.

Responsiveness

Responsiveness is another important feature that is a requirement for any useful scale. It is closely related to sensitivity, but relates to changes *within* patients. In particular, if a patient's health status changes over time can the instrument detect the changes? An instrument may be of limited applicability if it is not responsive to individual-patient changes over time. Responsiveness can also be regarded as providing additional evidence of validity of an instrument, since it confirms that the anticipated responses occur when the patient's status changes. A highly sensitive scale will usually also be highly responsive. An unreliable measurement (low test–retest *ICC*) will not be very responsive.

If the repeated measurements are highly correlated, as is frequently the case when assessing responsiveness, *ES* will be smaller than *SRM*. The *SRM*, on the other hand, is efficient for detecting change, which is why it is more closely related to the *t*-statistic and ANOVA. In line with most authors, we recommend using *SRM* in preference to *ES* when assessing responsiveness.

Sample size will in part depend on the degree of change that occurs. If a patient goes from a very severe state of poor health and high symptomatology to a complete cure, a small sample will suffice to detect this; if the changes are more subtle, a larger sample will be necessary. Many PRO instruments are developed for application in clinical trials, and it is common for responsiveness studies to evaluate change scores comparing on-treatment to off-treatment assessments. Stable estimates of responsiveness over two time points requires a sample size of at least 50 (King and Dobson, 2000).

Example from the literature

Homma *et al.* (2011) compared the responsiveness of the Overactive Bladder Symptom Score (OABSS) and a bladder diary when assessing symptoms of overactive bladder (OAB) in 79 Japanese patients. Patients were assessed before treatment (baseline) and at 12 weeks, after treatment with an antimuscarinic agent (Table 4.17). All changes from baseline were statistically significant with *p*-values uniformly < 0.001, and so the *p*-values do not aid identification of the most responsive items. Instead, the authors appropriately provide the *ES* and *SRM* values, and the most responsive OABSS items are 'urgency' and 'total score'. All of the ESs for the OABSS, except daytime frequency, were larger than those of the corresponding diary variables. Daytime frequency had almost the same values between the assessment tools (0.64 for the bladder diary and 0.60 for the OABSS). The authors' concluded that "OABSS can be an alternative to a bladder diary for symptom and efficacy assessment in daily clinical practice".

Table 4.17 Responsiveness of the Overactive Bladder Symptom Score (OABSS) instrument and a bladder diary, in 79 patients with overactive bladders

Assessment Item	Baseline	12 Weeks	Change	*p*-value	*ES*	*SRM*
OABSS (score)						
Daytime frequency	1.0 (0.5)	0.7 (0.5)	0.3 (0.6)	<0.001	0.60	0.50
Night-time frequency	2.2 (0.8)	1.8 (0.9)	0.4 (0.7)	<0.001	0.50	0.57
Urgency	3.4 (1.0)	1.4 (1.3)	2.0 (1.3)	<0.001	2.00	1.54
Urgency incontinence	1.9 (1.6)	0.6 (1.0)	1.3 (1.4)	<0.001	0.81	0.92
Total score	8.5 (2.6)	4.5 (2.6)	4.0 (2.6)	<0.001	1.54	1.57
Bladder diary (episode per day)						
Daytime frequency	9.0 (2.8)	7.2 (1.9)	1.8 (2.3)	<0.001	0.64	0.78
Night-time frequency	2.2 (1.4)	1.7 (1.1)	0.5 (1.0)	<0.001	0.36	0.50
Urgency	2.7 (2.4)	0.6 (0.9)	2.2 (2.2)	<0.001	0.92	1.00
Urgency incontinence	1.1 (1.8)	0.2 (0.7)	0.9 (1.6)	<0.001	0.50	0.56
Mean voided volume (mL)	155.1 (62.8)	184.4 (84.9)	29.1 (52.0)	<0.001	0.46	0.56

Values are mean (standard deviation). *p*-values were derived by Wilcoxon's signed-rank sum test.
Source: Homma *et al.*, 2011. Reproduced with permission of Elsevier.

4.8   Conclusions

This chapter has shown a variety of methods for examining the validity of measurement scores, to confirm that the scores appear to be consistent with their intended purpose. We also examined the assessment of the repeatability reliability, to ensure that the measurements appear to give consistent and repeatable results when applied to patients who are believed to be in a stable state. Finally, we showed ways of establishing that the scores are sufficiently sensitive or responsive to be able to detect differences between treatments or patients.

Sensitivity and responsiveness are amongst the most important attributes of a scale, because a non-sensitive scale is of little use for most practical applications. Furthermore, if a scale possesses face validity and is sensitive to the anticipated changes, it is likely to be measuring either the intended construct or something closely similar. However, a counter argument is that since many aspects of QoL are inter-correlated, sensitivity alone is not sufficient as confirmation of construct validity. If one dimension of QoL shows high sensitivity, it is likely that other scales correlated with this dimension will also show at least some degree of apparent sensitivity. Therefore, it is also important to consider other aspects of construct validity.

4.9   Further reading

There are many variations of the *ICC*, often – but not always – resulting in broadly similar values for the estimated coefficients. A distinction can be made between *ICC* for agreement or for consistency. It can also be shown that there are links between *ICC* and standard error of measurement, both being derived from analysis of variance. A taxonomy of six variants is provided by Shrout and Fleiss (1979), extended to 10 by McGraw and Wong (1996), and further reviewed by Weir (2005). Kottner *et al.* (2011) offer guidelines for reporting of ICC, reliability and agreement. Similarly, many interpretations of responsiveness (and sensitivity) exist, as described by Terwee *et al.* (2003) and Husted *et al.* (2000).

Kraemer *et al.* (2002) provide a useful review of the use and abuse of κ-coefficients, and discuss applications of the various versions.

5

Multi-item scales

Summary

In this chapter, we consider methods that are specific to multi-item scales. We examine ways of exploring relationships amongst the constituent items of a multi-item scale, and between the individual items and the scale to which they are hypothesised as belonging to. Most of these methods rely upon the examination of correlations. Do the items in a multi-item scale correlate strongly with each other? Do they correlate weakly with items from other scales? Do items correlate with the score of their own scale? Cronbach's α, multitrait-scaling analysis and factor analysis are three of the most frequently used methods for exploring these correlations.

5.1   Introduction

Many instruments contain one or more multi-item scales. For example, the HADS was designed with the intention that there would be anxiety and depression scales. Summary scores can be calculated for both scales. One of the reasons for using multiple items in a scale is that the reliability of the scale score should be higher than for a single item. For example, each of the seven items for anxiety in the HADS is assumed to reflect the same overall 'true' anxiety score. Thus although individual measurements are imprecise and subject to random fluctuations, an average of several measurements should provide a more reliable estimate with smaller random variability. Therefore, each item in a multi-item scale should contribute to an increase in reliability – but does it? We describe methods of assessing *internal consistency*, or *reliability for multi-item scales*. There is also the related assumption that the items in a scale reflect a single latent variable. We discuss how this *unidimensionality* can be examined.

Other aspects of *validation* can be explored when there are several multi-item scales in an instrument. The investigator should have a hypothetical model in mind when developing such instruments, and should be aware of the plausible relationships between the constructs and the items comprising them. Usually, items within any one scale should be highly correlated with each other (*convergent validity*), but only weakly correlated

Quality of Life: The Assessment, Analysis and Reporting of Patient-Reported Outcomes, Third Edition.
Peter M. Fayers and David Machin.
© 2016 John Wiley & Sons, Ltd. Published 2016 by John Wiley & Sons, Ltd.

with items from other scales (*discriminant validity*). These principles, which are part of *construct validity* as discussed in Section 4.4, apply also to items within a scale.

One important reason for constructing multi-item scales, as opposed to single-item measurements, is that the nature of the multiple items permits us to validate the consistency of the scales. For example, if all the items that belong to one multi-item scale are expected to be correlated and behave in a similar manner to each other, rogue items that do not reflect the investigator's intended construct can be detected. With single items, validation possibilities are far more restricted.

The methods of this chapter rely heavily upon the analysis of item-to-item correlations, and thus apply to Likert and other scales for which the theory of parallel tests applies. *Clinimetric* and *formative* scales containing *causal variables* follow different rules. These scales are discussed at the end of this chapter.

5.2   Significance tests

In statistical analyses we are frequently *estimating* values such as the mean value for a group of patients, the mean difference between two groups, or the degree of correlation (association) between two measurements. These estimates are invariably based upon patients in a study – that is, patients in a *sample* – and so the measurements observed and the estimated values calculated from them will vary from study to study. We might, for example, have carried out a randomised clinical trial (RCT) to compare two treatments, and wish to determine whether the observed difference in response rates is large enough for us to conclude that there is definitely a treatment effect. The problem is, of course, that if another investigator replicates the study they are bound to obtain somewhat different values for the treatment response rates since they will be dealing with a different sample of patients. Consequently, they may well obtain a very different value for the mean difference. Thus, if we have observed a fairly small difference in our study, there would not be very strong weight of evidence for claiming that we have definitely demonstrated that the treatments differ; it is quite possible that future trials could show that our findings were due to chance and not a treatment effect at all. The role of a statistical significance test is to quantify the weight of evidence, and we do so by calculating the probability that we could have observed at least as large a difference as that in our study purely by chance.

One problem is that even if the two treatments have identical clinical effect, we may well observe an apparent difference in our particular sample of patients. Furthermore, it is impossible to prove statistically that two treatments do have an identical effect; there is always a possibility that if measurements are taken more precisely, or if a larger number of patients are recruited, a difference (possibly very small) will eventually be detected. Hence it is convenient to start by assuming a *null hypothesis* of 'no difference' between the treatments, and we assess the observed data to decide whether there is sufficient evidence to *reject the null hypothesis*. If there is not, we continue to *accept the null hypothesis* as still remaining plausible. This procedure is in fact very similar to international law: we assume innocence (null hypothesis) unless there is sufficient weight of evidence to ascribe guilt (rejection of the null hypothesis).

The formal method that we use to weigh the evidence is a *statistical significance test*. This calculates the *probability*, or *p-value*, that we could have observed such extreme results even if the null hypothesis were true. If the *p*-value is very small, we conclude that there is very little chance of having obtained such extreme results simply because of patient-to-patient variability, and thus we would reject the null hypothesis as being fairly implausible. In practice, most investigators take a *p*-value of 0.05 or less (that is, a chance of 5 in 100, or 5%) as implying that the results are unlikely to be due to chance, and therefore reject the null hypothesis. A *p*-value less than 0.01 (that is, 1 in 100 or 1%) indicates far more convincing evidence, and many would regard $p < 0.001$ as fairly conclusive evidence. However, it is important to recognise that out of all the many studies published each year where investigators claim 'significant difference, $p < 0.05$', about 5% of publications will have reached this conclusion despite there being no treatment effect. This is because a *p*-value < 0.05 simply means that roughly 5% of studies might have observed such extreme data purely by chance.

Standard statistical books such as Campbell *et al.* (2007) or Altman (1991) provide extensive details of significance testing, and show how to calculate *p*-values for a variety of situations. Briefly, many tests take the form of

$$z = \frac{\text{Estimate}}{SE(\text{Estimate})}, \tag{5.1}$$

where 'Estimate' is, for example, the mean difference between treatments. *SE* is the standard error, or variability of the 'Estimate', that arises from the patient-to-patient variations. For many situations the calculated statistic, z, can be shown to be of one of the forms tabulated in the Appendix Tables T1 to T5. The most common of these is the Normal distribution (Tables T1 and T2), and from Table T1 we see that a value of 1.96 corresponds to $p = 0.05$. Thus, if the value of z is greater than 1.96, we could 'reject the null hypothesis with $p < 0.05$'.

5.3 Correlations

The methods described in this chapter make extensive use of correlations, both item-to-item and item-to-scale. For more extensive details about the use and misuse of correlations, readers are referred to Campbell *et al.* (2007).

Correlation coefficients are a measure of the degree of association between two continuous variables. The most common form of correlation is called Pearson's r, or the product-moment correlation coefficient. If there are n observations with two variables x_i and y_i (where i ranges from 1 to n),

$$r = \frac{\sum (x_i - \bar{x})(y_i - \bar{y})}{\sqrt{\sum (x_i - \bar{x})^2 \sum (y_i - \bar{y})^2}}, \tag{5.2}$$

where $\bar{x}$ and $\bar{y}$ are the mean values of x and y. The equation is symmetric, and so it does not matter which variable is x and which y. Pearson's r measures the scatter of the observations around a straight line representing trend; the greater the scatter, the lower the correlation.

The values of r lie between -1 and $+1$. For uncorrelated points $r = 0$, indicating no association between x and y. A value of $r = +1$ indicates perfect correlation with all points lying on a straight line from bottom left to top right, that is, positive slope. Similarly, $r = -1$ for points on a straight line with negative slope.

Range of variables

Many validation studies aim to include a heterogeneous group of patients with a variety of disease states and stages. However, correlations are greatly affected by the range of the variables. A homogeneous group of patients will have similar symptomatology to each other, and the ranges of their scores for PRO items and scales may be less than those from a more heterogeneous group. Consequently, item correlations for a homogeneous group of patients will usually be much less than for a more heterogeneous group. Thus increasing sample heterogeneity is an easy way to 'buy' higher correlations, but does not imply that the questions on the instrument are in any way more highly valid. Because of this, claims of high validity based upon correlations can be misleading, and may reflect merely sample heterogeneity; it is difficult to know what interpretation to place on the magnitude of the correlations. For instrument validation purposes, it is often easier to compare and contrast the *relative magnitude* of various correlations from within a single study than to interpret the absolute magnitude of correlations. Thus we emphasise such comparisons as whether an item correlates more highly with its own scale than with other scales. It remains appropriate to seek heterogeneous samples of patients for these comparisons.

Significance tests

The null hypothesis of no association between x and y implies that there is truly zero correlation ($r = 0$) between them. The significance test compares the quantity

$$z = \frac{r}{\sqrt{(1 - r^2)/(n - 2)}} \tag{5.3}$$

against a t-distribution with $n - 2$ degrees of freedom (df).

In many contexts we know, a priori, that two variables are correlated. In such a situation it is of little practical interest to test a null hypothesis of $r = 0$, since that hypothesis is already known to be implausible. If a significance test is carried out and the result obtained happens to be 'not significant', all we can say is that the sample size was too small. Conversely, if the sample size is adequate, the correlation coefficient will always differ significantly from zero. Thus a significance test for $r = 0$ should be carried out only when it is sensible to test whether r does indeed differ from zero.

Confidence intervals

Instead of significance tests, it is usually far more informative to estimate the confidence interval (*CI*). Although *r* itself does not have a Normal distribution, there is a simple transformation that can convert *r* to a variable *Z* that does. Writing $\log_e$ for the logarithmic function, this transformation is

$$Z = \frac{1}{2}\log_e\left(\frac{1+r}{1-r}\right). \tag{5.4}$$

Furthermore, it can be shown that, for a sample size of *n*, the standard error of *Z* is given by

$$SE(Z) = \frac{1}{\sqrt{n-3}}. \tag{5.5}$$

These equations assume that *n* is reasonably large – in practice, more than 50 observations.

Example

One correlation given by Silveira *et al.* (2010) and illustrated in Table 4.6 is $r = 0.63$ for the association between emotional functioning (QLQ-C30) and emotional well-being (FACT-G). Their sample size was $n = 102$ and so

$$Z = \frac{1}{2}\log_e\left(\frac{1+0.63}{1-0.63}\right) = 0.7414, \text{ and } SE(Z) = \frac{1}{\sqrt{102-3}} = 0.1005.$$

The *CI* for *Z* is

$$Z_{lower} = 0.7414 - (1.96 \times 0.1005) = 0.5444, \text{tc}$$

$$Z_{upper} = 0.7414 + (1.96 \times 0.1005) = 0.9384.$$

Therefore the 95% *CI* for *r* itself is

$$r_{lower} = (\exp(2 \times 0.5444) - 1) / (\exp(2 \times 0.5444) + 1) = 0.50, \text{ to}$$

$$r_{upper} = (\exp(2 \times 0.9384) - 1) / (\exp(2 \times 0.9384) + 1) = 0.73$$

Hence we would expect that the true value of *r* is likely to lie between 0.50 and 0.73.

A *CI* for Z can then be calculated as for any data that follow a Normal distribution. For example, a 95% *CI* is

$$Z_{lower} = Z - 1.96 \times \frac{1}{\sqrt{n-3}}, \text{ to } Z_{upper} = Z + 1.96 \times \frac{1}{\sqrt{n-3}} \tag{5.6}$$

Finally, Z_{lower} and Z_{upper} can be converted back to obtain the *CI* for r itself, using

$$r_{lower} = (\exp(2 \times Z_{lower}) - 1) / (\exp(2 \times Z_{lower}) + 1), \tag{5.7}$$

where exp is the exponential function, and with a similar expression for r_{upper}.

Significance test to compare two correlations

We can also use the Z-transformation and equations (5.4) and (5.5) for an approximate comparison of two correlation coefficients (r_1 and r_2) from two samples each of size n. The correlations r_1 and r_2 are converted to Z_1 and Z_2, and we calculate the difference of $Z_1 - Z_2$ (ignore the negative sign if $Z_2 > Z_1$). The standard error of this difference $Z_1 - Z_2$ is

$$SE(Z_1 - Z_2) = \sqrt{\frac{2}{n-3}}. \tag{5.8}$$

The difference $Z_1 - Z_2$ would be statistically significant ($p < 0.05$) if

$$z = \frac{Z_1 - Z_2}{SE(Z_1 - Z_2)} > 1.96. \tag{5.9}$$

Example

In the PROMIS CAT example of Table 4.7, the PROMIS pain behaviour correlates reasonably well with SF-36 bodily pain ($r = 0.66$), and slightly less well with FACIT fatigue ($r = 0.53$). With $n = 143$, the Z-scores are

$$Z_1 = \frac{1}{2}\log_e\left(\frac{1+0.66}{1-0.66}\right) = 0.7928, \quad Z_2 = \frac{1}{2}\log_e\left(\frac{1+0.53}{1-0.53}\right) = 0.5901,$$

Thus $Z_1 - Z_2 = 0.2027$, and $SE(Z_1 - Z_2) = 0.1195$.

Therefore $z = 0.2027 / 0.1195 = 1.70$.

This is less than 1.96, and so is not statistically significant at the 5% level. Therefore we conclude that the observed difference between the correlations (0.66 and 0.53) could be due to chance.

However, equation (5.9) assumes that r_1 and r_2 come from *independent* samples. This is clearly not true for the above example, where r_1 and r_2 are correlations between items measured on one sample of patients. This will also usually be the case in examples from multitrait-scaling analysis. In this situation, any test based on equation (5.9) only provides a very rough guide as to statistical significance. For multitrait-scaling analysis, precise comparisons are unimportant and this approach provides an adequate, simple approximation.

Intraclass correlation

Intraclass correlation was discussed in Chapter 4. When, instead of just one, there are k assessments for each of the n patients, Fisher (1925) showed that equations (5.4) and (5.5) can be extended to give

$$ Z = \frac{1}{2} \log_e \left(\frac{1 + (k-1)r}{1-r} \right), \tag{5.10} $$

with standard error

$$ SE(Z) = \sqrt{\frac{k}{2(k-1)(n-2)}}. \tag{5.11} $$

In the particular case of two observations ($k = 2$) per subject, as commonly collected in a test–retest study, Fisher recommended modifying the standard error:

$$ SE(Z) = \frac{1}{\sqrt{n-1.5}}. \tag{5.12} $$

The *CI*s can then be calculated using the methods of equations (5.6) and (5.7). Donner and Zou (2002) describe more powerful (and more complex) methods.

Rank correlation

The significance tests and *CI*s associated with Pearson's r require that at least one of the variables for the observations in the sample follow a Normal distribution. However, QoL and PRO items are frequently measured as categorical variables, often with a four- or five-point scale, and these will not have a Normal distribution form. Depending upon the nature of the sample, there may also be many individuals with extreme scores. For example, patients with advanced disease may have uniformly high symptomatology, implying asymmetrically distributed ordered categories. In these circumstances Spearman's rank correlation, $r_{Spearman}$, is preferable.

To calculate $r_{Spearman}$ the values of the two variables are each ranked in order, and then the calculation of equation (5.2) is performed using the values of the ranks in place of the original data. The distribution of $r_{Spearman}$ is similar to that of $r_{Pearson}$, and so the same methods can be utilised for confidence intervals and a test of whether two correlations differ significantly from one another. Svensson (2012) provides an example $r_{Spearman}$ and other ranking methods for exploring agreement and disagreement. For CIs and significance testing, Fieller et al. (1957) showed that Fisher's Z-transformation applies but with $SE(Z) = \sqrt{\frac{1.060}{(n-3)}}$ replacing equation (5.5).

Example from the literature

The validity and reliability of the Pediatric Cardiac Quality of Life Inventory (PCQLI) was evaluated in a multicentre study that recruited paediatric patients (8–18 years of age) with heart disease (HD) and their parents to complete the PCQLI and other PRO instruments (Marino et al., 2010). The PCQLI generates three scores: disease impact, psychosocial impact and total score. In total, the study enrolled 1605 patient-parent pairs, of which 803 of the patients were children (ages 8–12). Spearman correlations were reported for various comparisons. For example, child and parent-of-child PCQLI scores revealed moderate correlations for the three scales: disease impact, 0.55; psychosocial impact, 0.41; total scores, 0.50 ($p < 0.001$). In addition, test-retest correlations of these three scales were reported for 291 of the children: 0.82, 0.78 and 0.82; equivalent correlations for their parents were slightly higher: 0.87, 0.82 and 0.86. "Values of ≥0.70 were considered excellent."

As is customary, the authors reported p-values, testing the somewhat implausible null hypotheses that the true correlation is zero. Predictably, given the sample size, they rejected these hypotheses: "All Spearman correlation coefficients were statistically significant ($p < 0.001$)". Confidence intervals would have been more informative, as these indicate the uncertainty in the estimated values.

For example, applying the Z-transformation, the 95% CIs for parent-child disease impact ($N = 759$) is 0.49–0.60, and for child test–retest ($N = 291$) it is 0.78–0.86.

Polychoric correlation

The polychoric correlation was also introduced by Pearson as an alternative to $r_{Pearson}$. For $r_{Pearson}$, it is assumed that the variables being correlated are from a bivariate normal distribution, and are therefore continuous variables. For $r_{Polychoric}$, the assumption is that the observations are ordinal variables with an underlying joint bivariate distribution. For example, if two PROs are scored 1–4 for not at all, a little, quite a bit and very much, it is reasonable to assume that their discrete categories represent an underlying continuous bivariate distribution, even though we only observe a 'contingency table' with four-by-four categories. In this situation, $r_{Pearson}$ underestimates the true correlation. If there are five or more categories, and the variables are roughly symmetric, $r_{Pearson}$ is usually fine, but when there are only two or three categories or the data show marked asymmetry,

$r_{Polychoric}$ may be preferable for use with techniques such as factor analysis or structural equation modelling. The calculation of polychoric correlation is complex but is increasingly available as an option in statistical software packages, although it should be noted that most implementations assume an underlying bivariate normal distribution.

Correction for overlap

When exploring the correlation structure of the scales, we shall be interested in examining the relative magnitude of the correlations between the total scale score and each of the component items that form the scale. That will, for example, enable us to identify which items appear to be most consistent with the scale as a whole. However, when calculating the correlation between any one item, say x_1, and the total score of the scale in which the item is contained, a *correction for overlap* should be made. This is necessary because if the m items in a scale are x_1, x_2, ..., x_m, the correlation between, say, x_1 and the total $S = x_1 + x_2 + ... + x_m$ would be inflated since S also includes x_1 itself. Instead, x_1 should be correlated with the sum-score formed by omitting x_1 from the scale; that is, x_1 correlated with $S - x_1$.

Correcting for overlap is important. It can be shown that if two completely independent (i.e. uncorrelated, $r = 0.0$), randomly distributed variables from a Normal distribution are combined into a single scale, the correlation between either variable and the sum-score is approximately 0.71. However, this apparently high correlation is misleading. When the correction for overlap is applied, the 'corrected' correlations will be approximately zero, confirming that neither of the two variables contributes to the scale as defined by the remaining (other) item.

Example

The cognitive functioning scale (CF) of the EORTC QLQ-C30 comprises the sum of two questions, difficulty in concentrating (q20) and difficulty remembering things (q25). Although it may make clinical sense to group these into a single scale, it is arguable that they represent two different dimensions. In a sample of 900 patients, the correlation between q20 and the CF scale score was 0.87, while that between q25 and CF was 0.85. Both these correlations appear satisfactorily high. However, correcting for overlap, which amounts to correlating q20 with q25 because there are only two variables, the correlation is only 0.46.

5.4 Construct validity

Multi-item scales open up a whole new range of techniques for construct validity beyond those described in Chapter 4. For the main part, we shall be making use of correlations: correlations between items in the same scale, correlations between an item and items in other scales, correlations between a scale score and its constituent items, and correlations between items and external scales or other external variables. These enable us to check:

1. Dimensionality: do all items in a subscale relate to a single latent variable, or is there evidence that more latent variables are necessary to explain the observed variability?

2. Homogeneity: do all the items in a subscale appear to be tapping equally strongly into the same latent variable?

3. Overlap between latent variables: do some items from one subscale correlate with other latent variables?

Convergent and discriminant validity

Convergent and discriminant validity have been discussed in Chapter 4 in terms of relationships between different scales, or dimensions, of QoL or PROs. For multi-item scales, these concepts are extended to explore item-level relationships. In this setting, *convergent validity* states that items comprising any one scale should correlate with each other. This is closely related to internal consistency, and in effect declares that all items in a scale should be measuring the same thing. If theory leads us to expect two items to be similar, they should be strongly correlated; if they are not strongly correlated, that may imply that one or the other is not contributing to the scale score it was intended to measure. Convergence is often assessed by comparing the correlations between each item and the overall sum-score for the scale.

Equally important is *discriminant validity*, which states that if an instrument contains more than one scale, the items within any one scale should not correlate too highly with external items and other scales. Thus items that theory suggests are unrelated should not correlate strongly with each other. If an item correlates more strongly with those in a scale other than its own, perhaps the item is more appropriately assigned to that other scale. If several items, or all the items, correlate highly with items in another scale, this may suggest there are insufficient grounds for declaring that two separate scales exist.

Multitrait–multimethod analysis

Multitrait–multimethod (MTMM) analysis, described in Chapter 4, can also be used to explore the relationships between items and scales. For this, the traits represent the items and the postulated scales become the methods. However, the number of item-to-item correlations can become quite large and unwieldy to present. Thus for the SF-36 there are 36 items, and each of these could be correlated with the other 35 items. An alternative approach is to restrict the focus upon item-to-scale correlations, which is termed *multitrait-scaling analysis*.

Multitrait-scaling analyses

If an item *does not* correlate highly with the items from another scale, it may be expected to have a low correlation with the total score for that other scale. Similarly, if an item *does* correlate highly with other items in its own scale, it will also be correlated with the total sum-score for the scale. The principal objective of multitrait-scaling analysis is to examine these correlations, and thereby to confirm whether items are included in the scale with which they correlate most strongly, and whether the postulated scale structure therefore appears to be consistent with the data patterns. When calculating these correlations, the *correction for overlap* should be applied.

Widely used levels for acceptable correlation coefficients are the following. During initial scale development, *convergent validity* is supported if an item correlates moderately ($r = 0.3$ or greater) with the scale it is hypothesised to belong to, but when the instrument is undergoing final testing a more stringent criterion of at least 0.4 should be used; items with lower correlations are insufficiently related to other items within their domain, and should therefore be excluded. *Discriminant validity* is supported whenever a correlation between an item and its hypothesised scale is higher than its correlation with the other scales.

Unless there are clinical, other practical or theoretical grounds that outweigh the rules for convergent and discriminant validity, it is usually sensible to regard items that have poor convergent or discriminant properties as *scaling errors*. To allow for random variability and the sample size, the correlation coefficients may be compared using a statistical significance test. A *scaling success* is counted if the item to own-scale correlation is significantly higher than the correlations of the item to other scales. Similarly, if the item to own-scale correlation is significantly less than that of the item to another scale, a *definite scaling error* is assumed. If the correlations do not differ significantly, a *probable scaling error* is counted. Usually, a p-value less than 0.05 is regarded as 'significant' for this purpose.

Example from the literature

Blazeby *et al.* (2009) examined the convergent and discriminant validity of the QLQ-LMC21, a questionnaire that targets disease-specific issues in patients with colorectal liver metastases and supplements the more general cancer-specific QLQ-C30. The study recruited 356 patients who were about to commence treatment for their metastases.

Table 5.1 shows the correlations between the four hypothesised multi-item scales and their component items, with correction for overlap as appropriate. The three items comprising the fatigue scale (items numbered 7, 13 and 14) had corrected correlations of 0.76, 0.87 and 0.85 respectively with the fatigue scale (convergent validity). Each of these items had a significantly ($p < 0.05$) higher correlation with their own scale than with other scales (discriminant validity).

Table 5.1 Item-scale correlations for the EORTC QLQ-LMC21 questionnaire (a module to supplement the QLQ-C30), using data from 356 patients with colorectal liver metastases

| | | — Hypothesised scales — | | | |
Item	Description	Nutrition	Fatigue	Pain	Emotional problems
Nutrition					
lmc1	Trouble eating	0.70*	0.46	0.32	0.32
lmc2	Felt full up too quickly	0.70*	0.51	0.42	0.34
Fatigue					
lmc7	Less active than liked	0.49	0.76*	0.47	0.46
lmc13	Felt 'slowed down'	0.45	0.87*	0.52	0.47
lmc14	Felt lacking in energy	0.53	0.85*	0.51	0.47
Pain					
lmc9	Pain in stomach area	0.36	0.42	0.72*	0.29
lmc10	Discomfort in stomach area	0.35	0.44	0.66*	0.32
lmc12	Pain in back	0.32	0.46	0.43*	0.27
Emotional problems					
lmc17	Felt stressed	0.24	0.27	0.24	0.52*
lmc18	Less able to enjoy	0.47	0.67	0.44	0.53*
lmc19	Worried about future health	0.22	0.34	0.24	0.71*
lmc20	Worried about family's future	0.26	0.32	0.23	0.67*

*Correlations corrected for overlap.
Source: Data from Blazeby *et al.*, 2009.

Items that show definite scaling errors are usually candidates for excluding from a scale. It is less clear what to do about probable scaling errors. If the sample size is less than 100, estimates of the correlation coefficients will be imprecise and probable scaling errors may occur simply by chance – in which case the probable errors should be regarded as inconclusive. What sample size is necessary for multitrait-scaling analysis? Since a small sample size means that the correlations will be estimated imprecisely, resulting in non-significant *p*-values even when there are scaling errors, it is recommended that sample sizes be greater than 100 for scaling analyses. In the above example, the large sample size ($N = 356$) means that even small and unimportant differences in the level of correlations will be statistically significant, as shown in the column for scaling success. The magnitudes of the observed differences, their statistical significance and the size of the sample all have to be considered when interpreting the multitrait analysis results.

The selection of an appropriate sample of patients is also important. A heterogeneous sample, with patients from a variety of disease states and with a range of disease

> ### *Example from the literature*
>
> Blazeby *et al.* (2009) examined correlations between all 12 items and the four hypothesised scales of the QLQ-LMC21. Table 5.2 summarises the convergent and discriminant scaling errors, and the scale homogeneity and internal consistency values. For example, in Table 5.1 the three fatigue items had correlations with their own scale of between 0.76 and 0.87, and the nine correlations with other scales ranged from 0.45 (lmc13 with nutrition scale) to 0.53 (lmc14, also with nutrition). Also, for each fatigue item, its own-scale correlation was compared against the correlations with the three other scales, giving three tests per item and a total of nine tests for the fatigue scale; the results of these tests are summarised as 'scaling successes' in Table 5.2.
>
> Tests confirmed that QLQ-LMC21 items are more highly correlated with their own scales than with other scales. Thus in this sample the QLQ-LMC21 items satisfy scaling success criteria.
>
> **Table 5.2**   Item scaling tests: convergent and discriminant validity, scaling success and reliability (Cronbach's alpha) for the EORTC QLQ-LMC21 multi-item scales
>
> | Scales | No. of items | Convergent validity (range of correlations[a]) | Discriminant validity (range of correlations) | Scaling success[c] | Scaling success rate[d] | Reliability (Cronbach's α) |
> |---|---|---|---|---|---|---|
> | Nutritional problems | 2 | 0.70[b] | 0.32 to 0.51 | 6/6 | 100 | 0.80 |
> | Fatigue | 3 | 0.76 to 0.87 | 0.45 to 0.53 | 9/9 | 100 | 0.91 |
> | Pain | 3 | 0.43 to 0.72 | 0.27 to 0.46 | 7/9 | 78 | 0.76 |
> | Emotional problems | 4 | 0.52 to 0.71 | 0.22 to 0.67 | 9/12 | 75 | 0.79 |
>
> [a]Correlations of item with own scale are corrected for overlap.
> [b]For a two-item scale, this becomes the correlation between the two items.
> [c]Number of convergent correlations significantly higher than discriminant correlations/Total number of correlations.
> [d]Scaling success rate is the previous column as a percentage.
> *Source:* Blazeby *et al.*, 2009, Table 2. Reproduced with permission of John Wiley & Sons, Ltd.

severities, will result in a wide range of responses. This will tend to result in high correlations, especially for convergent validity. Thus most investigators aim to recruit a heterogeneous sample for their validation studies. To ensure that the instrument remains valid and sensitive for use with all types of patient, it is equally important to investigate performance in various subgroups and this will also affect the sample size requirements.

Example

The results presented in Table 5.2 are for all patients before commencing treatment. Blazeby *et al.* (2009) also checked convergent and discriminant validity of the QLQ-LMC21 during treatment and follow-up, and separately in the two subgroups hepatectomy and palliation. They report that convergent validity was excellent, and that scaling successes were high in all subgroups.

   These results, together with other data they present, lead to the conclusion that scaling assumptions are well met in the patients targeted by the QLQ-LMC21.

Multitrait-scaling analysis is a simple yet effective method for checking that the pattern of the correlations corresponds to expectations, and that items have been assigned to the scale that they are most strongly correlated with. It also identifies items that are only weakly associated with the rest of their scale. However, statistical correlation can point only to areas in which there may be problems and, as we note in Section 5.7, also assumes that the parallel tests model of Section 2.7 applies. Clinical sensibility should also be considered when interpreting seemingly inconsistent correlations.

   Although the necessary calculations for multitrait-scaling analyses can be performed using standard statistical packages, care must be taken to ensure that correction for overlap is applied where appropriate. The MAP-R program (Ware *et al.*, 1998) is a computer package that has been designed specifically for multitrait-scaling and provides detailed item-scaling analyses.

Factor analysis, dimensionality and multitrait scaling

Factor analysis is a form of structural equation modelling or SEM (not to be confused with *SEM*, the standard error of measurement). It is one of the most important and powerful methods for establishing construct validity of psychometric tests. Whereas the methods of the previous Sections rely to a large extent upon the scrutiny of inter-item and item-scale correlation matrices, factor analysis attempts to provide a formal method of exploring correlation structure. Although it provides a method for investigating the internal structure of an instrument, the results are difficult to interpret without a theoretical framework for the relationship between the items and scales. The simplicity of multitrait-scaling analysis, on the other hand, means that the results are easier to understand and more readily interpreted clinically.

5.5 Cronbach's α and internal consistency

A scale is *unidimensional* if the items describe a single latent variable. Thus, application of factor analysis (Chapter 6) should confirm that a single factor suffices to account for the item-variability in the scale, and factor analysis provides a means of examining and testing the dimensionality of scales. The term *homogeneity* is also often used as a synonym for unidimensionality. A related concept is *internal consistency* and, confusingly, many authors regard this as the same as homogeneity.

Internal consistency refers to the extent to which the items are inter-related. Cronbach's alpha coefficient, $\alpha_{Cronbach}$, is one method of assessing internal consistency, and is the method used most widely for this purpose. It is also a form of reliability assessment, in that for parallel and certain related tests it is an estimate of reliability, and even for other tests it provides a lower bound for the true reliability. It is a function of both the average inter-item correlation and the number of items in a scale, and increases as either of these increases. Although internal consistency is often regarded as a distinct concept, it is closely related to convergent validity. Both methods make use of within-scale between-item correlations.

If a scale contains m items that describe a single latent variable θ, and the observed total score is S, then the reliability is defined as $R = \dfrac{\sigma_\theta^2}{\sigma_S^2}$, which is the ratio of the true score variance to the observed score variance. Now θ, being the latent variable, is unknown and so we do not have an estimate of its variance σ_θ^2. Hence the reliability cannot be determined but has to be estimated. For summated scales of m items, Cronbach (1951) proposed the measure

$$\alpha_{Cronbach} = \frac{m}{m-1}\left(1 - \frac{\sum Var(x_i)}{Var(S)}\right). \tag{5.13}$$

Here, $Var(x_i)$ is the variance of the ith item in the scale, calculated from the sample of patients completing the QoL assessment, and $\sum x_i$.

The basis of Cronbach's α is that if the items were uncorrelated, $Var(S)$ would equal the sum of their individual variances, implying $\alpha_{Cronbach} = 0$. At the other extreme, if all the items are identical they would have perfect correlation; it can be shown that this results in $\alpha_{Cronbach} = 1$. Thus α is a measure of the consistency of the scale, and indicates the degree of inter-correlation of the items. However, it can also be shown that Cronbach's α underestimates the true reliability of θ, and is therefore a conservative measure.

Coefficients above 0.7 are generally regarded as acceptable for psychometric scales, although it is often recommended that values should be above 0.8 (good) or even 0.9 (excellent). For individual patient assessment, it is recommended that values should be above 0.9.

Perhaps one of the most useful applications of Cronbach's α is in the development of scales and the selection of items. If Cronbach's α changes little when an item is omitted, that item is a candidate for removal from the scale. Conversely, a new item may be worth including if it causes a substantial increase. However, as noted above, α increases as the number of items in the scale increases. Therefore, in order to assess the true benefit of adding one or more extra items, we first estimate the expected change in α that is attributable to lengthening the scale. This is expressed by the Spearman–Browne *prophecy formula*, which predicts the gain in α that is expected by increasing the number of items. If the original scale has n items, and the revised scale has m items,

$$\alpha_m = \frac{m\alpha_n}{n+(m-n)\alpha_n} = \frac{k\alpha_n}{k\alpha_n+(1-\alpha_n)}, \tag{5.14}$$

where $k = m/n$ and is the ratio of the number of items in the new scale over the number in the original scale. Thus merely having a longer scale automatically inflates Cronbach's α.

Example

If initially a scale has a Cronbach's α of $\alpha_n = 0.6$, then (assuming all items have approximately similar inter-item correlations) doubling the length of the scale by including additional items would give a value of $k = 2$. This results in an increase of Cronbach's α to $\alpha_m = 2 \times 0.6/[(2 \times 0.6) + (1 - 0.6)] = 0.75$.

In contrast, halving the number would result in $\alpha_m = 0.5 \times 0.6/[(0.5 \times 0.6) + (1 - 0.6)] = 0.43$.

Cronbach himself, in 1951, recognised the need to adjust for the number of items. He commented that a quart (approximately a litre) of homogenised milk is no more homogenised than a pint (approximately ½ litre) of milk, even though a quart is twice the volume of a pint. However, $\alpha_{Cronbach}$, the measure of homogeneity, does increase according to the size (number of items) of a scale. Since Cronbach's α increases as the number of items in the scale is increased, high values can be obtained by lengthening the scale. Even the simple expedient of adding duplicate items with closely similar wording will suffice to increase it. This has led many to question whether it is sensible to specify criteria for acceptable levels of Cronbach's α without specifying the number of items in the scale.

Another consequence of the Spearman–Browne formula, equation (5.14), is that if the individual items in the scale are good estimators of the latent variable in the sense that they estimate it with little error, they will have high correlations and few items are needed in the scale. On the other hand, if the items have much error, many items will be needed.

The theory behind Cronbach's α assumes that the scale relates to a single latent variable, and is therefore unidimensional. Although it is often assumed that $\alpha_{Cronbach}$ is itself a check for dimensionality, and that a high result implies a unidimensional scale, this is incorrect. Results can be misleadingly high when calculated for multidimensional scales. Therefore dimensionality should always be checked by, for example, using factor analysis.

The consequences of multidimensionality can be readily seen: consider a scale consisting of the sum of body weight and height. Although this would have very high test–retest repeatability, since neither measurement varies very much in stable subjects, Cronbach's α – supposedly an indicator of reliability – would not be correspondingly high because these items are only moderately correlated.

It can be shown that Cronbach's α is a form of intraclass correlation (*ICC*, Section 4.6), and thus it can also be estimated using ANOVA. Therefore the issues regarding correlations will also apply. Thus a wide and heterogeneous range of patients will tend to result in higher values, while the values will be low if the patients are similar to each other. Since it is almost always obvious that Cronbach's α must be greater than zero, significance tests of the null hypothesis that $\alpha_{Cronbach} = 0$ are usually irrelevant although often reported; provided the sample size is large enough, the p-value will invariably indicate statistical significance; a non-significant result indicates merely that the sample size is inadequate. More sensible, and far more informative, are confidence intervals. These are most conveniently estimated using the so-called bootstrap methods that are available in statistical packages such as STATA (StataCorp, 2013).

Example from the literature

Table 5.2 showed Cronbach's α for the QLQ-LMC21 obtained by Blazeby *et al.* (2009). The smallest value is 0.76 for the pain scale, and other values are 0.79, 0.80 and 0.91, indicating that the scales show good internal reliability.

Example from the literature

The EORTC QLQ-C30 (version 1.0) contained two items that assessed role functioning. These were 'Are you limited in any way in doing either your work or doing household jobs?' and 'Are you completely unable to work at a job or to do household jobs?' and took response options 'No' and 'Yes'. Low values of Cronbach's α had been reported, ranging from 0.52 to 0.66. There were also concerns about the content validity because it was felt that role functioning ought to encompass hobbies and leisure-time activities. Two new questions were introduced, replacing the original questions. These were 'Were you limited in doing either your work or other daily activities?' and 'Were you limited in pursuing your hobbies or other leisure-time activities?' The binary response options were changed into four-category scales.

Osoba *et al.* (1997) evaluated these modifications in patients who were assessed before, during and after chemotherapy or radiotherapy. With questions in the original format, Cronbach's α varied between 0.26 and 0.67. The revised items showed considerably higher internal reliability (0.78 to 0.88) and were accepted for the QLQ-C30 (version 2.0). While the rewording may have contributed to these changes in reliability, a more likely explanation is that increasing the number of categories from two to four accounted for the differences.

Alpha revisited

Cronbach's 1951 article was "a great success ... with approximately 325 social science citations per year ... [However,] I doubt whether coefficient α is the best way of judging reliability of the instrument to which it is applied." Those words were written by Cronbach himself some 50 years later, shortly before his death (Cronbach, 2004), when he cautioned against the excessive and uncritical use of the α coefficient. We also agree with Cronbach's comments that the standard error of measurement (*SEM*) is the most important single piece of information. Interpretation of the estimated *SEM* can be made by assuming the scale scores follow approximately a Normal distribution, in which case roughly 95% of individuals are expected to score within two *SEM* of their 'true' value. The *SEM* is obtained from a 'crossed-design' analysis of variance (ANOVA), which decomposes the overall variance into components due to patient-patient variability and the residual variability. When ANOVA is used to estimate α, it is assumed that the items are truly parallel with item-to-item variance of zero; then the *SEM* is estimated by the square-root of the residual variance. However, the generality of the ANOVA approach allows for items with differing means.

Cronbach also noted the importance of heterogeneity of content. "There is no reason to worry about scattered diversity of items ... It needs only to be recognised that an analysis that does not differentiate between the classes of items will report a larger *SEM* than a more subtle analysis." The example he uses is a mathematics test that contains both geometric-reasoning and numeric-reasoning items; there are obvious parallels with those QoL instruments that deliberately seek comprehensive content validity, and thereby report a lower α. Section 5.7 also shows that formative items affect heterogeneity, making α inappropriate.

In summary, α is overused, and better measures are available. An appropriate 'subtle' analysis using ANOVA and estimating the *SEM* is preferable. In Chapter 7 we shall also see that item response theory methods focus on the *SEM* as an indicator of test precision.

Modern trends

One consequence of the emphasis on Cronbach's α is that scales developed under the traditional psychometric paradigm have tended to be lengthy. If one feels that the α reliability is inadequate, the simplest expedient is to add more items to the scale. More recently, many investigators have found that for many purposes short scales are adequate, and in many cases one or two items suffice to provide the precision and reliability that is required. The developers of many instruments are introducing short-form versions, either as an alternative or as a replacement for their original questionnaire. As we shall see in Chapters 7 and 8, item response theory is effective for identifying the most efficient items, and another modern trend is to develop dynamic computer-based questionnaires that only ask as many items as are required for obtaining a pre-specified precision.

5.6 Validation or alteration?

Multitrait scaling and related analyses such as Cronbach's α are usually carried out in the later stages of instrument development, when field-testing. As described in Chapter 3, one of the aims of the field study is to determine and confirm the validity of the questionnaire, and the analyses we have presented are a key aspect of this. Thus the field study is usually intended as the final stage of developing and validating a new questionnaire. In theory, we hope to confirm that the hypothesised scale structure – which will have been specified before launching the field study – appears consistent with the observed data, supporting our claims of validity. In practice, all too frequently the analyses will reveal a few items (or even a few scales) that do not perform as well as expected. This can lead to revision of the scaling and scoring, and perhaps changes to the items in the questionnaire, after which reapplication of the multitrait scaling should produce improved results. Provided the alterations are minor, it may be reasonable to argue that the instrument appears to have acceptable validity. The problem is that when there are substantial changes it will become necessary to collect additional data from an independent sample in order to claim evidence of validity; often this is unrealistic in terms of funding and time. At the very least, reports of field studies must declare the hypothesised scale structure that was pre-specified in writing before the study was launched. All subsequent alteration to the scale structure, scale scoring or the items must also be clearly delineated. Then the readers are able to judge whether they feel claims of 'validity' are acceptable.

Example from the literature

Blazeby *et al.* (2009) described the QLQ-LMC21 module, which contains 21 items in a layout and response format similar to the QLQ-C30. They declared that preliminary qualitative investigations and interviews with patients had indicated that the relevant issues should be grouped into five multi-item scales (fatigue, nutrition, pain, social and emotional problems) and six single items (problems with taste, tingling hands, sore mouth, dry mouth, problems with jaundice and weight loss).

Following the multitrait analyses, it was found that item within-scale correlations in the nutrition and fatigue scales were at least 0.53 in all groups. These scales were not correlated with other scales in the module and were retained in their original form. Correlations in the hypothesised three-item pain scale demonstrated a small overlap with the fatigue scale, except in patients selected for palliative treatment. It was decided to retain this scale in its original form. The original hypothesised social problems scale demonstrated very poor scaling properties (within-scale correlations were less than 0.40 in all subgroups). This scale was therefore split into three single items. There was some overlap between the four-item emotional problems scale in patients undergoing palliative treatment, but in the surgical group this scale functioned well and it was retained in its original form. The final module (QLQ-LMC21), therefore, has four scales and nine single items. The internal consistency reliability of the scales (Cronbach's α coefficient) was high in most scales (at least 0.69).

If an item has poor correlation with the scale to which it is hypothesised to belong, there are several possible actions; the choice should depend on the quantitative analyses, the previous qualitative work from earlier stages of instrument development and discussion or debate among the researchers:

1. delete and discard the item;

2. remove the item from the scale but, if on qualitative grounds it is believed to be important, retain it as a stand-alone single item;

3. if it correlates more highly with another scale, perhaps it is appropriate to transfer it to that scale;

4. if upon review the item is considered important, perhaps the wording was inappropriate and it should be reworded;

5. perhaps the item should be retained in the original scale despite the poor correlations; this is most likely to arise with symptoms for a formative construct, as exemplified in Section 5.7.

If more than one item in a scale has poor correlation, more substantial changes to the constructs might be necessary, such as splitting one scale into two or more constructs, or changing the conceptual basis of a construct and renaming it accordingly.

If two items are highly correlated, or if Cronbach's α coefficient has very high value, another reason to discard an item is redundancy. At this stage of development it is less common to introduce new items, although this might be deemed necessary if one or more items are ineffective and are deleted, or if Cronbach's α is low.

5.7   Implications for formative or causal items

Most methods generally assume that the items in a scale are parallel tests – that is, that all the items in any one scale are selected so as to reflect the postulated latent variable, and each item is presumed to be measuring much the same thing. On that basis, the items should be correlated with each other. Sometimes this assumption is either untrue or inappropriate. In particular, many QoL scales contain PROs that are symptoms or other causal variables. As we have seen in Chapter 2, the correlations between such items can be misleading. These correlations do not indicate QoL constructs, but are often merely consequences of symptom clusters arising from the disease or its treatment. For example, in cancer patients, hair loss and nausea may both be associated with chemotherapy and therefore highly correlated, even though in terms of QoL concepts they may be unrelated to one another. The methods of this chapter are usually inappropriate for clinimetric or other scales containing items that are causal indicators, and are irrelevant for composite indicators.

Thus convergent and discriminant validity seem sensible criteria for instrument validity when one is considering scales made from items that are *reflective indicators*. When *causal indicators* are present, neither criterion need apply. It may be clinically sensible to retain certain formative items in a single QoL subscale even though they are only weakly correlated with each other and therefore have low convergent validity. Equally, it might make sound clinical sense to disregard some high correlations and treat some causal items as comprising two or more distinct scales, irrespective of discriminant validity. However, sometimes, even with causal indicators, very high correlations may be a sign that two items are measuring much the same concept and that one of the items is therefore redundant.

High internal consistency, as measured by Cronbach's α, is a fundamental requirement for instruments that are based upon reflective indicators and designed upon the principles of parallel tests. When scales contain formative items, there may be low convergent correlations and therefore low internal consistency. These scales exemplify Cronbach's comment: "There is no reason to worry about scattered diversity of items." Similarly, definitions of reliability do not work well for items that have a causal relationship with the latent variable of interest.

The implications for causal items and clinimetric scales are summarised in Figure 5.1.

Consequences for clinimetric and other scales containing formative items:

- Basic properties of measurement scales, such as content validity, sensitivity, responsiveness and test–retest reliability, are invariably important when devising any QoL instrument (both formative and reflective).

- Assessment of construct validity, including convergent and discriminant validity, is mainly based upon analysis of item-correlation structures, and is less relevant when formative items are involved.

- Cronbach's α is based upon item-to-item correlations, and is largely irrelevant for scales containing formative items.

Alternative criteria for clinimetric scales or scales with causal items:

- Clinical sensibility. This is equivalent to face validity.

- Comprehensive coverage of items.

- Emphasis upon items that patients rate as important.

- Emphasis upon items that patients experience frequently.

Figure 5.1 Clinimetric scales and scales with causal items.

Example

Whistance *et al.* (2009) developed a 29-item colorectal cancer module, the QLQ-CR29. They reported that the three items in the hypothesised pain scale consistently demonstrated weak correlations with the overall scale ($r < 0.40$) in many of the subgroups studied. The pain scale was, therefore, removed leaving three single items assessing anal/rectal pain, abdominal pain and pain when urinating.

An alternative approach would be to argue that disease-related pain is a meaningful construct, and that pain impacts on HRQoL. We could in principle have asked a single compound question: do you have pain in your abdomen, anus, rectum, or when urinating? It is cognitively less demanding to break this down into three separate items, and if pain *is* reported the individual items can be analysed or used to guide clinical management. Pain is a causal item, with severe pain, at any site, causing distress to the patient. The three-item construct is a formative scale, identifying the disease-related forms of pain that arise from colorectal cancer. The correlations merely indicate that many patients had one or another form of pain, according to the precise localisation of their tumour, but relatively few patients had multiple sources of pain. Since this is a formative construct, it is important that all potential sites of pain are covered.

Many studies have reported similar problems when constructing pain scales. For example, Baxter *et al.* (2010) developed an instrument for use on patients who are receiving home parenteral nutrition (HPN). The two pain items were 'aches or pains in your muscles or joints' and 'other pain', which only weakly correlated with each other ($r = 0.29$; Cronbach's $\alpha = 0.45$). The authors observed that "However, they were considered to be clinically important questions because it is well documented that HPN patients suffer from joint pain or cramps, and many have pain related to their underlying disease."

In clinimetric scales the items are chosen primarily from the perspective of high content validity, and the internal reliability can be low. Properties such as sensitivity and responsiveness are also of paramount importance.

Example

Apgar (1953) scores, mentioned in Chapter 2, are a well-known and useful index for the health of newborn babies. The items included (heart rate, respiratory rate, reflex responses, skin colour and muscle tone) were selected on the basis of being important yet distinct prognostic indicators. After many years of use, the Apgar score has been found to be an effective indicator of neonatal health. Despite this, the constituent items may have weak correlations and Cronbach's α is low.

It is also often inappropriate to use traditional psychometric methods when scales are designed on the basis of an item response model. In this case, items are deliberately chosen so as to be of varying difficulty, and the value of Cronbach's α, for example, may be misleading.

5.8 Conclusions

The methods described constitute a set of powerful tools for checking the validity of multi-item scales, to confirm that they appear to be consistent with the postulated structure of an instrument. However, confirming validity is never proof that the instrument, or the scales it contains, are really tapping into the intended constructs. Poor validity or reliability can suffice to indicate that an instrument is *not* performing as intended. Demonstration of good validity, on the other hand, is a never-ending process of collecting more and more information showing that there are no grounds to believe the instrument inadequate.

However, the techniques of this chapter rely upon analysis of inter-item correlations, and are suitable only for scales or subscales containing solely reflective indicators. When QoL scales contain causal indicators, the inter-correlations between these items arise mainly because of disease or treatment effects and not because of association with the latent variable for QoL. This renders correlation-based methods inappropriate.

However, sometimes it is possible to use clinical judgement to select a group of symptoms that are expected to be interrelated, and correlation methods may be suitable within this restricted subset of items. For example, several symptoms related to digestive problems could be selected. Even though these are causal items for QoL changes, they might also represent a coherent set of items reflecting, say, a disease-related symptom cluster. They can then be regarded as reflective indicators for disease state, and the methods of this chapter could be applied so as to produce a disease-based digestive function score. The validation methods for multi-item scales can therefore be used as a form of subscale validation, provided it is not claimed that this is evidence of a digestive construct indicating a QoL state.

For all instruments, clinical sensibility is crucial; this encompasses face and content validity, and comprehensive coverage of all important items. To be of practical value for clinical purposes or in randomised trials, sensitivity, responsiveness and test–retest repeatability are also extremely important. But the role of other aspects of validation is primarily to accrue evidence that the items behave in a sensible manner, and that the scales are consistent with the postulated constructs.

6
Factor analysis and structural equation modelling

Summary

Factor analysis and structural equation modelling are powerful techniques for exploring the item correlations during scale validation. We illustrate factor analysis techniques with a detailed example of its application to the HADS, showing interpretation of the typical output that is obtained from most computer packages. Factor analysis in scale development and scale validation are discussed, together with the limitations of this approach. Finally, we describe the more general approach of structural equation modelling.

6.1   Introduction

The methods of Chapter 5 were concerned primarily with examining item-to-item correlations in order to evaluate whether their patterns are consistent with the hypothesised scale structure. Factor analysis, on the other hand, can be used either as an automatic procedure to explore the patterns amongst the correlations (exploratory factor analysis, or EFA), or as a confirmatory method (CFA) for testing whether the correlations correspond to the anticipated scale structure. Thus factor analysis plays a major role in construct validation. Although CFA is the more flexible and powerful of the two, EFA is the form most commonly seen in outcomes research; EFA is simpler to implement, and does not require specification in advance of the details of the scale structures and the inter-item relationships. Structural equation modelling (SEM) is a more general technique that encompasses both CFA and EFA, and can be used to fit other complex models. All three approaches – EFA, CFA and SEM – are concerned with detecting and analysing patterns in the inter-item correlation (or covariance) matrix, and can be used to assess the dimensionality (number of factors) needed to represent the variability in the data. CFA and SEM can additionally test these patterns to confirm the validity of the postulated constructs. SEM can fit complex models involving both causal and indicator variables.

Item response theory (Chapter 7) provides powerful methods for scale calibration, but assumes that the items being scaled are from a single dimension. This assumption of unidimensionality is often tested using EFA or SEM (Figure 6.1).

Multitrait analysis

- Display of item–item correlations and item-scale correlations, using hypothesized scale structure.
- Uses arbitrary thresholds for convergent and divergent validity.
- Calculation of p-values for probable and definite scaling errors.

Exploratory factor analysis (EFA)

- Explores item-item correlations to identify clusters of highly correlated items (factors).
- Arbitrary rules to determine number of factors (for example scree plots, eigenvalues > 1.0).
- Factors may or may not coincide with meaningful constructs, as they only depend on the item-correlation matrix.

Confirmatory factor analysis (CFA)

- A construct model is pre-specified (e.g. from previous multitrait analysis or EFA), and is tested for adequacy of fit in a new dataset.
- CFA is usually implemented as a reduced form of SEM.

Structural equation model (SEM)

- A construct model is pre-specified and tested for goodness of fit.
- Complex models can be specified, including models with formative or causal items and scales.
- Controversy as to how to measure and test goodness of fit (all models are simplification of the complex constructs and if samples are large enough all models show statistically significant misfit; it is often unclear as to what constitutes adequate fit).
- Can compare two or more models to test whether there is evidence (p-value) that one provides better fit than another.
- Unfortunately, in many cases the parameterization of the models may be so similar in statistical terms that there is little power to discriminate between them.

Figure 6.1 Comparison of approaches to analysis.

6.2   Correlation patterns

Since correlations provide the basic information for factor analysis, it is appropriate to start by considering a correlation matrix in which the correlations between all pairs of items are displayed. Since the correlation of x against y is the same as the correlation of y against x, we only need to show the 'lower triangle' of correlations, as in Table 6.1.

The postulated structure of the HADS is relatively simple, with only two 7-item scales for anxiety and depression, and so it provides a convenient example for examining the techniques associated with factor analysis.

Example

The HADS questionnaire was completed by patients in many of the UK Medical Research Council (MRC) randomised clinical trials of cancer therapy. The results from six MRC trials have been pooled, yielding a dataset of 1,952 patients with bladder, bronchus, colorectal, head and neck, and lung cancers of varying stages from early to advanced. Table 6.1 shows the (Pearson) correlation matrix for all pairs of items. Since half of the HADS items are deliberately worded positively and half negatively, the 'negative' items have been recoded so that in all cases a response of 0 is the most favourable and 3 is the least favourable. By making the scoring consistent, it becomes easier to interpret the correlations: the highly related items should have high (positive) correlation.

There are clearly many fairly highly correlated items, with correlations between 0.4 and 0.6. Although from prior information we know that the odd-numbered questions (Q_1, Q_3, Q_5, ...) are the ones intended to reflect anxiety, it is difficult to see the pattern in this correlation matrix. However, rearranging the correlation matrix as in Table 6.2 makes the pattern very much clearer.

Items belonging to the two postulated scales are shown in cells in the grey-shaded triangles, anxiety being the upper area and depression the lower. It is now clear that there are fairly high (greater than 0.4, say) correlations amongst most items within the anxiety scale. The exception is Q_{11}, which is noticeably weaker. A similar pattern is seen amongst the depression scale items. It is also reassuring to note that the unshaded rectangular area has lower correlations, which is consistent with the hypothesis that the anxiety items are less strongly correlated with the depression items.

Table 6.1 Pearson correlations for the HADS questionnaire, from 1,952 patients in MRC trials BA09, CR04, CH01, CH02, LU12 and LU16

	Q_1	Q_2	Q_3	Q_4	Q_5	Q_6	Q_7	Q_8	Q_9	Q_{10}	Q_{11}	Q_{12}	Q_{13}	Q_{14}
Q_1	1													
Q_2	0.31	1												
Q_3	0.54	0.26	1											
Q_4	0.34	0.47	0.36	1										
Q_5	0.56	0.27	0.60	0.36	1									
Q_6	0.41	0.50	0.37	0.58	0.41	1								
Q_7	0.50	0.41	0.41	0.43	0.43	0.47	1							
Q_8	0.28	0.52	0.23	0.33	0.27	0.37	0.33	1						
Q_9	0.49	0.20	0.58	0.28	0.52	0.32	0.38	0.17	1					
Q_{10}	0.30	0.40	0.27	0.38	0.27	0.41	0.34	0.36	0.23	1				
Q_{11}	0.34	0.15	0.32	0.18	0.32	0.19	0.34	0.16	0.30	0.17	1			
Q_{12}	0.33	0.59	0.32	0.54	0.31	0.52	0.44	0.44	0.26	0.45	0.17	1		
Q_{13}	0.54	0.26	0.60	0.33	0.56	0.37	0.43	0.23	0.57	0.33	0.38	0.30	1	
Q_{14}	0.30	0.42	0.27	0.44	0.30	0.47	0.40	0.31	0.30	0.36	0.19	0.42	0.31	1

Table 6.2 Correlations from Table 6.1 rearranged corresponding to the HADS postulated subscales of anxiety (odd-numbered items) and depression (even-numbered)

	Anxiety							Depression						
	Q_1	Q_3	Q_5	Q_7	Q_9	Q_{11}	Q_{13}	Q_2	Q_4	Q_6	Q_8	Q_{10}	Q_{12}	Q_{14}
Q_1	1													
Q_3	0.54	1												
Q_5	0.56	0.60	1											
Q_7	0.50	0.41	0.43	1										
Q_8	0.49	0.58	0.52	0.38	1									
Q_{11}	0.34	0.32	0.32	0.34	0.30	1								
Q_{13}	0.54	0.60	0.56	0.43	0.57	0.38	1							
Q_2	0.31	0.26	0.27	0.41	0.20	0.15	0.26	1						
Q_4	0.34	0.36	0.36	0.43	0.28	0.18	0.33	0.47	1					
Q_6	0.41	0.37	0.41	0.47	0.32	0.19	0.37	0.50	0.58	1				
Q_8	0.28	0.23	0.27	0.33	0.17	0.16	0.23	0.52	0.33	0.37	1			
Q_{10}	0.30	0.27	0.27	0.34	0.23	0.17	0.33	0.40	0.38	0.41	0.36	1		
Q_{12}	0.33	0.32	0.31	0.44	0.26	0.17	0.30	0.59	0.54	0.52	0.44	0.45	1	
Q_{14}	0.30	0.27	0.30	0.40	0.30	0.19	0.31	0.42	0.44	0.47	0.31	0.36	0.42	1

Table 6.1 and Table 6.2 show the usual Pearson correlation coefficient, r. Since the HADS items take four-point responses, they are not strictly from a Normal distribution and other measures of correlation may be more suitable, as discussed in Section 6.8. Usually Pearson's r is adequate except in extreme situations, and similar results are in fact obtained when using the alternative methods with this HADS dataset.

A measure closely related to correlation is *covariance*. In equation (5.2), the numerator is the covariance of x and y, and the correlation is the covariance divided by the standard deviations of x and y. Most people find correlations easier to interpret since, unlike covariances, they are scaled from –1 to +1. However, factor analysis programs often use the corresponding covariances instead, and the underlying theory of factor analysis is more closely based upon covariances. One may draw an analogy with standard deviation (*SD*) versus variance; there is a direct relationship (square root) between *SD* and variance, but most people find *SD* to be the easier measure to interpret, even though variances are more convenient for generalisation and therefore used for ANOVA (analysis of variance). Hence we shall describe and illustrate the *correlation* structure of QoL data even though many factor analysis programs are in fact based upon analysis of covariances.

6.3 Path diagrams

One way to represent the many inter-relationships between the items is by means of a path diagram. Adopting standard conventions, we use circles to represent the latent variables or constructs, and boxes for the manifest variables or observable items. Lines link the items to their corresponding latent variable. Furthermore, if a construct is associated with particular items in the sense that a high value of the construct implies a high level for the item, we add directional arrows to the lines. Thus we regard the construct as implying a certain value of the item, or we might say the construct is *manifested* by the responses to the items. In extreme cases, the latent variable may be said to *cause* an outcome value for the item.

Example

The path diagram corresponding to the postulated structure of the HADS is shown in Figure 6.2. Thus if the anxiety has a high value, we would expect Q_1, Q_3, Q_5, Q_7, Q_9, Q_{11} and Q_{13} all to reflect this by manifesting high values. That is, we would expect reasonably strong correlations between these items and anxiety – although, since anxiety is a latent variable, we do not know its value and cannot calculate this correlation directly. Furthermore, in any dataset consisting of patients with a range of levels of anxiety, we would expect all of the corresponding items Q_1, Q_3, ..., Q_{13} to reflect those levels so that these items should show reasonably high correlations with each other. However, the lack of a direct link between, say, Q_1 and Q_3 indicates that if anxiety is constant (that is, if all patients have the same level of anxiety) then Q_1 and Q_3 would be uncorrelated; this is called *local independence*. As we shall see in Chapter 7, local independence is crucial for item response theory, although factor analysis appears somewhat more robust against violation of this assumption.

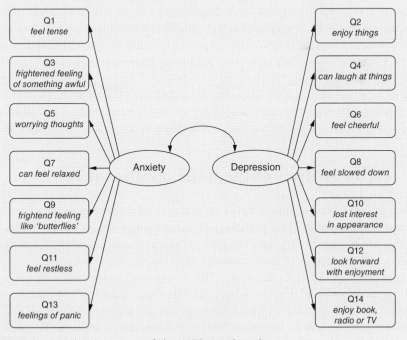

Figure 6.2 Postulated structure of the HADS questionnaire.

When two latent variables are correlated with one another, a curved line with arrows at both ends is used to link them. This is illustrated in Figure 6.2, where anxiety and depression are linked in this manner. Thus these variables are assumed to be correlated, since persons with higher levels of anxiety are more likely also to have higher levels of depression, and vice versa. Without this correlation between anxiety and depression, there would have been no link between, say, Q_1 and Q_2, and then we would have expected those items to have zero correlation with one another. Instead, given the relationship between anxiety and depression, we would expect some degree of correlation between Q_1 and Q_2.

This example is a relatively simple one, with only seven items for each of two postulated constructs. If we were analysing a more general QoL questionnaire there might be far more items and also more constructs.

6.4   Factor analysis

Factor analysis is a statistical technique that examines a correlation matrix, such as that in Table 6.2, and attempts to identify groups of variables such that there are strong correlations amongst all the variables within a group, but weak correlations between variables within the group and those outside the group. Thus, since the model assumed in Figure 6.2 implies that each of the seven anxiety items is correlated with each other, factor analysis should identify these as constituting one *factor*. If these items were indeed highly correlated, as we hope, the scale would be described as having 'strong internal structure'. Similarly, the seven depression items should form another factor. In principle one might be able to inspect a correlation matrix by eye, and verify whether this structure pertains. In practice this is usually difficult to do for all but the simplest of models, and so we often rely upon automatic techniques like factor analysis to explore the data for us.

Factor analysis as described here uses the correlation (or covariance) matrix as its staring point, and does not make use of any prior knowledge about the structure, or postulated structure, of the questionnaire. Therefore this is *exploratory* factor analysis.

6.5   Factor analysis of the HADS questionnaire

We explain how factor analysis works by using an illustrative example. The correlation matrix presented in Table 6.1 showed the inter-relationships of the HADS items. Although pre-treatment data were used for this example, we would expect to find very similar results if during- or post-treatment assessments were considered. A standard statistical program, STATA (StataCorp, 2013), was used to see how well the hypothesised factor structure is recovered. Very similar output would be obtained from most other packages. Most of the STATA default options are accepted. In general that might not be too wise; as will be discussed later, there are many choices to be made when carrying out factor analysis, and many of them can quite severely affect the analyses.

Eigenvalues and explained variance

Most computer programs start by assuming there might be as many factors as there are variables (items). If each item proved to be completely independent of all other items, we would have to regard each item as a separate construct or latent variable. In that case it would be inappropriate to construct any summary scale score, and the data would be summarised by factors that are the same as the original variables. This represents the 'full model' with the maximal number of factors. Thus factor analysis programs commence by calculating the importance of each of the possible factors.

The *eigenvalues*, or *latent roots*, are obtained by matrix algebra; their precise mathematical meaning need not concern us, but a rough interpretation is that the eigenvalues are a measure of how much of the variation in the data is accounted for by each factor.

Example

Table 6.3 shows the eigenvalues relating to the HADS data of Table 6.1, with one row for each of the $n = 14$ potential factors. The eigenvalues sum to n. The proportion of variance explained is then obtained by dividing the eigenvalue by n. Thus, for the first factor, $5.84/14 = 0.41$ or 41%. The first two factors account for 54% of the total variation. Using the eigenvalues-greater-than-one rule, there are assumed to be two factors. This conveniently confirms our prior expectation of two latent constructs.

Table 6.3   Factor analysis of Table 6.1: eigenvalues and proportion of the HADS variance explained

Factor	Eigenvalue	Difference	Variance explained: Proportion	Cumulative
1	5.84	4.08	0.41	0.41
2	1.76	0.94	0.13	0.54
3	0.82	0.07	0.06	0.60
4	0.75	0.07	0.05	0.65
5	0.68	0.07	0.05	0.70
6	0.61	0.04	0.05	0.75
7	0.57	0.06	0.04	0.79
8	0.51	0.07	0.04	0.83
9	0.44	0.00	0.03	0.86
10	0.43	0.03	0.03	0.89
11	0.40	0.00	0.03	0.92
12	0.40	0.03	0.03	0.95
13	0.37	0.00	0.03	0.98
14	0.37	—	0.02	1.00

Therefore the eigenvalues indicate the importance of each factor in explaining the variability and correlations in the observed sample of data. Usually these eigenvalues are scaled such that the total variability of the data is equal to the number of variables, and the sum of the eigenvalues will equal the number of items. The proportion of total variance explained by each factor is obtained by expressing the eigenvalues as percentages.

Most factor analysis programs will optionally use the eigenvalues to determine how many factors are present. A commonly used criterion is the so-called *eigenvalues greater than one* rule. Applying this rule, the number of distinct factors is assumed to be equal to the number of eigenvalues that exceed 1.0.

Factor loadings

Having decided upon the number of factors in the model, the next stage is to obtain the factor pattern matrix, or factor loadings, corresponding to the factor solution. These numbers indicate the importance of the variables to each factor, and are broadly equivalent to regression coefficients. The loadings are also equal to the correlations between the factors and the items.

Example

The output continues with Table 6.4, which gives the factor pattern matrix corresponding to a two-factor solution for the HADS data. At first sight Table 6.4 does not look too promising: the first factor has broadly similar loadings for all variables and is thus little more than an average of all 14 items. Factor 2 is difficult to interpret, although in this case it is noticeable that alternate items have positive and negative loadings.

Table 6.4 Factor loadings (unrotated) of two-factor solution for the HADS data in Table 6.1

Variable	Factor 1	Factor 2
Q_1	0.70	−0.31
Q_2	0.63	0.48
Q_3	0.69	−0.42
Q_4	0.67	0.29
Q_5	0.69	−0.36
Q_6	0.71	0.25
Q_7	0.70	−0.01
Q_8	0.54	0.38
Q_9	0.62	−0.46
Q_{10}	0.57	0.28
Q_{11}	0.44	−0.33
Q_{12}	0.67	0.42
Q_{13}	0.69	−0.41
Q_{14}	0.60	0.25

Rotation

It can be shown mathematically that the initial solution is not the only one possible. Other two-factor solutions are equally good at explaining the same percentage of the variability, and in fact there are an infinite variety of alternative solutions. In general the initial factor solution will rarely show any interpretable patterns. Therefore it is usual to *rotate*, or transform, the factors until a solution with a simpler structure is found. One of the most commonly used methods is *varimax*, although many alternatives have been proposed. Briefly, varimax attempts to minimise the number of variables that have high loadings on each factor, thereby simplifying the overall structure. Thus we hope to obtain a new set of loadings for the factors, with fewer items having high values for each factor, but with the same amount of the total variance still explained by the factors.

When there are only two factors, the pairs of factor loadings can be displayed in a scatter plot. This aids interpretation by displaying graphically the factor space and the inter-relationship of the items. Items that do not fit well into any factor can be easily identified, as can items that appear to relate to more than one factor. Multiple plots can be drawn when there are more than two factors, one for each pair of factors.

Example

If we proceed to use varimax rotation for the two-factor solution, we obtain Table 6.5 for the HADS data. To simplify the reading of Table 6.5, factor loadings above 0.4 have been shaded.

The anticipated relationships are apparent: the first factor relates to questions 2, 4, 6, (7), 8, 10, 12 and 14, while the second factor has questions 1, 3, 5, (7), 9, 11 and 13. Item 11 in Factor 2 is weaker than most other items (loading of 0.55), which corresponds to the low correlations that were noted in Table 6.2. However, most noticeable is item 7, which is included weakly in both factors. Inspecting Table 6.2 again, we see that Q_7 (fourth column in Table 6.2) has correlations above 0.4 with several depression items (Q_2, Q_4, Q_6, Q_{12} and Q_{14}), which explains its appearance in the depression factor. Apart from item Q_7, the fit may be regarded as extremely good and provides adequate confirmation of the postulated structure of the HADS. Others have found that Q_7, 'I can sit at ease and feel relaxed', is anomalous and does not appear to perform very well; it must be a candidate for revision in any future version of HADS.

Items 3 and 13 are almost overlapping, which is perhaps unsurprising given their similarity: 'I get a sort of frightened feeling as if something awful is about to happen' (item 3) and 'I get sudden feelings of panic' (13). Thus the results from factor analysis imply that one of these two items might be redundant.

Table 6.5   Rotated matrix of factor loadings from Table 6.4: varimax rotation

Variable	Factor 1	Factor 2
Q_1	0.27	0.71
Q_2	0.79	0.11
Q_3	0.19	0.78
Q_4	0.68	0.26
Q_5	0.23	0.75
Q_6	0.68	0.32
Q_7	0.49	0.50
Q_8	0.65	0.11
Q_9	0.11	0.76
Q_{10}	0.60	0.20
Q_{11}	0.07	0.54
Q_{12}	0.77	0.18
Q_{13}	0.19	0.78
Q_{14}	0.60	0.24

Example

Figure 6.3 shows the two varimax-rotated factors diagrammatically. The pairs of factor loadings of the 14 HADS items in Factor 1 and Factor 2 have been plotted against each other. The even-numbered items cluster together, demonstrating that the depression scale is coherent and contains consistent items. Most items of the anxiety scale are also clustered together, with the exception of Q_7 being closer to depression and Q_{11} being an outlier from the otherwise closely knit anxiety items.

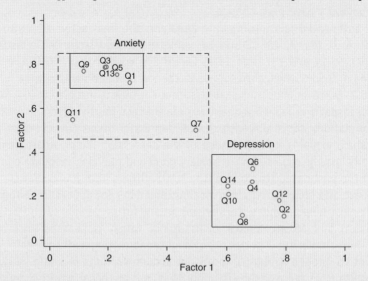

Figure 6.3   Plot of Factor 2 against Factor 1, using the rotated factors from Table 6.5.

6.6   Uses of factor analysis

Historical perspective

A useful insight into the role of factor analysis may be obtained by considering its origins; this also provides a useful background when discussing its limitations for validating QoL scales and complex PRO constructs.

Factor analysis was developed initially by Spearman around 1904 (Spearman, 1904), building upon earlier work by Karl Pearson. Spearman was interested in modelling intelligence, with a view to testing whether intelligence could be separated into two components. The first component would represent general ability, which was thought to be innate. The second component was specific ability which could vary according to subject (such as verbal skills or mathematics), and which could be influenced by education. Thus Spearman wished to show that the results from a battery of intelligence tests covering different school subjects would reveal one general factor, and that the remaining variability in the data could be explained by specific factors associated with each test. Although Spearman is commonly regarded as the father of factor analysis, over the years there has been much criticism of the way in which he used it. In particular, there has been recognition that unrotated factors almost invariably result in a model similar to that which Spearman was seeking, with the first factor being a general factor; this is an artefact of factor analysis as a statistical method, and does not serve to verify the model. Furthermore, there is now awareness that although rotation of factors is necessary it is also ill-defined, in that multiple solutions are possible. Therefore the current view of conventional factor analysis is that it is an exploratory technique, suitable for generating hypotheses about the structure of the data, and this is recognised by calling it *exploratory factor analysis* or EFA. The newer technique of *confirmatory factor analysis* (CFA) is better for testing whether a postulated model fits the data.

Another characteristic of the conceptual model underlying EFA is that intelligence tests, like most psychological tests, should follow the basic pattern shown in Figure 6.2. Hence, if the person being assessed has a high intelligence (anxiety or depression in our example), we would expect this to be reflected in corresponding high scores for each of the individual items comprising the test. Any item in the test that does *not* satisfy this requirement would, under the psychometric theory of tests, be regarded as a poor test-item and would be a candidate for removal from the questionnaire. Psychological, psychometric and educational tests are all typically constructed with the intention of measuring a few, possibly as few as one or two, subscales and contain a number of items that are expected to be homogeneous within each subscale. The HADS instrument is thus fully representative of such a test. This is rather different from many QoL instruments, which may contain a few items for each of many subscales. For example, the EORTC QLQ-C30 contains five functional scales, three symptom scales and a number of single items; furthermore, only three of the scales comprise more than two items.

Scale validation

The main objective of applying factor analysis to PRO measures is for construct validation, and two situations can be recognised. First, if there are strong preconceptions concerning the structure of the scale, factor analysis may

- confirm that the postulated number of factors are present (two in the example of the HADS)
- confirm the grouping of the items.

Secondly, when there is less certainty about the underlying model, an investigator may want to know:

- how many factors (or scales or constructs) are present
- how the individual items relate to the factors
- having identified the items that load on to each of the factors, whether this leads to definition of the substantive content or a meaning for the factors.

Scale development

Another role for factor analysis lies in the checking of new scales. An illustration of this can be seen in the example of the HADS. The intention was that seven questions related to anxiety, and seven to depression. However, as we have seen, Q_7 is associated with both scales and so perhaps the wording should be modified or a different and better-targeted item substituted. The factor analysis implies that Q_7 is as strongly associated with depression as with anxiety, and that either factor could influence the value of Q_7.

Factor analysis can also draw attention to items that appear to contribute little to their intended scale. That, too, can be seen in the HADS example. Item 11 loads relatively weakly upon the anxiety scale. This suggests that Q_{11}, 'I feel restless as if I have to be on the move', does not reflect anxiety as strongly as the other anxiety items and that a better question should be devised.

Thus factor analysis can draw attention to items that load on to more than one scale, and also to items that do not load convincingly on to any scale. It also facilitates the checking for excessively strong correlations between two or more items: if very high correlations are observed between two of the items included in one factor, it would be sensible to drop one item since all information is already contained in the other.

Scale scoring

When a scale or subscale is composed of several items, a scale score or summary statistic will be required; for example, individual patient scale scores for anxiety and depression are the natural summary from the HADS questionnaire. As we have seen, quite often a simple summated score is used, with the assumption of equal weighting being given to each item, which is perhaps a naïve way to combine items. Accordingly, various methods have been proposed for determining differential weights, and factor analysis is commonly advocated. Indeed, since factor analysis and related methods are commonly used to assess construct validity, a natural extension is to consider using the same techniques to ascribe weights to the items, based upon factor loadings. Applying the resultant weights to the observed item values results in *factor scores* for each patient, with scale scores corresponding to each factor.

Psychometricians, however, rarely use factor scores as a method of deriving outcome scores; more commonly, factor analysis is used only to identify those items that should be included in a particular factor or construct, and then either equal weights or weights derived from other investigations are used for scoring. The reason for exercising caution against using factor scores is that the scores are often neither very precise nor uniquely defined, and are affected by decisions made regarding the extraction and rotation methods. This instability is frequently described as *factor score indeterminancy*, and makes the use of factor scores from EFA controversial (for example, Grice, 2001; DiStefano *et al.*, 2009). Similar concerns affect CFA (Bollen, 1989; DiStefano *et al.*, 2009), and in addition the model specification – in particular the direction of the causality arrows (Section 6.11) – is also critical; for example, it is questionable whether pain affects the overall QoL or whether the state of a person's QoL affects their rating of pain. As found by Gundy *et al.* (2012), a variety of alternative models can provide approximately similar goodness of fit (Section 6.12), even though this implies substantial variation in their factor scores. Finally, any data-derived loadings based on one study may be inappropriate in the context of a different study drawn from another patient population. Thus, in general, we would advise against using factor analysis as anything other than a numerical process for exploring and reducing dimensionality for subsequent analyses, and we strongly caution against the use of factor loadings to compute scores.

6.7 Applying factor analysis: Choices and decisions

Factor analyses are rarely as simple and straightforward as the HADS example, in which

- there were few variables (14) and, more importantly, few factors (2)

- the postulated model was well defined and the HADS scale had been developed with each item carefully chosen to load on to one of the two factors

- the sample size was fairly large (1952 patients)

- the patients were likely to have a wide range of levels of anxiety and depression, making it easier to discern the relationships.

Thus it was a relatively easy task to obtain a convincing confirmation of the HADS scale using these data. However, the rest of this chapter explores the use of factor analysis in more detail, and discusses the range of decisions that must be made when carrying out analyses. Some of the choices can be quite crucial for obtaining a satisfactory solution.

Sample size

Sample size is important for all studies, and it has particular impact upon factor analysis. In factor analysis, where the factor structure is being explored, a small sample size will lead to large standard errors for the estimated parameters. Even more importantly, it may result in an incorrect estimation of both the number of factors and their structure. With a small sample size there will often be insufficient information to enable determination and extraction of more than one or two factors. On the other hand, with a very large sample size even trivial factors would become statistically highly significant, and so then there can be a tendency to extract too many factors. Therefore caution must be exercised in interpreting the results from large studies as well as small studies.

There is no general agreement about methods of estimating the suitable sample size. Sample size requirements will depend crucially upon the values in the between-item covariance matrix, and this is generally unknown before the study is carried out. Similarly, it will depend upon the distribution of responses to the questions, and this is likely to vary according to the population being studied and is rarely known in advance. Furthermore, many QoL items and PRO measures may be non-Normally distributed and strongly asymmetric, with high frequencies of subjects either reporting 'no difficulty' or 'very great difficulty' for individual items, thereby making simple approximations based upon Normal distributions of little practical relevance.

When the distribution of the variables and their correlation matrix is known or can be hypothesised, it is possible to carry out computer-based simulation studies to evaluate the effect of different sample sizes (Muthén and Muthén, 2002). Although some such studies have been reported, many have been for models with few factors, Normally distributed variables and simple correlation structures.

Many authors have provided conflicting recommendations and rules-of-thumb. Recommendations for the minimum number of subjects have ranged from 100 to 400 or more. Others have suggested five or 10 times the number of observed variables. Various functions of the number of factors and observed variables have also been proposed – for example, Kline (2010) suggests that, in the context of confirmatory factor analysis, 10 or even 20 observations per estimated parameter seem appropriate, where the number of identifiable parameters is, for the simplest of models encompassing k items, $N_p = k \times (k + 1)/2$. There is little theoretical basis for most of these rules. In addition, if the variables have low reliabilities or the inter-relationships are weak, then many more individuals will be needed.

Although these problems may make sample size estimation appear impractical, inadequate sample size has clearly been a problem in many studies, even though this is often appreciated only with hindsight either upon completion of the study or when other investigators report conflicting factor analysis results. Thus sample size calculations cannot be simply dismissed. The best advice is to be conservative and aim for large-sized studies. QoL scales frequently have five or more factors, and perhaps contain 30 or more items with few items per factor. The items are often discrete and form highly skewed scales with floor or ceiling effects. Then it seems likely that a minimum of a few hundred patients is required, and ideally there should be many hundreds.

Number of factors

The first step in factor analysis is to determine the number of factors that are to be extracted. This is one of the more important decisions to be made since a totally different and erroneous factor structure may be estimated if an incorrect number of factors is used. If too many, or too few, factors are mistakenly entered into the model, the analyses can yield solutions that are extremely difficult to interpret. On the other hand, it is frequently possible to ascribe plausible meanings to many combinations of variables, and it can be very difficult to identify whether factors are meaningful and which models are likely to be correct. Therefore much research has been carried out into methods for deciding the number of factors that are present.

One of the oldest and most widely used approaches is the Kaiser (1960) rule *eigenvalues greater than one*, as used in our example. Probably one (not very sound) reason for its near-universal application in computer packages is the simplicity of the method. Various foundations have been proposed for this rule, such as noting that the average eigenvalue is 1.0 and so the rule excludes all eigenvalues below the average. On the other hand, if there are 10 variables this rule will include factors that explain at least 10% of the variance, but if there were 50 variables then factors explaining as little as 2% would be retained. In general, this rule tends to include too many factors.

Another widely used method is the *scree plot*, which is simply a plot of successive eigenvalues (Cattell, 1966). The scree plot is fairly good at separating the important factors from the later 'factors', which are really little more than random noise; the scree is the random rubble of stones at the foot of the cliff face. Although interpretation of scree plots is subjective, frequently, as in Figure 6.4, a change in slope is fairly evident.

A third widely used method for estimating the number of factors is based upon *maximum-likelihood* (ML) estimation, although it has also been shown that for this purpose ML factor analysis is quite sensitive to the variability in the data ('residual' variance) and requires large sample sizes to yield reliable estimates. In our example, ML estimation produced closely similar results to the STATA default *principal-factor* estimates of Table 6.4, and successfully identified the two-factor solution.

Example

Figure 6.4 shows the scree plot for the HADS dataset, corresponding to the eigenvalues of Table 6.3. There is a clear elbow in the plot, with the first two factors lying above the sloping line formed by the eigenvalues for factors 3 to 14. This implies that a two-factor solution is appropriate. This conclusion is also in agreement with the eigenvalues-greater-than-one rule, as indicated by the horizontal straight line.

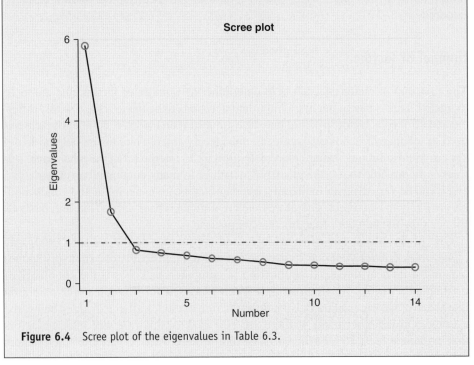

Figure 6.4   Scree plot of the eigenvalues in Table 6.3.

Despite reservations, in practice both the eigenvalues-greater-than-one rule and the scree plot seem to have reasonable characteristics. When the same number of factors is suggested by all three methods, as in this example, the solution is quite convincing.

Method of estimation

A variety of methods are available for estimating the factors, all leading to different solutions. Most statistical packages offer at least five or six methods for factor extraction. The only thing in common with all estimation procedures is that they define some arbitrary measure of goodness-of-fit, which is then maximised (or, if a measure of deviation from fit is used, minimised). Methods commonly used include ML, which produces estimates that are most likely to have yielded the observed correlation matrix under assumptions of Normal distributions. *Unweighted least squares* minimises the sum of the squared differences between the observed and model-predicted correlation matrices. *Alpha factoring* maximises the Cronbach's α reliability of the factors, so that (for example) the first factor has the maximum reliability or internal consistency. *Principal-axes factoring* maximises the accounted-for variance. *Minimum-residual factoring* minimises the off-diagonal residuals of the total variance–covariance matrix. Many further methods also exist, each with their proponents.

When the data possess a strongly defined factor structure, theoretical and empirical studies suggest that most methods of extraction will yield similar results. However, in other situations there may be considerable divergence in the factor solutions, especially when there are small sample sizes, few explanatory variables and a weak factor structure.

Statisticians generally prefer ML because it is based upon sound mathematical theory that is widely applicable to many situations. ML estimation also provides foundations for hypothesis testing, including tests for the number of factors. Furthermore, unlike other methods, ML yields the same results whether a correlation matrix or a covariance matrix is factored. Although it is commonly thought to be a disadvantage that ML estimation explicitly assumes that the sample is from a multivariate Normal distribution, ML estimation of factor structure is fairly robust against departures from Normality. However, under non-Normality the significance tests will be invalid; violation of the distributional assumptions can reduce ML to being no better than other techniques. Overall, we recommend ML estimation as the preferred method.

The role of the factor estimation step is to find an initial solution, which can then be rotated to provide a simpler structure. Although the initial factor estimates may appear to vary considerably according to the method used, it is often found that similar results are obtained after rotation, no matter which method of factor estimation was used.

Orthogonal rotation

Since there is no unique solution for the factor decomposition of a dataset, it is conventional to adopt an arbitrary procedure for rotation such that as many as possible of the items contribute to single factors. In other words, the aim of rotation is to simplify the initial factorisation, obtaining a solution that keeps as many variables and factors distinct from one another as possible. Thus rotation is an essential part of the factor analysis method, as the initial factor solution is frequently uninterpretable. The simplest rotations are *orthogonal*, which assumes that the underlying factors are not correlated with each other, and of these *varimax* is the most widely used and generally appears to yield sensible solutions. In mathematical terms, varimax aims to maximise the variance of the squared loadings of variables in each factor, and thus minimises the number of high loadings associated with each factor. In practical terms, varimax results in a 'simple' factor decomposition, because each factor will include the smallest possible number of explanatory variables. If there are preconceived ideas about the factor structure, it may be more appropriate to use goodness-of-fit tests to examine specific hypotheses, but for exploratory analysis the apparent simplicity and the sensible results following varimax have led to its near universal implementation in all computer packages.

However, many other methods do exist, most notably quartimax, which attempts to simplify the factor loadings associated with each variable (instead of the variable loadings associated with each factor). Orthomax and equamax are yet two other methods, and combine properties of both quartimax and varimax. If you are not satisfied with the arbitrary choice of varimax, there are plenty of alternatives.

Oblique axes

One assumption built into the model so far is that the factors are orthogonal and uncorrelated with each other. In many cases that is an unrealistic assumption. For example, there is a tendency for seriously ill patients to suffer from both anxiety and depression, and these two factors will be correlated. In statistical terms, we should allow *oblique axes* instead of insisting upon orthogonality. This leads to a whole set of other rotation methods and Gorsuch (1983) lists a total of 19 orthogonal and oblique methods out of the many that are available. Most statistics packages offer a variety of these methods. Unfortunately, different procedures can result in appreciably different solutions unless the underlying structure of the data happens to be particularly clear and simple.

Promax, which is derived from varimax, is the most frequently recommended oblique rotation method. Starting from the varimax solution, promax attempts to make the low variable loadings even lower by relaxing the assumption that factors should be uncorrelated with each other; therefore it results in an even simpler structure in terms of variable loadings on to factors. Promax is therefore simple in concept and results in simple factor structures. Not surprisingly, given its nature, promax usually results in similar – but simpler – factors to those derived by varimax. The most widely used alternative to promax is oblimin, which is a generalisation of earlier procedures called quartimin, covarimin and biquartimin; these all attempt to minimise various covariance functions.

As with so much of exploratory factor analysis, it is difficult – and controversial – to make recommendations regarding the choice of method. One procedure of desperation is to apply several rotational procedures to each of two random halves of the total pool of individuals; it is reassuring if different rotational procedures result in the same factors, and if these same factors appear in both random halves. In other words, rotation is a necessary part of the exploratory factor analysis procedure, but one should be cautious and circumspect whenever using rotation.

Example

Table 6.5 showed the effect of a varimax rotation, which revealed the two factors postulated to underlie the HADS questionnaire. However, as shown in Figure 6.2, it has been suggested that the anxiety and depression factors would be correlated. Therefore an oblique rotation is perhaps more appropriate. Table 6.6 shows the effect of oblique rotation using promax.

In this example, the strong factor structure of the HADS prevailed, and the oblique rotation yielded similar solutions to the varimax rotation. The negative signs attached to Factor 1 of the promax solution are immaterial, and reflect the arbitrary viewpoint from which the factors may be observed in geometrical space; the important features are the magnitudes of the loadings and the relative signs of the loadings within each factor. Perhaps the most noticeable difference from the varimax results in Table 6.5 is that the loading of variable 7 in Factor 1 has been reduced from 0.70 to 0.49, yet again emphasising that this variable does not perform satisfactorily.

Table 6.6   Oblique (promax) rotation of the factor loadings from Table 6.4

Variable	Factor 1	Factor 2
Q_1	−0.10	0.70
Q_2	−0.85	−0.11
Q_3	0.00	0.81
Q_4	−0.68	0.08
Q_5	−0.05	0.76
Q_6	−0.67	0.15
Q_7	−0.41	0.40
Q_8	−0.69	−0.07
Q_9	0.07	0.81
Q_{10}	−0.61	0.04
Q_{11}	0.06	0.58
Q_{12}	−0.81	−0.03
Q_{13}	−0.00	0.81
Q_{14}	−0.60	0.09

6.8   Assumptions for factor analysis

As with any statistical modelling technique, various assumptions are built into the factor analysis model and the associated estimation procedures. In many fields of research these assumptions may well be valid, but in the context of PRO measures there can be a number of problems arising from the frequently gross violation of the inherent assumptions.

Distributional assumptions

The standard factor analysis model makes no special assumptions about data being continuous and from a Normal distribution. Since the commonly used estimation procedures are based upon either ML or *least squares*, they assume continuous data from a Normal distribution. Furthermore, most methods of estimation of factors are based upon the Pearson product-moment correlation matrix (or, equivalently, the covariance matrix) with Normally distributed error structure. If these distributional assumptions are violated, any test for goodness-of-fit may be compromised. However, goodness-of-fit measures are central to ML factor analysis in order to determine the number of factors to be retained, and as noted above this number is crucial to the subsequent extraction of the factor loadings.

In reporting studies, it is important to specify the software that was used as well as the model and the methods of the fitting and rotation of factors. Although some published reports of QoL studies do indicate the software or model used, few discuss distributional properties of their data such as whether it is continuous and Normally distributed. Presumably the authors are unaware of the importance of these assumptions.

The two main types of departure from assumptions are that data may be discrete, possibly with only a few categories, or may be continuous but non-Normally distributed (e.g. highly asymmetrical or *skewed*). Many PRO measures are both categorical and highly asymmetrical at the same time.

Categorical data

Although a few QoL instruments use linear analogue scales, by far the majority contain questions taking discrete ordinal responses, commonly with as few as four or five categories. Mathematical theory for factor analysis of categorical data has been developed by, for example, Lee *et al.* (1995) and Bartholomew *et al.* (2011), and software is becoming widely available (e.g. Muthén and Muthén, 2010). However, this is largely an untested and unexplored area, and it remains unclear as to how effectively these techniques will be able to estimate the underlying latent structure and what sample sizes will be required in order to obtain stable and consistent estimation of factors.

Since many investigators use standard factor analysis even when they have four- or five-point scales, one should at least consider the effect of this violation of the assumptions. How robust is factor analysis? A few reports, based upon experience or computer simulations, have claimed that scales with as few as five points yield stable factors. However, it remains unclear whether factor analysis using Pearson's correlation coefficient is adequate provided the five-point scale can be regarded as arising from an underlying Normal distribution with cut-points. Furthermore, the situation regarding four-point scales remains even more dubious. At one extreme, it has been suggested that correlations are fairly robust and that even ordinal scales with at least three points can be included, but this has not been supported by others who generally recommend a minimum of five response categories. It also seems likely that sample size should be increased so as to compensate for the loss of information in shorter scales.

Since the numerical solution of factor analysis uses the correlation (or sometimes the covariance) matrix, it is natural to consider techniques intended for estimating correlations based upon discrete ordinal data. *Polychoric correlations* are formed by assuming that the discrete categorical observed values are a manifestation of data with an underlying (Normal) continuous distribution (see Section 5.3). The mathematical theory leads to relatively complex estimation procedures, but computer algorithms for their estimation are available. Few studies have made use of such methods, and again there are fears about the effect upon sample size. It is best to be very cautious about applying them to samples of fewer than 500–1000 observations.

Normality

We have commented on the effect of non-Normality upon ML estimation, but it can also prejudice other aspects of factor analysis. However, there are two reasons for anticipating highly non-Normal data in QoL research. Firstly, there is no reason to assume that categories labelled 'Not at all', 'A little', 'Quite a bit' and 'Very much' will yield equal-interval scales for patients' responses to any or all of the questions. Secondly, some of the items are likely to take extreme values depending upon the disease or the effects of its treatment. For example, cancer patients receiving certain forms of chemotherapy will almost invariably experience considerable nausea. Hence, for these patients, items such as nausea will have a highly asymmetric distribution with a ceiling effect of many responses towards 'Very much'. Thus QoL and PRO items frequently possess highly skewed non-Normal distributions. Unfortunately, little work has been done on the impact of this.

Example

Figure 6.5 shows the HADS data from cancer trials of the MRC, where many items are markedly skewed and no items appear to have Normal distributions. Several items also suffer from floor effects and tend to take minimum values for most patients, notably items Q_4, Q_6, Q_{10} and Q_{14}, and all items except Q_8 have very few patients with high responses.

Many other QoL scales may be expected similarly to contain items that deviate markedly regarding Normality.

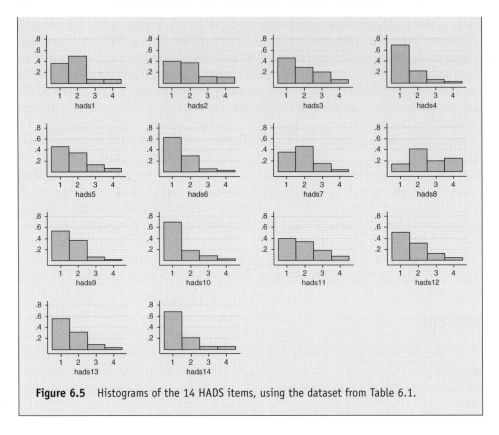

Figure 6.5   Histograms of the 14 HADS items, using the dataset from Table 6.1.

There have been attempts to develop so-called *asymptotically distribution-free* (ADF) factor analysis that makes no assumptions about the distribution of the data (for example Bartholomew *et al.*, 2011). However, results suggest that huge sample sizes may be necessary for acceptable performance – for example ADF on 15 variables with three 'strong' factors may require samples of between 2500 and 5000 observations.

Example from the literature

When Muthén and Kaplan (1992) simulated five-point variables of various degrees of skewness for four models (2–4 factors, 6–15 variables), with 500 and 1000 observations they found "Chi-squared tests and standard errors ... are not as robust to non-Normality as previously believed. ADF does not appear to work well."

Does the violation of assumptions matter?

Since most models for factor analysis assume continuous data with Normally distributed error terms, while many PROs depart substantially from this by being both categorical and non-Normal, what is the overall impact? The effect of these violations of assumptions is largely unknown, although empirical results and simulation studies suggest that the techniques may be relatively robust to reasonable degrees of departures. However, it seems likely that sample size, which in QoL studies is sometimes small by any standards, should be increased so as to compensate for this. As already noted for ML estimation, it is commonly found in practice that departures from Normality may have a marked effect upon testing goodness-of-fit and the estimation of the number of factors, but has rather less impact upon the factor extraction.

Unfortunately there is no simple rule of thumb to decide when ML estimation may be applied. Any sign of appreciable deviation from Normality will be claimed by critics as making analysis invalid, yet will be dismissed by the authors as of little consequence.

6.9   Factor analysis in QoL research

Given all the attendant problems and difficulties, it is perhaps surprising that factor analysis of QoL instruments so often results in apparently sensible factors. However, this may be simply a reflection of the strong and obvious correlation structure that underlies many 'constructs'; often the results, not surprisingly, confirm the expected QoL dimensions. Thus, provided there is adequate sample size, many studies do report finding factors that represent groupings of variables that could have been anticipated a priori to be correlated. However, many authors do also report major discrepancies in the factor structure when they repeat analyses with different datasets.

Example

Fayers and Hand (1997a) reviewed publications concerning seven studies reporting factor analysis of the RSCL. All publications agreed that the first factor represents general psychological distress and contains a broad average of the psychological items, and that other factors were combinations of various physical symptoms and side effects. However, there was considerable divergence about the details of the physical factors, with studies claiming to find two, four, five, seven or even nine factors. Several authors acknowledged that the extracted factors were curious and not easy to interpret. For example, one study combined dizziness, shivering, sore mouth and abdominal aches as a factor.

Instability of factors, especially after the first one or two factors have been extracted, is evidently a problem. Contributory reasons include the following:

1. Some variables have weak inter-correlations. This may occur because the underlying relationship really is weak, or because in a particular dataset the observed correlations are weak.

2. Some studies may be under-sized. This will tend to result in unreliable estimation of the number of factors, and in poor estimation of the factor structure.

3. Some studies may be so large that, if care is not exercised, too many factors will be identified because with very large numbers of measurements even weak inter-correlations will suffice to pull a few variables together into a less meaningful factor.

4. Different sets of data may yield different factor structures. For example, in a cancer clinical trial the chemotherapy patients may experience both nausea and hair loss, with these items appearing strongly correlated. In contrast, in a hormone therapy trial, the same items could be relatively uncorrelated. Thus they would form a single factor in the first study but would appear unrelated in the second. Factors for symptoms and side effects can vary in different subsets of patients and, for example in oncology, can depend upon site of cancer, disease stage, treatment modality, patients' gender and age.

5. Heterogeneous samples may yield strange factors. In a clinical trial comparing different treatment modalities, for example, factor analyses may produce factors that are essentially group differences (see the example in Section 6.10). These factors are non-obvious, difficult to interpret, and not consistent with the expectations of the latent structure. If it is known that there are separate subgroups, one possibility is to use the within-group correlation matrix of each subgroup and combine these to provide 'pooled within-group' estimates for the analyses.

6. Some symptoms may be uncorrelated and yet contribute to the same scale. For example, it might be thought clinically logical to regard eating problems as part of a single scale, even though some patients (e.g. with head and neck cancer) may be unable to eat because of an oral problem, while others (with oesophageal cancer) may be unable to swallow because of throat obstruction. A serious limitation with respect to either item can have a major impact upon the patient's eating, social functioning and QoL. Thus although the correlation between these two items might be low, for many purposes it could be appropriate to combine them into a single scale.

6.10   Limitations of correlation-based analysis

The reasons listed in the previous Section 6.9 are mainly a reflection of the fact that factor analysis is solely based on an examination of the correlation-structure of the observed data. Thus it is misleading to think of 'factors' as necessarily reflecting dimensions of QoL. Factors are merely groups of items that correlate more highly within themselves than with other items.

A particularly common example of misleading factors can be found whenever symptoms or side effects are included – as is commonly the case with disease-specific questionnaires. Clinicians recognise these groups of highly correlated symptoms: a *syndrome* is defined as 'a group of concurrent symptoms of a disease; a characteristic combination of emotions, behaviours, etc.' We should not be surprised if factor analysis identifies these syndromes, as it is an ideal statistical tool for doing so. But although the cluster of symptoms comprising a syndrome may be characteristic of the disease process, the symptoms may be unrelated in terms of their impact on QoL and need not necessarily form a logical dimension or QoL construct. The example in Section 6.11 illustrates these issues with a cluster of side effects that are typical of a particular treatment.

Nor do correlations between symptoms indicate that they are equally important in their impact on QoL; correlations merely tell us that patients with one severe symptom are also likely to experience the other symptoms severely, too. Factor analysis of symptoms and side effects can frequently be misleading. In Section 6.11 we explain how it *may* be possible to extend the basic factor analysis model to allow for these issues.

6.11   Formative or causal models

The models described so far have all been based upon the assumption that QoL scales can be represented as in Figure 6.2, with observed variables that reflect the value of the latent variable. For example, in the HADS, presence of anxiety is expected to be manifested by high levels of Q_1, Q_3, Q_5, Q_7, Q_9, Q_{11} and Q_{13}. However, many QoL instruments include a large number of PRO measures covering diverse aspects. For example, the RSCL includes 30 items relating to general QoL, symptoms and side effects; it also incorporates an activity scale and a global question about overall QoL. For simplicity, we restrict consideration to 17 items. Adopting a conventional EFA model, a path diagram such as that of Figure 6.6 might be considered.

This model assumes that a poor QoL is likely to be manifested by psychological distress, and that 'psychological distress' is a latent variable that tends to result in anxiety, depression, despair, irritability and similar signs of distress. This much does seem a plausible model. However, a patient with poor QoL need not necessarily have high levels of all treatment-related symptoms. For example, a patient receiving chemotherapy may well suffer from hair loss, nausea, vomiting and other treatment-related side effects that cause deterioration in QoL. However, other cancer patients receiving non-chemotherapy treatments could be suffering from a completely different set of symptoms and side effects that cause poor QoL for other reasons.

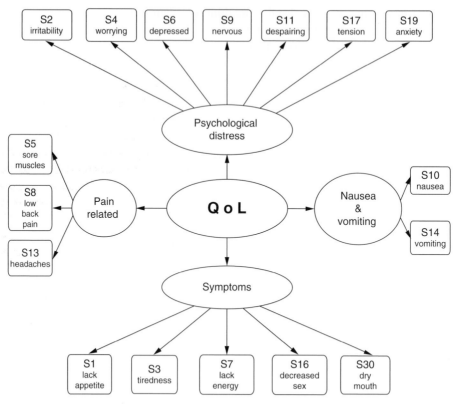

Figure 6.6 Conventional EFA model for the RSCL, showing factors for general psychological distress, pain, nausea/vomiting and symptoms/side-effects. Only 17 out of the 30 items on the main RSCL are shown.

Thus a poor QoL does not necessarily imply that, say, a patient is probably experiencing nausea; this is in contrast to the psychological distress indicators, all of which may well be affected if the patient experiences distress because of their condition. On the other hand, if a patient *does* have severe nausea, that is likely to result in – or cause – a diminished QoL. Hence a more realistic model is as in Figure 6.7, where symptoms and side effects are shown as *causal indicators* with the directional arrows pointing from the observed variables towards the 'symptoms and side effects' factor, which in turn causes changes in QoL. The observed items reflecting psychological distress are called *effect indicators*, to distinguish them from the causal indicators. Thus effect indicators can provide a measure of the QoL experienced by patients, while the causal indicators affect or influence patients' QoL.

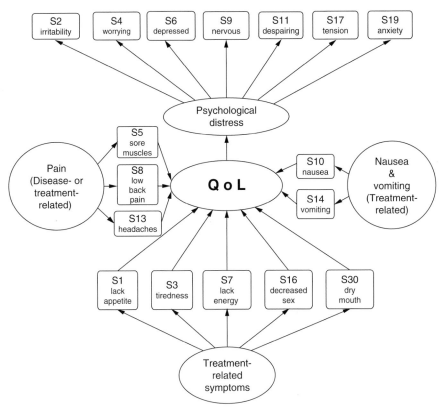

Figure 6.7 Postulated causal structure for 17 items on the RSCL. Treatment- or disease-related symptoms and side-effects may be causal rather than effect indicators.

Example from the literature

Fayers and Hand (1997a) analysed RSCL data from an MRC trial of chemotherapy with or without α-interferon for patients with advanced colorectal cancer. There appeared to be four factors, representing psychological distress, symptoms, nausea and vomiting, and pains and aches. At first sight the second factor, labelled 'symptoms', contained a strange combination of items: lack of appetite, decreased sexual interest, dry mouth, tiredness and lack of energy. However, these five symptoms were precisely the items that the study team had reported as the main treatment differences in the randomised trial. In other words, the second factor is an interferon-related cluster of symptoms, and the item correlations arise from treatment differences and not through any sense of this necessarily being a single meaningful QoL construct.

6.12 Confirmatory factor analysis and structural equation modelling

EFA is ill equipped to deal with causal variables. Instead, a more general approach has to be considered, with models that can represent structures such as those of Figure 6.7 and can estimate the coefficients and parameters describing the various paths. This approach is *structural equation modelling* (SEM). SEM models can be complex to specify. Some programs for SEM modelling are listed at the end of this chapter (Section 6.20), but SEM is also becoming widely available in many statistical packages. Although SEM is problematic for purely causal models, it is possible to obtain estimates for some models in which there is a combination of reflective and causal indicators, the so-called multiple indicator–multiple cause, or MIMIC, models.

One major difference between EFA and SEM is the emphasis that the latter places upon prior specification of the postulated structure. Thus one form of SEM is also known as *confirmatory factor analysis*, since a factor-analytic structure is pre-specified and one major purpose of the modelling is to test – or confirm – how well the data fit this hypothesised structure. Hence CFA focuses on goodness-of-fit tests, with the model being accepted as adequate provided there is no strong counter-evidence against it. Although such techniques have been widely used in areas such as educational and personality testing, they are as yet little practised in the field of QoL. However, given the many disadvantages associated with EFA, it should be apparent that SEM is likely to be a far more appropriate approach. Despite this, it must still be emphasised that many of the problems remain unresolved for SEM just as much as for EFA. In particular, criteria for goodness-of-fit are controversial, categorical data are hard to handle, non-Normality of data remains a major issue since Normality underpins most of the goodness-of-fit measures, and sample size is difficult to estimate in advance of carrying out the study.

Example from the literature

De Vet *et al.* (2005) carried out a systematic review of the use of factor analysis for validation of the SF-36. Twenty-eight studies were identified. In 15 of these studies – over half – EFA had been used when the appropriate method should have been CFA.

Although SEM is suitable for fitting causal models, it often cannot distinguish between causal and non-causal models; both may be found to provide a seemingly adequate fit to the dataset. This is because the underlying models that are appropriate for representing QoL constructs are rarely of sufficiently clear forms that enable SEM to reject the non-causal version while conclusively accepting the causal model as preferable. Thus SEM can rarely be used for inferring causality of individual QoL items.

Example from the literature

Gundy *et al.* (2012) explored the fit of seven alternative measurement models for the EORTC QLQ-C30. Data were obtained from 4,541 patients with cancers of various sites and with stages from early disease to advanced metastatic cancer. They suggested that the PhysicalHealth/MentalHealth model of Figure 6.8 seemed on balance to be the most promising, while acknowledging that the superiority of this model is "modest, and it remains to be seen whether its extra complexity – as compared to e.g., the simple HRQoL model – provides tangible (clinical) benefits".

In this model Physical and Mental health are two higher-order factors, with QLQ-C3 items 1 to 27 reflecting aspects of either or both of these higher-order factors. QoL is reflected by items 29 and 30, the two global items. QoL can also affect or be affected by Physical or Mental health.

One might speculate that Physical health would be affected by symptoms such as pain, nausea and vomiting, fatigue, constipation and dyspnoea, resulting in a causal model with arrows from the items to 'Physical' in Figure 6.8. However, Gundy *et al.* found no evidence of better fit for such a model.

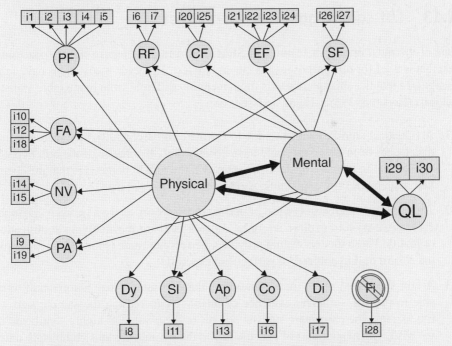

Figure 6.8 A PhysicalHealth/MentalHealth structural model for the EORTC QLQ-C30. *Source:* Gundy *et al.*, 2012, Figure 1(b). CC BY-NC 2.0 (http://creativecommons. org/licenses/by-nc/2.0/uk/). Reproduced commercially with permission of Springer Science+Business Media.

One of the largest hurdles for SEM in QoL research is that many models will inevitably be complex. For example, *feedback* mechanisms may be present, with many variables being a mixture of causal and effect indicators: difficulty sleeping may cause reduced QoL, which may in turn cause anxiety, which causes further sleeping problems and so further affects QoL. Diagrams such as Figure 6.6 and Figure 6.7 are a simplification of reality. In addition, it may be impossible with data from ordinary QoL studies to distinguish between alternative models: when variables can be both effect and causal simultaneously, there are estimation problems and sometimes the solutions cannot be determined uniquely. Many alternative models may all fit the observed data more-or-less equally well. In many cases this might be anticipated from the scale development process. Items that are highly correlated, whether causal or indicator items, most commonly form conceptually logical clusters – except in rare cases such as toxic side effects due to specific treatments, as illustrated in the examples above. More frequent problems can arise with formative items, as in the example in Section 5.7, where disease-related pain was assessed using weakly correlated items representing pain in each of the relevant locations; EFA and related techniques will interpret the low item-item correlations as indicating multiple factors.

6.13   Chi-square goodness-of-fit test

One of the most important features of SEM is testing goodness of fit. The statistical test that is used for this purpose is the chi-square test. However, statisticians have long recognised that the chi-square test is fundamentally different from many other statistical tests (Berkson, 1938). The main issues are:

1. A statistical significance test aims to estimate the probability that such extreme data as has been observed could have arisen purely by chance, if the null hypothesis is true. In the case of the chi-square test, the null hypothesis is that the specified model will fully explain the patterns in the observed data.

2. Thus the chi-square test is a test of perfect fit. However, as we have seen, the models that we wish to explore are only 'models' and are inevitably a simplification of reality. These models cannot provide a perfect fit. There is little point in testing the absurd null hypothesis of perfect and exact fit.

3. A non-significant result merely indicates that the sample size is too small to be able to provide sufficient evidence of misfit. By increasing the sample size we can increase the chi-square statistic and make the *p*-value as highly significant as we wish. The magnitudes of chi square and the *p*-value are thus completely uninformative.

4. As Berkson observed in 1938, what is the point of applying a chi-square test to a moderate or small sample if we already know that a large sample would show *p* highly significant?

5. A measure or index of model adequacy, or 'goodness of fit', is only valid if its magnitude is independent of sample size. If a model provides good (or poor) fit, the same measured level of fit should be found irrespective of the size of the sample. Chi-square is not a valid measure of goodness of fit.

6. As Berkson noted, the name 'Chi-square goodness-of-fit test' is misleading. It is a test of perfect fit, not adequacy or goodness.

7. Many of the problems associated with the chi-square test arise because we usually hope to accept the null hypothesis, as that would imply we have a model with adequate fit. However, most significance tests aim to reject the null hypothesis, thereby establishing that an effect is present. The chi-square test is arguably analogous to an equivalence test, as for example when comparing two treatments with the intention of establishing equivalence. In that setting, we usually start by defining a threshold below which we are willing to accept non-inferiority of the new treatment. Applying similar logic to testing adequacy of structural models, what we need is a prespecified goodness-of-fit threshold that indicates adequate fit to the model. For that, we require a goodness-of-fit index.

In summary, the chi-square test cannot be recommended as an indicator for or against good or adequate fit. A model may show statistically significant evidence of misfit, yet still be a useful and practical simplification of reality. Alternatively, if a model does not show significant evidence of misfit, we can only conclude that the sample size is too small.

Example from the literature

Use of the chi-square test continues to cause controversy. Gundy *et al.* (2012) found that none of the models they examined passed the stringent chi-square test of model fit ($p < 0.001$ for all models), indicating that none of these models captured all of the systematic variation in the data. They noted, however, that with 4,541 observations, a chi-square test is quite sensitive to detecting even the smallest of deviations. Using a number of goodness-of-fit indices, they decided that all of their models "demonstrated at least an 'adequate' approximation to the data". This provoked a commentary from McIntosh (2012), who cited a comment from Karl Joreskög: "the chi-square is all you really need". In their response, Fayers and Aaronson (2012) used the points listed above, and also noted that another (anonymous) reviewer had written "I'm glad you report the *df* and chi-square in Table 2, but please stop talking about it as a measure of fit. It is useless as such with the *N* that you have".

Thus the controversy about the appropriate goodness-of-fit measures was clearly in evidence in the reviews of the manuscript. Gundy *et al.* decided to report both chi-square and a variety of other approximate goodness of fit indices, but largely ignored the chi-square statistics and the corresponding *p*-values.

6.14   Approximate goodness-of-fit indices

Instead of using chi-square, conclusions should be based largely upon the magnitude of approximate goodness-of-fit indices, known as AGFIs. These are less sensitive to sample size. Unfortunately, many goodness-of-fit indices have been proposed, each with varying properties, and it is difficult to make a specific recommendation. We list a few of the more commonly used indices and thresholds (Kline, 2010; Browne and Cudeck, 1992; Hu and Bentler, 1999).

Comparative Fit Index (*CFI*) ranges from 0 (poor fit) to 1 (perfect fit), and is derived by comparing the chi-squares of a baseline (null) model against the target model. Values of *CFI* > 0.95 are commonly taken to indicate good fit, and values > 0.90 indicate acceptable fit. Some authors advocate more stringent 0.97 and 0.95 respectively.

The Tucker–Lewis Index (*TLI*), also known as the Non-normed fit index (*NNFI*) also measures relative fit of the model chi-squares, and similar thresholds to the *CFI* are commonly used. It is little affected by sample size, and has performed well in simulation studies.

The Goodness of Fit Index (*GFI*) uses a ratio of chi-squares to calculate the proportion of variance that is accounted for by the estimated population covariance matrix. It usually ranges from zero and one, with *GFI* > 0.95 indicating good fit, and *GFI* > 0.90 for acceptable fit.

Root Mean Square Error of Approximation (*RMSEA*) measures the discrepancy between the observed and model-implied covariance matrices, adjusted for degrees of freedom. It is an assessment of approximate fit to the population covariance matrix. A commonly used rule of thumb is that a *RMSEA* < 0.05 indicates close fit, while values between 0.05 and 0.10 indicate acceptable fit, and values > 0.10 indicate poor approximate fit. Confidence intervals can be calculated for *RMSEA*.

The Standardised Root Mean Square Residual (*SRMR*) is an overall badness-of-fit measure that is based on the fitted residuals, where the *residuals* are the differences between the observed values and those estimated by fitting the model. Thus, zero indicates perfect fit. An *SRMR* < 0.05 indicates good fit although it is not independent of sample size and so must be interpreted with caution.

Hu and Bentler (1999) have suggested a two-index presentation format. This always includes the *SRMR*, with one of the *NNFI* (*TLI*), *CFI*, *RMSEA* or a couple of others (not described here). Hu and Bentler also discuss the use of other thresholds for acceptable fit. Both the indices and the thresholds to be used must be prespecified in a protocol before any analyses are made. In the case of inadequate model fit, residuals and modification indices can be examined in order to detect possible causes. However, Barrett (2007) argues persuasively against the use of AGFIs, citing a number of examples that demonstrate the problems that can arise; a number of companion articles were published simultaneously, debating the quandary that this presents for SEM. Despite the controversial problems, most researchers continue to apply the recommendations of Hu and Bentler (1999), while regarding the thresholds as guidelines, not strict cut-offs, and assessing model fit on the indices collectively.

6.15   Comparative fit of models

So far we have assumed a single hypothetical model is being fitted to the data. In many cases, as in the example above, a number of models are proposed and the objective is to select the model that provides the best adequate fit. In such a case it makes sense to test whether there is sufficient evidence to claim one model superior to another; if there is no statistically significant difference, we must accept that there is a lack of evidence to support claims of model superiority. On the other hand, as with any statistical significance test, a significant p-value indicates that there is evidence supporting a claim of model superiority but provides no indication of the magnitude of the difference. For that, we must again resort to AGFIs.

The chi-square difference test is most commonly used for testing between two models. This is only valid if the models are nested, in the sense that the more complex model is the same as the simpler model but with additional constraints. For comparing goodness of fit, the AGFIs described above can be compared for the two or more models. In addition, the Akaike Information Criterion (*AIC*) is sometimes used (Burnham and Anderson, 2004). The *AIC* adjusts the chi-square value for the number of estimated parameters, and is a criterion for badness of fit. Publications commonly cite the *AIC* and *GFI* or variants of these indices. Differences greater than 0.01 between pairs of *TLIs*, *CFIs* or *RMSEAs* are typically considered to be substantial enough to merit attention (Cheung and Rensvold, 2002).

Example from the literature

Gundy *et al.* (2012) grouped their seven postulated models into three 'branches' of nested models, and presented a table of chi-square tests for each branch. In addition, they compared *CFI*, *TLI* and *RMSEA* for each model (Table 6.7). The PhysicalHealth/MentalHealth model was 'slightly' superior to the other models, although as noted above it remains unclear whether the differences are large enough to provide tangible clinical benefits.

Table 6.7   Tests of fit and approximate goodness-of-fit indices for various structural models of the EORTC QLQ-C30

Model	Chi-square*	df	CFI	TLI	RMSEA
1. 'Standard' Model	134	15	0.96	0.98	0.042
2. Physical Health, Mental Health, & QL	234	19	0.92	0.98	0.050
3. Physical Burden, Mental Function, & QL	248	18	0.92	0.97	0.053
4. Symptom Burden, Function, & QL	294	18	0.90	0.97	0.058
5. HRQL & QL	297	18	0.90	0.97	0.058
6. Formative Symptom Burden (free weights), Function, & QL	277	17	0.91	0.97	0.058
7. Formative Symptom Burden (fixed weights), Function, & QL	300	17	0.90	0.96	0.061

*All chi-square tests of model fit were significant at p < 0.001.
Source: Gundy *et al.*, 2012, Table 2. CC BY-NC 2.0 (http://creativecommons.org/licenses/by-nc/2.0/uk/). Reproduced commercially with permission of Springer Science+Business Media.

6.16   Difficulty-factors

Some scales contain items of varying difficulty or severity. For example, we have illustrated the physical functioning scale of the EORTC QLQ-C30, which in Section 3.8 we described as hierarchical or Guttman scale. Such scales, especially when formed by categorical items that have a limited range of response options – as is frequently the case when assessing PROs – can present problems for EFA and other analyses based on correlations (Ferguson, 1941). Consider a characteristic mobility scale: items such as run a long distance or carry heavy loads are aimed at discriminating between high performance patients, and these patients will presumably nearly all respond to items about standing up or getting out of bed using the single category 'no problem at all'. Conversely, the majority of those patients with very low performance are likely to choose the category 'not at all' for ability to run a long distance or carry heavy loads. Thus the most and least difficult items will have weak correlation with each other, largely because of attenuation caused by the coarseness of the categories. This is prone to result in EFA mistakenly identifying two distinct *difficulty-factors*: one scale (factor) for high-mobility items and another for low-mobility items. In some examples, more than two difficulty-factors may be reported.

In the next two chapters, on item response theory (IRT) and computer-adaptive testing, scales that are deliberately based on items of varying difficulty will be described. These methods usually assume unidimensionality. The difficulty-factors that are sometimes seen in this situation may appear confusing, even though the problems of difficulty-factors have long been recognised. As Gibson (1960) commented: "The dilemma of difficulty-factors has beset factor analysts for many years. When a group of tests quite homogeneous as to content but varying widely in difficulty is subjected to factor analysis, the result is that more factors than content would demand are required to reduce the residuals to a random pattern."

Example from the literature

Helbostad *et al.* (2011) describe the development of a computer adaptive assessment tool for evaluating the mobility of patients in palliative care. Since item response theory was being used for the item selection and scaling, the authors applied EFA to explore the dimensionality of the mobility scale. This suggested there were two underlying dimensions for mobility.

However, an alternative explanation is that one factor contained the least demanding items and reflected lower levels of functioning, and the other factor covered the most physically demanding items relating to higher functioning levels. Thus, the factors might be merely reflected the clustering of similar items in these areas rather than two essentially different factors. However, as Helbostad *et al.* observed, 'difficulty-factors' have been a long-recognised phenomenon in factor analysis. The items selected for the mobility item-bank certainly vary extremely widely in their difficulty, unlike the items most commonly seen in traditional psychometric tests where factor analysis is likely to be more appropriate.

The strikingly linear pattern of the item-loadings in Figure 6.9 may be compared to the clusters of items that are more commonly seen for EFA, as in Figure 6.3; this is consistent with difficulty-factors. The high internal consistency (Cronbach's alpha = 0.97) and a moderate to high correlation of items to the total scale further indicates good internal consistency of the scale. Thus, overall, the assumption of unidimensionality seems plausible.

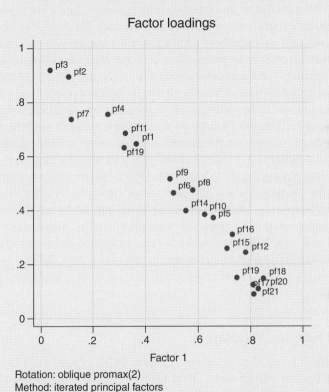

Rotation: oblique promax(2)
Method: iterated principal factors

Figure 6.9 Plot of Factor 2 against Factor 1, using the rotated factors from EFA of the mobility items. *Source:* Helbostad *et al.*, 2011, Figure 1. Reproduced with permission of Springer Science+Business Media.

6.17 Bifactor analysis

As noted in Section 6.16, IRT models usually assume unidimensionality, implying that a single latent variable suffices to explain the observed item-responses. The validity of IRT applications (including linking, adaptive testing, scoring) depends critically on the unidimensionality assumption. However, apart from simple homogeneous measures, few multi-item scales are likely to be strictly unidimensional. In many cases, multidimensionality is due to the heterogeneous item content that is required to properly represent the complexity of health constructs. Acknowledging this fact, researchers have focused on methods of exploring whether data are 'unidimensional enough' for application of IRT. Such scales may be termed 'essentially' or 'sufficiently' unidimensional. While various methods have been proposed, Reise *et al.* (2007) advocate the use of *bifactor analysis* and provide an illustration using PROs.

In essence, bifactor analysis consists of fitting a model in which each item is allowed to load on a 'common factor' and more specific 'group factors'. The common factor is formed as a general overall factor from all of the items. The group factors are the multiple dimensions that are hypothesised to exist, for example either derived from prior beliefs or as a result of EFA. In the simplest case, the comparison might assess whether the items represent two distinct dimensions with each item belonging to one and only one of the two group factors, or whether a single-dimension solution is adequate. The factors are constrained to be 'orthogonal' or mutually uncorrelated, so that all covariance is partitioned either into loadings on the common factor or onto the group factors. If the standardised loadings on the common factor are all salient (defined as > 0.30) and substantially larger than loadings on the group factors, the item pool is considered to be sufficiently homogeneous (McDonald, 1999). We are also interested in examining whether the loadings for the common factor (from the bifactor model) are only slightly reduced from the loadings obtained by fitting only a unidimensional factor; this would support claims for sufficient unidimensionality. When modelling patient-reported outcomes, the bifactor model has been suggested as having advantages over the closely related concept of higher-order factors (Chen *et al.* 2006).

Example from the literature

Pain is frequent in palliative cancer patients. Reliable pain assessment is necessary for patient management, treatment decisions, and clinical studies. In palliation, the most important dimensions of pain are intensity and interference. However, since pain interference is a consequence of and largely reflects pain intensity, Fayers *et al.* (2011) postulated that an overall summary measure of pain severity could be constructed by combining these two dimensions. Pain items, extracted from various validated questionnaires, were available from assessments of 395 cancer patients in palliative care and 168 chronic pain patients.

Experts reviewed the pain items, determining whether they assessed mainly pain intensity or pain interference (Table 6.8). EFA confirmed that both one- and two-dimension models (Models 1 and 2) were consistent with the observed data. The one-factor solution of Model 1 accounted for about 82%

Table 6.8 One-dimension, two-dimension and bifactor models: Factor loadings of 21 pain items, from 394 patients in palliative care and 168 patients with chronic pain

Item	Scale[1] a priori beliefs	Model 1: 1 dimension[2]	Model 2: 2-dimension[2] Intensity	Interference	Model 3: Bifactor[3] Common	Intensity	Interference	Variance explained[4]
maxp	I	0.88	0.83	.	0.72	0.57	.	0.86
bpi3	I	0.89	0.84	.	0.72	0.58	.	0.88
bpi5	I	0.87	0.83	.	0.71	0.57	.	0.84
resting	I	0.77	0.79	.	0.63	0.55	.	0.70
moving	I	0.80	0.77	.	0.65	0.53	.	0.72
SF36	I	0.67	0.60	.	0.55	0.41	.	0.48
pa1	I	0.91	0.76	.	0.75	0.52	.	0.87
pa15	I	0.65	0.59	.	0.53	0.41	.	0.46
pa10	I	0.79	0.65	.	0.65	0.45	.	0.65
pa8*	F	0.79	.	0.70	0.67	.	0.48	0.70
pa9*	F	0.74	.	0.80	0.63	.	0.55	0.71
pa14*	F	0.77	.	0.60	0.64	.	0.41	0.62
bpiB	F	0.75	.	0.69	0.63	.	0.48	0.64
bpiE	F	0.66	.	0.65	0.56	.	0.45	0.53
bpiG	F	0.73	.	0.69	0.62	.	0.48	0.62
pa4	F	0.85	0.50	0.46	0.70	0.35	0.32	0.71
pa5	F	0.74	.	0.68	0.63	.	0.47	0.63
pa6	F	0.83	.	0.70	0.70	.	0.48	0.76
pa11	F	0.82	0.52	0.42	0.68	0.36	.	0.67
pa12	F	0.83	0.52	0.43	0.69	0.36	.	0.69
pa13	F	0.67	.	0.49	0.56	.	0.34	0.47

[1]Experts judged pain items a priori to be assessing pain intensity (I), pain interference (F). Items marked with * were initially considered to reflect both I and F.
[2]Maximum likelihood factor analysis of polychoric correlations, followed by promax rotation. For clarity, only factor loadings of 0.4 or above are shown.
[3]The Bifactor model: loadings greater than 0.3 are shown for the lower-level factors.
[4]For each item, the proportion of its variance that is explained by the two-dimensional model.
Source: Fayers et al., 2011.

of the variation in the data, while the two-factor solution increases this by a modest amount to 89.8%, again providing but limited support to the presence of two factors. Model 3, the bifactor model, simultaneously fits a common factor as well as the intensity and interference factors. Factor loadings from Model 3 suggest that although it would be reasonable to regard the pool of items as unidimensional, it is preferable to retain two factors. This is shown by the loadings for the interference and the intensity items in the bifactor model, which are mainly above 0.3, while those for the common factor were rather lower than loadings shown for Model 1. This suggests that the intensity and the interference items do form separate clusters that are distinct factors or 'dimensions' of pain. However, the reduction from Model 1 is not substantial and thus the results of the bifactor analysis also imply that the two dimensions may be combined with little loss of information to form a single factor for overall pain severity.

Subsequent analyses also suggested that the two-factor solution might be simply an example of 'difficulty-factors', with the interference items predominantly indicating very high levels of pain.

6.18 Do formative or causal relationships matter?

Section 6.10 argued that there EFA should be used with caution when there are causal items, and Section 6.11 supported this with an example in which a factor was clearly a heterogeneous combination of treatment-related side effects that made little sense as a meaningful construct of QoL. On the other hand, in Section 6.12 the large study by Gundy *et al.* (2012) failed to find evidence that a causal model provided better fit. At first sight this may seem curious.

The technique of EFA was originally developed with parallel, reflective items firmly in mind (see Sections 2.6 and 2.7). In such a model, the items have been selected and developed as being independent characteristics of the postulated underlying latent variable, such as intelligence or personality. In contrast, in QoL research, for disease- or treatment-specific instruments we endeavour to identify *all* the symptoms that are relevant and impact on a patient's well-being. In the first case, EFA identified clusters of highly correlated items – factors – and these can reasonably be interpreted as constructs that underlie the latent variable. In the second case, EFA again identifies clusters of highly correlated items; that is what EFA is good at doing. This time, however, when symptoms are highly correlated and form 'symptom clusters', it is because they are closely related, both conceptually and through underlying biological mechanisms. For example, it is no surprise to find nausea and vomiting are highly correlated and form a 'factor'. Nor is it in the least surprising that items assessing pain severity and pain interference are correlated and form a 'factor'. Usually the factors from EFA will be conceptually sensible, because highly correlated items are usually closely related to each other.

Two examples where this fails have been provided. Firstly, Fayers and Hand (1997a), as described in Section 6.11, exemplified this by deliberately choosing a sample in which a control group of patients is contrasted against another group of patients receiving a treatment known to provoke a mixture of 'causal' side effects; a seemingly illogical combination of symptoms formed a factor. Secondly, EFA failed to produce the desired result in the example of items in the pain scale of Whistance *et al.* (2009), described in Section 5.7. Here, the three pain items are weakly correlated formative indicators, and EFA would not indicate a single factor even though the items can combine to form a scale for 'pain at any relevant site'.

When formative or causal items are included, any extrapolation of the EFA results to QoL constructs is dubious and relies upon additional assumptions that are frequently true but rarely spelt out. For example, if an instrument developer included some items that are irrelevant to QoL but are highly correlated with each other, EFA would correctly identify them as a 'factor' even though they are irrelevant to the construct supposedly being evaluated. But if we assume that the instrument developer has been thorough and sensible, such items would already have been thrown out before getting as far as EFA. Similarly, before even collecting data, instrument developers have usually selected and included items because they were deemed to have high impact on QoL.

So, with EFA we usually obtain the 'right' answers, but for the wrong reasons. The wrong theoretical model is being applied, but it may frequently appear to work well in practice. The factor loadings for causal indicators are difficult to interpret, and for composite indicators are meaningless.

6.19 Conclusions

Causal models, SEM and CFA hold great potential but have been little used in QoL research. There remain many controversial issues to be resolved before they can be recommended for routine usage. The simplest of the three, EFA, has many disadvantages, not the least of which is that it will frequently be an inappropriate model for QoL instruments because of the occurrence of causal indicators. Perhaps the principal attraction of EFA is its relative ease of application, and its ability to suggest possible factors in the data; but, as emphasised, these factors must be regarded as tentative and treated with circumspection. Also, provided one can be confident that only indicator variables are present, EFA offers convenient facilities for assessing the number of factors necessary to explain the data; dimensionality should always be explored before applying techniques such as item response theory. EFA is available through many of the commonly used statistical packages, and analyses using EFA can readily be carried out. On the other hand, SEM models are considerably more difficult to specify, even though most software is moving towards model specification using graphical path diagrams. The results output by the software packages are more difficult to interpret. Large sample sizes are required to fit or evaluate these models. But SEM does offer an appropriate means for confirming construct validity.

The emphasis with all three procedures is in testing goodness-of-fit of models. Alternative methods, such as item response theory, offer more justifiable methods for developing the scoring algorithms for questionnaires.

One overall conclusion should be that EFA, CFA and SEM are not black-box procedures that can be applied blindly. Before embarking on any such analysis, the investigator must consider the possible path structures for the relationships between the explanatory variables and the latent structures. Usually there will be a number of alternative models that are thought plausible. The role of the approaches we have described is to examine whether one or more of these models provides reasonable fit, and if it does the investigator may feel satisfied. But this neither 'proves' that the model is correct and unique, nor that the scale has been truly 'validated'; it confirms only that there is no evidence of bad fit.

6.20   Further reading, and software

Although dated, the book by Gorsuch (1983) is still recommended for a detailed description of factor analysis and related techniques. A more up-to-date and briefer text is Child (2006). Unlike many others on this topic, these books avoid detailed mathematics while covering factor analysis in depth; for example, Gorsuch has a whole chapter about selecting the number of factors, and two chapters about rotation methods. Nunnally and Bernstein (1994) contains extensive chapters about EFA and CFA, and has the advantage of greater emphasis on psychometric scales. Structural equation and latent variable models are fully described by Bollen (1989) and Kline (2010). Barrett (2007), and the many companion articles that were published simultaneously, make interesting reading about goodness-of-fit indices and the chi-square test of perfect model fit.

Widely used programs for fitting SEM models include AMOS (Arbuckle, 2009), EQS (Bentler, 1995), LISREL (Jöreskog and Sörbom, 2006) and MPLUS (Muthén and Muthén, 2010). Byrne (1998, 2006, 2009, 2011) has written practical books exemplifying the use of all these packages. Many statistical packages now implement SEM facilities.

7

Item response theory and differential item functioning

Summary

In contrast to the traditional psychometrics, item response theory introduces a different underlying model for the responses to questions. It is now assumed that patients with a particular level of QoL (or other PRO) will have a certain probability of responding positively to each question. This probability will depend upon the 'difficulty' of the item in question. For example, many patients with cancer might respond 'Yes' to 'easy' questions such as 'Do you have any pain?', but only patients with a high level of pain are likely to reply 'Yes' to the more 'difficult' question 'Have you got very much pain?' This chapter explains the role of item response models for instrument development, and how to fit them. Use of these models to examine the psychometric properties of items and scales, and in particular differential item functioning, is also described.

7.1 Introduction

As we have seen, under the traditional psychometric model of parallel test items with summated scales, it is assumed that each item is a representation of the same single latent variable. This is therefore a simple form of unidimensional scaling, in which it is frequently assumed that the items are of equal importance for measuring the latent variable, and that summated scales with equal weights can be used. It is also implicit to this model that the intervals between the levels (responses) for each category are equal, so that (e.g. on a typical four-category scale as used on QoL questionnaires) a change from 1 to 2 is of equal importance as a change from 2 to 3. Since it is assumed that each item is an equally strong estimator of the latent variable, the purpose of increasing the number of items is to increase the reliability of the scale and hence improve the precision of the scale score as an estimate of the latent construct.

Quality of Life: The Assessment, Analysis and Reporting of Patient-Reported Outcomes, Third Edition.
Peter M. Fayers and David Machin.
© 2016 John Wiley & Sons, Ltd. Published 2016 by John Wiley & Sons, Ltd.

In contrast, *item response theory* (IRT) offers an alternative scaling procedure. IRT was developed largely in fields such as education, and initially focused upon the simple situation of binary items such as those that are frequently found in educational tests and which are scored 'correct' or 'wrong'. There are a number of reasons explaining the importance of IRT in education. Firstly, the traditional psychometric theory of parallel tests tends to result in items of equal difficulty. In educational tests this is not appropriate, as it tends to polarise students into those who find all questions easy and those who do not have the ability to answer any question. IRT methods lead to examinations that include questions of varying difficulty, enabling students to be classified into levels of ability. Secondly, educational tests should not discriminate unfairly between students of equal ability but of different sex, race, culture, religious background or other factors deemed irrelevant. IRT provides sensitive methods for detecting differential item functioning (item bias) in different subgroups. Thirdly, in annual examinations the questions will have to change in each successive year to prevent students learning of the correct solutions. IRT provides methods for standardisation, to ensure that each year the examinations contain questions of similar difficulty and result in comparable overall scores. Fourthly, when students are faced by questions that are beyond their capability, if the valid responses are 'Yes' and 'No', it is likely that a proportion of the correct responses will be simply lucky guesses. IRT models can support adjustment for guessing, although this is less relevant in clinical applications. Thus IRT meets many of the demands of educational tests and much of the terminology such as *test difficulty* and *item bias* is most easily explained with reference to educational examinations.

Many aspects of IRT are equally pertinent to PROs and QoL. IRT is most clearly of relevance when considering scales that aim to classify patients into levels of ability, for example activities of daily living (ADL) or other physical performance scales. These scales usually contain questions describing tasks of increasing difficulty, such as 'Can you walk short distances?', 'Can you walk long distances?' and 'Can you do vigorous activities?' with 'Yes' or 'No' response items. As a consequence, the earliest examples of IRT in relation to PROs have been in the area of assessing ADL and mobility. Pain assessment is another natural field of application because level of pain may be regarded as analogous to level of ability, and many pain instruments contain items relating to severity or 'difficulty'.

From a modelling perspective, the main difference between IRT and traditional methods is that IRT considers the *probability* that a respondent selects particular categories of each item, whereas traditional methods focus on average scores; an obvious analogy can be made with linear regression versus logistic and ordered logistic regression. Historically, early applications of IRT focused on binary outcomes such as Yes/No or Correct/False while most PRO items permit responses at more than two levels and multicategory IRT is commonly applied.

Considering the practical aspects of item selection highlights the differences between the traditional parallel test and IRT approaches. A simple traditional test might consist of a single item, scored with multiple categories ranging from very poor (lowest category) to excellent (highest category). Then ability is assessed by the level of the response category. To increase precision and reliability, using traditional theory, additional parallel tests would be introduced and the average (or sum-score) used as the measure. In contrast, under the IRT model, items are chosen to be of varying difficulty, and to increase precision and reliability any additional items that are introduced are chosen so as to have difficulties evenly distributed over the range of the continuum that is of greatest interest. Although originally IRT-based tests included mainly dichotomous items, there has been a trend towards multicategory tests that can take three or four response levels.

In this chapter we primarily consider the application of IRT methods for validation of instruments, including the use of IRT to identify both the amount of information provided by each item in a multi-item scale and the extent of any differential item functioning. The next chapter describes how IRT can also be used for scoring of responses even when respondents complete different subsets of items, and how this can be exploited in the development of efficient computer-adaptive tests.

7.2   Item characteristic curves

The principal concept in IRT is the *item characteristic curve*, usually abbreviated as ICC (not to be confused with *ICC*, intraclass correlation). The ICC relates the probability of a positive response to the level of the latent variable. If we consider a questionnaire that is intended to measure physical functioning, the ICC for a single item is constructed as follows.

First, we require an estimate of the latent variable (overall physical functioning) for each patient. Ideally there would be an independent estimate of the 'true' value of their physical functioning, but in practice that is unknown. Possible choices include use of (i) a global question such as 'Overall, how would you rate your physical condition', (ii) an internally derived estimate based upon a number of items on the questionnaire, or (iii) another, possibly lengthier, questionnaire that has already been validated. For each level of the latent variable it is possible to calculate the percentage or probability of patients who respond positively to the item. When items have multiple response categories, it is customary to collapse them into two levels for estimating the probability of, for example, having 'no difficulty or limitations' versus 'some difficulty'. Usually the ICC obtained will look similar to those in Figure 7.1. The *global score* is assumed to be an estimate of the true value of a latent variable, θ, such as physical functioning. Thus patients with a global score of 3 will on average give a positive response to item A approximately half of the time, but have only a very small probability (less than 0.05) of responding positively on item B.

Item difficulty

In educational examinations there is the concept of *difficulty* when comparing items. The more intelligent or more successful pupils are able to answer even difficult questions successfully. In Figure 7.1, the two items shown vary in their difficulty. If the

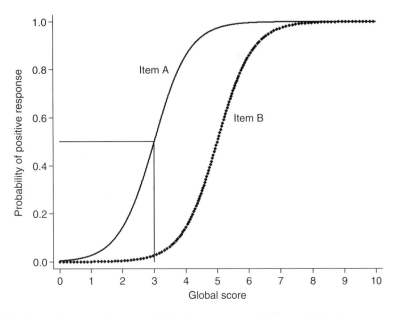

Figure 7.1   Item characteristic curves (ICCs) for two items of differing difficulty.

global score described educational attainment, item B would represent a more difficult question since for any particular global score the probability of answering B correctly is less than that for A. Although 'difficulty' is also a suitable word for describing ability to perform physical functions, it may be intuitively less obvious for describing some other aspects of PRO measures. It simply means that for a given value of the latent variable fewer patients will answer positively to a question related to a more advanced symptom or a more demanding task. Thus the difficulty parameter identifies the location of the item along the construct's continuum. In this chapter we adopt the widely used terminology '*item difficulty*', although some authors prefer the less specific or more neutral words '*item location*'.

One of the most useful features of IRT is that it provides a solid theoretical framework for estimating this item difficulty. Thus IRT facilitates the design of questionnaires containing items with a spread of levels of difficulty, and enables formal procedures to be used for selecting these items. It also leads to the development of scaling and scoring procedures for the aggregation of items into summary measures of ability. It provides methods for comparing different questionnaires and enables measures of patients' ability scores to be standardised across instruments.

Another important aspect of IRT is that it is 'sample free', because the *relative* item difficulties should remain the same irrespective of the particular sample of subjects. Thus the most difficult item remains the most difficult item irrespective of the sample and the mix of patient ability levels. It is this feature that enables IRT to be used for providing standardised tests.

Item discrimination

In Figure 7.1, a patient who responds positively to item A is most likely to have a global score of 3 or more; however, even about 10% of patients with a global score of 2 are expected to respond positively. Thus a positive response to A does not provide a clear indication of the global score. An ideal test item is one with an ICC nearly vertical, since the central sloping region of the S-shaped curve represents the region of uncertainty in which we cannot be certain whether patients with a specified value of the global score will respond positively or negatively to the item. Conversely, an extremely poor item would be one with an ICC close to the horizontal line corresponding to a probability of 0.5, for which all patients irrespective of their global score would answer positively half the time; this item would contain no information about the patients' ability.

The ability of a test to separate subjects into high and low levels of ability is known as its *discrimination*. Thus discrimination corresponds to the *slope* of the curve, and the steeper the slope the better. In Figure 7.2, item A discriminates between patients better than item B. Thus, for item A, patients whose global score is less than 2 will answer positively with low probability, and patients with a score greater than 4 will do so with high probability. Only those patients whose score is between 2 and 4 may or may not respond positively – a range of uncertainty of 4–2. In contrast, item B has a wider range of uncertainty of approximately 7–3.

Difficulty and discrimination are the two fundamental properties of binary items in questionnaires. If an item has poor discrimination, it may help to include several other items of similar difficulty so as to improve the reliability of the test. If an item has good discrimination, it is less necessary to have additional items with closely similar difficulty. An ideal test would consist of evenly spaced, near vertical ICCs that cover the range of abilities that are of interest.

7.3 Logistic models

Although IRT is a generic term for a variety of models, the most common form is the logistic item response model. It has been found that logistic curves provide a good fit to many psychological, educational and other measurements. If a patient, h, has an ability which is represented by the latent variable θ_h, then for a single item in a test the basic equation for the logistic model takes the form

$$P(\theta_h) = \frac{\exp\{\theta_h - b\}}{1 + \exp\{\theta_h - b\}}, \qquad (7.1)$$

where $P(\theta_h)$ is the probability of a positive response by patient h, exp is the exponential function, and b is the item difficulty that we wish to estimate. Alternatively, this equation can be rearranged and written in the so-called *logit* form

$$\log\left(\frac{P(\theta_h)}{1-P(\theta_h)}\right) = (\theta_h - b). \tag{7.2}$$

Thus b is the value of θ_h that has a probability of 0.5 for being positive (or negative). For example, in Figure 7.1, if the global score is 3 ($b = 3$) then item A has probability of 0.5 of being endorsed, and similarly when $b = 5$ for item B.

Since equation (7.1) requires only a single parameter b to be estimated, it is commonly described as the *one-parameter logistic model*. It is also often called the *Rasch model* in honour of the Danish mathematician who promoted its usage in this area (Rasch, 1960). This equation can be generalised by adding a second parameter, a. It then becomes

$$P(\theta_h) = \frac{\exp\{a(\theta_h - b)\}}{1 + \exp\{a(\theta_h - b)\}}. \tag{7.3}$$

The parameter a in equation (7.3) measures the slope of the ICC curve and is called the *discrimination* of the test. This is known as the *two-parameter logistic model*. Figure 7.2 shows ICCs with the same values of b as in Figure 7.1, but with a taking the values 1.75 for item A and 1.0 for item B. When there are n items on the questionnaire it is possible to fit a generalised form of equation (7.3), with different values of a and b for each item.

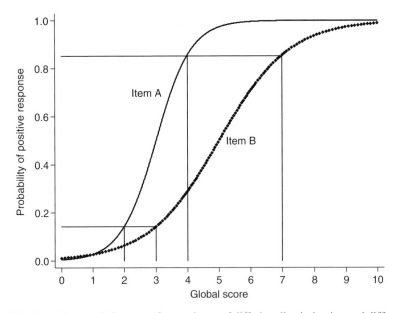

Figure 7.2   Item characteristic curves for two items of differing discrimination and difficulty.

One of the important properties of the logistic item response model is that it proves unnecessary to have estimates of the latent variable θ, provided one is interested only in the relative difficulties and discrimination of the items. The reason for this is that one can identify the relative positions of the curves without knowing the true values of the latent variable. These relative positions, corresponding to the relative sizes of the b-parameters, are usually expressed in terms of log odds-ratios (logits). A logit difficulty is the mean of the log odds that a patient of average ability will be able to move from one category to the next higher one. Typically the logits will range from −4 to +4, with +4 being the most difficult test.

Logistic regression

Although Rasch and other item response models are logistic models, there are crucial distinctions between estimation for IRT and standard statistical logistic regression. In logistic regression, θ is known and is the dependent or 'y-value'; in the Rasch model it is unknown. In the Rasch model, θ_h takes different values for each patient, h, leading to as many unknown parameters as there are subjects. Hence IRT is related to the so-called *conditional logistic regression*. For each item, i, one or more of the corresponding item parameters a_i and b_i have to be estimated according to whether the one- or two-parameter model is used.

Example from the literature

Haley *et al.* (1994) used IRT to examine the relative difficulty and the reproducibility of item positions of the 10-item physical functioning scale of the MOS SF-36, in a sample of 3,445 patients with chronic medical or psychiatric conditions. The Rasch one-parameter logistic model was used, with each item first dichotomised into 'limitations' or 'no limitations'.

The item difficulties of Table 7.1 were estimated in terms of Rasch logit values, and largely confirmed the authors' prior expectations. 'Bathing or dressing' was the easiest task (with a value −3.44), and 'vigorous activities' the most difficult (+3.67). The standard errors (*SEs*) of the b-values show the observed differences to be highly significant (greater than $2 \times SE$).

Item difficulties are clustered in the central region of the scale, with four items between −0.5 and +0.5. There is weaker coverage of the two extremes of the scale. The goodness-of-fit statistics (which we describe in Section 7.5) indicate that the Rasch model does not fit very well, with three items scoring item-misfit indices greater than +2, and another five items scoring less than −2.

Table 7.1   Rasch analysis of the PF-10 subscale in the SF-36

PF-10 items	b Item difficulty	SE	Item-misfit index
Vigorous activities	3.67	0.04	2.3
Climbing several flights of stairs	1.44	0.04	−3.4
Walking more than one mile	1.27	0.04	−0.2
Bending, kneeling, stooping	0.36	0.04	6.2
Moderate activities	0.18	0.04	−2.7
Walking several blocks	−0.11	0.04	−3.1
Lifting, carrying groceries	−0.36	0.04	0.0
Climbing one flight of stairs	−1.07	0.05	−5.1
Walking one block	−1.93	0.06	−3.2
Bathing or dressing	−3.44	0.07	8.9

Source: Hayley *et al.*, 1994. Reproduced with permission of Elsevier.

7.4   Polytomous item response theory models

The models described have been for binary or dichotomous items. Most QoL questionnaires use polytomous items. Creating dichotomous responses by grouping the response categories (as was done in the example of Table 7.1) results in loss of information. Appropriate models should be used according to the data. Although various other IRT models have been proposed for particular applications, such as psychomotor assessment, we focus on those models that are most commonly encountered in outcomes research. One approach that has been proposed for ordered categorical data involves dichotomising the data repeatedly at different levels, so that each g-category item is effectively decomposed into $g - 1$ binary questions. Thus an item that has three levels (such as 'not limited', 'limited a little', 'limited a lot') can be regarded as equivalent to two binary questions: 'Were you limited a little in doing vigorous activities?' (Yes or No), and 'Were you limited a lot in doing vigorous activities?' (Yes or No). In this way the PF-10, for example, is equivalent to 20 binary questions that can be analysed by a Rasch analysis. A number of models have been proposed that adopt this and other strategies. The most commonly used *polytomous* models are the graded response, partial credit, rating scale and generalised partial credit models, and these have all been used for modelling PROs that have ordered categorical response options. With these models it is usual to refer to *thresholds* rather than difficulties, where the threshold parameters identify the boundaries between successive categories; a response threshold is defined as the point at which a pair of consecutive response categories for an item are equally likely to be endorsed. Table 7.2 summarises the main models. Those that constrain the item slopes (discrimination) to be equal across all items belong to the 'Rasch family' of models.

Table 7.2 Characteristics of the main IRT models

Model		Item response format	Model characteristics	
			Discrimination	Difficulty/Threshold
Rasch Model (One Parameter Logistic Model)	1-PL	Dichotomous	Equal across all items*	Varies across items
Two Parameter Logistic Model	2-PL	Dichotomous	Varies across items	Varies across items
Nominal Response Model	NRM	Polytomous (no pre-specified ordering of response categories)	Varies across items	No ordering of category thresholds
Graded Response Model	GRM	Polytomous, ordered categories	Varies across items	Varies across items
Partial Credit Model	PCM	Polytomous, ordered categories	Equal across all items*	Varies across items
Rating Scale Model	RSM	Polytomous, ordered categories	Equal across all items*	Distance between categorical threshold steps is constant across items
Generalised Partial Credit Model	GPCM	Polytomous, ordered categories	Varies across items	Varies across items

*Models with equal discrimination across all items belong to the 'Rasch family'.

7.5 Applying logistic IRT models

Having seen the range of IRT models, how should we choose, fit and evaluate a suitable model?

Choosing IRT models

There is some controversy between those who favour the one-parameter Rasch model (and the corresponding generalisations for polytomous data), as opposed to those who advocate the more general two-parameter models. In education, where so much of the development of IRT has been carried out, there is a limitless choice of potential examination questions that can be coded 'right' or 'wrong'. The enthusiasts for the Rasch model point to the relative robustness of this model, and to a number of other desirable features to do with simplicity and consistency of scoring the scales. Thus they advocate selecting test items that fit the Rasch model, and rejecting all other candidate test items. In other words, they choose data that fit the model. In medicine, the choice of items is usually restricted to those that have high face and content validity, and there are finite choices for rephrasing any questions that do not fit the model. Thus it is common to find that one-parameter models are inadequate, and that to obtain reasonable fit we must use a two-parameter model. In medicine, we must choose a model that fits the data.

The choice of model can be tricky and is usually a combination of trial-and-error and evaluation of goodness-of-fit. Few software packages fit the full range of models and at the same time offer adequate diagnostics and goodness-of-fit measures.

Examples from the literature

Reeve *et al.* (2007) argued in favour of the graded response model (GRM): "The GRM is a very flexible model from the parametric, unidimensional, polytomous-response IRT family of models. Because it allows discrimination to vary item by item, it typically fits response data better than a one-parameter (i.e. Rasch) model. Further, compared with alternative 2-parameter models such as the generalised partial credit model, the model is relatively easy to understand and illustrate to 'consumers' and retains its functional form when response categories are merged. Thus, the GRM offers a flexible framework for modelling the participant responses to examine item and scale properties, to calibrate the items of the item bank, and to score individual response patterns in the PRO assessment."

In contrast, Petersen *et al.* (2011) chose the generalised partial credit model (GPCM) as the basis for developing a computerised adaptive test for the EORTC QLQ-C30 physical functioning dimension: "In the GPCM, each item has a slope parameter describing the item's ability to discriminate between subjects with different levels of PF, and a set of threshold parameters describing how likely it is to report problems on the item. An advantage of the GPCM is that it is a generalization of other well-known item models. If all items have the same slope, the model reduces to the partial credit model, which belongs to the family of Rasch models." However, Petersen *et al.* added: "To evaluate the effect of model choice on the item fit, we planned also to calibrate the graded response model, which has the same number of item parameters as the GPCM and often gives trace lines that are very similar to the GPCM trace lines."

Pallant and Tennant (2007) took another different approach, arguing that only Rasch models possess consistent measurement properties. They used the partial credit model (PCM) because it has equal slopes for all items and thus belongs to the Rasch family of models, explaining: "Note the orientation; because the model defines measurement, data are fitted to the model to see if they meet the model's expectations. This is opposite to the practice in statistical modelling where models are developed to best represent the data." This approach emphasises the testing of adequacy of fit of the model. Items are only accepted provided they have closely similar discrimination slopes and adequately satisfy the model.

Fitting the model

Fitting IRT models and estimating the item-parameters for difficulties and abilities is complex and usually requires iterative calculations. Most standard statistical packages have limited IRT-specific facilities for modelling although, as noted above, conditional logistic regression can in theory be used. However, specialised software incorporates better estimation facilities and display of results, and has the added advantage that IRT diagnostics such as goodness-of-fit indices are usually provided. Some programs for IRT modelling are listed at the end of this chapter (Section 7.15). Software for logistic IRT analysis usually displays estimates of the logit values and their accompanying standard errors. The estimated logits can be compared with each other, and their differences tested for significance using t-tests.

Graphical methods for goodness of fit

Graphical methods, and in particular the display of ICCs and item information curves, provide a useful overview of which items have the best fit and which are problematic; it is recommended that such displays form a starting point to any appraisal of item fit. Since most PROs are assessed by items that can have multiple response options, we shall assume polytomous IRT models are being used.

Item characteristic curves show which items contribute most effectively. The ideal item will have the following features. It should exhibit steep slope parameters, corresponding to very 'peaky' curves for each category on the ICC; such items have high discrimination. Successive categories should show distinct and uniformly spaced curves. The item should cover a distinct range of the continuum, complementing other items in the scale. An item with these properties contributes high levels of information to the dimension that is being evaluated. Conversely, poor items are those with weaker slopes that result in shallow curves. Four test items are shown in Figure 7.3, items A and C having steeper slopes than item B. Items A and C also cover different parts of the trait-level continuum, with A separating trait levels from approximately 0 to 2 and C from −2 to 0. Both are therefore useful. Although item B covers a similar range of trait levels as C, the less steep slopes of B tell us that it is less informative than C.

Response thresholds are an important feature of the ICC-plot. Since response thresholds are the points at which consecutive response categories of an item are equally likely to be endorsed, they are indicated on the ICC-plot by the points where the curves for adjacent categories intersect. A well-functioning item will have a response format that respondents use in a consistent manner. In particular, the response thresholds between successive categories should be ordered, such that the threshold between categories 1 and 2 falls below the threshold between categories 2 and 3, and so on. An item that shows one or more *disordered response* thresholds does not provide an adequate fit to an IRT model. The disordered responses indicate that responders are not able to discriminate sufficiently between the response categories they are asked to select from. Overlapping and disordered categories either indicate items with problems that should either be excluded or, at the very least, have categories that should be combined or reworded to produce a revised item with better performance. In Figure 7.3, category 2 of item D shows disordered thresholds because the intersection of categories 1 and 2 is to the right of the intersection of categories 2 and 3; respondents appear to be confused as to when to choose response 2. Thus this item has poor characteristics, and response

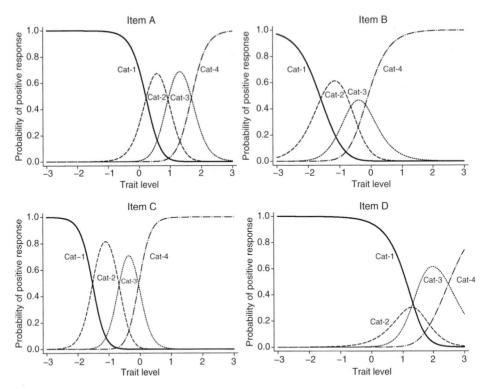

Figure 7.3 Item characteristic curves for four items, each with four categorical response options. The intersections between adjacent categories correspond to threshold parameters of the Generalized Partial Credit Model. Items A and C exhibit good properties, having steep slopes and covering different trait levels; item B covers a similar range of levels to C, but has weaker discrimination illustrated by less steep slopes; Item D is a weak item with disordered thresholds.

option 2 should either be combined with one of the adjacent categories, the options reworded, or the item excluded.

Item information functions can summarise the overall value of including individual items. Items that contribute little information are natural candidates for either removal or modification. *Test information functions* can also expose areas in the scale that are inadequately covered, and which would benefit by the addition of extra test items. Low levels of information imply high measurement error, because the test information function is inversely related to the square of the measurement error associated with the varying levels of the scale score:

$$SE = 1/\sqrt{InformationFunction}. \tag{7.4}$$

The reading material listed at the end of this chapter describes how to estimate and use information functions, and most IRT software has facilities for displaying them.

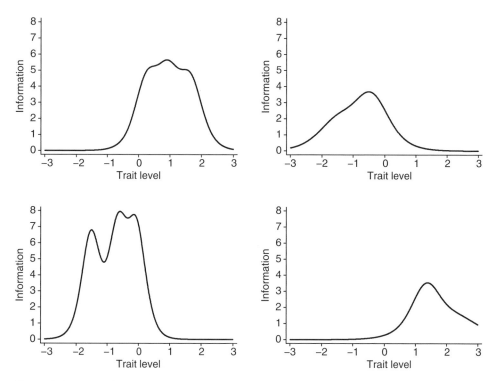

Figure 7.4 Item information curves corresponding to the four items of Figure 7.3. Items A and C are markedly superior to items B and D.

The item information curves corresponding to the items in Figure 7.3 are shown in Figure 7.4. Items A and C are more informative than B and D, and as already observed A and C target different levels of the trait being assessed.

Example from the literature

Fayers *et al.* (2005) explored the use of the 20-item Mini-Mental State Examination (MMSE) in palliative care patients. The MMSE is normally used as an interviewer-administered screening test for dementia, with a score of less than 24 out of the maximum 30 being regarded as the threshold implying cognitive impairment. It is also the most commonly used instrument for the assessment of cognitive impairment and delirium in palliative care. For these patients it is especially important to minimise the test burden, and it was found that between four and six items were sufficient when screening for delirium in these patients, with little loss of information compared to the full test. In Figure 7.5, a score of −3 corresponds to the MMSE threshold score of 24.

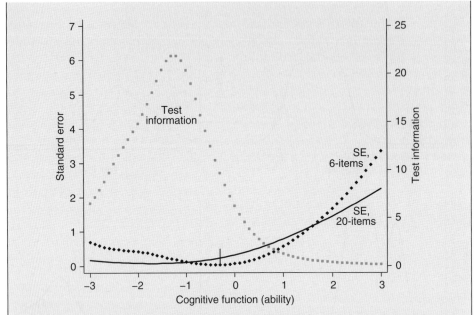

Figure 7.5   Standard error of MMSE score estimates in palliative care patients, showing that a 6-item test has similar properties to the full MMSE. *Source:* Adapted from Fayers *et al.*, 2005, Figures 2 and 4. Reproduced with permission of Elsevier.

Goodness-of-fit indices

Goodness-of-fit indices enable the adequacy of the model to be assessed, and a poor fit implies that one or more of the assumptions has been violated. Thus, a poor fit for a

Example from the literature

Pallant and Tennant (2007) examined responses to the HADS questionnaire made by from 296 outpatients attending a six-week musculoskeletal rehabilitation programme. The objective was to assess the appropriateness of a total score (HADS-14) as a measure of psychological distress. Initial testing revealed that responses to the two central options of the item 'dep2' seemed to be overlapping. This led to these response options being combined, leaving a three-category scale. Table 7.3 shows the results from fitting the PCM after item 'dep2' was recoded. The fit of the individual items was checked, and revealed two items (`dep2' and 'anx11', shaded) as showing misfit to the model. Both items showed fit-residual values above 2.5, and the *p*-value for item 'anx11' is highly significant even after allowing for multiple significance testing (Bonferroni correction). The positive fit-residual values obtained for these two items suggest low levels of discrimination. This was confirmed by inspection of the ICC plots.

Table 7.3 Fitting a Partial Credit Model to HADS data

Item	Location	SE	Fit-residual[1]	ChiSq[2]	p-value
Anxiety items					
anx1 I feel tense or 'wound' up	−1.197	0.089	−0.091	8.274	0.082
anx3 I get a frightened feeling as if something awful is about to happen	0.075	0.077	−0.142	7.701	0.103
anx5 Worrying thoughts go through my mind	−0.468	0.079	−1.332	10.029	0.039
anx7 I can sit at ease and feel relaxed	−0.817	0.093	0.829	3.447	0.486
anx9 I get a sort of frightened feeling like 'butterflies' in the stomach	0.785	0.091	−0.28	0.885	0.926
anx11 I feel restless as if I have to be on the move	−0.549	0.078	3.168	17.365	0.001
anx13 I get sudden feelings of panic	0.764	0.087	−0.715	2.946	0.566
Depression items					
dep2* I still enjoy the things I used to enjoy	−0.859	0.076	2.787	13.684	0.008
dep4 I can laugh and see the funny side of things	0.97	0.09	−1.408	6.357	0.174
dep6 I feel cheerful	1.331	0.097	−2.125	10.517	0.032
dep8 I feel as if I am slowed down	−1.716	0.085	1.179	3.313	0.506
dep10 I have lost interest in my appearance	0.796	0.084	0.098	1.298	0.861
dep12 I look forward with enjoyment to things	0.092	0.081	−1.227	4.243	0.374
dep14 I can enjoy a good book or radio or TV programme	0.794	0.085	0.514	5.724	0.221

*The item depression2 was recoded with the two central response options combined.
[1]The fit-residual statistic has 270.07 degrees of freedom.
[2]The chi-squared statistics have 4 degrees of freedom.
Source: Pallant and Tennant, 2007. Reproduced with permission of John Wiley & Sons, Ltd.

one-parameter model could imply that the two-parameter version may be more appropriate, that local independence is violated or that the logistic model is inappropriate. Usually, goodness-of-fit statistics will be produced for the overall model and 'misfit indices' may be given for individual items (item-misfit index) and for patients (person-misfit index).

Although the precise statistics used can vary, in general a large (positive or negative) value for the misfit statistic indicates that an item is frequently scored wrongly (item-misfit) or that a patient has given inconsistent responses (person-misfit). For example, the item-misfit index would be large for an item that is expected to be easy (low difficulty) if it cannot be accomplished by a number of patients with high overall levels of ability. Similarly, the value will be high if those with low overall ability are able to answer 'difficult' items. Most goodness-of-fit statistics follow an approximate χ^2 distribution (Appendix Table T4), and thus a significant p-value is evidence that the model does not provide a perfect fit.

Fit-residuals estimate the divergence between the expected and observed responses for each respondent or item response; fit-residuals are summed over all items (item fit-residuals) or summed over all persons (person fit-residuals). The residuals are standardised such that the mean item or person fit-residual should be approximately zero with a *SD* approximately equal to 1.0.

It is important, however, to remember that most models are nothing more than an approximation to reality. If the dataset is sufficiently large, even well-fitting and potentially useful models may fail to provide perfect fit to the observed dataset, and the p-value may be significant. On the other hand, if the dataset is small there will be insufficient information to detect poor fit even when the model is inappropriate. Statistical tests of goodness-of-fit should be used with caution.

Example from the literature

Petersen *et al.* (2011) collected data from 1,176 patients with cancer, on 56 candidate items for the development of a computerised adaptive testing (CAT) scale for physical functioning (PF). Fit of the GPCM model was appraised using item fit index. Because of multiple testing and a large sample, they used $p < 0.001$ as indicating misfit. Furthermore, they calculated the average difference between expected and observed item responses (bias) and the root mean square error (*RMSE*) of expected and observed item responses. Finally, they calculated the information function for the selected set of items to evaluate whether the items seemed to have acceptable measurement precision across the continuum.

Based on the evaluations of item fit, three items were deleted: item 2 had $p < 0.001$ for the fit test and the difficulty level and content of the item seemed to be covered by several better fitting items; item 48 had $p < 0.001$, *RMSE* = 0.63 (on a 0–3 scale) and for 13% of the patients, the observed and expected responses differed more than one response category; item 51 had $p < 0.001$ and disordered threshold parameters.

The GPCM was then recalibrated to the remaining 31 items, and the parameter estimates and fit statistics summarised (Table 7.4 provides a small excerpt).

Item 35 had $p < 0.001$, but since this was one of the few items relevant for patients with good PF, and the bias and *RMSE* were relatively small, Petersen *et al.* decided to keep the item. Otherwise, the fit of the 31 items appeared satisfactory. The 31 items appeared to provide good content coverage of the PF aspects of interest and there was good variability in the difficulties of the items, although the item pool has relatively few items at the upper extreme.

Table 7.4 Parameter estimates and fit statistics for a few items of the final IRT model for a physical functioning computer adaptive test

Item	No. of categories	Slope	Mean threshold	Item fit p-value	Bias	*RMSE*
1	2	2.29	−1.99	0.213	0.000	0.18
3	4	3.42	−1.33	0.003	0.004	0.39
4	2	1.99	−0.99	0.177	0.002	0.34
6	4	2.95	−1.21	0.054	0.004	0.45
7	4	2.99	−2.01	0.001	0.002	0.22
8	3	3.09	−1.91	0.130	0.001	0.19
11	4	3.05	−0.87	0.286	0.005	0.50
. . . . . .						
35	4	2.61	0.32	< 0.001	0.001	0.57

Source: Petersen *et al.*, 2011, Table 4. Reproduced with permission of Springer Science and Business Media.

Sample size

Large numbers of patients are required for the estimation procedure. Although it is difficult to be specific, sample sizes of 500 to 1,000 appropriately chosen respondents are recommended for item calibration, although in some simple cases as few as 250 may suffice (Thissen *et al.*, 2007). By 'appropriately chosen', it is implied that the sample should be representative of the full range of the target population and with at least some of the respondents selecting each response option of each item. Even with Rasch models, which are more robust than more general IRT models, it is advised to have sample sizes greater than 250 respondents for reliable fitting of the model and estimation of the parameters (Chen *et al.*, 2014).

7.6 Assumptions of IRT models

Latent variable models, including IRT models, are computationally more sensitive to their underlying assumptions than are models in which there is an observed dependent variable. Thus IRT models are less robust than logistic regression models. It is important to check the following assumptions before fitting an IRT model.

Monotonicity

Under the logistic IRT model, each ICC must be smoothly increasing. That is, the probability of a positive response should always increase as the ability increases, and thus the ICC curves should increase as the latent variable increases; this is called *monotonically increasing*. Confirming the monotonicity assumption is essential to the application of item response models. One way to assess monotonicity of an item is by regression of the item-score on the 'rest-score', where the rest-score is the scale score after omitting the item that is being examined (for example, the sum score of all items except the item in question). If an item complies with monotonicity, the average item score should not decrease for increasing values of the rest score (Junker and Sijtsma, 2000). Items that fail to show monotonicity should be rejected.

Unidimensionality

In addition, as with traditional psychometric scales, the latent variable should be *unidimensional*. This means that a single latent trait underlies all the items in the model and is sufficient to explain all but the random variability that was observed in the data. Section 6.17 illustrates the use of bifactor analysis for examining whether a scale is essentially unidimensional. After fitting the bifactor model, the standardised loadings of all items in the 'common factor' should exceed 0.30, and items with loading below this are candidates for removal. Alternatively, Rose *et al.* (2008) use confirmatory factor analysis to fit a single factor and eliminated all items with loadings below 0.40.

Local independence

Related to unidimensionality is the concept of *local independence*, which states that for patients with equal levels of ability there should be zero correlation between any pair of items within the scale. That is, although we would expect to observe a (possibly strong) correlation between any two items in a scale if we calculate the correlation for a group of patients, this correlation should arise solely because both items reflect the same latent trait. Therefore, if we take account of the value of the latent trait, all remaining variability should be attributable to random fluctuations and the correlation should become zero after the latent trait is 'held constant'. In practical terms of PROs, when two items appear to be correlated, that correlation should arise solely because both items are measuring the same single dimension or construct. Local independence is implicit in the reflective model (Section 2.6) and the assumption of parallel interchangeable items (Section 2.7), and is a crucial assumption for fitting and estimating the parameters of the logistic IRT model. Without local independence there would be too many unknown parameters to estimate and it becomes impossible to obtain a solution to the IRT equations. To test for local independence, after having decided that a factor (or bifactor) model indicates that the items belong to an essentially unidimensional scale, the residual correlations of the items after fitting the one-factor model can be examined. If local independence applies, the residual correlations between pairs of items should not differ from zero; correlations exceeding 0.2 are suggestive of dependence, and Rose *et al.* (2008) suggest eliminating an item when a pair of items have residual correlation > 0.25. Reeve *et al.* (2007) review several other methods for assessing local independence.

Examples from the literature

Fliege *et al.* (2005) used residual correlations to test the local independence of items in their computer-adaptive test for depression (D-CAT). They noted that research suggests that IRT models are fairly robust to minor violations of unidimensionality, and specified that one item would be eliminated from each pair of items with a residual correlation of 0.25 or more; in such pairs, the item with the higher number of residual correlations (> 0.15) with other items was deleted. Fliege *et al.* acknowledged that the choice of 0.25 was arbitrary; models of local independence are approximations of reality and the effect on parameter estimation of small departures from local independence is unclear.

In the study of Petersen *et al.* (2011), inspection of residual correlations for the 34 physical functioning items led the authors to comment that: "of the 561 possible correlations, seven (1.2%) were > 0.2 and three (0.5%) were >0.25 (details not shown). Since no clear pattern was observed in these correlations (i.e., they may just be random findings), all 34 items were retained in a unidimensional physical functioning model."

When causal indicators (Section 2.6) are involved, the IRT model becomes questionable. Firstly, local independence is usually strongly violated because causal variables are correlated by virtue of having been themselves caused by disease or treatment; they are not independent for given levels of the latent variable. Symptom clusters are, by definition, groups of highly inter-correlated symptoms and, for example, QoL instruments may contain many symptom clusters. Secondly, 'difficulty' is a central concept to the whole IRT approach. However, the frequency of occurrence of a symptom does not relate to its impact on a patient. Pain, for example, might occur with the same frequency as another (minor) symptom; yet for those patients with pain its affect upon QoL can be extreme. Also, if we consider patients with a given level of ability (QoL), the frequency of different symptoms does not reflect their 'item difficulty' or their importance as determinants of QoL. IRT is clearly inappropriate for use with composite indicators that form summary indexes (see Section 2.6).

Any scale consisting of heterogeneous symptoms associated with disease or treatments, and which may therefore contain causal variables that affect QoL, should be carefully checked. The most suitable scales for logistic IRT modelling are those in which there is a clear underlying construct and where the items are expected to reflect levels of difficulty. Hence we have used physical functioning as our prime example: in most disease areas, items such as 'walking short distances', 'walking long distances', 'climbing flights of stairs' and 'carrying heavy loads' are likely to reflect the overall level of physical functioning. Thus although these items may be causal variables with respect to levels of QoL, they are also indicators of the level of physical functioning.

7.7 Fitting item response theory models: Tips

IRT models place heavy demands upon datasets. The parameter estimates may be imprecise and associated with large standard errors, models may be unstable and computer programs may fail to converge to a solution. The tips in Figure 7.6 are analogous to those that can be applied to other forms of modelling, including linear regression, but they assume special importance for estimating IRT models.

1. Use large datasets!

2. Use purpose-built computer software with output that is tailored for IRT modelling and provides IRT-specific diagnostic information such as goodness-of-fit and misfit indexes.

3. Studies should be designed so that the observations cover the full range of item values. If there are few patients with extreme values, it can become unfeasible to obtain reliable estimates of the item difficulties. For example, when evaluating physical function in a group of elderly patients, the majority of patients may have poor overall physical function and respond 'No' to difficult questions, such as those about carrying heavy loads, walking long distances and going up stairs. It may then be impossible to estimate these item difficulties.

4. *Person-misfit indexes* identify individuals who fail to fit the model well. The stability of the model estimation can be greatly improved by excluding these patients from analyses. For example, some patients might state that they are unable to take a short walk, yet inconsistently also indicate that they can take long walks. Such conflicting responses cause problems when fitting IRT models.

5. *Item-misfit indexes* can identify items that should be excluded before rerunning the IRT analyses. For example, the question 'Do you have any trouble going up stairs?' might have a high level of misfit since some patients who cannot go up stairs will reorganize their lifestyle accordingly. If they believe that the questionnaire concerns the degree to which they are inconvenienced or troubled, they might truthfully respond 'no problems, because I no longer have any need to go upstairs'.

6. Item parameter estimates should be invariant if some of the other items are dropped.

7. Person scores should be relatively invariant even if some items are dropped.

Figure 7.6 Tips for fitting IRT models.

7.8   Test design and validation

One of the important uses of IRT is in aiding the design of PRO questionnaires. IRT can identify items that are not providing much information, perhaps because they have low discrimination, are of similar difficulty to other items and provide little extra information or because the response options result in disordered thresholds. If it is important to evaluate all levels of the latent variable, items should be spaced fairly uniformly in terms of their difficulty and should cover the full range of the latent variable. If, on the other hand, one were only interested in subjects with high levels of ability, it would be sensible to concentrate most items in that region of difficulty. Also, if existing items have poor discrimination levels, it may be necessary to add several parallel items of approximately equal difficulty so as to increase the overall reliability or discrimination of the scale. Alternatively, it may be possible to explore why certain items on the questionnaire have poor discrimination (e.g. by interviewing patients with extreme high or low ability and for whom the item response differs from that expected), and to consider substituting other questions in their place. When IRT is used for test design purposes, it can be useful to start with a large pool of potential or candidate items and estimate the difficulty and discrimination of each item. The questionnaire can then be developed by selecting a set of items that appear to provide adequate coverage of the scale and which have reasonable discrimination.

The graphical methods and goodness of fit indices described in Section 7.5 can be used for assessing the quality of items. Items that have poor performance should usually be revised or excluded, unless they fill an important gap in the scale and no better item is available.

7.9   IRT versus traditional and Guttman scales

Each item in a traditional psychometric scale will often be either multicategory or continuous, and the level of the item provides an estimate of the latent variable. A single item would be prone to errors, such as subjects incorrectly scoring responses, and would lack precision. Thus the main purpose of having multiple parallel items, in which all items have equal difficulty, is to reduce the error variability. This error variability is measured by reliability coefficients, which is why Cronbach's α is regarded as of fundamental importance in psychometric scale development and is commonly used in order to decide which items to retain in the final scale (see Section 5.5).

Scales based upon IRT models, in contrast, frequently use binary items. Estimation of the latent variable now depends upon having many items of *different* levels of difficulty. In this context Cronbach's α is largely irrelevant to the selection of test items, since a high α can arise when items have *equal* difficulty – which is of course the opposite of what is required.

IRT can also be useful for testing the assumption of parallel items. Logistic models can be fitted, confirming that the items are indeed of equal difficulty and have equal discrimination. To do this, the item categories can be grouped to reduce multi-category items into dichotomous ones. IRT then provides a sensitive statistical test for validation of traditional scales, confirming that the scales perform as intended.

Guttman scales are multi-item scales that require each successive item to be more difficult than its predecessor, and are thus conceptually closely related to IRT models. For example, the item 'Can you take short walks?' is easier than and therefore comes before 'Can you take long walks?', which in turn would be followed by even more difficult tasks. Although Guttman scales are seemingly similar to IRT models, they make a strong assumption that the items are strictly hierarchical. Thus, if a patient indicates inability to accomplish the easiest item, they *must* respond similarly to the more difficult items. Conversely, if a patient answers 'Yes' to a difficult question, all prior, easier questions must be 'Yes', too. Hence in a perfect Guttman scale the response pattern is fully determined by the subject's level of ability. Under this model the ICCs are assumed to have almost vertical lines, leading to nearly perfect item discrimination. Such extreme assumptions may occasionally be realistic, as for example in childhood physical development (crawling, walking and running), but are likely to be rarely appropriate for PROs. IRT, based upon non-perfect discrimination and logistic probability models, seems far more appropriate.

7.10   Differential item functioning

Differential item functioning (DIF) arises when one or more items in a scale perform differently in various subgroups of patients. Suppose a physical functioning scale contains a number of questions, one of which is 'Do you have trouble going to work?' Such a question might be a good indicator of physical problems for many patients but could be expected to be less useful for patients who have reached retirement age. They would not experience trouble going to work if they were no longer in employment. As a consequence, a summated scale that includes this question could yield misleading results. If retirement age is 65, say, there might appear to be an improvement in the average scale score at the age of 66 when compared with 64, simply because fewer 66-year-olds report trouble going to work. The item 'trouble going to work' could therefore result in a biased score being obtained for older patients.

One example of a PRO instrument that contains exactly this question is the Rotterdam Symptom Checklist (RSCL), although the RSCL prudently contains qualifying patient instructions that say: 'A number of activities are listed below. We do not want to know whether you actually do these, but only whether you are able to perform them presently.' Those instructions make it clear that the authors of the RSCL were aware of potential item bias and that they sought to eliminate the problem by using carefully worded instructions.

Example from the literature

It is difficult to be certain that all patients will read the instructions thoroughly and act upon them. The UK Medical Research Council (MRC) colorectal trial CR04 used the RSCL, and found that 88% of patients over the age of 65 reported trouble going to work, as opposed to 57% under that age. This is consistent with the suggestion of age-related DIF. It was also noted that 25% of patients left that item blank on the form, with most of these missing responses being among older patients. This further supports the idea of DIF, since it implies that those patients had difficulty answering that item or regarded it as non-applicable; by contrast, less than 6% of patients left any of the other physical activity items blank.

One particularly important application of DIF analysis in outcomes research is the detection of linguistic and cultural differences. It provides a powerful tool for detecting whether patients in one language group respond to an item differently from other patients; if an item shows DIF, it may be indicative of cultural differences or, more probably, a translation inadequacy.

Although the term *item bias* used to be widely used as a synonym for DIF, most authors prefer the latter as a less pejorative term. DIF simply assesses whether items behave differently within different subgroups of patients, whereas ascribing the term 'bias' to an item constitutes a judgement as to the role and impact of the DIF.

A more general definition is that items with DIF result in systematically different results for members of a particular subgroup. Rankings *within* the subgroup may be relatively accurate, but comparisons between members of different subgroups would be confounded by bias in the test item. In the colorectal trial example, subjects over the age of 65 were not directly comparable with those under 65, because those retired tended to interpret differently the question about trouble working.

DIF can be an issue whenever one group of patients responds differently from another group and may be associated with gender, age, social class, socioeconomic status and employment differences. It may also be associated with disease severity. For many questionnaires the extent of DIF problems is largely unknown. Fortunately, the problems may be less severe in treatment comparisons made within a randomised clinical trial, since randomisation should ensure that roughly similar proportions of patients from each relevant subgroup are allocated to each treatment arm. DIF may, however, distort estimates of the absolute levels of QoL-related problems for the two treatment arms.

Several methods have been developed for DIF analysis, including powerful approaches using logistic regression models or IRT models, but we shall first illustrate a robust nonparametric analysis using a chi-squared test.

Example from the literature

Groenvold *et al.* (1995) tested the EORTC QLQ-C30 for DIF, using data from 1,189 surgically treated breast cancer patients with primary histologically proven breast cancer. They examined each of the 30 items, using age and treatment (whether they received adjuvant chemotherapy or not) as the two external variables for forming patient subgroups.

The QLQ-C30 contains five items relating to physical activities. For the DIF analysis, each item was scored 0 (no problem doing activity) or 1 (unable to do, or only with some trouble), and so the summated scores of the physical functioning ranged from 0 to 5. When a patient scored 0 for physical functioning, all five of the items must have been zero. Similarly, those scoring 5 must have responded with 1 for each item. These patients provide no information about DIF and were excluded, leaving 564 patients to be examined for evidence of DIF.

Table 7.5 shows that the item 'Do you have to stay in a bed or chair for most of the day?' behaves differently from the other items in the same scale. At each level of the physical functioning scale, this particular item behaves differently in relation to age. Younger patients are more likely to reply 'Yes' to this question. A significance test confirmed that this was unlikely to be a chance finding ($p < 0.006$). This item was also biased in relation to treatment.

Groenvold *et al.* note that the bias seen here may reflect an effect of chemotherapy (mainly given to patients below 50 years of age): some patients may have been in bed owing to nausea, not to a bad overall physical function. They also found that the pain item 'Did pain interfere with your daily activities?' and the cognitive function item 'Have you had difficulty remembering things?' were biased in relation to treatment.

Table 7.5 DIF analysis of the EORTC QLQ–C30 physical functioning scale

Physical functioning score (PF)	Age	Have to stay in bed or a chair		Number of patients
		0 (no)	1 (yes)	
1	25–50	97.3	2.7	113
	51–60	99.0	1.0	104
	61–75	100	0	92
2	25–50	92.3	7.7	52
	51–60	96.7	3.3	61
	61–75	100	0	85
3 & 4	25–50	28.6	71.4	21
	51–60	46.7	53.3	15
	61–75	47.6	52.4	21

Source: Groenvold *et al.*, 1995. Reproduced with permission of Elsevier.

Mantel–Haenszel test

In the example of Table 7.5, age defined the subgroups in each two-way table and Groenvold *et al.* used a test statistic called *partial-gamma*. An alternative method is the Mantel–Haenszel approach for testing significance in multiple contingency tables, using a χ^2 test. This is easier to calculate by hand and is widely available in statistical packages. Whereas the partial-gamma test can analyse multiple levels of age, we now have to reduce the data to a series of 2×2 tables by creating age subgroups of 25–50 years and 51–75 years.

To apply this method, the data are recast in the form of a contingency table with $2 \times 2 \times G$ cells, where G represents the levels of the test score (physical functioning scores 1, 2, and 3 & 4). Thus at each of the G levels there is a 2×2 table of item score against the two age subgroups that are being examined for DIF.

Suppose each of the G 2×2 tables is of the form:

	Item score		
Subgroup	1	2	*Totals*
I	*a*	*b*	*r*
II	*c*	*d*	*s*
Totals	*m*	*n*	*N*

Then we can calculate the expected value of *a*, under the assumption of null hypothesis of no DIF. This is given by

$$E(a) = \frac{rm}{N}. \tag{7.5}$$

The corresponding variance and odds ratio are

$$Var(a) = \frac{mnrs}{N^2(N-1)}, \quad OR = \frac{ad}{bc}. \tag{7.6}$$

The Mantel–Haenszel statistic examines the differences between the observed *a* and its expected value, $E(a)$, at each of the G levels of the test score, giving in large-study situations

$$\chi^2_{MH} = \frac{\left\{ \sum_{j=1}^{G} \left[a_j - E(a_j) \right] \right\}^2}{\sum_{j=1}^{G} Var(a_j)}, \tag{7.7}$$

where $j = 1, 2, \ldots G$. This is tested using a χ^2 test with degrees of freedom $df = 1$.

Furthermore, an estimate of the amount of DIF is given by the average *OR* across the *G* tables, which is

$$OR_{MH} = \frac{\sum_{j=1}^{G} a_j d_j / N_j}{\sum_{j=1}^{G} b_j c_j / N_j}. \tag{7.8}$$

A value of $OR_{MH} = 1$ means no DIF, and other values indicate DIF favouring subgroup I ($OR_{MH} > 1$) or subgroup II ($OR_{MH} < 1$).

Example

The data of Groenvold *et al.* (1995), summarised in Table 7.5, can be collapsed into 2 × 2 tables ($G = 3$) as in Table 7.6.

Using equations (7.5) and (7.6) we calculate the expected value and variance of *a*, and the *OR* for each table, giving Table 7.7.

The three odds ratios are less than 1, reflecting that at all levels of PF there were fewer patients in the older age group who were limited to having to stay in a bed or chair. From equation (7.8), $OR_{MH} = 0.306$. Applying equation (7.7), the Mantel–Haenszel statistic is 6.65. Appendix Table T4 for χ^2, with $df = 1$, shows this to be statistically significant ($p = 0.0099$). Groenvold *et al.* report a slightly smaller *p*-value when using partial-gamma, but the Mantel–Haenszel test is regarded as more sensitive and the difference between the two results is small.

Table 7.6 DIF analysis of the number of patients having to stay in bed or a chair (Data corresponding to Table 7.5)

Physical functioning score (PF)	Age	Have to stay in bed or a chair		Number of patients
		0 (no)	1 (yes)	
1	25–50	110	3	113
	51–75	195	1	196
2	25–50	48	4	52
	51–75	144	2	146
3 & 4	25–50	6	15	21
	51–75	17	19	36

Table 7.7 Results for the Mantel–Haenszel test used to detect DIF

Physical functioning score (PF)	*a*	*E(a)*	*Var(a)*	Odds ratio
1	110	111.54	0.919	0.188
2	48	50.42	1.132	0.167
3 & 4	6	8.47	3.249	0.447

IRT and logistic regression for DIF analyses

Two other approaches to DIF involve fitting models and estimating parameters: logistic regression models, and IRT models. Three advantages of both these methods are that (a) other prognostic factors can be included in the models, and (b) patterns of DIF (uniform, non-uniform) can be explored, and (c) estimates of the magnitude of DIF are available.

IRT provides a natural method for examining DIF. In principle, the ICCs should be the same for all subgroups of patients, but DIF occurs if, for example, males of a given ability find a test more difficult than females of the same ability. Thus IRT approaches make use of the sample-free invariance implicit in the estimation of ICCs. The null hypothesis is that there is no DIF, and that therefore the ICCs are equal. Thus, for the two-parameter logistic model, this implies:

$$b_{\text{Male}} = b_{\text{Female}} \text{ and } a_{\text{Male}} = a_{\text{Female}}$$

The use of IRT for testing DIF has, however, been criticised (by, for example, Hambleton and Swaminathan, 1991). It should be used only when there is evidence that IRT models provide a good fit to the items and that all the assumptions for IRT are valid. We focus here on use of logistic regression, which is computationally simpler and more robust against violation of the assumptions.

Logistic regression

Although logistic regression may be less robust than the Mantel–Haenszel method described above, it possesses major advantages of flexibility and ease of application. As with the Mantel–Haenszel approach, the basis is to examine the observed data to see whether, for each level of overall scale score, the items perform consistently. In statistical terms, the analyses are 'conditioned' on the scale score.

We start by considering a scale that contains binary yes/no items; writing X for the item being examined for DIF, S for the scale score derived from all the items including X, and G for the grouping variable (in the previous example, G was the age group), the logistic model is

$$\log\left[\frac{P(X)}{1 - P(X)}\right] = \beta_0 + \beta_1 S + \beta_2 G, \tag{7.9}$$

where P is the probability of endorsing $X = 1$ for given levels of S and G. This is a standard logistic regression equation.

Applying this model, an item X does not exhibit DIF if it depends solely on the scale score S, with statistically significant values of β_0 and β_1. If S is insufficient to explain the value of X – as indicated by a significant value for β_2 – there is evidence of DIF across the groups G. Statistical significance only indicates that there is some evidence supporting the existence of DIF; the value of β_2 provides the log odds-ratio as a measure of effect size. Some authors have suggested that only log odds-ratios with absolute value exceeding 0.64 are important. Others use changes in R^2, the proportion of variance explained by adding G to the model, as an indicator of effect size; Zumbo (1999) proposes that an R^2 change of 0.13 to 0.26 is moderate, and above 0.26 is large.

When an item takes higher (or lower) values within one group, as we have been describing, it is called *uniform* DIF. *Non-uniform* DIF occurs when the level of discrepancy of an item varies according to the scale score; in an extreme case, this might be manifested by an item that only shows DIF between the G groups at high levels of S, but not at lower scale scores. Non-uniform DIF also implies that an item is less strongly related to the scale score in one of the groups.

In the logistic model, non-uniform DIF is represented as an interaction term and may be tested using the β_3 coefficient in

$$\log\left[\frac{P(X)}{1-P(X)}\right] = \beta_0 + \beta_1 S + \beta_2 G + \beta_3 (S \times G). \tag{7.10}$$

The logistic regression approach can also allow for other explanatory factors, such as patient characteristics. Ordered logistic regression can accommodate items with ordered or numerical response categories. Thus the logistic regression approach can be readily extended to cover various situations. Scott *et al.* (2010) review DIF analyses of PROs using logistic regression.

Although the summated scale score, S, is commonly used as the conditioning variable for logistic regression approaches, a hybrid approach is to use an IRT-based scale score instead (Crane *et al.*, 2006); this may be of advantage if IRT-based scores differ appreciably from the sum scores.

Examples from the literature

Martin *et al.* (2004) used logistic regression to assess DIF among the 13 translations of the short-form Headache Impact Test (HIT-6). Since the questionnaire was developed in the USA and then translated into other languages, US English was regarded as the reference group. Thirteen 'dummy variables' were created, corresponding to the 13 languages, and for each patient the appropriate dummy variable was set to 1 so as to flag the language, and all others set to 0. Since six items were evaluated for DIF in each of the translations, there were 78 comparisons. An arbitrary double criterion was used to reduce the impact of multiple testing: statistical significance of $p < 0.05$ and $R^2 > 0.20$.

No items showed uniform or non-uniform DIF causing concern, and so the translations were regarded as equivalent.

In contrast, Petersen *et al.* (2003) examined equivalence of nine translations of the EORTC QLQ-C30 emotional functioning scale, using log odds-ratio numerically larger than 0.64 with a p-value < 0.001. Two pronounced instances of DIF were the Norwegian translation of 'Did you worry?' (log $OR = 1.30$, $p < 0.001$) and the Swedish version of 'Did you feel depressed?' (log $OR = -1.18$, $p < 0.001$). Inspection of these items suggested possible sub-optimal translation. The Norwegian 'Har du vært engstelig?' is literally 'Have you been anxious?', and it seems likely that being anxious is more extreme than worrying. The Swedish word nedstämd is not only a possible translation of depressed, but has additional connotations of being dejected and feeling 'down'; 'nedstämd' was thought to be a more common state than 'depressed'.

If DIF is detected in a short scale, it may be difficult to ascribe the DIF to any particular item. This is because differential item functioning, as its very name implies, only shows that within the target group as opposed to the reference group the items behave differently *relative* to each other. Thus, considering the extreme case of a 2-item scale, if one item manifests true DIF in, say, a negative direction, the other item will inevitably show 'pseudo DIF' of comparable magnitude but in the opposite direction. Unless there are qualitative grounds for deciding that one of the items is responsible for the DIF, all one can say is that the two items behave differently relative to each other in this group of subjects. This is demonstrated in the next example. This example also illustrates the problems of selecting a reference group and focal groups.

Example from the literature

Scott *et al.* (2006) used logistic regression to explore DIF attributable to cultural differences in completing the EORTC QLQ-C30. It can be difficult to separate the effects of language/translation and culture, and so the approach adopted was to form geographical clusters that each included a number of countries and languages. Since the QLQ-C30 was developed in English and translated into other languages, these groupings were contrasted against each other and against UK English. Figure 7.7 shows the log odds-ratios for the two items ('severity' and 'interference') of the pain scale. Confidence intervals (95%) are shown, and log odds-ratios that were both significantly different from 0 and exceeded ±0.64 were regarded as important.

Pseudo DIF was apparent: for any given level of pain severity, many of the non-English groups reported significantly greater pain interference. But we cannot ascribe the DIF to the reporting of severity or the reporting of interference. All we can say is that these two items behave differently relative to each other in the different geographical clusters.

Scott *et al.* discuss the extent to which these somewhat arbitrary geographical groupings represent different cultures. For example, the East Asian group includes both South Koreans and Chinese speakers from China, Singapore and Hong Kong. Although countries such as Korea and China might be deemed culturally highly distinct, the patterns were similar across all these countries both for pain and for other scales that Scott *et al.* explored. Interestingly, a cohort of patients in Singapore completed the English language version of the questionnaire, yet their responses were consistent with the Chinese speakers.

QLQ–C30 Pain (PA)

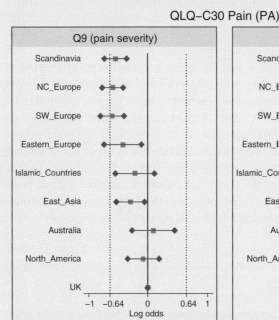
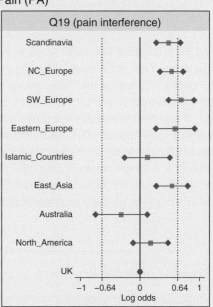

Figure 7.7 DIF analysis of EORTC QLQ–C30 2-item pain scale, by geographical region. *Source:* Scott *et al.*, 2007, Figure 4. Reproduced with permission of Springer Science+Business Media.

7.11 Sample size for DIF analyses

There are no established guidelines on the sample size required for DIF analyses, but the following recommendations are made by Scott *et al.* (2010). The minimum number of respondents will depend on the type of method used, the distribution of the item responses in the two groups, and whether there are equal numbers in each group. For binary logistic regression it has been found that 200 per group is adequate, and a sample size of 100 per group has also been reported to be acceptable for items without skewness. For ordinal logistic regression, simulations suggested that 200 per group may be adequate, except for 2-item scales. As a general rule of thumb, we suggest a minimum of 200 respondents per group as a requirement for logistic regression DIF analyses.

7.12 Quantifying differential item functioning

It can be difficult to quantify how much of a problem the issue of DIF is in practice. Although DIF has the potential to bias international comparative studies that use PROs, it may be less of a problem in clinical trials. Randomised treatment allocations in trials are usually stratified by country or centre, and many of the biases due to uniform DIF ought to occur in each group equally. For example, the consequences of DIF due to language or cultural effects are likely to be diminished in a trial that has been stratified by country. This would not necessarily apply to non-uniform DIF, nor to observational studies that are unable to make comparisons against a randomised control group. Although it is unclear how frequently substantial non-uniform DIF occurs, most authors suggest it is less common than uniform DIF. It may also be noted that DIF in an individual item will have much less impact on a long scale (for example, containing more than twenty items) than on a short one. Issues of DIF may affect all instruments, but its true extent and impact remains unknown.

When DIF is expressed as a log odds-ratio, the results can be translated into a clinically meaningful scale in the context of a specific scenario. Practical details of an approach for calculating the impact of the observed DIF effect are provided by Scott *et al.* (2009b).

Example from the literature

Scott *et al.* (2006) illustrate the impact of their results by considering a real study. Compared to the original English version, the Norwegian translation of the EORTC QLQ-C30 fatigue scale showed significant DIF in one of the three items, with Norwegians less likely to endorse the question 'Were you tired?' (log odds-ratio = −0.58). Scott *et al.* observed that, if it were assumed this item showed DIF, the FA scale scores would be around six points higher if the study had been carried out in an equivalent group of English patients, which corresponds to a difference that is generally regarded as small but clinically important. Since the patients in this randomised clinical trial were stratified by country, this DIF would not have affected the conclusions regarding the treatment comparison.

7.13 Exploring differential item functioning: Tips

DIF, like so many psychometric techniques, has been most extensively researched in fields such as education – because it is crucial that examinations should not contain questions that favour one ethnic group over another or one gender over the other.

1. Logistic regression is easier to use than most other forms of tests for DIF, and has the advantage of considerable flexibility. However, unlike IRT-based approaches, it makes use of the observed scale score as the conditioning variable.

2. Sample sizes should usually be at least 200 patients per group, and appreciably larger samples are required for using two-parameter IRT models.

3. Ordered logistic regression for items with multiple categories requires larger sample sizes.

4. Many investigations of DIF involve a considerable degree of multiple testing, and so it is commonly recommended to demand p-values of at least 0.01, or even $p < 0.001$, as a requirement for statistical significance. Alternatively, p-values may be adjusted using Bonferroni or other corrections.

5. Both statistical significance and effect size should be considered when deciding whether an item displays DIF. When using logistic regression, log odds-ratios with absolute value greater than 0.64 have been suggested. Other authors have used odds ratios outside the range 0.5 to 2.0. Another widely used criterion for logistic regression is the combination of $p < 0.01$ with a multiple correlation coefficient R^2. Moderate DIF is indicated by $R^2 > 0.13$, and large DIF by $R^2 > 0.26$.

6. It is generally thought that non-uniform DIF occurs less frequently than uniform DIF, but that it should be routinely tested for.

7. Test purification has been recommended by many authors. This is an iterative process that consists of recalculating the scale score (used as the conditioning variable) after deleting items that were most strongly identified as showing DIF, and then repeating the analyses.

8. The item being studied for DIF should be included when calculating the scale. Several papers have shown that type-I errors may be inflated if it is omitted.

9. Patients should be matched as accurately as possible; this implies that categories of the scale score should not be collapsed to form larger groups.

10. Care should be taken in defining the focal group. When evaluating translations, the original language version will normally form the reference group and the translated versions will be the focal groups.

Figure 7.8 Tips for exploring DIF.

Therefore much of the extensive theoretical work that has been carried out and most of the empirical studies into the effectiveness of DIF techniques have focused on educational and similar examinations. These examinations commonly contain large numbers of questions. In contrast, little is known about the effect of using DIF analyses on short scales of, say, fewer than 10 items. However, it seems likely that IRT-based methods may perform poorly under these situations, whereas the assumptions underlying the application of logistic regression imply that it is likely to be relatively robust.

Theory from educational psychometrics not only focuses on lengthy multi-item scales but also frequently assumes items are scored dichotomously as correct/incorrect, in which case floor and ceiling effects are generally not an issue. In contrast, PRO scales may be short, with items taking multi-category responses, and there may be serious floor/ceiling effects. Bearing these reservations in mind, we provide a list of tips culled mainly from Scott *et al.* (2010) (Figure 7.8).

7.14 Conclusions

IRT is becoming widely applied to PROs, despite the mathematical complexity of many of the models, the need for large sample sizes, the problems of including multi-category items, and the need for specialised computer software. Unfortunately, IRT makes strong assumptions about the response patterns of the items, and is sensitive to departures from the model. Patient outcome data are not as tidy and homogeneous as the items in educational examinations. The example that we considered by Haley *et al.* (1994) found that a Rasch model did not fit items in the physical functioning scale of the SF-36 very well. Perhaps this is not surprising: the assumption of local independence is a very demanding requirement, yet it is crucial to the estimation procedures used for IRT. Scales that include causal variables influencing QoL, such as treatment- or disease-related symptoms, will usually violate this assumption because the external variable (treatment or disease) introduces correlations that cannot be fully explained by the latent variable (QoL). Although scales such as physical functioning may appear to be homogeneous and contain items that are more closely hierarchical (increasing difficulty), the requirements for IRT are still highly demanding. For example, tasks such as bending and stooping may usually be related to physical functioning, but some patients who can walk long distances may have trouble bending and others may be able to bend but cannot even manage short walks. Thus the seemingly hierarchical nature of the items may be violated, with some patients providing apparently anomalous responses.

One important feature of IRT is that the mathematical nature of the model enables the inherent assumptions to be tested, and goodness-of-fit should always be examined. The logistic models can help to identify items that give problems, but when items do not fit the model it becomes difficult to include them in subsequent IRT analyses. Estimates of relative difficulty of items appear to be reasonably robust, but caution should be used when extending the model to other analyses. Tests of DIF are probably most easily applied using non-IRT approaches such as logistic regression conditioning on the computed scale score.

IRT is a useful tool for gaining insights that traditional techniques cannot provide. DIF analyses provide another powerful tool to complement the methods we have described in earlier chapters. Both IRT and DIF analyses are particularly useful in screening items for inclusion in new questionnaires, and for checking the validity of assumptions even in traditional tests. For these purposes alone, both techniques certainly deserve wide usage. The most exciting roles for IRT in outcomes research, however, lie first in the standardisation of different instruments so that PROs as assessed by disease- and treatment-specific instruments can be compared across different groups of patients and, secondly, in the development of computer-administered adaptive testing – as discussed in the next Chapter. Both of these objectives require extremely large databases for the exploration of IRT models.

7.15   Further reading, and software

IRT is a complex subject, and a good starting point for further reading is the book *Fundamentals of Item Response Theory* by Hambleton *et al*. (1991). For a comprehensive introduction, *Item Response Theory for Psychologists* by Embretson and Reise (2000) provides an excellent review while still avoiding complex mathematics. The Rasch model is described in detail by Andrich in *Rasch Models for Measurement: RUMM2030* (2010). Reeve *et al*. (2007) lay out in detail the plans used by the Patient-Reported Outcomes Measurement Information System (PROMIS) group.

There have been a number of recent advances in methods for assessing DIF, which are comprehensively covered in *Differential Item Functioning* by Osterlind and Everson (2009). Item bias is also the subject of the extensive book edited by Holland and Wainer (1993). A review of a wide range of methods, parametric and non-parametric, for assessing DIF, measurement equivalence and measurement invariance are reviewed by Teresi (2006), while Scott *et al*. (2010) review the choices that must be made when using logistic regression.

Examples of programs for IRT modelling include the following: PARSCALE (Muraki and Bock, 2003) can estimate parameters for one- and two-parameter models containing dichotomous and polytomous items, using graded response and generalised partial credit models. It can display item and test information functions. PARSCALE can use IRT to test for DIF. MULTILOG (Thissen, 2003), which focuses on multiple-category and polytomous models, can also fit graded response and generalised partial credit models, and in addition offers the nominal response model for polytomous items. However, it provides less information about item analysis and goodness-of-fit. RUMM (Andrich *et al*., 2010) and WINSTEPS (Linacre, 2011) both fit Rasch models and provide comprehensive facilities for test and scale development, evaluation and scoring. In the spirit of Rasch modelling, these packages assume common slopes and estimates the thresholds (difficulties) for dichotomous and polytomous items. IRTPRO (Cai *et al*., 2011) is a program with graphical interface and extensive modelling and graphics facilities. There are also packages that focus on specific functions, such as SIBTEST (Stout and Roussos, 1996) for IRT-based DIF analysis. Finally, general statistical packages increasingly provide facilities for comprehensive IRT modelling.

8

Item banks, item linking and computer-adaptive tests

Summary

Self-administered questionnaires have traditionally been paper-based. Apart from groups of items that are skipped over as not applicable, all patients complete the same questionnaire items. Computer-adaptive testing, in contrast, enables questions to be tailored to the individual patient, thereby maximising the information gathered. This offers two advantages: questionnaires can be shorter and the scale scores can be estimated more precisely for any given test length. Computer-adaptive testing involves accessing a large item bank of calibrated questions, and when a new patient is being assessed the computer program selects the most appropriate and informative items. Thus no two patients need complete the same set of items, and the computer-adaptive test imitates a clinical interview in that the choice of successive items to use depends on interpreting the accruing information from responses to previously asked items. In this chapter we show how IRT enables us to calibrate a collection of items, select the most informative items on a dynamic basis, and generate consistent scores across all patients.

8.1 Introduction

Computer-adaptive tests (CATs) concern the development of 'tailored' or adaptive tests. If a group of patients are known to be severely limited in their physical ability, it may be felt unnecessary to ask them many questions relating to difficult or strenuous tasks. Conversely, other patients may be fit and healthy, and it becomes less relevant to ask them detailed questions about easy tasks. Thus specific variants of a questionnaire may be more appropriate for different subgroups of patients. In a few exceptional cases, this approach can be adopted even when using traditional questionnaires. For example, if a question about physical functioning were to ask 'Can you walk a short distance?' and the respondent answers 'No', it would not be informative to ask next 'Can you run a long distance?' as we already know what the answer will be. In this simple example an experienced

Quality of Life: The Assessment, Analysis and Reporting of Patient-Reported Outcomes, Third Edition.
Peter M. Fayers and David Machin.
© 2016 John Wiley & Sons, Ltd. Published 2016 by John Wiley & Sons, Ltd.

interviewer might complete the answer without asking the item. However, in the more general case, such as when the response to the question about walking is 'with a little difficulty', we may suspect that the question about running will not add much information, but we cannot predict the exact response. Therefore, in a conventional interview setting, we would ask the full set of questions so as to be able to calculate the overall scale score.

An alternative is to use a dynamic procedure known as *computer-adaptive testing*. The principle of CAT is to make use of a previously generated pool of items, termed an *item pool* or an *item bank*. When assessing a patient, at each stage of the test process we evaluate the responses that have been made so far, and we draw the most informative item from the pool of those remaining. This process continues until we have a sufficiently precise estimate of the scale score. Thus the aim is to attain a precise score while asking the patient to answer as few questions as are necessary. Wainer (2000) has shown that CAT questionnaires are typically 30–50% shorter than conventional questionnaires with the same measurement precision.

The key to CAT is the use of logistic item response theory (IRT) modelling, which was introduced in the previous chapter. IRT enables each item to be calibrated along a single continuum that represents the latent trait, or scale score. Thus a consistent scale score can be calculated, irrespective of which set of items was completed by an individual patient. In effect, we have a single ability scale and can identify and exploit those items that relate to the segments of interest along the scale. After each item has been answered, the computer dynamically evaluates the respondent's location on the ability continuum. Then, according to the previously calibrated item difficulties, the maximally informative item to present next is selected. Continuing the above example, if the respondent has very much difficulty walking a short distance, the computer might have selected for the next question an item about walking around the house. In contrast, if the response were that there is no difficulty at all in walking, far more informative items might concern walking long distances or running.

Figure 8.1 shows the principles of the CAT algorithm. IRT provides the essential features that enable CATs. In this chapter, we shall explore each of the issues indicated in Figure 8.1 and illustrate the implementation of CATs.

8.2   Item bank

The first stage in developing a CAT is the creation of a comprehensive *item bank*. An item pool, or item bank, is a collection of items that represent and define a single dimension (domain) (Figure 8.2). The aim of item banking is to gather together a number of items that are positioned along the full range of the continuum being addressed. That is, the items should be of varying difficulty and should cover all levels of ability or functioning that are of relevance for measurement. If the objective of the instrument is screening for symptoms needing treatment, the emphasis might be on having a comprehensive set of items with difficulties either side of the threshold for therapy; on the other hand, for most research applications, a wider segment of the continuum – or even the entire range – may be of interest.

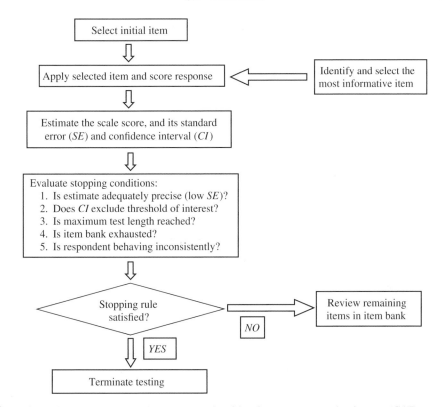

Figure 8.1   Chart representing the computer algorithm for a computer adaptive test (CAT).

- **Item banking and item calibration**
  The difficulty of each item can be evaluated, providing estimates of the item positions along the ability continuum.

- **Scale standardisation and test equating**
  Once the items have been calibrated for difficulty, consistent scale scores may be calculated irrespective of which particular set of items have been used. This approach can also be used when comparing similar subscales in different instruments, when it is known as *test linking or test equating*.

- **Test information**
  As already outlined, we can evaluate the amount of information in a test, and also the additional information contributed by each item (Section 7.5). This enables us to identify which item is optimally informative and should be selected for the next stage of the test procedure.

- **Precision of scale scores**
  The test information function is inversely related to the SE of the estimated score. Thus at the same time as evaluating the test information, we can calculate the SE that applies to the current estimate of the patients scale score. When the SE becomes sufficiently small, we know that we have attained sufficient precision and can terminate the test.

Figure 8.2   Item banking.

When building an item bank, a common initial approach is to review the literature on existing instruments and assemble a number of items from these questionnaires. Also, at an early stage of the development, thought should be given to any gaps in the continuum or segments that are not well covered. Although the subsequent data collection and quantitative analyses will in due course reveal any gaps, frequently an early qualitative review will indicate whether there is need for additional items, for example at the high and low ends of the continuum. Items may come from many different sources and will inevitably have a variety of formats, phrasing and response options. To produce a coherent instrument such idiosyncrasies will have to be standardised, although care should be taken to ensure that this does not compromise the conceptual basis of those items.

Examples from the literature

Fatigue is a common symptom both in cancer patients and in the general population. It is commonly regarded as difficult to assess effectively and efficiently, and is frequently under-treated. Lai *et al.* (2005) developed an item bank for assessing cancer-related fatigue. The preliminary item bank consisted of 92 items. Fourteen came from the authors' existing FACIT questionnaires and another 78 were written following a review of the literature, to cover the continuum in terms of content and item difficulty and to eliminate ceiling and floor effects.

    Another example of an item bank was the development of the Headache Impact Test (HIT) for assessing the burden of headaches (Bjorner *et al.*, 2003). These authors began by selecting items from four widely used measures of headache of impact, which resulted in 53 items in total. These items were standardised to have five-category rating scales, and the items were reworded to specify a recall period of 30 days.

8.3 Item evaluation, reduction and calibration

After developing the list of candidate items (Figure 8.3), the next step is to test them on patients and collect response data. Patients, representative of the diversity of the target groups at which the measurement scale will be directed, should be recruited and asked to complete the items. The aim is to establish that

1. all items relate to a single unidimensional scale,

2. the assumptions of local independence and monotonicity are satisfied,

3. an IRT model provides adequate fit for each item,

4. there is no evidence of substantial DIF across the patient subgroups,

5. item difficulty can be assessed.

    The first three points are interrelated. Essentially, they concern ensuring that the items perform equally across all subgroups of patients, and that all items represent the

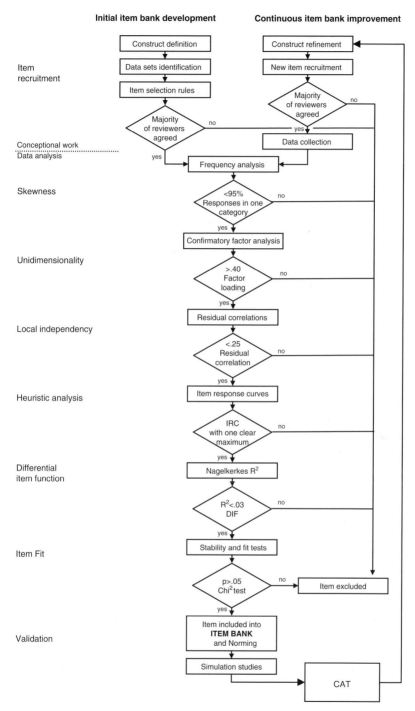

Figure 8.3 Stages in the development of an item bank, for use in a computer adaptive test (CAT).
Source: Rose *et al.* 2008, Figure 1. Reproduced with permission of Elsevier.

same single dimension. Methods of the previous chapters provide the means for making these tests – for example, dimensionality may be assessed by the factor analysis methods of Chapter 6 (exploratory-, confirmatory- or bi-factor analysis). Items that fail to meet the dimensionality requirements should be reviewed and possibly revised or reworded. Alternatively, they might be excluded from the item bank. The IRT methods of Chapter 7 can then be applied, to assess the validity of the assumptions (Section 7.6). After fitting an IRT model, the items are tested for fit to the IRT model, and those that do not show adequate fit should be modified and retested, or considered for removal from the item bank. Poorly performing items, with weak discrimination or disordered response categories (Section 7.5) should be deleted. Finally, the possibility of DIF with respect to major socio-demographic and clinical factors should be explored (see Section 7.10), leading again to further items that may have to be rejected.

After this 'winnowing' or pruning of the item bank, the remaining items should be calibrated according to the IRT model. The aim is to calibrate along a single latent trait the difficulties of all items, providing estimates of their location and discrimination. Not only are these parameters required for the application of CAT, but they also reveal any gaps in the item bank where there may be a lack of items targeting a particular range of difficulties. New items may be required to address these gaps; after testing, they may be added to the item bank.

Example from the literature

To evaluate and calibrate the 53 candidate items of the HIT, Bjorner *et al.* (2003) used a national survey to interview 1,016 randomly selected persons in the USA. First, dimensionality was explored using confirmatory factor analysis (CFA). Three alternative factor models were considered and the authors decided that, despite poor model fit, it would be justifiable to apply a unidimensional IRT model to the data. Then, initial evaluation of the item characteristic curves (ICCs) indicated that for some items adjacent categories were non-informative, and so these were combined to give fewer distinct categories. Next, the generalised partial credit IRT model (see Section 7.5) was applied for a more extensive exploration of the characteristics of each item, and to estimate the item thresholds. Logistic regression DIF analyses confirmed that there were no major signs of DIF and that the items performed similarly in all patients. The authors concluded that the item pool could be considered as a basis for a CAT test (this example is continued in Section 8.5).

8.4   Item linking and test equating

Item linking

So far we have been describing the situation where all patients complete the full set of items that will be included in the item bank. This may not be feasible for several reasons. Sometimes the item bank will be too large, and the burden on patients would either be too great or might be likely to lead to poor compliance; it may be preferable to divide the items into smaller 'testlets' or sub-tests. Sometimes there may be existing data available for some items, which can contribute to the estimations. Also, if the item bank is deemed inadequate in places, it may be desired to add further items at a later date.

Fortunately it is not necessary for all patients to give responses to the full set of items – indeed, it is possible to fit the IRT models even if no patients receive all of the items. All that is required is that there should be a sufficient overlap of items administered to different patients so that the estimated scale scores can be *anchored* and the item difficulties estimated. Thus when considering existing sets of data, the important thing is that there should be *anchor items* that are the same as items used in other questionnaires. Without such anchor items, the problem of different respondent samples being likely to have different underlying trait levels would make the analyses and the estimates difficult, or even impossible, to interpret.

When constructing large item banks, the usual solution is to divide the items across two or more separate and shorter questionnaires, with each questionnaire including a common set of questions as anchor items. Thus all respondents receive the anchor items. These anchor items are chosen to be broadly representative of the item bank and roughly uniformly spaced across the latent trait continuum. Optimally, these should include items towards both the upper and lower limits of the scale. Ten or more anchor items are frequently advocated, although for linking a large number of items some authors recommend that as many as 20% of the total should be anchors (Cook and Eignor, 1989).

This study design is known as the *common item design*. There are then several methods for calibrating the items onto a common continuum, or *item linking*. One method is *concurrent calibration*, in which IRT software is used to calibrate the combined set of items onto a single standard metric. The assumption is that there is a 'true' underlying score (the latent trait) that is being estimated by all items.

A variant of concurrent calibration is to first estimate only the parameters of the common items, and then while holding them fixed (anchored) the parameters of the remaining items are estimated for each questionnaire. A linear transformation function can then be derived from the parameter estimates.

Alternatively, using *separate calibration*, each respondent sample is analysed separately, and the parameter estimates of the anchor items are used to identify an appropriate linking transformation. This approach allows items from a number of samples to be transformed to the metric defined by a single specified base sample.

Usually, linear transformation functions are used, and one test or questionnaire is defined as the *base* to which others will be transformed. The equating of questionnaires can be accomplished either by identifying a function for transforming the scores, or by determining a function that transforms the IRT parameter estimates from one test to the other. A simple approximate procedure for matching is in terms of how many *SD*s the scores, or parameter estimates, are above the mean for the test – this is known as the *mean and sigma* method. Details of all these procedures are given in Kolen and Brennan (2010).

A number of other study designs have been proposed for item linking. For example, a sample of respondents can be randomly allocated to receive one of two (or more) instruments. Then we can assume that all differences in overall trait level are random and that the groups are randomly equivalent. These, and other more complex designs, are outlined by Embretson and Reise (2000) and discussed by Kolen and Brennan (2010).

Test equating

A topic related to item linking is the *linking of scale scores*, known as *test equating*. The aim here is to calibrate different instruments against each other. Similar procedures to those mentioned above can be used. Strictly, however, two scales can only be equated if they satisfy the following conditions:

• *Equal construct requirement*

They should measure the same construct and refer to the same continuum.

• *Equal reliability requirement*

They should have the same reliability.

• *Symmetry requirement*

If a score on one questionnaire is equated to a score on the second questionnaire using a transformation procedure, the second scores can also be equated to the first by using the inverse transformation procedure. Note that this is unlike solutions from linear regression, in which a regression of x on y is not the inverse function of the regression of y on x.

• *Equity requirement*

The scales must be equally effective so that it is immaterial which is used.

• *Population invariance requirement*

They must have the same relationships for different populations.

These requirements are clearly mandatory for equity in educational testing. In a medical context, however, it is perhaps more common to use regression methods for *prediction* of the scores that would have been expected if another instrument had been used (see Section 17.7); this is frequently the aim when comparing results across studies. However, Fayers and Hays (2014b) show that regression-based methods for test-linking result in artificially reduced estimates of the standard deviations and must be used with caution for group comparisons and clinical trials. *Calibration* is used when questionnaires measure the same construct but with unequal reliability (for example when less reliable short-form instruments are used instead of the longer and more precise standard versions), or unequal difficulty (an example of the latter would be a difficult version of a questionnaire for healthy people and an easier version for those with severe illness).

Example from the literature

McHorney and Cohen (2000) constructed an item bank with 206 functional status items, drawn from a pool of 1,588 potential items. Even 206 items was considered too lengthy for a mail survey of the elderly, and also it was thought that some closely similar items would be perceived by the respondents as redundant duplicates. Therefore three questionnaires were constructed, each containing a common set of 89 anchor items and 39 unique items. The response options to all items were standardised to have six categories.

A graded response IRT model was fitted using the package MULTILOG (Thissen, 2003). Concurrent calibration was used for all groups. First, the anchor items were tested for DIF, as it is essential that these items should function in the same way within all the groups. A total of 28 items exhibited DIF and were excluded as anchors. Another 18 items were excluded because they exhibited little variability in participants' responses. The remaining items were used as anchors for equating the three forms. As output from the equating, the authors presented a four-page table of the IRT thresholds and discriminations for all items.

Although no items were 'very, very easy', about two-thirds were located at the easier end of the continuum. Only six items were rated as 'very difficult' (such as 'climbing more than 30 steps', 'carrying large bags of groceries', 'scrubbing the floor'). Items with highest discrimination were those associated with clearly defined explicit activities, including 'put underclothes on', 'move between rooms', 'get into bed', 'take pants off'. Poorly discriminating items tended to be those that could be ambiguous. For example, the response to 'difficulty using a dishwasher' would be unclear if the respondent does not have a dishwasher, and similar ambiguities apply to items such as 'difficulty driving in the dark'.

8.5 Test information

Test information functions, as described in Section 7.5, can be evaluated for the full item pool, to assess the adequacy of coverage of the items. Also, as we have seen in Figure 7.5 and equation (7.4), the standard error of measurement is estimated by the square root of the inverse of the information function. Any inadequate coverage should be addressed by creating new items to complement the existing pool.

The test information function is also used after the CAT has been developed and is being applied to individual patients. During each cycle of the algorithm in Figure 8.1, the test information function is evaluated for the set of items that have been currently included in the test. The corresponding *SE* is calculated and the *CI* (confidence interval) can be computed.

Example from the literature

Bjorner *et al.* (2003) examined the information content of the items used in the Headache Impact Test (HIT). Figure 8.4 shows the information function for the HIT item pool, together with the *SE* of measurement. The scale has been defined such that the population mean is zero and the *SD* is one. It can be seen that the item pool is most informative at two *SD*s above the mean, where there are relatively few headache sufferers. The items in the pool are less informative for patients with little headache.

Bjorner *et al.* (2003) conclude that the item pool shared the weakness of the original instruments in providing inadequate information for people with little or average headache. Therefore they investigated additional items that clinical experts proposed as suitable for discriminating amongst people with mild headache.

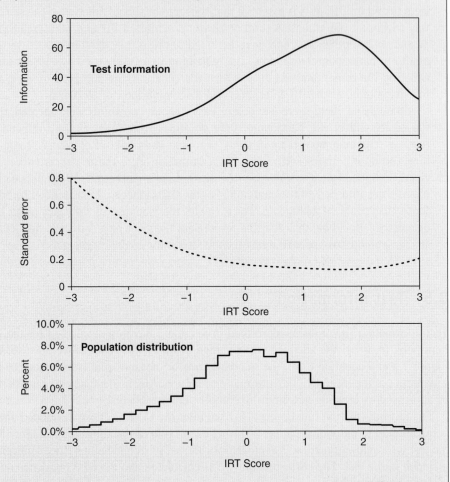

Figure 8.4 Information function and standard error of measurement for the HIT item pool compared with the population distribution of headache impact. *Source:* Bjorner *et al.*, 2003, Figure 3. Reproduced with permission from Springer Science and Business Media.

8.6   Computer-adaptive testing

After constructing the initial item bank and calibrating the items, the preliminary CAT test can be developed and tested on patients. The outline of the CAT procedure was shown in Figure 8.1. Each patient will receive a different set of questions. These questions are chosen with difficulties that should be challenging to the patient, and are therefore maximally informative when estimating a precise scale score. For these scale scores, simple summated scores would be inconsistent and are inappropriate. Instead, since the individual questions have been calibrated along the continuum and their item difficulties estimated, IRT-based scoring makes use of these item difficulties to calculate scores that reflect the patient's position on the continuum. This is a complex calculation, and hence adaptive testing is invariably computer based.

When a patient commences the test, the initial item is usually chosen as one of medium difficulty. From the patient's response, the current (initial) estimate of their scale score is made. Being based on a single item, this will not be a very precise score. Therefore the next (second) item is selected, chosen to have difficulty (or thresholds) in the region of this current estimate of the patient's scale score. The response to this item enables the score to be recalculated with greater precision. The precision of this revised estimate is calculated using IRT, and the *SE* and *CI* are determined. If the *SE* is not considered sufficiently small or the *CI* is too large, another question is selected from the item bank. This process continues, as shown in Figure 8.1, until satisfactory values are obtained for the *SE* and the *CI* (or until the items have been exhausted or the patient has answered the maximum permitted number of items).

We have presented the development and calibration of the item bank as being a separate and distinct phase from the application of the CAT. However, the CAT data that is subsequently collected on patients can be also added to the information already in the item bank, enabling a more precise computation of the item characteristics. New items may also be added as necessary to the item bank. Thus there may be overlap between the development and application phases, with the item bank that feeds into the CAT model continuing to be expanded and modified.

Figure 8.5 summarises the main advantages and disadvantages of CAT over conventional questionnaires.

Advantages

- The number of questions presented to each respondent is minimised.
- Selection of items is individually tailored, and irrelevant items omitted—potentially enhancing responder compliance.
- Floor and ceiling effects can be minimised.
- The user can specify the desired degree of precision, and the test continues until the precision is attained.
- Individuals making inconsistent response patterns can be identified.
- Items and groups of respondents showing DIF are readily identified.

Disadvantages

- Comprehensive item pools have to be developed and tested.
- Item calibration studies require large numbers of patients.
- The methodology is more theoretically complex than that of traditional psychometrics.
- Implementation in hospital and similar settings may present practical difficulties.
- Ideally, item banks will have continued expansion and refinement even after the CAT has been released.

Figure 8.5 Advantages and disadvantages of CAT.

Examples from the literature

Lai *et al.* (2003) illustrate how the precision increases as successive items from their fatigue CAT are applied to an example patient. Initially, a screening item ('I have a lack of energy') was applied. The patient responded 1 on the 0–4 scale, indicating 'quite a bit' of fatigue. From the previously calibrated item bank, it was known that this meant the patient's score on the 0–100 fatigue scale was expected to be between 29.6 and 47.3, with the midpoint value of 38.5 being the best estimate. However, the range of uncertainty is 47.3–29.6 = 17.7, which is very wide. Therefore another item was selected, with difficulty (mean threshold value) close to 38.5; this item was 'I have trouble finishing things because I am tired.' The patient endorsed 1 on this item, too, which led to a more precise score estimation of 38.5 to 47.3, with a midpoint estimate of 42.9. The test continued until four items had been applied, when the predicted scale score was 44.9 plus or minus 2.0.

Figure 8.6, adapted from Ware *et al.* (2003), compares the CAT scores against the scale scores based on the full item pool of 54 headache impact items. The agreement and precision improve as the number of items in the CAT increases from 6 to 10, 13 and 20.

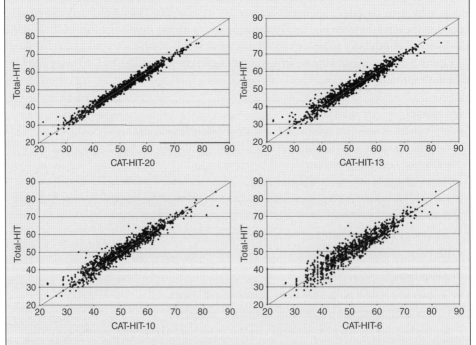

Figure 8.6 Relation between HIT scores based on the full 54-item pool and the CAT based on 6, 10, 13 or 20 items. *Source:* Ware *et al.*, 2003, Figure 2. Reproduced with permission of Springer Science and Business Media.

8.7   Stopping rules and simulations

The CAT continues until terminated by a *stopping rule*, as shown in Figure 8.1. The choice of stopping rule is a compromise between the wish to obtain high precision and the desire to keep the test short. The most effective way to review the consequences of various stopping rules is by computer-based simulations. Simulations generated from the patient-response data already collected for the item bank are called *real simulations* (McBride, 1997). The principle is to apply the algorithm shown in Figure 8.1 to each of the previously observed patients that are in the database. The computer only uses the responses that would have been obtained during a live CAT, and the responses that the patient made to other items is ignored.

This simple approach is less useful when item-linking of multiple questionnaires has been used, as many respondents may not have answered some of the items that become selected when the CAT is applied. Instead, the IRT model that has been fitted can be used to simulate responses that would be representative of a random sample of respondents (simulees).

Example from the literature

Fliege *et al.* (2005) adopted both these simulation approaches when developing a CAT for depression (D-CAT). After calibrating the items, the CAT algorithm was applied and the stopping rule of $SE \leq 0.32$ was evaluated. For 'real simulations', the response data collected for calibrating the CAT was used. For IRT simulations, 100 virtual persons were simulated at each 0.25 interval along the latent trait continuum from −3.5 to +3.5, resulting in a sample of 2,900 'simulees'.

Most of the respondents had depression scores within two SDs of the mean value, that is, over the latent trait continuum of −2.0 and +2.0. The real simulations indicated that over this range an average of 6.12 items ($SD = 2.11$) was needed to obtain estimates with an $SE \leq 0.32$. Using simulees, an average of 7.15 items ($SD = 1.39$) were needed over this range.

It was concluded that there is little difference in information between the total 64-item test score and the CAT score, which is based on an average of approximately six items. Fleige *et al.* comment: 'The considerable saving of items without a relevant loss of test information is in line with previous studies.'

The example of Fliege *et al.* is interesting, as this is one of the few studies that has been able to create an item pool with item locations so effectively spread across the full continuum. However, Reise and Waller (2009) observe that this was accomplished by treating depression as a bipolar continuum marked by happiness items (optimistic) on one end and depression items on the other; they question this, firstly suggesting that the lower end of a depression scale should not be 'happiness' but 'lack of depression', and secondly citing the findings of Stansbury *et al.* (2006) that positively worded items on a well-known depression measure needed to be eliminated to achieve adequate fit to an IRT model.

8.8   Computer-adaptive testing software

Many investigators have found it necessary to develop their own CAT programs, as commercially available software for handling polytomous responses is limited. First, standard IRT software is frequently used to estimate the item parameters, and this calibration process is repeated at intervals whenever an appreciable number of additional patients have been accrued to the central database. Recalibration would also occur whenever new items are being written and added to the item pool. Then when a new patient is being tested, CAT software can use these stored item parameters and their associated IRT models. The algorithm of Figure 8.1 is used, with the CAT program calculating the individual patient scores and *SE*s. Further items are selected and applied, until the stopping rule is satisfied.

Some questions and issues that should be considered when developing or purchasing software include those in Figure 8.7.

- Patients have varying computer skills, and software should be robust and 'user friendly', with an effective human-computer interface.
- What input device or devices should be supported? Possibilities include touch sensitive PC tablets, mobile phones and voice input.
- Many patients may be old, have poor eyesight, or have limited dexterity. Therefore the questions should be written in a large bold font, with large boxes for tapping the response.
- Should several items be displayed on the screen simultaneously, or should they be presented one at a time? The decision may partly depend on the complexity of the questions being used.
- Should there be a facility for patients to go back and either review their responses or correct them?
- Are translations of the item bank needed, and if so can the software support all of them?
- How will the data be saved? Is it desired to integrate or link the CAT results with hospital information systems or other databases?
- Are individual patient scores to be calculated and made available to the patient's clinician? In what format will these be displayed or printed?
- Will patient responses be accumulated for subsequent analyses and improvement of the item bank? Monitoring of patients' responses (such as recording the time taken for responding to each item) can also be useful for improving the item bank and the CAT.
- Checks of data quality should be implemented, with detection of inconsistent responses and 'patient misfit'.
- The usual needs for data security and data protection of confidential medical data will apply.
- Comprehensive backup facilities in case of system failure are essential.

Figure 8.7   Issues to be considered for CAT software.

8.9 CATs for PROs

Major benefits from using CAT have been found in other fields, such as educational testing. Similar gains should be attainable for PRO and QoL instruments, although there are some challenges:

- *Items should have varying difficulty*

  In educational examinations it is easy to identify test items that have major differences in difficulty levels. Similarly, it is easy to demonstrate the efficiency of CAT for outcomes such as physical functioning, or the impact of pain on daily activities. For many other PROs the advantages may be far smaller.

- *Length of questionnaires*

  In educational examinations, the students are clearly motivated to respond to as many questions as they can – the issues of examination length are of less concern than in health-related applications. In contrast, the usual requirement for QoL studies to assess multiple dimensions means that for many applications the maximum number of items per scale will be tightly limited. This may reduce the benefits of CAT. On the other hand, the efficiency of CAT should offer major advantages over traditional paper-based questionnaires.

- *Dimensionality/local independence*

  As emphasised in previous chapters, concerns about dimensionality, and especially local independence, may be more severe in health assessment than in education. This may be particularly important for symptoms of disease and side effects of therapy, which may constitute formative scales.

- *Item sequencing*

  The developers of almost all traditional questionnaires rigidly emphasise that the order of questions must remain fixed and that no new items may be inserted. This is because of fears that responses to earlier items may influence later ones in some unspecified manner. In CAT, each patient will receive different items and in varying sequences. The impact of changes in item order remains largely unknown.

- *Cost and practicality*

  In educational settings, the provision of computer facilities is more easily structured than in busy hospital environments. Costs and delivery are important considerations for any test, and the implementation of CAT in hospital settings and in multicentre clinical trials needs further investigation.

Given these considerations, careful evaluation of the benefits of CAT in outcomes research is called for.

Multidimensional CAT

Since QoL is, by definition, multidimensional, it has been suggested that multidimensional CAT should be used (Petersen *et al.*, 2006). The principle here is that since many of the dimensions are strongly correlated they are informative about each other, and so either the total number of items that are presented can be further reduced or extra precision derived by making maximum use of all the information collected. For example, a person who is very fatigued will tend to report a correspondingly poor physical functioning. Thus, when assessing levels of fatigue, the CAT ought to make use of information from dimensions such as physical functioning. Petersen *et al.* found that by using multidimensional CAT for the EORTC QLQ-C30 about half the items sufficed to obtain comparable precision to the standard QLQ-C30 version 3.

DIF and CAT

Although items exhibiting DIF are generally deprecated, CAT may also offer a potential to correct for DIF effects. In some scales it may be difficult to avoid item bias, and the investigators may decide to overcome DIF by including different items for different subgroups of respondents. For example, suppose an instrument is required for use in a clinical trial that will be recruiting patients aged from 10 to 70. It might be desired to obtain a single indicator of physical function even though 'good physical functioning' will take on a different meaning for children as opposed to adults. In such a situation the investigator might have one question for adults about going to work, a different question for children about going to school, and possibly other questions aimed at other subgroups of patients such as the retired. Then each question would be relevant only for its own target subgroup, and would not be valid for other patients. The results could be analysed by calibrating the individually targeted questions onto the overall physical functioning continuum. In this simple example one could in principle have considered instead using a compound question, such as: 'Do you have trouble going to school/work or doing housework/performing retirement activities?' However, this could be confusing and easily misunderstood, and the listed activities might have different relevance in the various subgroups; IRT and CAT offer greater potential for a consistent scaling.

8.10 Computer-assisted tests

This chapter is mainly about the use of IRT to develop CATs – computer-*adaptive* tests. However, another important use of computers is in computer-assisted testing. In clinical and related settings it is standard practice for the nurse, clinician or other interviewer to adapt the questions according to the relevant issues. For example, if a patient says they have a particular symptom, the interviewer may inquire about severity and duration. Some symptoms may be intermittent, in which case frequency may be

relevant. Sometimes significant questions may concern impact on the patient or interference with activities. Computer-assisted tests can be developed, mimicking the traditional patient–clinician interview. The objective of these tests is to expand out the
reported symptoms, as appropriate in each case, by exploring the relevant aspects and
issues surrounding each specific symptom.

This form of testing is most useful when the assessments are intended for routine
patient management, but may also be of value when collecting information in clinical
trials: an obvious situation concerns the detection and reporting of unusual adverse
effects.

A useful combination of testing may be CAT for measuring the main QoL dimensions, and tailored questions for expanding out relevant symptomatology.

8.11   Short-form tests

The methodology of IRT and CAT can also be used to generate efficient so-called
short-form (SF) versions of questionnaires, in which an optimal set of items is selected
from the item bank such that maximum precision over a specified range is obtained
when using the minimal number of items. The benefit of adding items can be assessed
in terms of the impact on precision of the estimated scores; either the maximum number of items or the desired precision may be prespecified when developing the SF
instrument. Many instrument developers offer brief SF versions, frequently developed
in parallel with a full CAT approach. Since these SF versions consist of fixed sets of
items, all respondents complete the same questionnaire, and it may for example be
presented in a traditional paper-and-pencil format.

One particular aspect of an IRT-based SF approach is that separate SF versions of a
questionnaire may be developed for specific populations. For example, when assessing
physical functioning of severely ill hospital in-patients the range of interest is different
from that in a relatively healthy population. In terms of IRT, we can search for items
that yield an information function covering the required population distribution. Thus
different SF versions, all calibrated to provide scores on a single common metric, may
be generated for specific populations that are expected to have different mean scores,
ranges or *SD*s. Also, for some applications brevity (fewer items, less burdensome) may
be more important than precision. IRT and CAT provide the tools for deriving such SF
questionnaires.

8.12   Conclusions

CAT potentially presents major advantages over traditional testing. In particular, it
offers the possibility of gaining greater precision while presenting fewer questions to
the patient. It also results in tailored tests that avoid asking patients irrelevant – and
therefore possibly irritating – questions. Scores from CAT also have the advantage that

their precision is automatically determined as part of the computational process, which is rarely the case with traditional methods. But, on the other hand, the development process is more complex and involves the development, validation and calibration of large item banks.

The benefit of the CAT approach is that it is less burdensome for the respondents. Fewer items are required for any given level of precision. For any given number of items, the estimated scores from a CAT are more precise than for a traditional questionnaire with a fixed set of items.

Although CATs are theoretically more efficient than traditional tests, the greatest gains are apparent only when dimensions are amenable to evaluation using items of varying difficulty. Thus the assessment of physical functioning and activities of daily living offer ideal examples – even traditional instruments resort to questions regarding from easy tasks, such as ability to get out of bed, through to more difficult activities such as running a long distance. Similarly, 'impact' scales readily offer items of varying difficulty. Examples include the impact of fatigue on daily activities, the interference of pain on activities, and the headache impact test that we have described. For other types of scale it may be more difficult to devise items of appreciably varying difficulty, in which case the benefits of CAT are less clear.

8.13   Further reading

The book by Wainer (2000) provides a comprehensive discussion of the development of CATs. Examples of papers setting out principles and methodology for developing item banks and CAT systems for PROs are Reeve *et al.* (2007), Rose *et al.* (2008), Thissen *et al.* (2007) and Petersen *et al.* (2010). The special issue of *Quality of Life Research* (2003) volume 12, number 8, contains several papers illustrating the development of the headache impact test. Two groups have developed CATs for cancer-related fatigue, and both provide comprehensive details: the reports of the Functional Assessment of Chronic Illness Therapy (FACIT) group (Lai *et al.*, 2003, 2005) may be compared against those of the EORTC group (Giesinger *et al.*, 2011; Petersen *et al.*, 2013). Test equating, scaling and linking are detailed by Kolen and Brennan (2010).

PART 2
Assessing, Analysing and Reporting Patient-Reported Outcomes and the Quality of Life of Patients

9
Choosing and scoring questionnaires

Summary

Previous chapters have reviewed the aims, principles and psychometric techniques of questionnaire design, validation and testing. We have emphasised that developing a questionnaire is a lengthy and time-consuming process; it is recommended that investigators make use of existing questionnaires whenever appropriate. This chapter discusses how to identify and select a suitable questionnaire. We also describe the principal methods of scoring the results.

9.1   Introduction

There is a wide diversity of instruments for assessing QoL and measuring PROs, and the choice of instrument may be crucial to the success of a study. Although many questionnaires exist, not all have been extensively validated. The selection must be made with care, and expert advice is important. The choice of questionnaire will depend on the study's objectives and the characteristics of the target population. For some studies, it will be most natural to seek a generic instrument that enables comparisons to be made against other groups of patients, possibly from other disease areas. This might be the case when an expensive intervention is being explored in a clinical trial and the study results are to be used in a health-economic evaluation. In other studies, it may be more important to identify areas in which a new treatment affects the QoL of patients, and patient-reported side effects may be the principal objective. In this chapter, we explore how the study objectives may influence the choice of questionnaire.

A large part of the instrument selection process consists of checking and verifying that the candidate instruments have been developed with full rigour and that there is documented evidence to support claims of validity, reliability, sensitivity and other characteristics. In effect, the investigator who is choosing an instrument will need to

Quality of Life: The Assessment, Analysis and Reporting of Patient-Reported Outcomes, Third Edition.
Peter M. Fayers and David Machin.
© 2016 John Wiley & Sons, Ltd. Published 2016 by John Wiley & Sons, Ltd.

judge the extent to which formal development procedures have been followed, and will then have to decide how important any omissions may be. We present a checklist to aid the evaluation of instruments.

Clinical trials or clinical practice?

This chapter focuses on clinical trials. QoL instruments are also being increasingly used in clinical practice, for individual patient monitoring and management. This raises other issues, which are not covered here. The comprehensive review by Snyder *et al.* (2012) is recommended reading.

9.2   Finding instruments

There are a number of books providing extensive collections of reviews, both for general and disease-specific questionnaires. Examples include Bowling (2001, 2004), McDowell and Newell (2006) and Salek (2004).

Many disease-specific reviews of QoL instruments exist. These reviews may report the results of literature searches, describing all generic and disease-specific questionnaires that have been used for a particular condition, and sometimes debate the contrasting value of the approaches. It can be worth searching bibliographic databases for articles containing the keywords 'review' together with 'quality of life' and the disease in question. Unfortunately, some of these reviews are likely to have been written as part of a justification for developing a new instrument, in which case they may conclude that no satisfactory tool exists for assessing QoL in this population – and declare the author's intent to fill the gap.

The Patient-Reported Outcome and Quality of Life Instruments Database (PROQOLID) is an Internet resource at <http://www.proqolid.org/>. PROQOLID is indexed by pathology/disease, targeted population and author's name, and has general search facilities. It is a useful aid for identifying disease-specific instruments. For subscribers, it additionally contains descriptions and review copies of a growing number of instruments.

Special populations

Standard instruments may not be suitable for particular populations. For example, instruments intended for children present a set of challenges. Children have age-dependent varying priorities that are frequently misunderstood by adults. Younger children may need help completing questionnaires, while proxy assessment may be necessary for the youngest ones. Landgraf (2005) and Solans *et al.* (2008) provide reviews of the issues and thoughts about how to assess QoL in children, and describes the more prominent questionnaires.

Another example is the assessment of patients with dementia, which may pose challenges both in understanding what causes distress and in the measurement of the pertinent issues. Again, proxy assessment may be necessary. Ettema *et al.* (2005) provides a review, although more recent instruments have been developed since then.

9.3   Generic versus specific

Generic instruments focus on broad aspects of QoL and health status, and are intended for use in general populations or across a wide range of disease conditions. If it is considered important to compare the results of the clinical trial with data from other groups of patients, including patients with other diseases, a generic instrument will be appropriate.

A generic instrument is required when making health-economic assessments that cover a range of disease areas, or when contrasting treatment costs versus therapeutic gains across different diseases. However, for the valid application of health-economic methods, it will be necessary to use an instrument that has in addition been developed or calibrated in terms of utilities, preferences or a similar system of values.

In contrast, disease-specific instruments are usually developed so as to detect more subtle disease and treatment-related effects. They will contain items reflecting issues of importance to the patients. In some clinical trials, the objective of the QoL assessments is to detect patient-reported differences between the test and the control treatment. In these trials, the instrument of choice will frequently be disease-specific and therefore sensitive to the health states that are likely to be experienced by patients eligible for the study. Disease-specific instruments may also provide detailed information that is of clinical relevance to the management of future patients.

When evaluating new treatments, or novel combinations of therapies, the possible side effects and consequent impact on QoL may sometimes be uncertain. An instrument that is sensitive to the potential side effects of therapy may be required, and this will generally indicate the need for a disease- or treatment-specific instrument. Even so, not all disease-specific instruments have the full range of appropriate treatment-specific items that are relevant for the particular form of therapy under investigation, and at times multiple questionnaires must be used, or supplementary items devised, to address the pertinent issues of interest.

The separation of instruments into generic and specific can function at different levels. Thus the EORTC QLQ-C30 and the FACT-G are examples of instruments that are generic for a class of disease states. These instruments are core modules that are intended for use with supplementary modules focusing on particular subcategories of disease and specific treatments. Since they were designed to be modular, both the core and a supplementary module can be used together on each patient.

Other instruments assess individual aspects of QoL, with PROs for symptoms such as pain, fatigue, anxiety and depression, and if these dimensions are of particular interest in the trial the questionnaires may be used alongside disease-related or generic instruments. Thus a trial investigating the use of erythropoietin (EPO) for fatigue in cancer patients might use an instrument such as the EQ-5D for health-economic purposes, to evaluate the cost-effectiveness of treating the fatigue in cancer patients, with the EORTC QLQ-C30 to assess QoL and a fatigue questionnaire to explore the benefits of EPO on individual patients.

Although it may occasionally be possible to use a combination of generic, disease-specific and dimension-specific instruments, the result may be a questionnaire package that takes an unacceptably long time to complete and which contains questions that are more or less repeated in different formats.

9.4   Content and presentation

When one or more potentially suitable instruments have been identified, ostensibly covering the same issues, the next stage is to consider the whether it addresses all the relevant issues in a suitable manner. The content – and even the style of presentation – of instruments can vary considerably. For example, the two most widely used generic cancer instruments, the FACT-G and the EORTC QLQ-C30, differ appreciably. The developers of the FACT-G placed emphasis on psychosocial aspects, whereas the team designing the QLQ-C30 included a far greater proportion of clinicians. This is reflected in the nature of the two questionnaires. However, there is sufficient overlap that it would seem inappropriate to use both questionnaires in a treatment comparison study. A choice has to be made.

Example from the literature

Holzner *et al.* (2001) studied a heterogeneous group of 56 patients who were treated with bone marrow transplant (BMT), and 81 who were diagnosed as having chronic lymphatic leukaemia (CLL). All patients completed both the FACT-G and the EORTC QLQ-C30. Holzner *et al.* show that the two instruments have substantial differences even in the four major domains.

In the physical domain, the QLQ measures basic physical functions and efficiency ('physical functioning'), while the FACT focuses primarily on symptoms such as fatigue and pain ('physical well-being'). This was reflected in lower QLQ scores in the CLL patients compared to the BMT patients, partly because the CLL patients are on average 30 years older; there was no such difference between CLL and BMT with the FACT.

In the emotional domain, BMT patients had lower FACT scores than CLL patients, but the QLQ scores showed no differences. This was attributed to the QLQ emotional functioning scale referring to mood states (irritability, tension, depression, worry), whereas the FACT emotional well-being scale emphasises existential issues (worries about the future, death) – and thus patients under-going life-threatening BMT scored lower.

In the social domain, the FACT is directed at aspects of social support, while the QLQ focuses on how physical condition interferes with family and social life. It is suggested that this explains why the QLQ shows lower scores for BMT than for CLL, while there is no difference between the FACT scores.

Finally, the QLQ defines 'role functioning' in terms of work and leisure activi-ties, but the equivalent FACT dimension is many-faceted and includes aspects of working, enjoyment, coping and satisfaction.

Holzner *et al.* note that:

a. when selecting a QoL instrument, investigators should not rely on names of subscales and domains but must take into account the contents of individual items,
b. similarly, interpretation and comparison of study results should be based on the content of items and not rely on names of subscales,
c. similar differences could probably be found among other QoL instruments.

9.5 Choice of instrument

Criteria for choosing

How should one select an instrument for use? Assuming that you have formed a shortlist of potentially suitable instruments that purport to address the scientific issues that are relevant to your study, the next steps are first to review the content of the instruments and, secondly, to check whether the instruments have been devel-oped rigorously.

Points to consider are included in the checklist shown in Box 9.1. It is likely that few, if any, instruments will be found to satisfy all these requirements – and, for many instruments, much of the required information may be unreported and unavailable. A judgement must be made as to the adequacy of the documented information and the suitability of the instruments.

The checklist has a brief section titled validation. The topics from Part 1 of this book provide a basis for checking the validity and related aspects, such as sensitivity, responsiveness and reliability. Terwee *et al.* (2007) have produced a checklist of crite-ria for measurement properties of instruments, and the COSMIN group extend this in a very thorough and comprehensive checklist covering the full range of psychometric issues (Mokkink *et al.*, 2010). Valderas *et al.* (2008) also provide a general checklist. Validation of translations is outlined in Part 1 (Section 3.14), and further details are also provided in Wild *et al.* (2005).

The reasons for selecting a particular instrument should be documented in the study protocol, and may be referenced when later reporting the results of the study.

Box 9.1 Choosing an instrument – a checklist

Documentation
1. Is there formal written documentation about the instrument?
2. Are there peer-reviewed publications to support the claims of the developers?
3. Is there a user manual?

Development
1. Are the aims and intended usage of the instrument clearly defined?
2. Is there a clear conceptual basis for the dimensions assessed?
3. Was the instrument developed using rigorous procedures? Are the results published in detail? This should include all stages from identification of issues and item selection through to large-scale field-testing.

Validation
1. How comprehensive has the validation process been, and did the validation studies have an adequate sample size?
2. Do the validated dimensions correspond to the constructs that are of relevance to your study?
3. Is there documented evidence of adequate validity?
4. Is there evidence of adequate reliability/reproducibility of results?
5. What is the evidence of sensitivity and responsiveness? How do these values affect the sample size requirements of your study?

Target population
1. Is the instrument suitable for your target population? Has it been tested upon a wide range of subjects from this population (e.g. patients with the same disease states, receiving similar treatment modalities)?
2. If your population differs from the target one, is it reasonable to expect the instrument to be applicable? Is additional testing required to confirm this?
3. Will your study include some subjects, such as young children or cognitively impaired adults, for whom the instrument may be less appropriate?

Feasibility
1. Is the method of administration feasible?
2. How long does the instrument take to complete (patient burden)?
3. Are the questions readily understood, or is help necessary?
4. Are there any difficult or embarrassing items?

5. Is the processing of questionnaires easy or do items require coding, such as measurement of visual analogue scales?
6. If multiple questionnaires are to be used (e.g. generic- and disease-specific questionnaires), are they compatible with each other? Many instruments come with the advice: 'If more than one questionnaire is to be used, our one should be applied first'—which is clearly impractical when several make the same demand.

Languages and cultures
1. Has the instrument been tested and found valid for use with patients from the relevant educational, cultural and ethnic backgrounds?
2. Are there validated translations that cover your needs, present and future?
3. If additional language versions are required, they will have to be developed using formal procedures of forward and backward translation and tested on a number of patients who also complete a debriefing questionnaire.

Scoring
1. Is the scoring procedure defined? Is there a global score for overall QoL?
2. Are there any global questions about overall QoL?

Interpretation
1. Are there guidelines for interpreting the scale scores?
2. Are there any reference data or other guidelines for estimating sample size when designing a trial?
3. Is there a global question or a global measure of overall QoL?
4. Is there, or is it necessary to provide, an open-ended question about 'other factors affecting your QoL, not covered above'?
5. Are treatment side effects covered adequately?

Adding ad hoc items

Sometimes an existing instrument may address many but not all of the QoL issues that are important to a clinical investigation. In such circumstances, one can consider adding supplementary questions to the questionnaire. These questions should be added at the end, after all the other questions of the instrument, to avoid any possibility of disturbing the validated characteristics of the instrument. Interposing new items, deleting items and altering the sequence of items may alter the characteristics of the original questionnaire. The copyright owners of many instruments stipulate that new items may only be added at the end of their questionnaire.

Sometimes it may be thought possible to extend a questionnaire by adopting an item taken from other sources and thus known to have been tested. Commonly, however, the wording of both the item and its response options will have to be changed, making the new item consistent with the rest of the questionnaire. Thus, ideally, each additional item should be tested rigorously to ensure that it has the desired characteristics. In practice, this is frequently not feasible. For example, a clinical trial may have to be launched by a specific deadline. However, as a minimum, all new items should be piloted upon a few patients before being introduced to the main study. Debriefing questions similar to those we have described (Part 1, Sections 3.6 and 3.15) should be used.

Although the use of ad-hoc items to supplement a questionnaire may readily be criticised, in many situations it is better to devise additional questions, with care, than to ignore completely issues that are clearly relevant to a particular illness or its treatment.

9.6   Scoring multi-item scales

There are three main reasons for combining and scoring multiple items as one scale. Some scales are specifically designed to be multi-item, to increase reliability or precision. Sometimes items are grouped simply as a convenient way of combining related items; often this will follow the application of methods such as factor analysis, which may suggest that several items are measuring one construct and can be grouped together. Also, a multi-item scale may arise as a clinimetric index, in which the judgement of a number of clinicians and patients is used as the basis for combining heterogeneous items into a single index.

In the following descriptions it is assumed that all items in a scale are scored in the same direction. For example, in a symptom scale it is usual for high scores to represent a high level of symptoms, in which case it would be necessary to recode any items in the scale for which high scores indicate a favourable outcome, fewer symptoms or less severe symptoms.

Summated scales

The simplest and most widely practised method of combining, or *aggregating*, items is the method of *summated ratings*, also known as *Likert summated scales*. If each item has been scored on a k-point ordered categorical scale, with scores either from 1 to k, or 0 to $k - 1$, the total sum-score is obtained by adding together the scores from the individual items. For a scale containing m items, each scored from 0 to $k - 1$, the sum-score will range from 0 to $m \times (k - 1)$. Since different scales may have different numbers of items or categories per item, it is common practice to *standardise* the sum-scores to range from 0 to 100. This is done by multiplying the sum-score by $100/(m \times (k - 1))$. As noted above, if some questions use positive wording and others negative, it will be necessary to reverse the scoring of some items so that they are all scored in a consistent manner with a high item score indicating, for example, a high level of problems.

Example

The emotional functioning scale of the EORTC QLQ-C30 (Appendix E6) consists of questions 21–24. These four items are scored from 1 to 4. A patient responding 2, 2, 3 and 4 for these items has a sum-score of 11. The range of possible scores is from 4 to 16. Thus we can standardise these scores to lie between 0 and 100 by first subtracting 4, giving a new range of 0 to 12, and then multiplying by 100/12. Hence the standardised score is $(11-4)\times100/12 = 58.3$. However, the Scoring Manual for the EORTC QLQ-C30 (Fayers *et al.*, 2001) specifies that high scores for functioning scales should indicate high levels of functioning, whereas high responses for the individual items indicate poor functioning. To achieve this, the scale score is subtracted from 100 to give a patient score of 41.7.

The main requirement for summated scales is that each item should have the same possible range of score values. Usually it would not be sensible to sum, for example, an item scored 1–3 for 'not at all', 'moderately', 'very much' with another item scored from 1 ('none') to 10 ('extremely severe'). One way to correct for this is to standardise the items so that they have similar means and variances. However, it is usually best to develop questionnaires so that they have uniformly rated items with similar numbers of categories and similar ranges of score values.

Likert summated scales are optimal for parallel tests because the foundation of these is that these each item is an equally good indicator of the same underlying construct (see Part 1, Section 2.7). Perhaps surprisingly, summated scales have in practice also been found to be remarkably robust and reliable for a wide range of other situations. Thus when scoring a number of items indicating presence or absence of symptoms, a simple sum-score could represent overall symptom burden. Similarly, hierarchical scales – although totally different in nature from parallel tests – are also often scored in the same way, and a high score indicates a high number of strong endorsements. Occasionally multi-item scales are comprised of items that are neither consistently parallel nor hierarchical; perhaps summated scales will still be a reasonable method of scoring.

Example from the literature

The items of the physical functioning scale of the EORTC QLQ-C30 are clearly not parallel items. However, using the property of summated scales that higher scores correspond to greater numbers of problems, this is the approach recommended by the EORTC Quality of Life Study Group for scoring the physical functioning scale (Fayers *et al.*, 2001).

Section 15.5 explains methods of calculating sum-scores when some of the items are missing. Essentially, the most common approach is that if at least half of the items are present, the mean of those items is calculated and it is assumed that the missing items would have taken this mean value.

Weighted sum-scores

It is sometimes suggested that *weights* should be applied to those items that are regarded as most important. Thus, for example, an important item could be given double its normal score, or a *weight* of 2, so that it would have values from 0 to $2 \times (k - 1)$. If there are three items in a scale, and one is given double weight, that is equivalent to saying that this item is just as important as the other two combined. If the ith item has a score x_i, we can assign weights w_i to the items and the sum-score becomes $\sum w_i x_i$. However, empirical investigations of weighting schemes have generally found them to have little advantage over simple summated scales.

Other methods for aggregating items into scores have been proposed, including Guttman scalogram analysis, the method of equal-appearing intervals and multidimensional scaling. These methods are now rarely used for PRO scales. In the past, factor weights derived from exploratory factor analysis have occasionally been used when aggregating items; in Part 1, Section 6.6, we showed that the use of factor loadings to produce weights for scale scoring is unsound. For indicator variables, the principal alternative to summated scales is item response theory, or *IRT-scoring* (see Part 1, Chapters 7 and 8). IRT-scoring is most pertinent when items are chosen from an item bank specifically because they are of varying difficulty, and becomes essential when computer-adaptive tests are used.

For scales containing *causal variables*, or '*formative scales*', there are other considerations. Although summated scores are frequently used, causal variables should only be included in Likert summated scales with caution. There is no reason to expect that symptoms such as, for example, pain, dyspnoea and appetite loss will have equal impact on patients; many investigators argue that it is more likely that some issues are more important than others in terms of their impact, and that therefore items should 'weighted' to reflect their relative importance. Thus, Fayers *et al.* (1997a) argue that if a scale contains several causal items that are, say, symptoms, it is surely inconceivable that each symptom is equally important in its effect upon patients' QoL. While some symptoms, even when scored 'very much', may have a relatively minor impact, others may have a devastating effect upon patients. Instead of a simple summated scale, giving equal weight (importance) to each item, symptom scores should in theory be weighted, and *the weights should be derived from patients' ratings of the importance and severity of different symptoms*. In practice, most well-designed instruments will only contain causal items if they that are deemed to have an important impact on patients' QoL. Also, for those instruments that ask about the intensity of symptoms, it is likely that many patients may rate a symptom less severe if it impacts to a lesser extent on their QoL (i.e. the distinction between severity and impact may become blurred). In any event, experience suggests that summated scales are surprisingly robust to causal items, and it has been observed that weighting makes little difference in practice (for example, Hsieh C-M, 2012; Russell *et al*, 2006; Wu CH, 2008). From empirical studies, it has repeatedly been observed that performance of the ensuing scale scores is relatively insensitive to the choice of weights; this has been termed the flat maximum effect (Von Winterfield and Edwards, 1982). Hand (2004) uses a mathematical argument to explain this: if the constituent items are moderately highly correlated, scale scores formed by equal weights (i.e. unweighted) will be fairly highly correlated with scales that use optimal weights and will thus have similar performance properties (Hand, 2004, pp. 171–172). By performance, we mean for example that weighted and unweighted scores will generally be found to be equally discriminative in known-group comparisons and equally responsive to changes over time.

In an extreme case the causal variables might be *sufficient causes*, such that a high score on any one of the sufficient-cause symptoms would suffice to reduce QoL, even if no other symptoms are present. Linear models, such as Likert summated scales and weighted sum-scores, will no longer be satisfactory predictors of QoL. Non-linear functions may be more appropriate. A maximum of the symptom scores might be a better predictor of QoL than the average symptom level. Utility functions are another possibility (see, for example, Torrance *et al.*, 1996), and these lead to an estimation of QoL by functions of the form $\Sigma w_i \log(1 - x_i)$, where x_i lies between 0 and 1.

Although also described as *formative*, scales such as activities of daily living (ADL) are solely defined by their component items, and these items are *composite indicators* that do not have a causal impact on the latent variable (see Part 1, Chapter 2 for discussion of causal and composite indicators). Such scales are usually summarised as an *index* score formed by a linear sum-score. Most commonly equal weights are assumed, although in some cases weighted sum-scores, with weights based on judgement of item contribution to the index that is being formed, might be better able to reflect the definition of the index (Bollen and Bauldry, 2011).

Norming systems: *Z*-scores and *T*-scores

A variety of norming systems have been used for psychological, personality and educational tests, to standardise both individual measurements and group means. First a reference group is defined, which is typically a national sample of the random population. This is used to derive the normative data, which is commonly divided by age and gender strata. National reference samples are available for many of the most widely used generic questionnaires, covering an increasing number of countries. The data from clinical trials and other studies can then be scored by comparison with these normative data.

One of the simplest methods is *percentile rank*. Each subject can be given a percentile ranking in comparison with the reference sample. Thus a percentage-rank score of 75 would indicate that a subject has a raw score or response that is greater in magnitude than 75% of the reference group. A patient with a percentile rank of 50 would have a raw score equal to the median. Percentile ranks are easily understood and communicated: 'Your quality of life is as good as that of the top 10% of the population'. However, they suffer the disadvantage that the scale is non-linear: if we assume an underlying Normal distribution, a change from 50% to 55% corresponds to a much smaller change in raw score than a change in the extreme values, such as from 5% to 10% or 90% to 95%.

Z-scores are raw scores expressed in standard deviation units, and indicate how many *SD*s the raw score is above or below the reference mean. If the reference sample has a mean of Z_{Pop} and a standard deviation SD_{Pop}, to transform the raw score X_i of the ith patient in a trial, we use

$$Z_i = (X_i - Z_{Pop}) / SD_{Pop}.$$

Thus Z-scores have a mean of zero, and an SD of 1. If the raw scores follow a Normal distribution, the Z-scores will too, and it becomes easy to translate between percentile-ranks and Z-scores.

More commonly used, T-scores are similar to Z-scores but with a mean of 50 and an SD of 10 (although, curiously, some well-known intelligence tests use an SD of 15). Thus a patient's T-score can be derived from

$$T_i = (Z_i \times 10) + 50.$$

Example from the literature

Linder and Singer (2003) used T-scores to show the health-related QoL of adults with upper respiratory tract infections (Figure 9.1). The SF-36 was used, and the T-scores were calculated using reference values from the 1998 USA general population National Survey of Functional Health Status. The patients with urinary-tract infections were also contrasted against adults with self-reported chronic lung disease, osteoarthritis and depression drawn from the same survey. p-values are indicated, but it would have been more informative to provide exact p-values and show 95% confidence intervals.

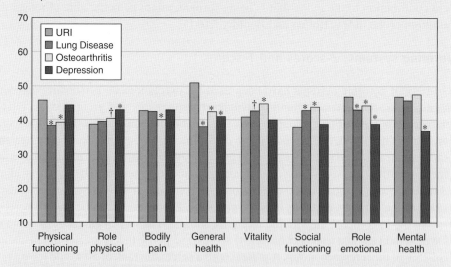

Figure 9.1 The SF-36 health status of 318 adults with upper respiratory tract infections (URIs). T-scores were calculated using the general USA population. The URI patients were also contrasted against patients with lung disease, osteoarthritis and depression. *Note:* *$p < 0.001$, †$p < 0.05$ for comparisons with URI. *Source:* Reproduced with kind permission of Springer Science and Business Media. Linder JA and Singer DE (2003) Health-related quality of life of adults with upper respiratory tract infections. *Journal of General Internal Medicine* 18: 802–807.

There is inconsistency over the use of the terms Z-score and T-score. Many authors – but by no means all – reserve the use of Z-scores to refer to data that do have a Normal distribution, if necessary by the prior application of a suitable *normalising transformation*. For some psychometric tests this is achieved by making use of extensive look-up percentile tables that provide the T-score. Unfortunately, many PRO scales have a limited number of possible categories. This, together with floor and ceiling effects, may make it impossible to obtain a Normal distribution.

However, frequently the distributions are at least moderately close to a Normal distribution. Then, since a T-score of 30 is two SDs below the reference mean of 50, patients with scores below 30 are outside the 95% Normal range and are in the lower 2.5% of the population. The same applies to all scales that are converted to the T-scores metric, making it possible to draw comparative inferences regarding which scales show the largest departure from the population values.

IRT-based scoring

When instruments have been developed using IRT models, it is natural to use IRT-based scoring. The process is complex, and makes use of computer software. One major advantage of IRT models is that the relative difficulties of the items are estimated, enabling valid scale scores to be calculated for patients who may have answered different subsets of items. This means that allowance is automatically made when there are missing items within a scale; it also provides the basis for computer-adaptive tests.

Examples from the literature

Norquist *et al.* (2004) compared Rasch-based (one-parameter IRT) scoring versus sum-scores, for the Oxford Hip Score (OHS) questionnaire. Data were collected on 1,424 patients receiving total hip replacement surgery. The OHS contains two 6-item scales, representing pain and functional impairment. Each item has five response categories. Using the summated-scale method as the base (1.0), the relative precision of the Rasch scores was estimated. These varied between 0.96 and 1.48, with most of the values not representing a statistically significant improvement over the use of summated scales. Higher relative precisions were found for the changes in scores from baseline to one year. The authors conclude that there may be some gains in sensitivity from using Rasch-based scoring, although they also suggest that in some situations there may be substantial gains, such as when comparing groups of patients.

In contrast, Petersen *et al.* (2005) report no gains when using IRT methods to score the physical functioning, emotional functioning and fatigue scales of the EORTC QLQ-C30.

Since IRT scoring is so powerful, several authors have explored using these methods on conventionally designed instruments. In particular, scales such as those for physical functioning will typically have items of varying difficulty, ranging from 'easy' tasks such as being able to get out of bed and get dressed, through to the more difficult activities such as running long distances. These scales theoretically appear ideally suited to IRT scoring. In practice, the gains appear to be at best modest. Perhaps this is because in most instruments these scales are short, and the few items they do contain have multi-category response options. Also, since the items have presumably been selected using traditional psychometrics, they are less likely to be optimal for IRT scaling.

Health-economics scores

The scoring methods described above are intended to produce a score for each patient, summarising their overall QoL or individual dimensions and issues. These scores may then be used for individual patient management, or averaged across patients to provide group means.

In contrast, the aim in health-economic assessments is rather more to obtain a single summary index that encapsulates a patient's QoL, such that this can be combined with other outcomes such as survival and cost, enabling the estimation of overall treatment cost–benefit for groups of patients. This leads to fundamentally different approaches to scoring, using utilities, as discussed in Chapter 17.

9.7   Conclusions

Designing and developing new instruments constitutes a complex and lengthy process. It involves many interviews with patients and others, studies testing the questionnaires upon patients, collection of data, and statistical and psychometric analyses of the data to confirm and substantiate the claims for the instrument. The full development of an instrument may take many years. If at any stage inadequacies are found in the instrument, there will be a need for refinement and retesting. Many instruments undergo iterative development through a number of versions, each version being extensively reappraised. For example, the Appendix shows version 3.0 of the EORTC QLQ-C30 and version 4 of the FACT-G. Instruments in the appendices, like many other instruments, will have undergone extensive development along the lines that we have described.

In summary, our advice is: Don't develop your own instrument – unless you have to. Wherever possible, consider using or building upon existing instruments. If you must develop a new instrument, be prepared for much hard work over a period of years.

Similarly, scoring should usually follow the recommendations of the instrument developers. Unless otherwise specified by the developers, simple summations serve well for a wide variety of scales.

9.8 Further reading

The books listed in Section 9.2 for finding instruments (Bowling, 2001, 2004; McDowell and Newell, 2006; Salek, 2004) also contain advice about the criteria that should be used to inform choices. Reeve *et al.* (2013) recommends minimum standards for PRO measures used in patient-centred outcomes research or comparative effectiveness research. Lohr (2002) provides a useful checklist of 'attributes and review criteria', as does also the EMPRO group (Valderas *et al.*, 2008). Terwee *et al.* (2007) describe criteria for measurement properties of instruments; the COSMIN group provide a thorough and comprehensive checklist for validity and other psychometric issues (Mokkink *et al.*, 2010).

6.6 Further reading

10

Clinical trials

Summary

The inclusion of PROs in clinical trials, and especially multicentre clinical trials, presents a number of difficult organisational issues. These include standardisation of the procedures for assessment and data collection, specification of measurement details to ensure consistent assessment, methods for minimising missing data and the collection of reasons for any missing responses. In particular, many trials report serious problems of compliance, and there are problems for interpretation of results when data are missing. Hence it is important to seek methods of optimising the level of compliance, both of the participating institution and of the patient. In this chapter we describe a number of methods for addressing these issues, which should be considered when writing clinical trial protocols involving QoL assessment. A checklist is provided for points that should be covered in protocols.

10.1   Introduction

The success or failure of the trial will depend on how well the protocol was written. A poorly designed, ambiguous or incompletely documented protocol will result in a trial that will not be able to answer the questions of interest. The protocol must be concise, yet detailed and precisely worded with all the requirements clearly indicated so that the trial is carried out uniformly by all participants. Protocols should contain a statement about the rationale for assessing QoL or PROs, justifying their importance to the participating clinician. Sometimes this may be brief, although a more detailed discussion might be appropriate when QoL is a major endpoint of the study.

Poor compliance bedevils randomised clinical trials with PROs, leading to serious problems of analysis and interpretation. In some instances the potential for bias in the analyses could even render the results uninterpretable. Compliance can be greatly enhanced by ensuring that all those involved in the trial, from medical staff to patients, are aware of, and agree with, the relevance of PROs as a study endpoint.

Quality of Life: The Assessment, Analysis and Reporting of Patient-Reported Outcomes, Third Edition.
Peter M. Fayers and David Machin.
© 2016 John Wiley & Sons, Ltd. Published 2016 by John Wiley & Sons, Ltd.

Equally, it is important to recognise that QoL assessment should be incorporated in a clinical trial only when it really is relevant to do so. This may depend on the aims of the trial and the precise objective in including a QoL assessment. PROs are not necessarily relevant to all clinical trials. It may be unnecessary to measure overall QoL in small early phase I or phase II trials, although it can be useful on an exploratory basis or as a pilot study when developing instruments for subsequent studies. On the other hand, PROs for particular domains of QoL may be more pertinent in early trials, and in some cases may be the primary outcome (for example, when the objective is to treat pain). Overall QoL is mainly of importance in phase III clinical trials. The following situations can be identified:

1. Trials in which the new treatment is expected to have only a small impact on such clinical endpoints as long-term survival, cure or response and any small improvement in the primary clinical endpoint may have to be weighed against the negative aspects upon QoL of an intensive therapy. This appears to cover the majority of long-term chronic diseases, including cancer.

2. Equivalence trials, where the disease course in both arms is expected to be similar but there are expected to be QoL benefits or differences in morbidity. QoL may be a primary endpoint in these trials.

3. Trials of treatments that are specifically intended to improve QoL. This includes trials in palliative care, for example palliative radiotherapy for cancer and bisphosphonates for metastatic bone pain. QoL is most often the primary endpoint in these studies.

4. Studies involving health-economic cost-effectiveness balanced against QoL gain.

10.2   Basic design issues

Type of study

The choice of study design is always crucial. However, in most situations the assessment of QoL or PROs will have to be repeated with each subject on two or more occasions, and hence the study will be both prospective and longitudinal in nature. The design options are therefore limited in number. It could either be a follow-up study of a single cohort of subjects with any comparisons made between subject types within the cohort, or a two (or more) group comparison of which the randomised parallel group trial is a specific example. Crossover designs are less frequently appropriate in QoL studies, and in this chapter we focus on parallel-group randomised trials.

Organisational issues

There are often choices within a QoL study as to when and by who the instrument is to be completed. Even in the context of self-completed QoL instruments there will be occasions when help is needed, perhaps for an elderly person who can comprehend but not easily complete a questionnaire, or for someone with vision difficulties. It is often important to specify whether the instrument is to be completed before or after a clinic appointment with the responsible physician, and whether or not the physician has any knowledge of the patient responses when conducting the medical examination. Some of these options may influence the responses.

Mode of administration

Traditionally, questionnaires have been paper-based. Electronic approaches are also available, such as computer touch-screens, web-based data capture and smart-phone methods. Computer-adaptive testing, as the name implies, is founded on electronic capture. Most studies that compare different modes of administration find small or negligible impact on the results (e.g. McColl and Fayers, 2005; Gundy and Aaronson, 2010), although others disagree: Hays *et al.* (2009) report that telephone administration is associated with more-positive scores, with differences of up to a half-*SD*.

Protocol

As with any clinical study, it is important to describe the details of the study in a protocol. In any event, this will often be a mandatory requirement of the investigators' local ethics committee. The protocol should describe the main purpose of the study and the target subjects or patient group. It should also address specific issues, including the principal hypotheses and the QoL outcomes to which they relate, the definition of 'clinically important differences' used for sample size estimation, and strategies for minimising the number of missing QoL forms.

Sample size

The sample size necessary for a good chance ('power') of detecting a realistic target difference should be calculated during the study design stage, and full details must be specified in the protocol. This calculation is usually based on a PRO that is pre-specified as the primary outcome. It depends on aspects of the analysis, which should also be specified in the protocol, including the statistical test to be used. Examples of sample size estimation are provided in Chapter 11.

Defining multiple endpoints

By its nature, QoL assessment tends to incur problems of endpoint multiplicity – multiple PROs (items/domains), assessed at multiple time points. Chapter 11 discusses how *p*-values are affected by multiple significance testing. One approach that avoids much of the complexity of correcting *p*-values is to pre-specify a hierarchy of endpoints, identifying one or more PRO measures as the primary outcomes of interest and a few additional outcomes as secondary. The analysis of all other PRO measures is then regarded as exploratory. Similarly, if it is intended to carry out a cross-sectional analysis, a single assessment time can be pre-specified for the primary analysis; alternatively, for a longitudinal analysis, details of the statistical methods should be provided. It is essential that the clinical trial protocol defines the endpoint measures and the criteria for the statistical analysis and interpretation of results. Decisions about the handling and analysis of endpoints should be made and recorded before recruiting patients; failure to do this may jeopardise the creditability of a trial. Later chapters discuss in greater detail the analysis and reporting of PROs in clinical trials.

10.3   Compliance

When QoL is assessed in a clinical trial, it is important to ensure that the information collected is representative of the patients being studied. However, when data are missing for some patients, a question arises as to whether the patients with missing data differ from those who returned completed forms. As a consequence, missing data present severe problems with the analysis and interpretation of results. Therefore the amount of missing data in a trial should be minimised. Data may be unavailable for two principal reasons:

- unavoidable reasons, of which the most common in some disease areas is patient attrition due to early deaths.

- low compliance, in which forms that should have been completed by patients and returned to the trials office may be missing; this has frequently been a serious problem in clinical trials.

Example from the literature

The Lung Cancer Working Party of the UK Medical Research Council (MRC) assessed aspects of QoL with a five-item daily diary card that patients completed at home (Fayers et al., 1997b). Only 47% of the expected patient daily diary cards were returned, and a third of the patients provided no data at all. It was noted that there were major differences in compliance rates according to the centre responsible for the patient, providing strong support for the belief that much of the problem is institution compliance rather than patient compliance.

Compliance has continued to be a problem in later MRC trials, when other instruments have also been used, and when assessments have been made while patients attended the clinic.

Measuring compliance

Compliance is defined as the number of QoL questionnaires actually completed as a proportion of those expected. The number of patients alive at each protocol assessment point represents the maximum number of QoL forms, as patients must be excluded upon death.

It is important to verify that the forms received have indeed been completed at the scheduled times. For example, if the scheduled QoL assessment is on day 42 and the corresponding QoL form is not completed until (say) day 72, the responses recorded may not reflect the patient QoL at the time point of interest. However, it is necessary to recognise the variation in individual patient's treatment and follow-up, and so a time frame, or *window*, may be allowed around each scheduled protocol assessment time. The exact definitions will depend upon the nature of the trial, but the initial assessment will usually be given a tight window such as no more than three days before randomisation, to ensure that it represents a true pre-treatment baseline. During the active treatment period, the window may still have to be narrow, but it should allow for treatment delay. Similarly, if an assessment is targeted at, say, two months after surgery, a window of acceptability must be specified. Later, during follow-up assessments, the window may widen, particularly in diseases for which there is a reasonable expectation of long survival and follow-up. Finally, since it is unlikely that many patients will continue to complete forms until the day of death, when analysing and reporting the results it may be appropriate to impose a cut-off point at some arbitrary time prior to death.

Example from the literature

In a trial comparing two chemotherapy regimens (labelled IF and CF) for palliative treatment of patients with cancer of the stomach or oesophagogastric junction, QoL assessments were required at baseline, every eight weeks until disease progression and then every three months until death (Curran, 2009). To be considered evaluable at baseline, a questionnaire must have been filled in within 15 days before randomisation. To be considered evaluable on treatment, a questionnaire had to be filled in more than four days after the completion of the latest infusion so as not to take into account the immediate toxicities following infusion. Data were to be analysed according to time windows of eight-week periods, i.e. plus/minus four weeks of the theoretical assessment date for assessments before progressive disease. Compliance was calculated as the ratio of the total number of subjects with at least one evaluable questionnaire per time window over the total number of expected questionnaires.

Table 10.1 indicates the compliance within these windows for the first five assessment periods. The overall compliance rates were low, at 60% (IF) and 56% (CF).

Table 10.1 Compliance for QLQ-C30 questionnaires by protocol-planned assessment during the first 9 months, in a trial comparing two chemotherapy treatments for advanced adenocarcinoma of the stomach or oesophagogastric junction

	IF ($N = 170$)			CF ($N = 163$)		
Assessment	Number of patients	Patients with at least one questionnaire	Rate (%)	Number of patients	Patients with at least one questionnaire	Rate (%)
Baseline	170	145	85.3	163	143	87.7
Week 8	162	97	59.9	149	79	53.0
Week 16	138	76	55.1	126	57	45.2
Week 24	106	55	51.9	91	35	38.5
Week 32	73	27	37.0	63	26	41.3

Source: Curran *et al.* 2009, Table 1. CC NC 4.0 (<http://creativecommons.org/licenses/by/4.0/>). Reproduced commercially with permission from Springer Science and Business Media.

Various trials groups use different definitions of windows, making it difficult to compare reported compliance rates. Clearly, a group using a window of plus or minus a week from the time of surgery might expect to report worse values for compliance than if they used a window of plus or minus two weeks. Given this variation in defining compliance, it is slightly surprising to find that the reported experience of several study groups has been similar.

Causes and consequences of poor compliance

Serious problems in compliance with QoL assessments have been reported in many multicentre clinical trials, especially in palliative trials involving poor-prognosis patients. In some trials only about half the expected post-baseline QoL questionnaires were returned. In the palliative setting many patients are frail, and it is perhaps not surprising that there will be a lack of enthusiasm for completing questionnaires when death is imminent. However, poor compliance is not necessarily attributable to a lack of patient compliance. Compliance rates have repeatedly been found to vary widely according to institution, which has often led, perhaps unfairly, to poor compliance being attributed to the lack of commitment by clinicians; in busy clinics, the lack of resources for assisting patients, for example, can be an equally important institution-related component. Thus single-centre trials can frequently achieve better compliance, especially if a research nurse is assigned solely for the purpose of QoL collection.

When patients become increasingly ill with progressive disease, they can find it difficult to continue completing questionnaires. This poses a methodological problem for investigators who wish to assess effects in settings such as palliative care during the terminal stages of disease, because it is highly likely that the patients who do complete their assessments will be those with the better QoL. Thus it is well recognised that the consequence of missing questionnaires may be biased estimates both of overall levels of QoL and of treatment differences, and that this bias may be sufficiently severe to invalidate the conclusions of a study.

Example from the literature

Hopwood *et al.* (1994) describe a trial in which information was provided by 92% of patients who the clinician assessed as having good performance status (normal activity, no restrictions), compared to only 31% of those assessed as very poor (confined to bed or chair).

It was concluded: "At present, given the rapid attrition in lung cancer trials and the rather low levels of compliance in completing questionnaires, there is no entirely reliable way of analysing data longitudinally."

In general, one might anticipate that the patients with missing forms are those that have the lowest performance status and the poorest QoL, but this may not always be the case.

Examples from the literature

Trials in palliative care often have high rates of attrition from death and poor rates of compliance because of declining health of patients, and compliance can be particularly challenging if questionnaires are posted for self-assessment at home. Fielding *et al.* (2006) describe a trial of 434 palliative care patients randomised to standard care or to comprehensive palliative care at a specialised unit. The EORTC QLQ-C30 was used. All patients completed questionnaires at baseline, but at the each of the five following monthly assessments between 68% and 73% of patients returned questionnaires by post. Fielding *et al.* (2006) noted that baseline Karnofsky performance status was significantly different ($p < 0.001$), with a higher proportion of the non-responders having a baseline Karnofsky score of 70 or lower (low scores represent poorer functioning). In addition, at each follow-up visit the previous month's overall QoL score was a significant predictor of compliance.

In contrast, Cox *et al.* (1992) found the reverse effect when using the Nottingham Health Profile (NHP) on heart transplant patients: those about to die or to be lost to follow-up tended to have poorer QoL scores than those who missed their next follow-up. Cox *et al.* suggest that one reason for poor compliance is that: "Those experiencing fewer problems may not be so diligent in returning questionnaires."

Improving compliance

It is important to make every effort to maximise compliance, both to avoid bias and to avoid reduction of sample size. In some studies, it may be necessary to use homecare staff or home-visit nurses to assist the patients in completing questionnaires. Compliance may also be greatly improved by providing reminder letters or phone calls. It is also possible to make major enhancements to compliance rates by suitable training of the healthcare staff involved in the trial, and by ensuring that patients are fully informed about the usefulness of the information being collected.

Example from the literature

Sadura *et al.* (1992) developed and implemented a comprehensive programme specifically aimed at encouraging compliance. They report an overall compliance of above 95% in three Canadian trials, which they attribute to their programme.

However, they acknowledged that it is unclear whether similar success can be obtained with different questionnaires, in different types of trials, in different institutions and during long-term follow-up. Also, the Canadian group used a level of resources that may not be available to other groups conducting international multicentre randomised trials: in one study, "nurses called the patients at home on the appropriate day to remind them to complete the questionnaire". Given careful planning, and provided adequate resources are made available, it *is* possible to achieve high compliance.

Acceptable levels of compliance

At best, low compliance raises questions about whether the results are representative, and at worst it may jeopardise any interpretation of the treatment comparisons. This is especially so when compliance rates differ according to treatment group and patients' performance status. In addition, poor compliance means that there are fewer data items available for analyses, and thus there may be questions about the adequacy of the sample size. However, if this were the only issue one solution would be to recruit extra patients so as to compensate for the losses owing to non-compliance. Unfortunately, this does not address the more serious issue of potential bias in the results; if compliance rates stay the same then, no matter how much patient numbers are increased, the bias will remain.

Thus the answer to the question of what is an acceptable rate of loss to follow-up is: 'Only one answer, 0%, ensures the benefits of randomisation.' Schulz and Grimes (2002), writing about clinical trials in general, comment that this is obviously unrealistic at times. They note that some researchers have suggested a simple *five-and-twenty* rule of thumb in which less than 5% loss is thought probably to lead to little bias, while greater than 20% loss potentially poses serious threats to validity, and in-between levels leading to intermediate levels of problems. Some journals refuse to publish trials with losses greater than 20%. Schulz and Grimes advise that "Although the five-and-twenty rule is useful, it can oversimplify the problem … Expectations for losses to follow-up depend on various factors, such as the topic examined, the outcome event rate, and the length of follow-up." These conclusions, although written with reference to outcomes in general, might be applicable QoL outcomes too.

Example from the literature

Despite publications in the 1990s demonstrating that missing QoL data may cause bias in the analyses of a clinical trial, and that the amount of missing data can be reduced by taking simple precautions, it continues to be a serious problem.

Fielding *et al.* (2008) searched four leading medical journals to identify clinical trials published in 2005 or 2006. QoL outcomes were reported in 61 (21%) trials. Six (10%) reported having no missing QoL data, 20 (33%) reported $\leq$ 10% missing, eleven (18%) 11–20% missing, and 11 (18%) reported > 20% missing. Missingness was unclear in 13 (21%).

The majority of trials (82%) did provide flow diagrams and reasons for missingness such as withdrawal, death or other medical problems. However, there was no detailed discussion of these reasons and the impact they may have had on the analysis and subsequent results.

The authors concluded that there should be a clearer reporting of the methods used and the amount of missing data, which should be described separately for each treatment arm. The impact that missing data potentially has on results should always be discussed and a sensitivity analysis provided. Where imputation is used to estimate the most likely values of the missing data (see Chapter 15), the reason for the choice of method should be given.

Recording reasons for non-compliance

Missing data, and hence low compliance, may arise from many causes, including clinicians or nurses forgetting to ask patients to complete QoL questionnaires, and patients refusing, feeling too ill or forgetting. Low 'compliance' does not necessarily imply fault on the part of the patient or their medical staff.

One advantage of studying QoL as an integral part of a clinical trial is that additional clinical information about treatment or disease problems can be collected at each visit of the patient, and this information can indicate why QoL data have not been collected. The reasons for not completing the questionnaire should be collected systematically, for example as in Figure 10.1. This information should be summarised and reported, and may also be used as an indication of whether particular missing data are likely to have occurred at random, in which case the imputation of the corresponding missing values may be improved.

Has the patient filled in the scheduled quality of life questionnaire?
0 = no, 1 = yes ☐

If **no**, please state the main reason:
☐   1 = patient felt too ill
☐   2 = clinician or nurse felt the patient was too ill
☐   3 = patient felt it was inconvenient, takes too much time
☐   4 = patient felt it was a violation of privacy
☐   5 = administrative failure to distribute the questionnaire to the patient
☐   6 = (at baseline) patient didn't speak the language or was illiterate
☐   7 = other, please specify ....

Figure 10.1   Questionnaire to ascertain the reason why a patient has not completed the current QoL assessment.

10.4   Administering a quality-of-life assessment

For QoL to be successfully incorporated into a clinical trial, practical steps have to be taken to ensure good standards of data collection and to seek as many methods as possible for improving compliance.

Because of heavy workloads, many clinicians are unable to give the necessary attention to data collection in a QoL study. Responsibility for explaining about QoL assessment and distributing questionnaires is often allocated to research nurses or other staff associated with the clinical trial. As pivotal members of the research team, nurses and data managers need a clear view of their job-specific tasks to improve efficiency and the quality of data. Research nurses play a major role in the education of patients and therefore may be influential in generating interest in the QoL part of the study. Suitably trained personnel can ensure better compliance of QoL data through standardisation and continuity of working procedures, and comprehensive programmes of training are important. These should be supplemented by written operating procedures and guidelines for the administration of QoL assessments in clinical trials. One example of detailed guidelines for improving data quality and compliance in clinical trials is the manual written by Young *et al.* (2002).

The patient

Most patients are willing to complete QoL questionnaires, especially if they are assured that the data will be useful for medical research and will benefit future patients. Therefore patients should be given full information about the procedures, and any of their concerns should be answered.

- Patients should be given a clear explanation of the reason for collecting QoL data.

- Information sheets should supplement the verbal information given to patients, detailing the rationale for collecting QoL data and explaining aspects of the procedure. The information sheet should include the frequency and timing of assessments, the need to answer all questions, and the importance of completing the questions without being influenced by the opinions of others.

- Patients should be told how their questionnaires will be used. In particular, they should be told whether the information will be seen by the clinician or other staff involved with their management, or whether it will remain confidential and used solely for scientific research purposes.

- The questionnaire should not be too lengthy and should contain clear written instructions.

- Patients should be thanked for completing the questionnaire and given the opportunity to discuss any problems. They should be encouraged to help with future assessments. For example, patients could be asked to remind staff if later questionnaires are not given out.

The medical team

Similarly, the medical team deserves to receive an explanation of the value of QoL assessment in the particular study. Sceptical staff make less effort, and will experience greater difficulty in persuading patients to complete questionnaires.

- The role of QoL assessment should be emphasised. If it is a primary endpoint for the study, patients should be randomised only on condition that relevant QoL assessments have been or will be completed.

- It is useful to assign a research assistant or a research nurse to QoL studies. Clinicians may be engaged in other tasks when patients come for their treatment.

- Named individuals at participating institutions should be identified for specific roles, especially if the clinical trial is multicentre. At some institutions this might involve several individuals for the different tasks. Responsibilities include:

    a. explaining to the patient the rationale for QoL assessment and its implications

    b. giving QoL questionnaires to patients (one possibility is that questionnaires should be completed while waiting to be seen by the clinician)

    c. providing a quiet, private and comfortable place for the patient to complete them

    d. ensuring that help is readily available for patients who require it

    e. collecting and checking questionnaires for completeness

    f. sending reminders and collecting overdue or missing questionnaires

g. forwarding completed questionnaires to the clinical trial office and responding to queries arising.

- It is important to consider the provision of systematic training to accompany the written instructions for staff responsible for administering the questionnaires.

- Regular feedback should be given, to maintain motivation. This might include reports of data quality (numbers of completed forms, compliance rates, details of missing items) and tabulation of baseline, pre-randomisation data.

- Finally, the medical team should be reminded that experience shows that most patients are willing to complete QoL questionnaires.

Example from the literature

Hürny *et al.* (1992) report that compliance in a trial of small-cell lung cancer varied between 21% and 68%, with larger institutions having the highest rates of compliance. Institution was the only significant factor for predicting compliance. Patient age, gender, education and biological prognostic factors at randomisation were not found to be predictors.

It was suggested that smaller institutions might be at a disadvantage, as they usually do not have the resources to dedicate a full-time staff member to data management and quality assurance. However, with an organised effort at the local institutional level, high-quality data collection could be achieved. It was also recommended that to achieve good-quality QoL data there is a need for the systematic training and commitment of staff at all institutions.

10.5 Recommendations for writing protocols

Protocols should aim to be concise, practical documents for participating clinicians, covering all aspects of the day-to-day running of the clinical trials. It is to be hoped that brevity encourages reading and observance of the content of the protocols. There is no consensus as to the optimal way of presenting all the relevant background information and justification of QoL study design. Different approaches are used by different trials organisations, according to their needs and preferences and according to the nature of individual trials. Thus while it is important to consider the study's objectives and details of the design, it is unclear how much of this should be incorporated in the working protocol or whether it should be recorded separately. One possibility is to mention these issues briefly in the main study protocol, and to address them in greater detail in written accompanying supplementary documents. These additional documents should comprise part of the package that is also sent to the Protocol Review Committee and to the local Ethics Committees (Institutional Review Boards). The following examples are taken from a range of protocols, with specific illustrations of text that has been used in MRC protocols (Fayers *et al.*, 1997b).

Rationale for including QoL assessment

A section in the protocol should explain the reasons why QoL is being assessed. Some clinicians are less committed to QoL evaluation than others, and so it is important to justify the need for the extra work that the participants are being asked to carry out.

> ### *Quality of life follow-up*
>
> *Quality of life is an important endpoint of this study. The timing of treatment may have a considerable impact on patients. The long-term palliation and prevention of symptoms are important factors in the treatment of relapsed disease. It is important therefore that all centres participate in this study.*

Emphasising good compliance

The need for good compliance should be stressed to participants, telling them that a serious effort is being made to ensure completeness of QoL data collection. In trials where QoL is a major endpoint or the principal outcome measure, optimal compliance is clearly essential: patients who fail to return QoL data do not contribute information for analysis. In extreme cases a trial Data Monitoring Committee (DMC) could recommend early closure of the trial if the level of QoL compliance is unacceptable. Thus protocols should emphasise the importance of QoL assessment, and should also encourage doctors to emphasise this to patients.

> *Such data will be an essential source of information for comparison between the two arms in this study.*
> *Emphasise to the patient that completion of these forms helps doctors find out more about the effects of treatment on patients' well-being.*

Identify contact persons

We have described the need to identify personnel within the medical team, to take responsibility for the various tasks associated with administering QoL questionnaires. It is recommended that one named person be identified to serve as the contact at each centre. This person is responsible for collecting the QoL data and ensuring that the forms are checked and returned to the trials office. This might or might not be the clinician responsible for the patients, although in general it is recommended that a person other than the responsible clinician should administer the questionnaire to the patient, so that the form may be completed prior to consultation with the doctor. In addition, it has been suggested that patients try to please their doctor or nurse, and thus the responses may be distorted if the person responsible for managing their treatment is present while they complete the forms.

> *A named person in each centre must be nominated to take responsibility for the administration, collection and checking of the QoL forms. This may or may not be the clinician responsible for the patients.*

Written guidelines for administering QoL questionnaires

There should be written guidelines aimed at those administering the questionnaires in the clinical setting. These address the issues of poor compliance at the level of the participating institute. The topics covered should range from suggestions about adopting a sympathetic approach towards patients who may be feeling particularly ill or may have just been informed about the progression of their disease, for example, through to instructions about the need to ensure back-up staff for times when the normal QoL personnel are on leave or absent.

There should be instructions about the checking of forms, including procedures for patients who fail to complete answers for all questions, such as how to handle patients who have not understood what is required or who do not wish to respond to particular questions (e.g. 'Explain to the patient the relevance and importance of these particular questions and the confidentiality of the information'). The guidelines should indicate any questions that are anticipated to present particular problems. For example, staff might be warned: 'Some patients omit to answer the question about sexual interest, because they find it embarrassing and consider it irrelevant. However, it is included as an indicator of the general health and well-being of the patient.' Similarly, for a question about loss of appetite: 'Patients may be confused between inability to eat due to symptoms such as dysphagia or inability to eat because of lack of appetite; it is the latter meaning that is intended.'

> An information pack is sent to all participating centres detailing the procedures for quality of life assessment and providing guidelines for ensuring optimal compliance.

Checking forms before the patient leaves

When clinical data are missing from a form, it is frequently possible to retrieve the information from hospital notes. QoL is different; once the patient has left the hospital, it will be too late to retrieve missing data or clarify unclear information, except by contacting the patient by telephone, email or post. Therefore there should be statements about the need for the QoL forms to be checked before the patient has left the clinic and any action to be taken in the event of missing data. There should also be instructions regarding procedures to follow when questionnaires are missing: should the patient be contacted, possibly by post with a pre-paid envelope or by telephone/email, or should the data be accepted as missing and only the reason recorded?

> The questionnaire must be collected before the patient leaves and **checked to ensure that all questions have been answered.** *If necessary, go back to the patient immediately and ask him or her to fill in any missing items.*
>
> If a questionnaire assessment is missed because of administrative failure, the patient should be contacted by telephone, *email or letter and asked to complete and return a mailed questionnaire as soon as possible.*

Baseline assessment

There will usually be a *baseline assessment*, taken before randomisation. In addition to providing a pre-treatment baseline against which the patient's subsequent changes can be compared, this also enables a baseline comparison between the randomised study groups. If differences are present, it may be necessary to make compensatory statistical adjustments when subsequently analysing the data. When follow-up data are missing, the baseline information can also allow examination of the patterns of loss, and can often be used to minimise the systematic biases that may arise from missing data.

The baseline assessment should be made before the patient has been informed of the randomised treatment allocation; otherwise, knowledge of the treatment assignment may cause different levels of, for example, anxiety within the two treatment groups. Furthermore, by ensuring that QoL is assessed before randomisation and made an eligibility criterion for randomisation, we can try to ensure that form completion is 100%.

> ### Randomisation
>
> *Patients should be randomised by telephoning the Trials Office. The person telephoning will be asked to confirm that the eligibility criteria have been met, and that the patients have completed their initial quality of life questionnaires.*

Assessment during therapy

Some trials have used a daily diary card, obtaining a complete picture of the changing symptomatology and QoL before, during and after therapy. More commonly, and especially in large multicentre clinical trials, it is necessary to identify specific time points when a QoL questionnaire should be used. Since administering and completing questionnaires imposes burdens on the patient, it is desirable to limit the number and frequency of questionnaires.

Often, for administrative convenience, assessment times during treatment will be chosen to coincide with patient visits to the clinic. For diseases requiring long-term treatment, for example hypertension, a patient's condition may be expected to be relatively stable and so the precise time point may not be critical. In this situation, the timing of QoL assessment becomes relatively easy. For other diseases, such as cancer, patients commonly attend at the start of each course or cycle of chemotherapy treatment, with the patient completing the QoL questionnaire while waiting to be reassessed by the clinician. However, some QoL instruments specify a time frame of 'during the last week ...', and will therefore only collect information about how the patient recalls feeling during the week preceding the next course of therapy. If treatment courses are, for example, pulsed at intervals of three to four weeks, this may or may not be what is ideally wanted, as the impact of transient toxicity might remain undetected. That is, the investigators will have to decide whether temporary toxicity-related reductions in QoL are of importance, or whether the longer-term effects as seen later during each cycle are more important. Sometimes it may be appropriate to assess QoL at, say, one week after therapy.

Another point to be considered is that sometimes treatment may be delayed, possibly because of toxicity, in which case if assessments are made immediately preceding the next (delayed) course of treatment, the impact of the toxicity upon QoL may not be noticed.

In principle, it is desirable to use the same timing schedule in all treatment arms, with QoL assessments being made at times relative to the date of randomisation. In practice, this may be difficult in trials that compare treatments of different modality or where the timing of therapy and follow-up differs between the randomised groups. In these settings, patients may attend the clinic at different times and therapy in the treatment arms may also be completed at different times. This leads to differences in the timing of assessments within the arms of the study, which can make any interpretation of results difficult if patients are deteriorating as a consequence of their disease progressing from the time of randomisation.

In summary, there are compromises to be made in those studies that investigate QoL in the context of treatment events such as surgery and intermittent courses of chemotherapy and radiotherapy. Assessments may be made relative to the treatment events or relative to the randomisation date. They may also be timed to occur after, but relative to, the date of the previous course of treatment or immediately preceding the following course. Sometimes a combination of strategies can be used.

Clearly the general timing of the assessments must be specified, for example 'two weeks after surgery'. However, a more precise specification might specify a window within which assessments are valid, for example 'at least two, but not more than three, weeks after surgery'.

> The quality of life questionnaire *should be completed by the patient **before** randomisation, at 6 weeks, 12 weeks, 6 months and 1 year.*
>
>   Most patients are expected to keep to their protocol treatment time schedule, but to allow for occasional delays a wind*ow of one week around each time point will be accepted.*

Follow-up (post-treatment) assessment

There may also be follow-up assessments after completion of treatment. Sometimes the primary scientific question concerns QoL during therapy, and if post-treatment assessment is thought necessary perhaps one suffices. In other studies, it may be important to continue collecting data in order to explore treatment-related differences in the long-term impact of therapy and control of disease progression. Sometimes it is relevant to continue assessment until and after any relapses may have occurred, and in some studies, such as those of palliative care, assessments may continue until death. In all these situations, to eliminate bias, long-term assessments in both treatment groups should normally be at similar times relative to the date of randomisation. If the questionnaires are mailed to patients, any appropriate schedule can be used; if they are to be handed out at clinics, the choice of times may be restricted for logistic reasons.

Specifying when to complete questionnaires

Generally it is advisable for QoL to be assessed before the patient is seen by the clinician. Then the patient will not have been affected by anything occurring during their consultation. Furthermore, it is usually convenient for the clinic to administer the assessment while the patient is waiting to be seen. This also enables the clinical follow-up form to include the questions: 'Has QoL been assessed? If not, why not?'

> ### *Follow-up*
>
> *The patient should complete the questionnaires while waiting to be seen in the clinic – this should be done in a quiet area.*

Patients should also be encouraged to request their QoL forms upon arrival at the clinic, since this will help to prevent QoL assessments being forgotten and there is usually suitable time to complete the forms while waiting to be seen by the clinician.

> If you are not given a questionnaire to complete when you think it is due, please remind your doctor. You can, of course, decline to fill in a questionnaire at any time.

Some instruments relate to 'the past week'. In many trials, the patient attends hospital three or four weeks after the previous cycle of chemotherapy or radiotherapy, and thus assessments at these times may not always include the period during which therapy was received. It is important that patients be aware of the time frame of the questions.

> *It is important to explain to the patient that the questionnaire refers to how they have been feeling **during the past week**.*

Help and proxy assessment

Nurses, doctors and family members often underestimate the impact of those items that most distress the patient. Therefore it is important that the patients should complete the QoL questionnaire themselves. Similarly, patients may be influenced by the opinions of others if either helped to complete questionnaires or if interviewed.

> ### *Example from the literature*
>
> Cook *et al.* (1993) compared the same questionnaire when interviewer- or self-administered, on a sample of 150 asthma patients. When using the self-administered version, patients recorded more symptoms, more emotional problems, greater limitation of activities, more disease-related problems and a greater need to avoid environmental stimuli. On average, 47% of items were endorsed when self-administered, but only 36% when interviewed.

Similar patterns have been observed by others; patients tend to report fewer problems and better QoL when interviewed by staff. It is advisable that patients should receive help only when it is absolutely necessary, and doctors, nurses and partners should all be discouraged from offering help unless it is really needed.

However, some patients may be unable to complete the questionnaire by themselves or have difficulty understanding the questions. Examples range from vision problems and forgotten glasses to cognitive impairment. In these cases, help should be provided, as assisted completion is better than either a total absence of data or incorrect information through misapprehension. Similarly, if a few patients are too ill or too distressed to complete the forms, someone familiar with their feelings may act as a proxy. *Proxies* are typically a 'significant other' such as a partner, partner or close family member but may include staff, such as a nurse who knows the patient well. For some trials, such as those in psychiatry or advanced brain malignancies, it might be anticipated that the majority of patients will be unable to complete questionnaires and it may be appropriate to make extensive – or even exclusive – use of proxy assessment. Proxy assessment may also be needed for young children who are unable to complete questionnaires, even though parents and other adults usually have a very different set of priorities from children and value emotional and physical states differently. Sometimes it can be anticipated that a large proportion of the patients will become unable to complete questionnaires as the trial progresses, for example in trials of palliative care that involve rapidly deteriorating patients. In these cases the use of proxy respondents could be considered as an integral part of the trial. In general, however, proxy assessment should be avoided whenever possible.

Despite this, the differences between proxies and patients tend to be small, with proxies rating patients as having slightly lower levels of functioning and more symptomatology (McColl and Fayers, 2005; Gundy and Aaronson, 2008). It is better to use proxy raters rather than have either missing data or unreliable data from cognitively impaired patients. Gundy and Aaronson further suggest it may be better to ask proxies to make their own assessment rather than attempt to predict the patient's self-assessment.

The instructions to the patients should normally ask them to complete the forms on their own, that is, without conferring with others. The study forms should collect details of any assistance or use of proxies.

The patient should complete the questionnaire without conferring with friends or relatives, and all questions should be answered even if the patient feels them to be irrelevant. Assistance should be offered only *when the patient is unable to complete the questions by him/herself.*

Will QoL forms influence therapy?

There are differing opinions as to the value of having QoL forms available for use by the treating clinician, or whether they should be confidential. For example, those patients who are keen for their therapy to be continued may be reticent about revealing deterioration in QoL or side effects of treatment if they believe that their responses might cause treatment reduction. Also, some patients try to please their clinician and nursing staff, and may respond overly positively. Although evidence for this remains scant, there is support from studies showing differences between QoL assessments completed by self-administered questionnaire versus interview-administered questionnaire, in which interview-assisted completion resulted in a reduced reporting of impairments. A tendency for yea-saying, or *response acquiescence*, when filling in

QoL questionnaires has also been noted (Moum, 1988). Thus it can be an advantage to assure patients that the QoL information is confidential and will not be seen by the clinician; some trials supply pre-paid envelopes addressed to the Trials Office, in which the questionnaires may be returned.

On the other hand, in some hospitals the clinicians and nurses use the QoL forms to assist with patient management – which is of advantage to the trial organisation in that it may increase compliance with form completion. In addition, there are considerations of individual and collective ethics. From the point of view of guaranteeing bias-free interpretation, there are arguably grounds to maintain – and assure the patient of – confidentiality. Thus there are both advantages and disadvantages to keeping the forms confidential and not using them to influence therapy, but in either case the procedures should be standardised and specified.

> You will be given a folder of questionnaires and some pre-paid envelopes in which to return them. We would like you to complete one of these questionnaires just before you go to the hospital for the start of each course of chemotherapy, for other treatment or at a routine check-up.
>
> (Pre-paid envelopes are addressed to the Trials Office.)

Patient information leaflets

An initial leaflet may be provided prior to requesting informed consent from the patient. This can either be combined with the general information leaflet that the patient receives when completing QoL questionnaires, or may be a separate brief document that is specifically given out during the consent process. In addition to describing the nature of randomised trials and discussing issues of relevance to consent, it should explain the reasons for evaluating QoL and indicate what this involves. It should mention the frequency and timing of assessments.

If QoL is the primary endpoint in a trial, it may be included as a condition on the patient consent form. Patients who are unwilling to contribute towards the primary endpoint of a trial should be ineligible for randomisation.

> We will also ask you to fill in a form, which assesses your quality of life, before you receive treatment and at 3, 6, 12 and 24 months after your *treatment starts. The quality of life questionnaire is a standard form that is used for other patients and allows us to compare quality of life across various diseases. Because of this, there are some questions that may not seem relevant to your disease and its treatment. **However, please try to answer them all.***

QUALITY OF LIFE QUESTIONNAIRE

About your questionnaires

We are concerned to find out more about how patients feel, both physically and emotionally, during and after different treatments. In order to collect this information, brief questionnaires have been designed that can be completed by patients themselves. We would like you to complete questionnaires before, during and after your treatment at this hospital.

The questionnaires refer to how you have been feeling **during the past week** and are designed to assess your day-to-day well-being, as well as to monitor any side-effects you may be experiencing. Your questionnaires will be sent to the Medical Research Council where they will be treated in confidence and analysed together with those from patients in other hospitals to help plan future treatments.

We enquire about a wide range of symptoms as the questionnaires are designed for use in many different areas of research, but please feel free to discuss any symptoms or concerns with your doctor.

Completing the questionnaires

If possible, complete the questionnaires on your own. Please try to answer all the questions but do not spend too much time thinking about each answer as your first response is likely to be most accurate. If a question is not applicable to you, please write alongside 'not applicable' or 'N/A', but do not leave any question blank.

When you attend the hospital for the first time, you will be asked to complete a questionnaire. We would like you to complete further questionnaires each time you come into the hospital for an assessment. If you are not given a questionnaire to complete, please remind your doctor. You can, of course, decline to complete a questionnaire at any time without affecting your relationship with your doctor. The questionnaire will help us to acquire the knowledge to improve the treatment of patients with your condition.

Thank you for your help

Figure 10.2   Patient QoL Information Leaflet.

The Patient QoL information leaflet is a detailed document that the patient may take away for reference. It should introduce the reasons for using questionnaires, explain aspects of the QoL assessment, and attempt to answer queries that patients commonly ask. Figure 10.2 shows an example.

Randomisation checklist

Completion of the initial QoL assessment is often made a prerequisite for randomisation. This not only provides baseline QoL data for all patients but also ensures that patients understand the procedure and, by implication, agree to participate in the study of QoL.

Randomisation checklist

ELIGIBILITY *(please tick to confirm)*

☐ *Patient consents to participate in the trial, and patient is willing and able to complete QoL questionnaires.*
☐ *Patient has completed the first QoL questionnaire.*

(TO RANDOMISE, TELEPHONE THE TRIALS OFFICE.)

Clinical follow-up forms

The question 'Has patient completed QoL forms?' serves as a reminder to the clinician and should protect against patients leaving the hospital before completing the questionnaire. Furthermore, in the event of refusal or other non-compliance, for example if the patient feels too ill to complete the questionnaire, it is important to obtain details regarding the reasons. There should be a question 'If no, give reasons'. This information helps decide how to report and interpret results from patients for whom QoL data are missing.

The follow-up forms should also document whether significant help was required in order to complete the questions, or whether a proxy completed them.

Follow-up form

Has patient completed Quality of Life form?   ☐ Yes ☐ No
*If **NO**, please state reason:*

· ·
· ·
· · · · · · · · · · · ·
*If **YES**, indicate whether the patient required help completing the form, and if so please give details:*

· ·
· ·
· · · · · · · · · · · ·

10.6 Standard operating procedures

Although not usually part of the main clinical trial protocol sent to participating clinicians, there is also a need for documentation of the standard operating procedures (SOPs) at the Trials Office, and an outline of the intended analysis plan. This should be specified at the inception of the trial and covers all aspects of the clinical trial. In particular, for QoL it should detail the statistical analysis and interpretation of the clinical trial results when there are missing data. Nowadays, the SOP is a standard part of Good Clinical Practice (GCP).

10.7 Summary and checklist

There are many considerations when incorporating QoL assessment into clinical trials. The most readily apparent of these is compliance. However, compliance is but one of the issues that need to be addressed in a protocol and it remains far too easy to omit other necessary details. Hence the use of checklists is important. By ensuring that all the details are covered, and provided there are adequate resources and training, it should be possible to optimise the quality of the information collected and the level of compliance achieved.

1. During the design stage of a study, sufficient financial resources should be available to provide an adequate infrastructure to manage the study and to integrate the QoL assessment into the normal daily practices of a clinic.

2. Objectives of the study should be presented clearly in the protocol, including the rationale for QoL (and particularly if it is a main study endpoint).

3. It is preferred that QoL not be an optional evaluation.

4. Based on the objectives of the study, an appropriate valid instrument should be selected and if necessary additional treatment-specific questions should be developed, tested and added as appropriate. However, the number of items should be kept to a minimum.

5. The QoL questionnaire should be available in the appropriate languages in relation to potential participants in the clinical trial. If additional translations are required, they should be developed using tried and tested translation procedures.

6. The schedule of assessments should not be too much of a burden for the patient, yet at the same time it should be frequent enough and at appropriate time points to provide a relevant picture of the patient's QoL over the study period. For practical reasons, the schedule of QoL assessments should coincide with the routine clinical follow-up visits for the trial.

7. Statistical considerations in the protocol, including anticipated effect size, sample size and analysis plan, should be clear and precise.

8. Protocols should include guidelines on QoL data-collection procedures for clinicians, research nurses and data managers.

9. There should be a policy of education for all those involved, from training for staff through to information documents for patients.

10. A cover form should be attached to the questionnaire. This should be completed if the patient did not complete the questionnaire, providing reasons for non-completion.

Figure 10.3 summarises the issues discussed in this chapter. A protocol for a clinical trial should normally address all of the points enumerated here.

CHECKLIST

Are the following points addressed in the protocol?

☐ Is rationale given for inclusion of QoL assessment?
☐ Is importance of good compliance emphasized?
☐ Is a named contact-person identified as responsible in each participating centre?
☐ Are there written guidelines for the person administering the questionnaires?
☐ Are all forms checked for completion whilst patient still present?

Timing of assessments:
　a. ☐　Are baseline assessments specified to be pre-randomisation?
　b. ☐　Is timing of follow-up assessments specified (valid window)?
　c. ☐　Is timing of follow-up assessments specified (before/whilst/after seeing clinician)?

☐ Is it specified whether help and/or proxy assessment are permitted?
☐ Will QoL forms be used to influence therapy or patient management?

Are the following forms and leaflets available?
PATIENT CONSENT INFORMATION LEAFLET (Pre-Consent Form):
　☐ Is QoL assessment explained?

PATIENT QOL INFORMATION LEAFLET:
　☐ Is there a leaflet for the patient to take home? (See specimen in Figure 10.2)

RANDOMISATION CHECKLIST:
　☐ Is QoL completion a pre-randomisation eligibility condition?

CLINICAL FOLLOW-UP FORMS:
　a. ☐ Do follow-up forms ask whether QoL assessment has been completed?
　b. ☐ Do follow-up forms ask about reasons for any missing QoL data?
　c. ☐ Do follow-up forms ask whether help was needed?

Figure 10.3 Checklist for writing clinical trials protocols.

10.8   Further reading

The drug regulatory bodies provide useful guidelines about the implication of collecting PROs in clinical trials (European Medicines Agency, 2005b; United States Food and Drug Administration, 2009). These cover various aspects of the design of trials, such as protocol considerations and the frequency of assessment, as well as the handling of missing data and the analysis of multiple endpoints.

The Center for Medical Technology Policy (CMTP) has produced a guidance document with recommendations for the appropriate inclusion of patient-reported outcome (PRO) measures in the design and implementation of effectiveness studies and clinical research in adult oncology; much of their recommendations are equally applicable to other disease areas (Basch *et al.*, 2011).

11
Sample sizes

Summary

This chapter describes how sample sizes may be estimated for QoL studies. To obtain such sample sizes it is necessary to specify, at the planning stage of the study, the size of effect that is expected. The type of statistical test to be used with the subsequent data needs to be stipulated, as do the significance level and power. Situations in which means, proportions, ordered categorical and time-to-event outcomes are relevant are described. Sample size considerations are included for the difference between groups, comparison with a reference population and non-inferiority studies, as well as unpaired and paired situations. The consequences of comparing more than two groups or simultaneously investigating several endpoints are discussed.

11.1 Introduction

In principle, there are no major differences in planning studies using QoL assessment compared with using, for example, a comparison of blood pressure levels between different groups. The determination of an appropriate design and study size remains as fundamentally important in this context as in others. A number of medical journals, including those specialising in QoL, subscribe to the CONSORT statement and stipulate in their statistical guidelines that a justification of sample size is required (Schultz et al., 2010). A formal calculation of the sample size is an essential prerequisite for any clinical trial, and, for example, guidelines from the Committee for Proprietary Medicinal Products (CPMP, 1995) have made it mandatory for all studies in the European Union since 1995. However, it must be recognised that one is usually designing a study in the presence of considerable uncertainty – the greater this uncertainty, the less precise will be our estimate of the appropriate study size.

This chapter focuses on clinical trials and observational studies. However, the methods described are general and applicable to other situations, including questionnaire validation.

Quality of Life: The Assessment, Analysis and Reporting of Patient-Reported Outcomes, Third Edition.
Peter M. Fayers and David Machin.
© 2016 John Wiley & Sons, Ltd. Published 2016 by John Wiley & Sons, Ltd.

11.2   Significance tests, *p*-values and power

Later chapters refer extensively to statistical significance tests and p-values, for example when comparing two or more forms of therapy. Since patients vary both in their baseline characteristics and in their response to therapy, an apparent difference in treatments might be observed due to chance alone, and this need not necessarily indicate a true difference due to a treatment effect. Therefore it is customary to use a significance test to assess the *weight of evidence* and to estimate the probability that the observed data could in fact have arisen purely by chance. The results of the significance test will be expressed as a p-value. For example, $p < 0.05$ indicates that so extreme an observed difference could only be expected to have arisen by chance alone less than 5% of the time, and so it is quite likely that a treatment difference really is present. Although results of a significance test are expressed in terms of p-values, when designing a study the equivalent value is instead referred to as α, the risk of a *false positive* or *type 1 error*. If we decide that $p < 0.05$ will suffice to denote statistical significance, we set $\alpha = 0.05$.

If few patients were entered into the trial, then even if there really is a true treatment difference, the results are likely to be less convincing than if a much larger number of patients had been assessed. Thus the weight of evidence in favour of concluding that there is a treatment effect will be less in a small trial than in a large one. In particular, if a clinical trial is too small, it will be unlikely that one will obtain sufficiently convincing evidence of a treatment difference, even when there really is a difference in efficacy of the treatments. Small trials frequently conclude 'there was no significant difference', irrespective of whether there really is a treatment effect or not. In statistical terms, we would say that the sample size is too small, and that the 'power of the test' is very low. The *power*, $1 - \beta$, of a significance test is a measure of how likely a test is to produce a statistically significant result, on the assumption that there really is a true difference of a certain magnitude. Thus β is the probability of failing to obtain a significant test result when there really is a true treatment effect as large as the specified target; β is the *false negative* rate, or *type 2 error*. The larger the study, the more likely it is to detect treatment effects that may exist, and so the higher its power.

Suppose the results of a treatment difference in a clinical trial are declared 'not statistically significant'. Such a statement indicates only that there was an insufficient weight of evidence to be able to declare that the observed data are unlikely to have arisen by chance. It does not mean that there is no clinically important difference between the treatments. If the sample size was too small, the study might be very unlikely to obtain a significant p-value even when a clinically relevant difference is present. Hence it is of crucial importance to consider sample size and power both when planning studies and when interpreting statements about 'non-significance'.

11.3   Estimating sample size

To estimate the required sample size it is necessary to specify the significance level α (also, perhaps confusingly, called the *test size*), the power $1 - \beta$, and the anticipated difference (*effect size*) in QoL that may be expected between alternative groups.

The effect size, which we write as Δ, is the target value that we hope to be able to detect expressed in units of standard deviation; that is, if we wish to detect a difference $(\mu_T - \mu_C)$ between two means μ_T and μ_C and if the standard deviations of these two PROs is assumed equal and written as σ, then the standardised difference is $\Delta = (\mu_T - \mu_C)/\sigma$. Ideally we would like to be able to detect a small value of Δ with low rates of false positives (α small) and with high power (β small). Unfortunately, the smaller the values of α, β and Δ, the larger the necessary sample size.

Choosing the type 1 error

Convention often dictates that tests are two-sided and of at least 5% significance level, represented by a type 1 error of $\alpha = 0.05$. Clearly it would be preferable to aim for a more convincing 1% level if possible, with $\alpha = 0.01$. In most settings, values higher than $\alpha = 0.05$ are unacceptable.

Choosing the power

Usually the power is set to a minimum of 80%. However, assuming there really is a true difference as large as the anticipated target, Δ, this represents a one-in-five risk of failing to obtain statistical significance. It is time consuming, expensive and hard work to write a protocol, obtain funding and execute a clinical study. Are you willing to accept a 20% risk of failure? We recommend wherever possible aiming for 90% power, with $\beta = 0.10$. If $\alpha = 0.05$, aiming for $\beta = 0.10$ instead of 0.20 typically results in an increase of 34% in total sample size, as shown in Table 11.3.

Choosing the target effect size

The target effect size should be both *realistic* and *clinically relevant*. It should be realistic in the sense that it would be futile to design a study comparing two very similar treatments on the assumption that there will be a huge treatment effect; there is no point in designing a small trial that does not have the power to detect differences that are plausible. Thus the target difference should be a realistic difference based on current knowledge. The target effect should also be large enough to be deemed clinically relevant, that is, noticeable by the patient and considered an important change; again, there is no point in designing an extremely large study to have the power to detect trivial and unimportant differences in PROs. Hence in addition to being a realistic difference, the target should also be an important difference as judged by the stakeholder – usually the patient. Chapter 18 on clinical interpretation discusses various methods for determining clinical relevance and *minimally important differences*.

Frequently there is insufficient prior experience to quantify the anticipated differences with much precision. In addition, QoL is often summarised in terms of more than one outcome variable; for example, the EORTC QLQ-C30 has 30 questions that are combined to produce essentially 15 different outcomes. Not only are there 15 different outcomes, but also they will often all be assessed on different occasions throughout the study thereby generating a longitudinal profile for each patient. Typically, in a clinical trial setting, assessments start immediately before randomisation, are at relatively frequent intervals during active therapy, and perhaps extend less frequently thereafter until death.

As already indicated, in order to estimate the appropriate sample size the anticipated effect size must be determined for each study based on experience, published data or pilot studies. First, the PRO variables (scales or items) should be identified and ranked in order of importance for the specific study under consideration. For instance, the investigators may know, from previous observation of patients with the specific disease and receiving standard therapy for the condition, that patients experience considerable fatigue. If one objective of the new therapy is to alleviate symptoms, fatigue might be regarded as the most important aspect of QoL and, in the context of a clinical trial, could be used for sample size determination purposes. The remaining PROs would then play a secondary role.

Once the principal endpoint variable has been established, it is necessary to identify how this is to be utilised to assess the outcome on a patient-by-patient basis. This may not be easy. There are likely to be several (perhaps many) assessment times for each patient. One possible approach is to create a summary of each patient's profile. Thus Matthews *et al.* (1990) recommend that a series of observations be analysed through summary measures obtained from each patient, for example the change from baseline QoL assessment to that at the end of active therapy, the time above a certain level, or the *area under the curve (AUC)*.

After this summary is determined, an average of this for each of the study therapies needs to be estimated. In the context of planning a randomised trial of two alternative therapies, these might be a standard or control treatment (C) and a test treatment (T). The control average can be obtained from previous experience of other or similar patients; for some instruments, such as the EORTC QLQ-C30, published reference data are available (Scott *et al.*, 2008). It is then necessary to specify the benefit in QoL that is anticipated by use of the test therapy in place of the control. This too may be obtained from previous experience or may have to be elicited in some way using clinical opinion.

This benefit or effect size, Δ, has been variously defined as the 'minimum value worth detecting' or a 'clinically important effect' or 'quantitatively significant' (see the Chapter 18 on clinical interpretation). Sometimes there may be neither the experience of nor agreement on what constitutes a meaningful benefit to the patient. Cohen (1988) suggests that, when there is an absence of other information about relevant sizes for effects, a small effect usually corresponds to $\Delta = 0.2$, a moderate effect to $\Delta = 0.5$ and a large effect to $\Delta = 0.8$ (see also Chapter 18). The smaller the effect, the larger the study. Figure 11.1 illustrates this for the two-sample t-test used to compare two unpaired means (details are given in Section 11.4). The figure shows the total sample size required when applying a two-sided test with significance level $\alpha = 0.05$, for powers $1 - \beta = 80\%$ and 90%. An effect size of 0.2 calls for a large study of between 800 (80% power) and over 1000 (90% power). In contrast, if the effect size is above 0.8, relatively small sample sizes are sufficient. In practice, one rarely has a precise effect size in mind, and the degree of variation in sample size shown in Figure 11.1 makes it clear that it is foolish to regard sample size estimations as exact requirements; statisticians routinely round the estimates upwards to a convenient higher number, as is done in Table 11.3.

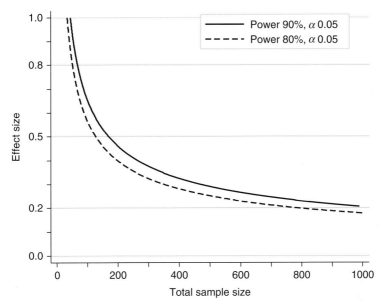

Figure 11.1 The total sample size required to detect an effect of a specified size, using a two-sample *t*-test to compare two unpaired means with α of 0.05 and powers of 80% and 90%.

Example from the literature

Julious *et al.* (1997) describe HADS anxiety and depression data generated from 154 patients with small-cell lung cancer in a randomised trial conducted by MRC Lung Cancer Working Party (1996). The data for the anxiety scores are given in Table 11.1.

A practical advantage of the HADS instrument is that an estimate of clinically important levels of distress can be made using recommended cut-off scores for each subscale. Thus a score of 15 or more is regarded as a potential clinical case, perhaps signalling more detailed clinical examination and possibly treatment; a score between 8 and 10 is borderline, and one of ≤7 is regarded as normal. As a consequence, sometimes the actual score may be ignored and the analysis may be based upon comparison of the proportions in these three categories for the different treatment groups.

Suppose we assume that the HADS domain for anxiety is the more important of the two domains and that the summary measure of most relevance is the HADS assessment two months post-randomisation. Then the endpoint of interest becomes one of the simplest possible.

Table 11.1   Frequency of responses to the HADS anxiety scale, for patients with small-cell lung cancer two months post-randomisation

Category	Anxiety score	Number of patients
Normal	0	7
(0–7)	1	5
	2	20
	3	11
	4	11
	5	11
	6	11
	7	17
Borderline	8	13
(8–10)	9	7
	10	13
Case	11	7
(11–21)	12	2
	13	6
	14	4
	15	5
	16	2
	17	1
	18	0
	19	1
	20	0
	21	0
Total		154
Normal	0–7	93 (60.39%)
Borderline	8–10	33 (21.43%)
Case	11–21	28 (18.18%)
Median anxiety score	6	
Mean anxiety score	6.73	
SD	4.28	

Source: Julious *et al.*, 1997, Table 2. Reproduced with kind permission of Springer Science and Business Media.

Sample size formulae

There are several possible approaches to calculating the sample size required for data such as those of Table 11.1. One is to assume the data have (at least approximately) a Normal distribution. The second is to categorise the data into binary form, for example 'case' or 'not case'. A third is to categorise into more than two categories, for example 'case', 'borderline' or 'normal' – or to consider the full form of the data as an ordered categorical

Table 11.2 The values of $(z_{1-\alpha/2} + z_{1-\beta})^2$ for commonly encountered values of α and β

Significance level α		Power $1 - \beta$	
2-sided	1-sided	0.80	0.90
0.01	0.005	11.679	14.879
0.02	0.010	10.036	13.017
0.05	0.025	7.849	10.507
0.10	0.050	6.183	8.564

variable with, in our example, $\kappa = 22$ levels. Each statistical significance test or method of analysis has an associated formula for sample size and power calculations. We provide formulae and example calculations for the most common statistical tests used in QoL studies.

In the formulae given below, we give the total number of subjects required for a clinical study for a two-sided test with significance level α and power $1 - \beta$. In these formulae, $z_{1-\alpha/2}$ and $z_{1-\beta}$ are the appropriate values from the standard Normal distribution for the $100(1 - \alpha/2)$ and $100(1 - \beta)$ percentiles, obtained from Appendix Table T1. Since many of the equations involved the term $(z_{1-\alpha/2} + z_{1-\beta})^2$, Table 11.2 gives its value for some of the most commonly used combinations of significance level and power. For example, the illustrative calculations mostly use a two-sided significance level of 5% and a power of 80% or 90%. From the Appendix Table T1, $z_{1-\alpha/2} = 1.96$ and for 80% power $z_{1-\beta} = 0.8416$, or for 90% $z_{1-\beta} = 1.2816$, so the term $(z_{1-\alpha/2} + z_{1-\beta})^2$ equals 7.849 and 10.507 respectively.

11.4 Comparing two groups

Means – unpaired

In a two-group comparative study where the outcome measure has a Normal distribution form, a two-sample t-test would be used in the final analysis (see Campbell *et al.*, 2007). In this case the (standardised) anticipated effect size is $\Delta_{Normal} = (\mu_T - \mu_C)/\sigma$, where μ_T and μ_C are the anticipated means of the two treatments and σ is the *SD* of the PRO measures and which is assumed the same for both treatment groups. On this basis, the total number of patients to be recruited to the clinical trial, is

$$N_{Normal} = \frac{4\left(z_{1-\alpha/2} + z_{1-\beta}\right)^2}{\Delta_{Normal}^2} + \frac{z_{1-\alpha/2}^2}{2}. \tag{11.1}$$

Figure 11.1 uses this equation to show the sample size requirements when $\alpha = 0.05$, for powers $1 - \beta = 80\%$ and 90%. Table 11.3 also shows some commonly used effect sizes, and the resultant study size for these values of α and $1 - \beta$. The final term of equation (11.1) is important only in small samples and usually may be omitted. For example, in the case of $z_{1-\alpha/2} = 1.96$ the final term is $1.96^2/2 \approx 2$.

Table 11.3 The total sample size* required to detect an effect of a specified size, using a two-sample t-test to compare two unpaired means with a significance level of 5% and powers of 80% and 90%

Effect size Δ	0.2	0.3	0.4	0.5	0.6	0.7	0.8	0.9	1.0
Power									
$1 - \beta = 80\%$	790	360	200	130	90	66	52	42	34
$1 - \beta = 90\%$	1060	470	270	180	120	88	68	54	44

*Sample sizes of 100 and above have been rounded upwards to a multiple of 10.

Example

The mean HADS anxiety score is $\bar{x} = 6.73$ with a large $SD = 4.28$, indicating a rather skew distribution far from the Normal form, as does the full anxiety distribution in Table 11.1. Consequently, it may not be advisable to use equation (11.1) directly to calculate sample size.

However, if the data are transformed using a logarithmic transformation, the transformed variable may have a distribution that approximates better to the Normal form. To avoid the difficulty of a logarithm of a zero score, each item can be coded 1–4 rather than 0–3. Each scale is the sum of seven items, giving sum scores from 7 to 28, so this is equivalent to using $y = \log_e(x + 7)$ where x is the HADS anxiety score on the original scale. In this case, the data of Table 11.1 lead to $\bar{y} = 2.5712$ and $SD(y) = 0.3157$.

Unfortunately, there is no simple clinical interpretation for the y-scale, and so the inverse transformation is used to obtain scores corresponding to the HADS scale. Thus, the value corresponding to $\bar{y}$ is $x = \exp(\bar{y}) - 7 = 6.0815$, and this is closer to the median anxiety score of 6 than the original $\bar{x}$ of 6.73. Importantly, the distribution has a more Normal form on this transformed scale and equation (11.1) can be applied once the effect size Δ_{Normal} is specified.

The therapy aims to reduce anxiety in the patients, that is, to increase the proportion classified as 'normal' – and this corresponds to a desired reduction in HADS. We may postulate that the minimum clinically important difference to detect is a decrease in this equivalent to 1 unit on the HADS, that is, from 6.0815 to 5.0815. This is then expressed as an anticipated effect on the logarithmic y-scale as $\Delta_{Normal} = (\mu_T - \mu_C)/\sigma = [\log_e (5.0815 + 7) - \log_e (6.0815 + 7)]/0.3157 = (2.4917 - 2.5712)/0.3157 = -0.25$. This would be regarded as a small effect size, using the guidelines proposed by Cohen (1988). Using equation (11.1) with $\Delta_{Normal} = -0.25$ gives $N_{Normal} = 504$ patients or approximately 250 patients in each group.

The sample size depends only on the absolute value of the anticipated difference between treatments. It is independent of the direction of this difference. Thus, the same sample size would be obtained if $\Delta_{Normal} = +0.25$, for example if a new but potentially more toxic therapy was being investigated and an increase in anxiety is likely.

Means – paired

Some QoL studies may be designed in a matched case–control format. In this situation, patients with a particular condition may be of interest and we may wish to compare their QoL with a comparative control (non-diseased) group. This could be a comparison of elderly females with rheumatism against those without the disease. Thus, for every patient identified, a control subject (female of the same age) is chosen and their QoL determined. The paired or matched difference between these two measures then gives an indication of their relative difference in QoL. These differences are then averaged over all N_{Pairs} of the case–control pairs, to provide the estimate of group differences.

On this basis, the number of patient-control pairs to be recruited to the clinical trial is

$$N_{Pairs} = \frac{\left(z_{1-\alpha/2} + z_{1-\beta}\right)^2}{\Delta^2} + \frac{z_{1-\alpha/2}^2}{2}. \tag{11.2}$$

This expression is of a similar form to equation (11.1), but here there is a major difference in how $\Delta = \delta/\sigma_{Difference}$ is specified. Thus $\sigma_{Difference}$ here is the anticipated SD of the N differences between the case-control pairs. It is neither the SD of the case values themselves nor the SD of the corresponding control values (which are often of similar magnitude).

Machin *et al.* (2008) point out that there is a relationship between the SD for each subject group, σ, and the SD of the difference, $\sigma_{Difference}$. Thus:

$$\sigma_{Difference} = \sigma\sqrt{2(1-\rho)}, \tag{11.3}$$

where ρ is the correlation coefficient between the values for the cases and their controls. An exploratory approach is to try out various values of ρ to see what influence this may have on the proposed sample size. It should be noted that when the values are weakly correlated, with ρ less than 0.5, equation (11.3) implies that a *larger* sample size will be required than if an unpaired test were used. Paired matching is only beneficial when the outcomes have a correlation greater than 0.5.

Example

Regidor *et al.* (1999) give the mean physical functioning (PF) measured by the SF-36 Health Questionnaire in a reference group of 1,063 women aged 65 years and older as 55.8 with $SD \approx 30$. The SD is large relative to the size of the mean, which suggests that the distribution of the PF score may be rather skewed.

Suppose we are planning a case–control study in women 65 years or older who have rheumatism. It is anticipated that these women will have a lower PF by as much as five points. How many case–control pairs should the investigators recruit?

It is first worth noting that even if the distribution of PF scores is not itself of the Normal distribution form, the differences observed between cases and controls may approximate to this pattern. This is what is assumed.

In this example $\delta = 5$, and in order to determine the anticipated effect size $\Delta = \delta/\sigma_{Difference}$ we need a value for $\sigma_{Difference}$ itself, although we can first assume $\sigma = 30$. Table 11.4 shows the different values for $\sigma_{Difference}$ depending on the value of ρ. For each of these values there is an effect size Δ and finally the number of case-control pairs required is calculated from equation (11.2). Various options are summarised in Table 11.4, which show that there is a wide range of potential study size that depends rather critically on how ρ effects $\sigma_{Difference}$ and hence Δ and ultimately N_{Pairs}. The numbers in this table have been rounded upwards to the nearest 10 subjects to acknowledge the inherent uncertainty in the sample estimation process.

Table 11.4   Variation in the size of a case–control study (two-sided $\alpha = 0.05$ and power $1 - \beta = 0.8$), assuming $\delta = 5$ and $\sigma = 30$

ρ	0.0	0.2	0.4	0.6	0.8	0.9	0.95
$\sigma_{Difference}$	42.4	37.9	32.9	26.8	19.0	13.4	9.5
Δ	0.12	0.13	0.15	0.19	0.26	0.37	0.53
N_{Pairs}	570	460	350	230	120	60	30

Proportions – unpaired

The statistical test used to compare two groups when the outcome is a binary variable is the Pearson χ^2 test for a 2×2 contingency table (see Campbell *et al.*, 2007). In this situation the anticipated effect size is $\delta_{Binary} = (\pi_T - \pi_C)$, where π_T and π_C are the proportions of 'normals', however defined, with respect to depression in the two treatment groups. On this basis, the number of patients to be recruited to the clinical trial, is

$$N_{Binary} = \frac{2\left(z_{1-\alpha/2} + z_{1-\beta}\right)^2 [\pi_T(1-\pi_T) + \pi_C(1-\pi_C)]}{\delta_{Binary}^2}. \tag{11.4}$$

Alternatively, the same difference between treatments may be expressed through the odds ratio (OR), which is defined as

$$OR_{Binary} = \frac{\pi_C / (1-\pi_C)}{\pi_T / (1-\pi_T)}. \tag{11.5}$$

This formulation leads to an alternative to equation (11.4) for the sample size. Thus

$$N_{OddsRatio} = \frac{4\left(z_{1-\alpha/2} + z_{1-\beta}\right)^2 / \left(\log OR_{Binary}\right)^2}{\bar{\pi}(1-\bar{\pi})}, \tag{11.6}$$

where $\bar{\pi} = (\pi_C + \pi_T)/2$. Equations (11.4) and (11.6) are quite dissimilar in form, but Julious and Campbell (1996) show that they give, for all practical purposes, very similar sample sizes, with divergent results occurring only for relatively large (or small) OR_{Binary}.

Example

Table 11.1 indicates that there are approximately 60% of patients classified as 'normal' with respect to anxiety. Suppose it is anticipated that this may improve to 70% in the 'normal' category with an alternative treatment. The anticipated treatment effect is thus $\delta_{Binary} = (\pi_T - \pi_C) = (70 - 60)\% = 10\%$. This equates to a total sample size of $N_{Binary} = 706$ from equation (11.4).

Alternatively, this anticipated treatment effect can be expressed as $OR_{Binary} = (60/40)/(70/30) = 0.6428$. Using this in equation (11.6), if $\alpha = 0.05$ and $1 - \beta = 0.8$, with $\bar{\pi} = (0.70 + 0.60)/2 = 0.65$, also gives a total sample size of $N_{Odds-Ratio} = 706$ patients. As noted, the difference between the calculations from the alternative formulae is usually small and inconsequential.

Proportions – paired

In the matched case–control format discussed above, the comparison of elderly females with rheumatism to those without the disease may be summarised as 'Good' or 'Poor' QoL. Thus the possible pairs of responses are (Good, Good); (Good, Poor); (Poor, Good) and (Poor, Poor). The McNemar test for such paired data (see Campbell *et al.*, 2007) counts the number of the N_{Pairs} which are either (Good, Poor) or (Poor, Good). If these are s and t respectively, the odds ratio for comparing cases and controls is estimated by $\psi = s/t$, and the proportion of discordant pairs by $\pi_{Discordant} = (s + t)/N_{Pairs}$. To estimate the corresponding study size, anticipated values for ψ and $\pi_{Discordant}$ need to be specified. Then

$$N_{Pairs} = \frac{\left\{ z_{1-\alpha/2}(\psi + 1) + z_{1-\beta}\sqrt{(\psi + 1)^2 - (\psi - 1)^2 \pi_{Discordant}} \right\}^2}{(\psi - 1)^2 \pi_{Discordant}}. \tag{11.7}$$

Just as we saw for paired means, it is often difficult to anticipate the impact of pairing upon sample size estimates because the calculations require more information than for unpaired designs. Usually, the purpose of pairing or matching is to obtain a more sensitive comparison; that is, to reduce sample size requirements. Thus the sample size needed for a paired design should usually be less than for an unpaired one, and may often be appreciably less.

Example

Suppose in the previously discussed case-control study of women who have rheumatism that their overall QoL is to be summarised as 'good' or 'poor' and so is that of their controls. It is anticipated that a major difference in the odds ratio will be observed; so a value of $\psi = 4$ is specified. It is further anticipated that the discordance rate will probably be somewhere between 0.5 and 0.8. How many case-control pairs should be recruited?

In this example $\psi = 4$, which is itself the anticipated effect size, we also need to specify $\pi_{Discordant}$. Table 11.5 shows some options for the study size for differing values of $\pi_{Discordant}$ calculated using equation (11.7).

The numbers in this table have been rounded upwards to the nearest 10 subjects in recognition of the inherent imprecision in the sample estimation process.

Table 11.5 Variation in the size of a matched case–control study, assuming $\psi = 4$ (two-sided $\alpha = 0.05$ and power $1 - \beta = 0.8$)

$\pi_{Discordant}$	0.5	0.6	0.7	0.8
N_{Pairs}	50	40	30	30

Ordered categorical data

The transformation of data when dealing with a variable that does not have a Normal distribution leads to difficulties in interpretation on the transformed scale and, in particular, the provision of an anticipated effect size. It would be easier if the original scale could be preserved for this purpose. In fact the data of Table 11.1 are from an ordered categorical variable and the statistical test used when the outcome is ordered categorical is the Mann–Whitney U-test with allowance for ties (see Sprent and Smeeton, 2007). Thus it would be more natural to extend from the comparison of two proportions, which is a special case of an ordered categorical variable of $\kappa = 2$ levels, to $\kappa = 22$ levels for the HADS data. Formulating the effect size in terms of OR_{Binary} rather than δ_{Binary} enables this extension to be made. The estimated sample size is given by Whitehead (1993) as

$$N_{Categorical} = \frac{12\left(z_{1-\alpha/2} + z_{1-\beta}\right)^2 / (\log OR_{Categorical})^2}{\left[1 - \sum_{i=0}^{k-1} \bar{\pi}_i^3\right]}, \quad (11.8)$$

where the mean proportion expected in category i ($i = 0$ to $\kappa - 1$) is $\bar{\pi}_i = (\pi_{Ci} + \pi_{Ti})/2$, and π_{Ci} and π_{Ti} are the proportions expected in category i for the treatment groups C and T.

The categories are labelled as 0 to $\kappa - 1$, rather than 1 to κ, so that they correspond directly to the actual HADS category scores of Table 11.1. Here, the $OR_{Categorical}$ is an extension of the definition of OR_{Binary} given in equation (11.5) and is now the odds of a subject being in category i or below in one treatment group compared with the other. It is calculated from the cumulative proportion of subjects for each category 0, 1, 2,…, $(\kappa - 1)$ and is assumed to be constant through the scale.

The effect size in equation (11.8), as summarised through $OR_{Categorical}$, implies an assumption of proportional odds. This means that each adjacent pair of categories for which an OR can be calculated, that is OR_1, OR_2,…, OR_{21} for the HADS, all have the same true or underlying value $OR_{Categorical}$. Thus the odds of falling into a given category or below is the same, irrespective of where the HADS scale is dichotomised. This appears to be a very restrictive assumption but, for planning purposes, what is of greatest practical importance is that, although the ORs may vary along the scale, the underlying treatment effect should be in the same direction throughout the scale. Thus all ORs are anticipated to be greater than 1 or all are anticipated to be less than 1.

When using an ordered categorical scale, the ORs are a measure of the chance of a subject being in each given category or less in one group compared with the other. For the HADS data there are 21 distinct ORs. However, the problem is simplified because the OR anticipated for the binary case, that is the proportions either side of the 'caseness' cut off, can be used as an average estimate of the OR in the ordered categorical situation (Campbell *et al.*, 1995). Thus, if the trial size is to be determined with a Mann–Whitney U-test in mind rather than the χ^2 test for a 2×2 table, the anticipated treatment effect is still taken to be OR_{Binary}.

Julious *et al.* (1997) illustrate the evaluation of equation (11.8). First Q_{Ci}, the cumulative proportions in category i for treatment C, are calculated using, for example, tables of reference values. Then, for a given (constant) $OR_{Categorical}$, the anticipated cumulative proportions for each category of treatment T are given by

$$Q_{Ti} = \frac{OR_{Categorical}Q_{Ci}}{OR_{Categorical}Q_{Ci} + \left(1 - Q_{Ci}\right)}. \tag{11.9}$$

After calculating the cumulative proportions, the anticipated proportions falling in each treatment category, $\bar{\pi}_{Ti}$, can be determined from the difference of successive Q_{Ti}. Finally, the combined mean of the proportions of treatments C and T for each category is calculated.

We have assumed here that the alternative to the binary case ($\kappa = 2$) is the full categorical scale ($\kappa = 22$). In practice, however, it may be more appropriate to group some of the categories but not others to give κ categories, where $3 \le \kappa < 22$. For example, merging the HADS scores into the caseness groups defined earlier would give $\kappa = 3$, while $\kappa = 5$ if the caseness categories are extended in the manner described below.

Although there are 22 possible categories for the full HADS scales, it is reasonable to ask whether the full distribution needs to be specified for planning purposes. In many situations it may not be possible to specify the whole distribution precisely, whereas it may be easier to anticipate the proportions when there are fewer categories. The HADS scale is often divided into three categories for clinical use: 'normal' (≤ 7), 'borderline' (8–10) and 'clinical case' (≥ 11). For illustration purposes only, we define two additional categories: 'very normal' (≤ 3) and 'severe case' (≥ 16). Thus HADS scores 0–3 are 'very normal', 4–7 'normal', 8–10 'borderline', 11–15 'case' and finally 16–22 'severe case'.

Example

Table 11.6 gives, for the data of Table 11.1, the number of cases and cumulative proportions anticipated in each category for the anxiety dimension if we re-categorised the HADS anxiety scale into five categories as above.

Assuming $OR_{Categorical} = OR_{Binary} = 1.5556$ as we calculated above, then, for example, the anticipated proportion for category 2 of treatment T is from equation (11.9):

$$Q_{T2} = OR_{Categorical} \, Q_{C2}/[OR_{Categorical} \, Q_{C2} + (1 - Q_{C2})]$$

$$= 1.5556 \times 0.6039/[1.5556 \times 0.6039 + (1 - 0.6039)] = 0.7034.$$

The remaining values are summarised in Table 11.6. Values of π_{Ti} are calculated from the difference of successive Q_{Ti}. For example, $\pi_{T2} = 0.7034 - 0.3760 = 0.3274$. The final column of the table gives the corresponding values of $\bar{\pi}_i = (\pi_{Ci} + \pi_{Ti})/2$. The denominator of equation (11.5) is therefore

$$1 - [0.3276^3 + 0.3260^3 + 0.1929^3 + 0.1320^3 + 0.0214^3]$$
$$= 1 - 0.0793 = 0.9207,$$

and finally from equation (11.8), if $\alpha = 0.05$ and $1 - \beta = 0.8$, $N_{Categorical} = 524$.

Repeating the calculations with the three categories for HADS ('normal', 'borderline', 'case'), the corresponding sample size is $N_{Categorical} = 680$. Finally, reducing the categories to normal versus the remainder (borderline and cases), $N_{Binary} = 712$. The increasing sample size suggests that the less we can assume about the form of the data, the larger the study must be.

Table 11.6 Patients with small-cell lung cancer two months post-randomisation, categorised for anxiety 'caseness' following assessment using HADS. Cumulative proportions observed on standard therapy C and anticipated with test therapy T

				Cumulative proportion			
Category	Anxiety score	Number of C patients	π_{Ci}	Q_C	Q_T	π_{Ti}	$\bar{\pi}_i$
Very normal	0–3	43	0.2792	0.2792	0.3760	0.3760	0.3276
Normal	4–7	50	0.3246	0.6039	0.7034	0.3274	0.3260
Borderline	8–10	33	0.2143	0.8182	0.8750	0.1716	0.1929
Case	11–15	24	0.1558	0.9740	0.9831	0.1081	0.1320
Severe case	16–22	4	0.0260	1	1	0.0169	0.0214
Total		154					

Source: Data from Medical Research Council Lung Cancer Working Party, 1996.

Time-to-event data

Sometimes the endpoint of interest can be the time from randomisation until a patient achieves a particular value of their QoL or PRO. For example, suppose patients with a HADS of 10 or less (normal and borderline) will be recruited into a trial, and that it is also known that many of these patients will experience deterioration (increasing HADS) while receiving active therapy, but may then achieve improvement over their admission values. If a clinically important improvement is regarded as a HADS decrease of two points, then, with repeat assessments, one can observe if and when this first occurs. For those patients who experience the defined improvement, the time in days from baseline assessment to this outcome can be determined. For those who do not improve sufficiently, perhaps deteriorating rather than improving, their time to improvement will be censored at their most recent QoL assessment. The eventual analysis will involve Kaplan–Meier estimates of the corresponding cumulative survival curves, where here 'survival' is 'time to improvement', and comparisons between treatments can be made using the logrank test (Machin *et al.*, 2006).

To estimate the size of a trial, one can utilise the anticipated proportion of patients who have improved at, say, 12 weeks in the C and T groups respectively. However, in the actual study we will be determining as precisely as possible the exact time that the patient shows the QoL improvement specified.

In this situation the size of the anticipated effect is determined by the hazard ratio, Δ, the value of which can be obtained from

$$\Delta = \frac{\log_e \pi_C}{\log_e \pi_T},\qquad(11.10)$$

where, in this case, π_C and π_T are the anticipated proportions improving (here by 12 weeks) with C and T therapy respectively. Once the anticipated effect size Δ is obtained, the number of patients that are required for the study is given by

$$N_{Survival} = \frac{2\left[\dfrac{\left(z_{1-\alpha/2} + z_{1-\beta}\right)(1+\Delta)}{(1-\Delta)}\right]^2}{(2 - \pi_T - \pi_C)}.\qquad(11.11)$$

Example

Suppose for the HADS $\pi_C = 0.65$ but it is anticipated that the test treatment will be effective in improving this to $\pi_T = 0.75$ at 12 weeks. In this case, $\Delta = \log_e 0.65/\log_e 0.75 \approx 1.50$. Substituting these values in equation (11.11) with $\alpha = 0.05$ and $1 - \beta = 0.8$ gives $N_{Survival} = 660$.

One aspect of a trial, which can affect the number of patients recruited, is the proportion of patients who are lost to follow-up during the trial. Such patients have censored observations determined by the date last observed, as do those for whom the event of interest (here decreasing HADS anxiety score of 2 points) has not occurred at the end of the trial. If the anticipated proportion of censored patients is w, the sample sizes given in equation (11.11) should be increased to compensate by dividing by $1 - w$.

11.5   Comparison with a reference population

If a study is comparing a group of patients with a reference population value for the corresponding PRO, effectively one is assuming that the reference population value is known. As a consequence, this is not estimated from within the study and so subjects are not needed for this component. Hence fewer subjects will be required overall.

Means

In this case, when the population or reference mean QoL is known, the sample size necessary is given by equation (11.1), but with the 4 removed from the numerator in the first term, giving equation (11.12). This effectively reduces the sample size required, compared with a two-group comparison, by one-quarter:

$$N_{Normal} = \frac{\left(z_{1-\alpha/2} + z_{1-\beta}\right)^2}{\Delta_{Normal}^2} + \frac{z_{1-\alpha/2}^2}{2}. \tag{11.12}$$

Proportions

If a study is comparing the proportion of patients with, say, good QoL with a reference population value for the same QoL measure, effectively one is assuming that the reference population proportion is known and is not estimated from within the study. In this case, provided the proportions are close, the sample size necessary is approximately one-quarter that given by either equation (11.4) or (11.6).

11.6   Non-inferiority studies

Sometimes, in a clinical trial of a new treatment for patients with, say, a life-threatening disease such as cancer, it may be anticipated that the new treatment (Test) will at best bring only modest survival advantage over the current (Standard). Or, perhaps a new treatment is more convenient or cheaper. However, in such circumstances, any gain in efficacy might be offset by a loss of QoL. If there is a loss, then we may regard the Test as an acceptable replacement for the Standard provided any loss is no greater than η units of QoL. The quantity η is termed the level of non-inferiority between the QoL measure in the two treatment groups, and is the maximum allowable difference between the QoL measure in the two groups. If we ultimately observe an actual difference no greater than η, we accept that the two groups are essentially equivalent.

Earlier, when comparing two means or two proportions, we implied a null hypothesis of the form $\theta_{Standard} = \theta_{Test}$, where $\theta_{Standard}$ and θ_{Test} are the parameters we wish to estimate with our study. Thus in the conventional test of significance we seek to test $\delta = \theta_{Standard} - \theta_{Test} = 0$. In testing for non-inferiority this is modified to testing $\theta_{Standard} - \eta = \theta_{Test}$ against the alternative one-sided hypothesis $\theta_{Standard} - \eta < \theta_{Test}$ or alternatively expressed as $\delta = \theta_{Standard} - \theta_{Test} < \eta$.

These considerations lead to a $100(1 - \alpha)\%$ CI for $\delta = \theta_{Standard} - \theta_{Test}$ of

$$LL \text{ to } [\text{Difference} + z_{1-a} \times SE \text{ (Difference)}]. \tag{11.13}$$

Here the value of LL (the lower confidence limit) depends on the context but not on the data (see below). Note that this is a so-called one-sided CI and uses $z_{1-\alpha}$ not $z_{1-\alpha/2}$.

At the design stage, we need to specify the non-inferiority limit, η (> 0), and also the significance level α and the power, $1 - \beta$, such that the upper confidence limit (UL) for δ, calculated once the study is completed, will not exceed this pre-specified value η.

In the formulae given previously, we gave the total number of subjects required in a clinical study for a two-sided test with significance level α and power $1 - \beta$. In this section all calculations use a one-sided significance level.

In most applications, θ_{Test} is assumed to equal $\theta_{Standard}$. Further since η is likely to be small, such that a difference of η or less is clinically unimportant, the sample size required for a non-inferiority trial may be substantially larger than for the more usual superiority trial. The choice of η is critical, and the drug regulatory bodies emphasise this in documents about non-inferiority trials (European Medicines Agency, 2000, 2005a; United States Food and Drug Administration, 2010). Similarly, as in the two examples below, when a one-sided confidence limit is used the coverage probability should be 97.5%, that is, $\alpha = 0.025$.

Means

When two means are compared, the lower limit for the CI of equation (11.13) is $LL = -\infty$, that is negative infinity. The total sample size, $N_{Non-inferiority}$, required for a comparison of means from two groups of equal size and anticipated to have the same population mean and SD, σ, is

$$N_{Non-inferiority} = \frac{4\left(z_{1-\alpha} + z_{1-\beta}\right)^2}{\Delta^2}, \tag{11.14}$$

where $\Delta = \eta / \sigma$ can be thought of as the effect size.

> ### Example from the literature
>
> A non-inferiority study was used by Lee *et al.* (2011) to compare two methods of pain relief during labour. The primary outcome was decrease in pain measured by a VAS at 30 minutes post intervention. The authors specified 90% power with a one-sided α of 0.025. The non-inferiority margin was set at 1.0, and the true difference was assumed to be zero. Citing results from a meta analysis, the authors assumed a standard deviation of 2.5 on the VAS. From equation (11.14), this leads to a sample size of 132 patients per group, or 264 in total. The authors also assumed a 20% attrition rate, and estimated approximately 54 patients might be lost from the study; although they suggested increasing the sample size by 54 patients accordingly, this ignores the fact that the additional patients will also themselves be subject to attrition at the same rate. Equation (11.17), below, implies that the correct total should be approximately 330 patients.

Proportions

We assume that the outcome of the trial can be expressed as the proportion of patients with good QoL. After testing for non-inferiority of the treatment, we would wish to assume the probabilities of 'good' QoL are for all practicable purposes equal, although we might have evidence that they do in fact differ by a small amount. For this comparison $LL = -1$ in equation (11.13), as that is the maximum possible difference in the proportion of responses in the two groups.

The total sample size, $N_{Non\text{-}inferiority}$, required for a comparison of proportions from two groups of equal size and anticipated to have response proportions $\pi_{Standard}$ and π_{Test} with mean $\bar{\pi}$ is

$$N_{Non-inferiority} = \frac{4\bar{\pi}(1-\bar{\pi})\left(z_{1-\alpha} + z_{1-\beta}\right)^2}{\eta^2}. \qquad (11.15)$$

> ### Example from the literature
>
> Urodynamic studies (UDS) are routinely obtained prior to surgery for stress urinary incontinence in women, despite a lack of evidence that this has an actual impact on outcome. Nager *et al.* (2009) carried out a non-inferiority trial to ascertain whether preoperative UDS is of any value. The primary outcome was twelve-month patient reported response to the Urogenital Distress Inventory (UDI) and the Patient Global Index-Improvement (PGI-I), with the women classified into success if UDI decreased by 70% and PGI-I was rated 'much better' or higher. One-sided $\alpha = 0.025$ and power $= 80\%$ were used. The true proportion

of successes was assumed to be equal in the two groups, and from previous reports this was estimated to be 70% giving $\pi_{Standard} = \pi_{Test} = \bar{\pi} = 0.70$. The equivalence margin 'was chosen based on the belief that 11% was the largest amount that we would allow the success rate to differ and still deem the no UDS group non-inferior, while still producing a realistic sample size'. Thus $\eta = 0.11$. Using these assumptions, equation (11.15) indicates that a total 544 patients are required. Allowing for a 10% dropout rate, 608 women should be recruited.

11.7 Choice of sample size method

It is important when designing any study to obtain a relevant sample size. In so doing it is important to make maximal use of any background information available. Such information may come from other related studies and may be quite detailed and precise, or it may come from a reasonable extrapolation of observations from unrelated studies, in which case it may be regarded as very imprecise. It is clear that the more we know, or realistically assume, of the final outcome of our trial at the planning stage, the better we can design the trial. In our example, we have detailed knowledge of HADS outcome at two months, based on more than 150 patients. We may be fairly confident, therefore, that provided the treatment C in a planned new trial remains unaltered and the patient mix remains the same, we can use this distribution for planning purposes. If the trial is to test a new therapy T then, possibly apart from some very preliminary data, we may have little information about the effect of T on QoL. In this case, we suggest that the investigator has to decide if he or she wishes to detect, say, a one-, two- or three-point change in the average HADS score. This change has then to be expressed as an anticipated effect size before the sample size equations given here can be applied. The smaller the anticipated benefit, the larger the subsequent trial. If an investigator is uncomfortable about the assumptions, it is good practice to calculate sample size under a variety of scenarios so that the sensitivity to assumptions can be assessed.

In general, when designing a clinical trial, there will often be other variables (covariates), apart from allocated treatment itself, such as gender, age, centre or stage of disease. These may or may not affect the clinical outcome. Such variables may be utilised to create different strata for treatment-allocation purposes, and can also be used in the final analysis. If the QoL variable itself can be assumed to have a Normal distribution, the final analysis may adjust for these variables using a multiple regression approach. If a binary type of measure of QoL has been used, the covariates can be assessed by means of a logistic regression model (Campbell *et al.*, 2007). Similarly, if a time-to-event measure of QoL is being used, the covariates can be assessed by means of a Cox proportional hazards model as described by Machin *et al.* (2006).

11.8   Non-Normal distributions

Several of the formulae that we have presented assume that the target effect (such as the difference in means of two groups) follows a Normal distribution, and that t-tests can be used. We used a transformation approach for non-Normal data, illustrated by the logarithmic transformation, and made sample size calculations accordingly. Logarithms are typically suitable whenever we are more interested in percentage changes rather than absolute changes, because they convert multiplicative effects into linear effects; thus $\log(x \times y) = \log(x) + \log(y)$. Thus for depression scored 0–100, we might decide that a change from 10 to 20 (doubling of the score, or 100% increase) is a more noticeable change than going from 80 to 90, which is also a 10-point absolute change but only a 12.5% increase. More generally, whenever the data distribution is skewed with a tail extending to the right, a logarithmic transformation may well be beneficial in converting the numbers into a more Normal shape. The inverse transformation of the logarithm is the exponential function, and so we can readily convert back to the original scale after calculating confidence intervals or mean scores. Logarithms only apply to numbers greater than zero and so the example using the HADS also illustrated that the HADS items were coded 1–4 instead of 0–3 and corresponding changes made to the thresholds. Other common transformations for the purpose of converting continuous data with a skew distribution to a symmetrical Normal shape are the reciprocal and the square root. In addition, for other types of data (such as the number of events observed to occur in a given time) there are many other transformations available.

As we have indicated, it is not uncommon that, when designing a trial where a PRO is the primary measure of interest, there is little prior knowledge of the full distribution of the scores. Thus the very detailed information provided by Table 11.1 might not be available. However, this need not necessarily present a major problem for the full ordered categorical approach to sample size calculation. Whitehead (1993) indicates that knowledge of the anticipated distribution within four or five broad categories is often sufficient. This information, which may be solicited from experience gained by the clinical team, can then be used to aid the design of studies using HADS and other QoL instruments.

Both t-tests and analysis of variance are remarkably robust against violations of Normality. Walters and Campbell (2005) observed that QoL data tends to have discrete, bounded and skewed distributions. Using 'bootstrap' computer simulations, they found that despite this conventional methods of sample size estimation performed well. Norman (2010) argued that analyses "examining differences between means, for sample sizes greater than 5, do not require the assumption of Normality and will yield nearly correct answers even for manifestly non-normal and asymmetric distributions like exponentials", although Fayers (2011) responded that claims for robustness of significance tests refer to type I errors and that non-Normality can greatly affect the estimation of the standard error, resulting in a serious loss of power and this will also be associated with misleading sample size estimation. Thus we conclude overall that substantial deviations from Normal distribution should *not* be ignored.

11.9   Multiple testing

The *p*-value of a significance test is the probability of observing such extreme data purely by chance alone. However, if one carries out a large number of significance tests the *p*-value becomes distorted as there is a greatly increased risk that at least one test will be associated with an extreme *p*-value, purely by chance. As we discuss in later chapters about analysis, this *multiple testing* can present problems for the analysis of PROs. Three situations can be identified: repeated assessments leading to multiple testing at different time points, comparisons of several groups of patients resulting in multiple pairwise comparisons, and the analysis of multiple PROs.

Repeated QoL assessments over time

In Chapter 14 we illustrate the use of generalised estimating equations and multilevel models, as two methods for analysing repeated measures data. When QoL assessments are repeated, the within-patient measurement values will be correlated most highly for assessments that are closest in time. In theory, if the correlation structure is known, it would be possible to make a formal sample size calculation. In practice, this is rarely feasible. For sample size purposes, when repeated measures of the same QoL item are involved, one recommended approach to design is to choose either a key observation time as the endpoint observation or to use a summary statistic such as the *AUC*. A summary of these basic observations will then provide the values for the groups being compared and the basis for the sample size determination.

Comparing multiple groups of patients

In circumstances where three or more groups are being compared, we recommend calculating the sample size appropriate for each possible comparison. This will provide a range of possible sample sizes per treatment group. It is then a matter of judgement as to which should be used for the final study – the largest of these will be the safest option but may result in too large a study for the resources available. If the number of groups is large, some note may have to be taken of the resulting numbers of significance tests. One possibility is to use a Bonferroni adjustment (see the next section) for the sample size. In some circumstances, the different groups may themselves form an ordered categorical variable; for example, intervention may be graded as 'none', 'limited' or 'intensive'. In this case there is a structure across the intervention groups, and a test-for-trend may be appropriate. Then no Bonferroni adjustment need be considered.

Multiple endpoints

Earlier in this chapter we indicated that it is very important to identify a single PRO as the principal QoL endpoint. If there are additional endpoints, it is advisable to rank these in order of importance. We recognise that in many situations there may be a very long list of QoL variables but would urge that those which are to be included in a formal analysis should be confined to at most four or five. The remainder should be consigned to exploratory hypothesis-generating analyses or descriptive purposes only. However, if analyses of the four or five outcomes are to be made, some recognition of the multiple statistical hypothesis testing that will occur should be taken into account during the planning process.

In practice, it is very unlikely that the associated anticipated effect sizes would be of the same magnitude or direction. Thus, for example, $k = 4$ endpoints denoted (in rank order of importance) by $\Omega_{(1)}$, $\Omega_{(2)}$, $\Omega_{(3)}$ and $\Omega_{(4)}$ might be used separately in four sample size calculations, and four different estimates are likely to result. The final study size is then likely to be a compromise between the sizes so obtained. Whatever the final size, it should be large enough to satisfy the requirements for the endpoint corresponding to $\Omega_{(1)}$ as this is the most important endpoint and hence the primary objective of the trial.

To guard against false statistical significance as a consequence of multiple testing, it is a sensible precaution to consider replacing the significance level α in the various sample size equations by an adjusted test size using the *Bonferroni correction*, which is

$$\alpha_{Bonferroni} = \alpha / k. \qquad (11.16)$$

Thus $\alpha_{Bonferroni}$ is substituted instead of α in the equations given above. For $k = 4$ and $\alpha = 0.05$, $\alpha_{Bonferroni} = 0.05/4 = 0.0125$. Such a change will clearly lead to larger sample sizes; for example, from Table T1, $z = 1.96$ when $\alpha = 0.05$, whereas for $\alpha = 0.0125$ the value of z is approximately 2.50 and the numerators of, for example, equation (11.1) will both be larger. In this case, the overall sample size must be increased by a multiplication factor of about 1.36. Figure 11.2 shows the multiplication

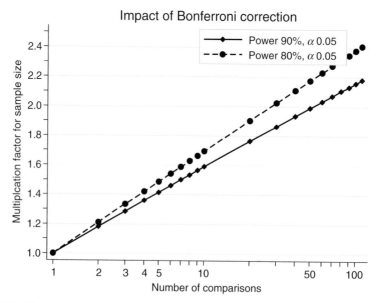

Figure 11.2 Sample size multiplication factors to compensate for multiple comparisons when applying a Bonferroni correction.

factors that are required so as to compensate for multiple comparisons when using the Bonferroni correction, for $\alpha = 0.05$ and power of 80% or 90%.

Use of the Bonferroni correction remains controversial. It assumes that the tests are independent of each other, which is equivalent to the unrealistic assumption that the outcomes are uncorrelated; consequently it is a conservative, or over extreme, correction of the p-values. As we discuss in the Chapter 16 on practical and reporting issues, another compromise is to report unadjusted p-values while adopting a cautious approach of, say, $p < 0.01$ when making claims of statistical significance.

11.10 Specifying the target difference

Figure 11.1 makes it clear that one of the most important determinants of sample size is the magnitude of the effect size. When planning a study, we might be tempted to aim for a modest effect size, since experience indicates that investigators tend to be over-enthusiastic and optimistic about the benefits of new therapies. But a small-to-modest effect size will necessitate a large study – and, frequently, a study that is totally unrealistic. This leads to a re-examination of the target difference: is it realistic to anticipate a larger effect size? There is no point in setting unrealistically large targets, as this would merely mean that the true effect, if there is one, is likely to be smaller than planned for, and so the study becomes unlikely to obtain a statistically significant result. At the other extreme, it is equally futile to specify a target effect that is so small that patients and clinicians would fail to discern any benefit. Thus it is important to consider the range of effect sizes that would be scientifically realistic as well as clinically worthwhile. There will be an element of iteration, exploring the impact of different effect sizes on the required sample size, and – one hopes – eventually obtaining a compromise that results in a potential study design. The chosen target effect size, and the consequent sample size, will then have to be justified to the funding body, to the ethical review panel and eventually to the journal in which one aspires to publish.

11.11 Sample size estimation is pre-study

It must be emphasised that it is only meaningful to make a sample size or power calculation when designing a study, *before* recruiting patients. Thus medical journals specifically demand to know whether the sample size estimations were pre-study. Post hoc power calculations are of little value; if an observed effect is not statistically significant, we know that the power of detecting such a difference is less than 50%. Conversely, if an effect is found to be very highly significant, we know that the power is high enough to have detected that effect. If power calculations were not carried out pre-study, the only meaningful way to present the results is using confidence intervals to reflect the implications of the sample size on the estimated parameters.

11.12   Attrition

As discussed in the Chapter 10 on clinical trials and subsequently Chapter 15 on missing data, QoL studies frequently have major problems regarding compliance and missing data. It is rare that a study will have 100% of forms completed and returned. In some clinical trials there may also be severe attrition due to deaths. The effective sample size may be markedly less than the number of patients recruited. When planning a study, adequate allowance must be made for all forms of attrition – and, we find through experience, there is a strong tendency to underestimate the levels of attrition. Estimated sample sizes should be inflated by an appropriate compensatory factor. If the calculated sample size was n and it is anticipated that the proportion of patients lost might be ω, the appropriate sample size is $n_{Adjusted}$ where

$$n_{Adjusted} = \frac{n}{1 - \omega}.$$

(11.17)

11.13   Circumspection

We have emphasised the importance of making the best possible estimate of sample size when designing a study. However, it must also be apparent that there are lots of choices that must be made and that many of these are very arbitrary or based on parameters that are unknown or uncertain. As Senn (2003) comments: "There is a considerable disparity between the mathematical sophistication involved in a sample-size determination and the practical basis from which it must proceed, namely the choice of a 'clinically relevant difference' (or some other treatment difference) and a 'guesstimate' of the variability in the experiment to be performed." We have great sympathy with his suggestion that: "In many cases it is a more sensible approach to sample-size determination to have a look at what sort of trial has been run in the past in a particular area and see what sort of inferences were possible rather than going through some complicated power calculation: often this is no more than a ritual." A similar view is expressed by Norman (2012).

11.14   Conclusion

When designing any study, there is usually a whole range of possible options to discuss at the early design stage. We would therefore recommend that various anticipated benefits be considered, ranging from the optimistic to the more realistic, with sample sizes being calculated for several scenarios within that range. It is a matter of judgement, rather than an exact science, as to which of the options is chosen for the final study size.

In QoL studies, there are many potential endpoints. As we have stressed, it is important that a clear focus be directed to identifying the major ones (at most five). This is clearly important for sample size purposes, but it is also necessary to state these end-points clearly in the associated study protocol and to ensure that they are indeed the main focus of the subsequent report of the completed study.

We would recommend, when an ordered categorical variable such as HADS is the QoL outcome measure, that equation (11.6) is utilised directly. This is preferable to seeking a transformation that enables the formula for a Normal variable (equation 11.1) to be used. The major reason is that this retains any treatment benefit on the original QoL scale and therefore will be more readily interpreted. Although the associated methods of analysis are less familiar, statistical software is available for these calculations.

Finally, it should be noted that if time-to-event endpoints are to be determined with any precision, there must be careful choice of the timing of QoL assessments. This is to ensure that for each patient the date when the event occurs can be determined reasonably precisely. Time-to-event techniques are unlikely to be useful if the assessment intervals are lengthy.

11.15   Further reading

There is extensive literature about sample size estimation, and many books on the subject. Machin *et al.* (2008) provide detailed consideration of sample size issues in the context of clinical studies and also provide a PC-based program for the calculations. For less common tests, it may be necessary to make bibliographic searches. Computer-intensive simulations or 'bootstrap methods' are useful alternatives that may be used to generate sample size estimates when formulae are unavailable; these are described by Walters and Campbell (2005).

Drug regulatory agencies have taken the lead in setting standards in this area, and the documents about non-inferiority testing (European Medicines Agency, 2000 and 2005a; United States Food and Drug Administration, 2010) and multiplicity issues (European Medicines Agency, 2002) make interesting reading. These documents also cover other study designs such as equivalence testing which, while in some ways similar to non-inferiority testing, raises additional issues not covered in this chapter.

12

Cross-sectional analysis

Summary

This chapter describes the types of analysis and graphical methods appropriate to the comparison of groups of patients with QoL assessment at a common time point. The methods described are thus cross-sectional in nature. We describe some basic ideas for assessing statistical significance when comparing two groups, such as z- and t-tests, and the associated confidence intervals (*CIs*) and the extension of these to the comparison of several groups using analysis of variance (ANOVA). These ideas are then generalised to enable differences to be adjusted for covariates, such as baseline patient characteristics (for example age and gender), using regression techniques. The relationship between ANOVA and linear regression is illustrated. Modifications to the methods for binary and ordered categorical variables are included, as well as methods for continuous data that do not have the Normal distribution form. Finally, some graphical methods of displaying cross-sectional data are introduced.

12.1 Types of data

As we have seen, QoL data are usually collected using a self-assessment instrument containing a series of questions. The answers to some of these questions may be analysed directly or be first combined into a number of scales or domains, such as physical, emotional or cognitive, for the subsequent analysis. The variables from these questionnaires are of various types: they include binary, categorical, ordered categorical, numerical discrete or, less frequently, continuous variables. The statistical methods required for summarising and comparing groups of patients depend on the type of variable of concern.

Nominal data

Nominal data are data that one can name. They are not measured but simply counted. They often consist of 'either/or' type observations, for example dead or alive. At the end of the study, the proportion or percentage of subjects falling into these two binary

Quality of Life: The Assessment, Analysis and Reporting of Patient-Reported Outcomes, Third Edition.
Peter M. Fayers and David Machin.
© 2016 John Wiley & Sons, Ltd. Published 2016 by John Wiley & Sons, Ltd.

categories can be calculated. In the SF-36, question 4c asks subjects to answer 'Yes' or 'No' to: 'Were [you] limited in the *kind* of work or other activities?'

However, nominal data may have more than two categories – for example ethnic group or marital status – and the percentages falling into these categories can be calculated. The categories for nominal data are regarded as unordered since, for example, there is no implication that Chinese, Indian and Malayan ethnicity are ranked in order on some underlying scale.

Example from the literature

Scott *et al.* (2009a), in investigating the impact of cultural differences on PROs, explored the impact of language on responses to items on the EORTC QLQ-C30. Since the questionnaire was developed in English and translated into other languages, English was the reference group. In the absence of any meaningful ordering, results for the other languages were presented in alphabetical sequence.

Nominal data with more than two categories are rarely used as PROs, but are more frequently encountered for covariates such as marital status, place of treatment, living conditions and (for cancer patients) histology.

Ordered categorical or ranked data

In the case of more than two categories, there are many situations when they can be ordered in some way. For example, the SF-36 question 1 asks: 'In general, would you say your health is: Excellent, Very good, Good, Fair, Poor?' In this case there are five ordered categories ranging from 'Excellent' to 'Poor'. The proportion or percentage of subjects falling into these five categories can be calculated, and in some situations these categories may be given a corresponding ranking 1, 2, 3, 4 and 5, which may then be used for analysis purposes. An example is the test-for-trend as alluded to in Table 12.2. However, although numerical values are assigned to each response, one cannot always treat them as though they had a strict numerical interpretation, as the magnitude of the differences between, for example, Excellent (Rank 1) and Very good (2) may not necessarily be the same as between Fair (3) and Poor (4).

The majority of questions on QoL instruments seek responses of the ordered categorical type. Unless item response theory (IRT) scoring is used, these items are commonly described as Likert scales and scored by assigning sequential integers starting from either 0 or 1. Other variables, in addition to PROs, may also be scored using ranks.

Numerical discrete/numerical continuous

Numerical discrete data consist of counts; for example, a patient may be asked how many times they vomited on a particular day, or the number of pain relief tablets taken.

On the other hand, numerical continuous data are measurements that can, in theory at least, take any value within a given range. Thus a patient completing the EuroQol questionnaire is asked to indicate: 'Your own health today' on a 10-cm vertical scale whose ends are defined by 'Worse imaginable health state' with value 0 cm and 'Best imaginable health state' with value 10 cm.

In certain circumstances, and especially if there are many categories, numerically discrete data may be regarded as effectively continuous for analytical purposes.

Continuous data: normal and non-normal distributions

A special case of numerical continuous data is that which has a Normal distribution – see, for example, Campbell *et al.* (2007). In this case special statistical methods such as the *t*-test are available, as we shall describe. Frequently, however, QoL data do not have even approximately a Normal distribution. For example, many items and scales, especially when applied to healthy subjects or extremely ill patients, may result in data with a large number of maximum *ceiling* or minimum *floor* scores, which is clearly not of a Normal distribution form. Then alternative statistical methods, not based upon the assumption of a Normal distribution, must be used.

Aggregating continuous data

The usual method of analysing continuous data involves calculating averages or means, or possibly mean changes or mean differences. This is the standard approach to aggregating continuous data into summary statistics, and is applied to continuous data of nearly all sources, from weights and heights through to blood pressures. However, as has been stressed in earlier chapters, many regard this as being questionable when applied to QoL data because it assumes inherently that the scores are on equal-interval scales. In other words, it assumes that since the mean of two patients both scoring 50 on a scale from 0 to 100 equals the mean of two patients scoring 25 and 75, these pairs of patients have, on average, equivalent QoL.

Clearly, the data should be analysed and reported in a manner that allows for the distribution of patient responses. If there is concern that low scores are particularly important, overall means may be inadequate to reflect this and, for example, it may be appropriate in addition to consider percentages of patients below a threshold value. When data follow a Normal distribution, the means, *SD*s and *CI*s provide an informative way to describe and compare groups of patients, and usually suffice to reflect any overall shift in response levels due to treatment differences. However, when the distributions are non-Normal, and especially when the shape of the distributions is not the same in all treatment groups, care must be taken to describe these distributions in detail as the reporting of a simple mean or median may not be adequate.

12.2   Comparing two groups

The essence of statistical analysis is to *estimate* the value of some feature of the patient population, derived from the data that have been collected. This may be the sample mean, the sample proportion, the slope of a linear regression relationship, or the difference between two such quantities calculated from distinct groups. In all these circumstances, what we observe is regarded as only an estimate of the true or underlying population value. The precision associated with each estimate is provided by the corresponding standard error (*SE*).

In very broad terms, the majority of statistical significance tests reduce to comparing the estimated value of the quantity of interest with its *SE* by use of an expression of the form

$$z = \frac{\text{Estimate}}{SE(\text{Estimate})}. \tag{12.1}$$

The value of z so obtained is sometimes called a *z-statistic*, and the corresponding *p*-value can be read from tables of the Normal distribution (Appendix Table T1). Large values lead one to reject the relevant null hypothesis with a certain level of statistical significance or *p*-value. Statistical significance and the null hypothesis are discussed in detail in basic statistics books but, in brief, the *p*-value is the probability of the data, or some more extreme data, arising by chance if the *null hypothesis* of *no difference* were true.

The associated (95%) *CI* takes the general form of

$$\text{Estimate} - 1.96 \times SE(\text{Estimate}) \text{ to } \text{Estimate} + 1.96 \times SE(\text{Estimate}) \tag{12.2}$$

The general expressions (12.1) and (12.2) will change depending on circumstances, and may have to be amended radically in some situations. Precise details are to be found in general textbooks of medical statistics, including Campbell *et al.* (2007) and Altman (1991). Altman *et al.* (2000) focus on *CI*s in particular.

Binomial proportions

If there are two groups of patients, the proportions responding to, for example, the SF-36 question 4a, relating to the '… kind of work or other activities' can be compared. Thus if there are m and n patients respectively in the two groups, and the corresponding number of subjects responding 'Yes' are a and b, the data can be summarised as in Table 12.1.

Here the estimate that we are focusing on is a difference in the proportion answering 'Yes' in the two treatment groups. This estimate is

$$d = p_I - p_{II} = \frac{a}{m} - \frac{b}{n}, \tag{12.3}$$

Table 12.1 Proportion of patients in two treatment groups responding 'Yes' to SF-36 question 4a

Category	Treatment group I	II	Total
'Yes'	a	b	r
'No'	c	d	s
Total	m	n	N
Proportion 'Yes'	$p_I = a/m$	$p_{II} = b/n$	$p = r/N$

and the standard error (SE) is

$$SE(d) = \sqrt{\frac{p_I(1-p_I)}{m} + \frac{p_{II}(1-p_{II})}{n}}. \qquad (12.4)$$

The null hypothesis here is that there is truly no difference between the treatments being compared, and that therefore we expect d and hence z to be close to 0.

Categorical data

In Table 12.1 there are $R = 2$ rows and $C = 2$ columns, giving the $G = 4$ cells of a 2×2 contingency table. An analysis of such a table can also be conducted by means of a χ^2 *test*. The general expression is

$$\chi^2_{\text{Homogeneity}} = \sum_{i=1}^{G} \frac{(O_i - E_i)^2}{E_i}, \qquad (12.5)$$

where O_i and E_i are the observed and expected number of observations. For the $G = 4$ cells of Table 12.1, the observed values are $O_1 = a$, $O_2 = b$, $O_3 = c$ and $O_4 = d$ with expected values $E_1 = mp = rm/N$, $E_2 = np = rn/N$, $E_3 = m(1-p) = ms/N$ and $E_4 = n(1-p) = ns/N$.

This test has now moved away from the format described by equation (12.1) but gives exactly the same results. Although in common use, a disadvantage of the χ^2 approach is that it does not provide a statistic that describes the magnitude of the effect, and so a CI cannot be calculated in any obvious way.

In more technical language, the quantity z^2 follows a χ^2 distribution with $df = 1$. In general, a χ^2 test has $df = (R-1) \times (C-1)$, where R and C are the numbers of rows and columns of the corresponding $R \times C$ contingency table. *Fisher's exact test*, referred to by Temel *et al.* (2010), is another approach that is appropriate whenever the total sample size is small. This makes a slight difference here, especially for the PHQ-9 comparison in which only two of the early palliative care patients showed signs of major depressive disorder; whereas the χ^2 value of 5.41 implies $p = 0.02$, Fisher's more

Example from the literature

Temel *et al.* (2010) compared early palliative care with standard oncologic care, and carried out a randomised trial in 151 patients with metastatic non-small-cell lung cancer. Mood was assessed using the Hospital Anxiety and Depression Scale (HADS) and the Patient Health Questionnaire 9 (PHQ-9). For the HADS, which has two subscales (anxiety and depression) with values ranging from 0, indicating no distress, to 21, indicating maximum distress, the authors defined a score higher than 7 on either HADS subscale to be clinically significant. The PHQ-9 is a 9-item measure that evaluates symptoms of major depressive disorder, which was diagnosed if a patient reported at least five of the nine symptoms of depression on the PHQ-9, with one of the five symptoms being either anhedonia or depressed mood.

The authors reported the percentages of patients with mood symptoms, assessed on the basis of each of these three measures, in the group assigned to standard treatment and the group assigned to early palliative care, were as follows: HADS-depression, 38% (18 of 47 patients) versus 16% (9 of 57), $p = 0.01$; HADS-anxiety, 30% (14 of 47 patients) and 25% (14 of 57), respectively; $p = 0.66$; and PHQ-9, 17% (8 of 47 patients) versus 4% (2 of 57); $p = 0.04$. The analyses were performed with the use of a two-sided Fisher's exact test.

Replicating the calculations using equation 12.5, we obtain χ^2 values of 6.7895, 0.3576 and 5.4119. Considering the first of these, use of Table T4 with $df = 1$ and $\chi^2 = 6.79$ leads to a p-value < 0.01. However, since the values in Table T4 with $df = 1$ are in fact equivalent to those of Table T1 squared, a more precise p-value can be obtained. Thus Table T1 with $z = \sqrt{6.79} = 2.61$ gives the p-value $= 0.0091$. Since a small p-value is taken as an indication that the null hypothesis may not hold, we conclude that there is a difference between the two groups with respect to depression.

precise exact test indicates $p = 0.04$. This is the value quoted by Temel *et al.* In broad terms, Fisher's test would be appropriate if any of the four shaded cells of Table 12.1 has an expected value of less than 5.

For a categorical variable of k (> 2) categories, there will be a $2 \times k$ table. The corresponding test is χ^2 of the form of equation (12.5), but now there are $G = 2k$ cells, and the calculated value is referred to Table T4 with $df = k - 1$.

This *test for homogeneity* asks a general question as to whether there are any differences between the two treatments – it is very non-specific. However, in the situation of an ordered categorical variable as is common with QoL data, a *test-for-trend* with $df = 1$ can supplement the homogeneity χ^2 test of equation (12.5). This makes use of the category ordering by assigning numerical values to the respective ranks, as in

Example from the literature

Islam *et al.* (2010) carried out a comparative cross-sectional study in a cohort of adult patients to assess the association between traumatic facial injury and the presence of anxiety and depressive disorders. Fifty consecutive adult patients attending the maxillofacial outpatient clinic following facial trauma were compared to 50 adult control subjects who were under follow-up following elective oral and maxillofacial surgery. Table 12.2 shows the HADS depression assessments, categorised as normal (no depression), borderline or case (probable depression). These three categories are ordered and given the ranks labelled $i = 1, 2$ and 3. Thus 10/50 (20.0%) are regarded as cases of depression with facial trauma, while the corresponding figure for the control group is 0/50 (0%).

Ignoring first the fact that depression is an ordered categorical variable, direct calculation of equation (12.5) is possible. Here, $k = 3$, $O_1 = 36$, $O_2 = 4$, . . . , and $O_6 = 0$ and the corresponding expected values (in italics in Table 12.2) are $E_1 = 40.0$, $E_2 = 5.0$, . . . , and $E_6 = 5.0$. If all these values are substituted in equation (12.5), then $\chi^2_{\text{Homogeneity}} = 11.20$ with two degrees of freedom. The corresponding entry in Table T4 for $\alpha = 0.01$ is 9.21, and so this result is statistically significant; the actual p-value is approximately 0.004. This test indicates that there is no evidence of real differences in the proportion of normal, borderline and cases within the two treatment groups.

Table 12.2 HADS depression score for 50 patients with facial trauma and 50 matched controls at the first follow-up after oral and maxillofacial surgery. The table shows observed (Obs) and expected frequencies. Because the depression states of no, borderline and probable are increasingly severe grades, a test for trend is suitable

| | | Patient group | | | |
| | | Facial trauma | Control | Total | |
Depression*	Rank (*i*)	Obs (Expected)	Obs (Expected)	*N*	*q*%
No depression	1	36 (40.0)	44 (40.0)	80	45.0
Borderline	2	4 (5.0)	6 (5.0)	10	40.0
Probable depression	3	10 (5.0)	0 (5.0)	10	100.0
Total		50	50	100	

*No depression = score 0–7, borderline = score 8–10, probable >11.
Obs; Number observed.
Source: Adapted from Islam *et al.*, 2010. Reproduced with permission of Elsevier.

Table 12.2, and checks if there is any evidence of increasing or decreasing changes over the categories. In terms of Table 12.2, this test checks for trend in the values of q, the proportion of patients within each trauma group for each of the three levels of HADS depression.

Following the necessary calculations (see Altman, 1991), $\chi^2_{Trend} = 7.90$. In this case direct use of Table T4 with $df = 1$ gives the p-value < 0.01 rather than the more precise 0.005 if one had referred $z = \sqrt{7.90} = 2.81$ to Table T1.

One can also check to see whether the assumption that the proportion q changes in a linear way with x is a reasonable assumption. This test for departure from trend compares χ^2_{Trend}, which will always be the smaller of the two, with $\chi^2_{Homogeneity}$. The difference between them $\chi^2_{Homogeneity} - \chi^2_{Trend} = 11.20 - 7.90 = 3.30$ has $df = k - 2 = 3 - 2 = 1$, and from Table T4 the p-value < 0.1. More precisely, since $df = 1$, $z = \sqrt{3.30} = 1.82$ and the p-value is 0.069.

In summary, albeit not statistically significant, in this dataset there was fairly strong evidence of more depression in the trauma group, and this could be explained by a linear trend.

Normally distributed data

If the data can reasonably be assumed to have an approximately Normal distribution, an appropriate summary statistic is the mean. This may be the case for data that are continuous, numerically discrete or ordered categorical. However, before analysis, checks should be made to verify that the assumption of a Normal distribution is reasonable.

Examples from the literature

Islam et al. (2010) also show a table comparing the mean HADS scores in the facial trauma and control groups (Table 12.3). The authors write "The distribution of data was deemed to be relatively normal overall. A two-sample t-test was used to evaluate difference in anxiety and depression scores between facial trauma and control groups."

However, assuming the data are indeed Normal, then the distribution should be symmetrical and the mean plus-and-minus twice the SD would cover most of the 'normal range' of the data (more precisely, this should be 1.96 × SD for a large sample or, in this example, the value from the t-distribution with $N - 1 = 49$ degrees of freedom; and in theory approximately 95% of the observations should lie within the normal range, with 2.5% outside the upper and lower limits). Here, the respective lower limits for the normal range of the HADS scores are for the control group 3.92 − (2 × 2.8) = − 1.7 and 4.33 − (2 × 3.5) = − 2.7, and for the facial trauma patients 5.94 − (2 × 3.1) = − 0.3, and 5.91 − (2 × 4.5) = −3.1. These values are well below the lowest possible HADS sores of 0. Thus, based on this rough and simple calculation, one might question the assumption of a Normal distribution.

Table 12.3 Comparison of mean HADS scores in 50 patients with facial trauma and 50 matched controls

Variable	Facial trauma group (N = 50) Mean (SD)	Control group (N = 50) Mean (SD)	Mean difference (95% CI)	p-Value	Effect size
HADS depression	5.94 (3.1)	3.92 (2.8)	−2.0 (−3.4 to −0.6)	0.006	0.68
HADS anxiety	5.91 (4.5)	4.33 (3.5)	−1.6 (−3.5 to 0.2)	0.07	0.39

Source: Adapted from Islam et al., 2010. Reproduced with permission of Elsevier.

It is usually prudent to check whether the mean $\pm 2 \times SD$ has this property of corresponding roughly to the normal range. In this example there are presumably quite a few patients with very low or zero anxiety and depression, indicating that the data might be skewed and not of the Normal distribution form; this would lead to an inflated SD and to the absurd lower limits that lie outside the valid range of HADS scores. Fortunately, as noted below, the t-test is remarkably robust against deviation of the assumptions.

Assuming the QoL data have an approximately Normal form, the two treatments are compared by calculating the difference between the two respective means $\overline{x}_I$ and $\overline{x}_{II}$. Thus the true difference, δ, is estimated by

$$d = \overline{x}_I - \overline{x}_{II}, \tag{12.6}$$

where

$$SE(d) = \sqrt{\frac{SD_I^2}{n_I} + \frac{SD_{II}^2}{n_{II}}}, \tag{12.7}$$

and SD_I and SD_{II} are the standard deviations within each group. Provided SD_I and SD_{II} are not too dissimilar, an approximate test of significance for the comparison of two means is then provided by equation (12.1), as before. However, a better estimate of the SE is obtained by assuming that, although the means may differ, the SDs of each group are both estimating a common value, denoted by σ. Therefore the two estimates SD_I and SD_{II} can first be combined to obtain a pooled estimate of σ. This is given by

$$SD_{Pooled} = \sqrt{\frac{(n_I - 1)SD_I^2 + (n_{II} - 1)SD_{II}^2}{(n_I - 1) + (n_{II} - 1)}}. \tag{12.8}$$

The corresponding SE is then

$$SE_{Pooled}(d) = SD_{Pooled}\sqrt{\frac{1}{n_I} + \frac{1}{n_{II}}}. \tag{12.9}$$

There will usually be very little difference in the numerical values calculated here from those by equation (12.7).

Then the test of significance for the comparison of two means is provided by the *t-test*:

$$t = \frac{d}{SE_{Pooled}(d)}.$$
(12.10)

This is referred to Table T1 of the standard Normal distribution to obtain the corresponding significance level, or *p*-value.

In order to ascertain the *p*-value in *small* samples, however, *t* of equation (12.10) is referred to Table T3 of the *t*-distribution with $df = (n_I - 1) + (n_{II} - 1) = (n_I + n_{II}) - 2$ rather than Table T1. Similarly, the expression for the $100(1 - \alpha)\%$ *CI* of equation (12.2) replaces $z_{1-\alpha/2}$ by $t_{1-\alpha/2}$ where the particular value of *t* to use will depend on the degrees of freedom. From Table T1 for $\alpha = 0.05$ we had $z_{0.975} = 1.96$ and this value remains fixed whereas, in small sample situations, $t_{0.975}$ will change with differing *df*. One recommendation is always to use Table T3 in preference to Table T1 since the final row of the former contains the entries of Table T1. As a rule if the degrees of freedom are less than 60 Table T3 should be used.

Example from the literature

Table 12.3 from Islam *et al.* (2010) shows the mean differences due to treatment effects, with their 95% *CI*s and *p*-values. Their calculations can readily be replicated by using equation 12.8 which provides the pooled *SD*, followed by equations 12.9 and 12.10 to obtain the value of the *t*-statistic and hence the *p*-value. The effect size is given by the mean difference divided by SD_{Pooled}.

The authors concluded that there was substantially more depression in the facial trauma group, but although the higher levels of anxiety were also observed the result was not statistically significant.

Non-normally distributed data

In many situations, QoL data do not have even approximately the Normal distribution form. As noted in Chapter 11 on sample size estimation, *t*-tests and many other statistical tests are remarkably robust – to the extent that some authors suggest that for most PROs one can with impunity ignore even quite severe violations of the Normality assumption (Norman, 2010). However, as noted by Fayers (2011), 'robustness' implicitly refers only to α, the type I error; the power of the test can remain severely compromised.

When assessing the distribution of data and the applicability of the Normal distribution, the most important aspect is symmetry. If the distribution is asymmetric, and especially if there is a long tail to the right-hand side ('skewed to the right'), the estimates of the *SD* can become very inflated. This is manifested by unreasonable results when the normal range is calculated: for a Normal distribution, the mean value $\pm (2 \times SD)$ should include approximately 95% of the observed data. In extreme cases either the upper value of the normal range will exceed the maximum possible value for the scale or, more frequently, the lower value for the range may be negative even when minus values are impossible. In such cases, alternative significance tests may be more reliable and more sensitive.

Examples from the literature

The use of the normal range as a rough check for the plausibility of a Normal distribution was illustrated in the previous example for Table 12.3. However, in that example we did not have access to the raw data. The departure from Normal may well be small and, as we note, the *t*-test has robust properties. A more extreme illustration of departure from a Normal distribution is seen in the HADS data from Julious *et al.* (1997), where Table 12.4 has 22 categories that are formed from the summed responses of seven items on the HADS depression scale. The data are numerically discrete, with a far from Normal distribution form. Consequently, the median rather than the mean provides a better summary, and 'non-parametric' statistical tests such as the Wilcoxon or Mann–Whitney test may be more appropriate.

Table 12.4   Frequency of responses on the HADS for depression

Category	Depression score	Number of patients
Normal	0	4
	1	16
	2	12
	3	13
	4	12
	5	10
	6	19
	7	13
Borderline	8	11
	9	9
	10	4
Case	11	5
	12	11
	13	4
	14	2
	15	3
	16	4
	17	0
	18	0
	19	1
	20	0
	21	1
	Total	154

Source: Julious *et al.*, 1997, Table 2. Reproduced with permission of Springer Science and Business Media.

In situations where the data are clearly non-Normal the usual procedure is to replace individual data values, which are first ordered or ranked from smallest to largest, by the corresponding rank. Thus each value now has one of the values 1 to N, where N is the total number of observations. If there are two groups of exactly equal size, $N/2$, and the null hypothesis of no difference between the groups is valid, the sums of the sets of ranks for each group separately would be approximately equal. Otherwise, the sums would differ. This test is termed the *Mann–Whitney test* and is often denoted by U. Full details are provided by Altman (1991).

In contrast, the *test-for-trend* of the Table 12.2 data from Islam *et al.* (2010) compares the mean values of the variable x, which can take only the values 1, 2 and 3, in the two treatment groups. Here:

$$\bar{x}_{\text{Trauma}} = \frac{(36 \times 1) + (4 \times 2) + (10 \times 3)}{50} = 1.48 \text{ and}$$

$$\bar{x}_{\text{Control}} = \frac{(44 \times 1) + (6 \times 2) + (0 \times 3)}{50} = 1.12,$$

where the smaller mean from the control group indicates lower depression levels in this group. Note that the median of each group is 1, demonstrating that here the medians provide too coarse a summary to distinguish the two groups.

Although the standard method for comparing two means is the two-sample z- or t-test, this is strictly only appropriate if the variable (here x, the rank) has an approximately Normal distribution. This is clearly not the case here. As a consequence, the Mann–Whitney distribution free test may be preferable for these categorical responses.

Example from the literature

Glaser *et al.* (1997) compare the school behaviour and health status of 27 children after treatment for central nervous system tumours with school-age controls using, amongst others, teacher assessment by the Health Utilities Index (Mark III).

The authors used the Mann–Whitney U-test and state that the children "were perceived to have impaired emotion ($z = 2.64$, $p = 0.01$)." In their report they have used the notation z in place of U, but the latter would usually be preferable as it is then clear exactly which test procedure has been used in the calculation.

Morton and Dobson (1990) show how the differences in the response patterns can be summarised using the average ranks $\bar{R}_I$ and $\bar{R}_{II}$ for groups I and II. Thus

$$\theta = \frac{(\bar{R}_I - \bar{R}_{II})}{\bar{N}}, \tag{12.11}$$

where $\bar{N}$ is the average number of observations per group.

Example

We illustrate the calculation of θ using the data of Table 12.2. All observations from both groups of 50 are first numbered from 1 to 100, so that observations in category $x = 1$ have the numbers from 1 to $(36 + 44 =)$ 80, those in category $x = 2$ from 81 to 90 and those in category $x = 3$ from 91 to 100 (Table 12.5). The median rank for category 1 is the mean of the smallest and largest numbers for the category, which is 40.5. Similarly, the median rank for category 2 is 85.5 and for category 3 is 95.5.

Table 12.5 Ranked observations of HADS depression from the facial trauma study of Table 12.2, deriving a median for each of the three categories

Category	Ranked observation number	Category median rank
1 (No depression)	1–80	40.5
2 (Borderline)	81–90	85.5
3 (Probable depression)	91–100	95.5

Then, making use of Table 12.2, the rank total for the trauma group is $(36 \times 40.5) + (4 \times 85.5) + (10 \times 95.5) = 2755.0$ and its average is $2755.0/50 = 55.1$. The rank total for the control group is $(44 \times 40.5) + (6 \times 85.5) + (0 \times 95.5) = 2295.0$ and its average is $2295.0/50 = 45.91$. The average number of subjects in the groups is $(50 + 50)/2 = 50.0$. Therefore using equation (12.11), $\theta = (55.1 - 45.9)/50.0 = 0.184$.

This estimator is a measure of the difference between the two groups. If all the observations in the control are larger than any in the trauma group, $\theta = -1$; conversely, if all of the trauma group observations are larger than the control group observations, $\theta = +1$; and if they have similar total rankings, $\theta = 0$.

One possible approach if data do not have a Normal distribution is to use a *transformation*, for example using the logarithm of the data for analysis rather than the actual data. However, as we have pointed out, this may complicate the interpretation of the results. Bland and Altman (1996) provide further details.

Computer-intensive *bootstrap* methods provide a general approach to estimating confidence intervals when there is uncertainty about the distribution of the data (Altman *et al.*, 2000). An increasing number of statistical packages offer bootstrap estimation. The principle is that a large number of repeated *samples with replacement* are taken from the original dataset, enabling the sampling variability to be reflected in the calculation of the confidence limits.

Time-to-event

We will see in Chapter 13 that, in certain circumstances, it may be appropriate to summarise longitudinal QoL data such that the repeated values from each subject are reduced to a single measure, such as the *area under the curve (AUC)*. Once summarised in this manner, the analysis then proceeds in a cross-sectional manner. An alternative approach that also converts longitudinal data to a single summary for each patient is *time-to-event* analysis. Examples are the time until deterioration in health, or the time until improvement or relief; in these cases the 'event' is the deterioration or the attainment of relief. Sometimes the event can be easily defined, but care must be taken when, for example, an endpoint is time until pain relief and some patients may report a brief period of no pain followed by worse pain: should we use time until, first reported relief, no matter how brief that may be? Clear definitions should be indicated in the study protocol.

Often, time-to-event data do not have a Normal distribution and are much skewed, and so the methods described in this chapter are not immediately applicable. Although a logarithmic transformation of the data may improve the situation, it does not provide the solution because time-to-event studies may have *censored* observations: censoring occurs when patients discontinue providing information after a certain time. This may happen for various reasons, including patient withdrawal and patient death. Thus time-to-event studies generate times (often termed *survival times* since the statistical techniques were developed in studies measuring times to death), some of which are censored. It is beyond the scope of this text to describe the associated statistical techniques for summarising such data, but they can be found in Machin *et al.* (2006).

Example from the literature

Cicardi *et al.* (2010) describe two trials assessing the use of a bradykinin-receptor antagonist in hereditary angiodema. Based on preliminary investigation, one of the three main symptoms (cutaneous swelling, cutaneous pain, or abdominal pain) was defined in each patient as the index symptom. The primary end point was the median time to clinically significant relief of the index symptom, where clinically significant symptom relief was defined as a decrease in the score on a visual-analogue scale (VAS) of at least 20–30 mm, depending on the initial symptom severity. Therefore, the decrease in severity necessary to achieve the primary end point was at least 30% (i.e. 30-mm decrease from a baseline score of 100 mm). This decrease had to have been sustained for three consecutive measurements on the VAS, with the first measurement being the time point at which clinically significant relief was achieved. Groups were compared using the log-rank test. The antagonist made an appreciable and statistically significant reduction in the median time until pain relief, particularly in the second trial where median time to relief was two hours with antagonist versus 12 hours on the other arm ($p < 0.001$).

In this study, pain relief was rapid and within hours. In other settings, such as the treatment of trigeminal neuralgia, we may be concerned with pain relief lasting several years. Then, some patients may die and there will be censoring due to death. In particular, if the death rates differ in the randomised groups, the comparison could become biased. A solution is to define the endpoint not simply as duration of pain relief, but 'pain-free survival'. Han and Kim (2010) used this approach in an observational study when assessing the role of alcohol nerve blocks. Pain recurrence was defined as the return of any pain, regardless of whether it was controlled by medication or required another procedure. 'Survival curves' were constructed for the censored pain-free survival observations, and the log-rank test was used to compare these curves. The probabilities of remaining pain free at one, two, three and seven years after a successful alcohol block were 90.4, 69.0, 53.5 and 33.0%, respectively.

Cumulative distribution functions

The results from time-to-event analyses can be summarised in a few numbers, as in the example of the angiodema trial above, where the medians are given. Frequently such data is also illustrated by survival curves, which are appropriate for both censored and (as here) uncensored data. The paper by Han and Kim (2010), with censored data, did display survival curves. These show the entire profile of the results, supplementing the summary values provided in the text.

A similar approach can be used for other data, showing the cumulative distribution functions of the responses for groups being compared. This has the advantage that it avoids any suspicion that the authors might have selected a favourable threshold for judging patient changes. It is a potentially preferable method to depict the effect of treatment across the entire study population by showing all magnitudes of change and the proportion of individuals within a trial achieving each level.

Example from the literature

Figure 12.1 is an example provided by Wyrwich *et al.* (2013), and shows separate curves for the two treatment groups and the placebo in a trial of treatment for Alzheimer's disease. The Alzheimer's Disease Assessment Scale-Cognitive subscale (ADAS-Cog) was used as the outcome measure. The horizontal axis shows the change in ADAS-Cog score from baseline, and the vertical axis shows the cumulative percentage of patients achieving that level of change; a negative change indicates improvement. Although the frequently used thresholds of 0, 4 and 7 change reductions are tabulated and marked, the advantage of this figure is that percentages of patients can be viewed over the full range of possible changes.

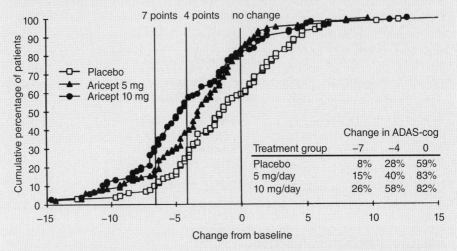

Figure 12.1   Cumulative distribution function of responses for Aricept® 5 and 10 mg doses compared to placebo. Important change thresholds considered for ADAS-cog score decreases over 24 weeks are 7, 4 and 0 points. *Source:* Reproduced from ARICEPT® Oral Solution (Donepezil Hydrochloride) [approval label, Figure 2]. Available at: http://www.accessdata.fda.gov/drugsatfda_docs/label/2004/21719lbl.pdf.

12.3   Adjusting for covariates

Normally distributed data

In most circumstances the QoL measure of primary interest will be affected by characteristics of the subjects under study. In a clinical trial, these could include the treatment under study and the age of the patient. We can relate the value of the QoL observed to one of these variables (e.g. age) by the following *linear regression model*:

$$\text{QoL} = \beta_0 + \beta_{Age} Age, \qquad (12.12)$$

where the constants β_0 and β_{Age} are termed the *regression coefficients*. In particular, β_{Age} is the slope of the regression line that relates QoL to age.

If b_{Age}, the estimate of β_{Age} that is obtained by fitting this model, is close to 0, we conclude that QoL does not change with age. The mean QoL then provides an estimate b_0 of β_0.

Example from the literature

Greimel *et al.* (1997) use a linear regression model to relate activities-of-daily-living (ADL) scores to various characteristics of 227 cancer patients who had been discharged from hospital. In particular, they regressed ADL on patient age and estimated the slope of the regression line as $b_{Age} = -0.006$. They do not give the estimate of β_0.

The negative value of b_{Age} here suggests, as one might anticipate, that the ADL scores decline slowly with age. The decline over the age range in the study of 21 to 88 years is estimated by $-0.006 \times (88 - 21) = -0.402$. This is less than half a point on the ADL scale.

However, such a linear regression model implies that the rate of decline is constant over the more than 60-year age span, which is very unlikely so that the model of equation (12.12) would be unsuitable to describe these data. A sensible precaution, before embarking on a regression analysis in this and any situation, is to make a scatter plot of QoL against the variable in question. In this example, we would examine how ADL changes with age to verify whether the relationship is, approximately at least, linear.

The analysis for comparing the means of two treatments by the *z*- or *t*-tests can also be formulated using a linear regression model of the form

$$QoL = \beta_0 + \beta_{Treatment}v, \tag{12.13}$$

where v is coded 0 for the first treatment group and 1 for the second. Then if $v = 0$ in this equation, $QoL = \beta_0$, and this can be thought of as the true, or population, mean value of the QoL score for the first treatment group. Similarly, when $v = 1$, $QoL = \beta_0 + \beta_{Treatment}$ represents the population value of the QoL score for the second treatment group. Hence the difference between the groups is $(\beta_0 + \beta_{Treatment}) - \beta_0 = \beta_{Treatment}$. This was estimated

Example

The data of Islam *et al.* (2010) in Table 12.2 can also be used to estimate the slope of the relationship. This gives $b = 0.2195$ with $SE(b) = 0.0757$. From these, $z = b/SE(b) = 0.2195/0.0757 = 2.90$ and, using Table T1, the *p*-value is 0.004 which is a similar result to the χ^2_{Trend} test.

The positive slope, $b = 0.1010$, indicates that the relative proportion of patients with trauma tends to increase as the category changes from normal through borderline to case. This trend suggests that controls have less depression. The corresponding 95% *CI* for the slope using equation (12.2) is 0.069–0.370.

by d of equation (12.6). The equivalent null hypothesis of no difference between treatments can be expressed as $\beta_{Treatment} = 0$. This leads to $z = b_{Treatment}/SE(b_{Treatment})$ where $b_{Treatment}$ is the corresponding estimate derived from the data.

The test-for-trend described earlier is equivalent to fitting the linear regression line of QoL on the variable v.

Suppose a study were investigating the relative merits of two types of intervention on QoL and the outcome measure was ADL. Since it is known that ADL declines with increasing age, one might ask whether a difference in mean ADL observed between the two intervention groups at the end of the study is explained by a different spectrum of subject ages within each intervention group. This can be assessed by combining equations (12.12) and (12.13) into the multiple regression equation

$$\text{ADL} = \beta_0 + \beta_{Treatment} v + \beta_{Age} Age. \tag{12.14}$$

This equation can then be fitted to the data using standard computer packages. The process is best done in two stages.

First we can fit the model $\text{ADL} = \beta_0 + \beta_{Treatment} v$, to obtain estimates of β_0 and $\beta_{Treatment}$. Then we fit the full model, equation (12.14), to obtain new estimates of β_0 and $\beta_{Treatment}$ together with an estimate of β_{Age}. If the second value corresponding to $\beta_{Treatment}$ remains effectively unchanged from the first obtained, then, despite any imbalance of age within the two groups, the estimate of the difference between treatments remains unaffected. However, if the value corresponding to $\beta_{Treatment}$ is markedly different, the imbalance of age within the two groups does affect the estimated difference between the interventions. This adjusted-for-age estimate is then a better measure of the treatment difference.

If other variables, such as age and gender, also influence QoL, the regression equation (12.14) can be extended to include them:

$$\text{QoL} = \beta_0 + \beta_1 v_1 + \beta_2 v_2 + \ldots + \beta_u v_u. \tag{12.15}$$

These regression models can all be fitted using standard statistical packages. A careful description of multiple regression is given by Tai and Machin (2014).

In randomised controlled trials, through the randomisation process, variables such as age and gender are usually fairly balanced between the treatment groups. It is often more critical to adjust for these factors in non-randomised studies.

Example from the literature

Al-Ruthia *et al.* (2015) evaluated the impact of adjuvant atypical antipsychotics (AAPs) on HRQoL among patients who had been using of antidepressants for at least a year. Patients were classified into users of antidepressants plus adjunctive AAPs ($N = 306$) and users of antidepressants only ($N = 3,332$). Multivariate linear regression analyses were conducted to examine the association between the utilisation of AAPs and HRQoL measured using the SF-12v2 physical and mental summaries. Al-Ruthia *et al.* suggested that the following factors were likely to impact on HRQoL, and showed that their frequency distributions differed across the AAP users and non-users: age, sex, race, annual total personal income, marital status, employment status, insurance status, years of education, Charlson Comorbidity Index (CCI) score after being dichotomised into (0 and ≥ 1), number of prescription medications associated with the depression diagnosis, patients' satisfaction with their health care quality and a measure of depression, the Patient Health Questionnaire-2 (PHQ-2 scores being dichotomised into ≥ 3 versus < 3). Therefore they used multiple linear regression to control for these 12 covariates.

Table 12.6 shows the regression-adjusted comparisons of AAPs versus no AAPs, for the SF-122v2 Mental Component Summary (MCS) scores. AAP utilisation was associated with lower MCS scores ($b = -1.55$, 95% $CI = -3.0247$ to -0.0827, $p = 0.0385$), suggesting that use of adjunctive AAPs is associated with a worse mental quality of life than use of antidepressants alone. However, we observe that the result is not very highly significant ($p = 0.038$) and these authors made no allowance for multiple testing (mental and physical components were reported, each with 12 covariates).

Table 12.6 Multiple regression analysis of results from the Mental Component Summary scores of the SF-12v2, in patients taking antidepressants with or without adjuvant atypical antipsychotics. The main comparison is adjusted to allow for twelve covariates

Variable (reference group)	*b*-Coefficient	95% CI	*p*-value
Main comparison:			
Atypical antipsychotics (AAPs)	−1.55	−3.02 to −0.08	0.038*
Covariates:			
Race (non-Hispanic White)	−0.0539	−1.270 to 1.162	0.93
Marital status (married)	0.895	0.187 to 1.603	0.014*
Educational status (education years)	0.0637	−0.058 to 0.185	0.30
Age (years)	0.110	0.0839 to 0.1358	< 0.0001**
Sex (female)	0.0749	−0.643 to 0.792	0.84
Employment status (employed)	1.084	0.186 to 1.981	0.018*
Income (total personal income)	0.000012	−0.000001 to 0.000024	0.064
Insurance status (uninsured)	−0.558	−1.964 to 0.849	0.44
Quality of Health Care Rating (high rating of health care ≥7)	0.514	−0.486 to 1.514	0.31
Patient Health Questionnaire-2 (PHQ2-score ≥3)	−16.12	−16.98 to −15.27	< 0.0001**
Charlson Comorbidity Index (CCI ≥1)	0.327	−0.363 to 1.017	0.35
Prescription medications associated with depression	−0.282	−0.481 to −0.083	0.0057**

*p <0.05; **p <0.01.
Source: Adapted from Al-Ruthia *et al.*, 2015. Reproduced with permission of Elsevier.

Example from the literature

In randomised clinical trials, if properly conducted, the randomisation process should ensure that all pre-treatment characteristics are more-or-less balanced out and any differences can be ascribed to chance alone. It can still be important to adjust for prognostic factors, and especially so for any factors used to stratify the randomisation. However, the word-count restrictions of many journals can make it difficult to present full details of the analyses and often only scant summary details are provided.

For example, Knols *et al.* (2011) report an RCT the effects of an outpatient physical exercise program on the HRQoL of hematopoietic stem-cell transplantation recipients. The authors comment that "The covariates used in the models are indicated in the footnotes of Tables 4–6", and a typical footnote is "The covariates used in the model for knee extension, grip strength, walking speed and 6-MWT were age, gender, type of SCT and body mass index."

Non-normally distributed data

If the data have a binary form, for example if the responses are 'Yes' or 'No', the regression methods described require modification. Previously we assumed that the QoL scale was a categorical variable that for practical purposes has a Normal distribution form. This is clearly not the case if the variable is binary. For technical reasons, because the proportion, denoted p, has a restricted range from 0 to 1 and not from $-\infty$ to $+\infty$ as is the case for a variable with a Normal distribution, $\log[p/(1 - p)]$ is used on the left-hand side of the corresponding regression model such as equation (12.12). The right-hand side remains unchanged. The expression $\log[p/(1 - p)]$ is usually abbreviated as $\text{logit}(p)$ – hence the terms *logit transformation* and *logistic regression*.

The logit transformation of p leads to summarising the relative merits of two treatments by the *odds ratio* (*OR*) rather than by the difference between two proportions. Thus from Table 12.1, where p_I is the probability of a response 'Yes' with treatment I, then $(1 - p_I)$ is the probability of responding 'No'. This gives the odds of the responses as p_I to $(1 - p_I)$, or $p_I/(1 - p_I)$. For example, if $p_I = 0.5$ then the odds are 1 since the 'Yes' and 'No' responses are equally likely. Similarly, for treatment II, the corresponding odds are $p_{II}/(1 - p_{II})$. The ratio of these two odds is termed the *OR*, that is

$$OR = \frac{p_{II} / (1 - p_{II})}{p_I / (1 - p_I)}. \tag{12.16}$$

The value under the null hypothesis of no treatment difference corresponds to $OR = 1$ since the odds will then be the same in both treatment groups. It is estimated, using the notation of Table 12.1, by $OR = (a/c)/(b/d) = ad/bc$.

If we are investigating differences between two treatments in this context, an equation of the form (12.13) is replaced by the logistic regression equation

$$\mathrm{logit}(p) = \beta_0 + \beta_{\mathrm{Treatment}} v. \tag{12.17}$$

Again, if the treatment group is I, $v = 0$ and logit $(p) = \beta_0$, whereas if the treatment group is II, $v = 1$ and logit $(p) = \beta_0 + \beta_{Treatment}$. The difference between these two is $(\beta_0 + \beta_{Treatment}) - \beta_0 = \beta_{Treatment}$. From this the OR is estimated by $OR = \exp(\beta_{Treatment})$. As indicated earlier, the null hypothesis of no treatment difference is expressed through $\beta_{Treatment} = 0$, since $OR_{Null} = e^0 = 1$.

Example

Suppose the principal interest in the trial described by Islam *et al.* (2010) is the proportion of patients without depression as indicated by HADS in the two groups, then Table 12.2 can be reduced to Table 12.7.

Using the *z*-test for the difference in proportions with no depression levels, here 0.72 for trauma and 0.88 for control, gives $z = 2.041$ ($p = 0.041$). The estimate of $OR = (36 \times 6)/(44 \times 14) = 0.3506$.

The corresponding logistic regression model fitted to these data using STATA (StataCorp, 2013) is logit(p) = 0.1035 − 1.0480v, so that $b_{Treatment} = -1.0480$ and $OR = \exp(-1.0480) = 0.3506$, which is the same as the value we calculated before.

For this example, there is no advantage to the more complex logistic approach. However, in addition to the HADS score itself and the treatment received, patient-specific variables such as age, gender, severity of trauma and so on are routinely recorded in such studies. Without the use of logistic regression, their influence on the observed treatment differences would be difficult to assess.

Table 12.7 HADS depression score for 50 patients with facial trauma and 50 matched controls at the first follow-up after oral and maxillofacial surgery, derived by combining the borderline and probable depression categories of Table 12.2. The table shows observed frequencies

	Patient group		
Depression*	Facial trauma	Control	Total
No depression	36 (72.0%)	44 (88.0%)	80
Borderline/case	14	6	20
Total	50	50	100

*No depression = score 0–7. Borderline or probable case = score >8.

Choosing covariates

Factors that are strongly prognostic of outcome should normally be considered as potential covariates in a clinical trial, irrespective of whether the means of these factors are statistically different in the treatment arms. Thus the baseline (i.e. at randomisation) QoL assessment is frequently a candidate – as discussed in the next section. It is also recommended that factors used for stratifying the randomisation or minimising the allocation imbalance should be used as covariates (Kahan and Morris, 2012).

12.4   Changes from baseline

Many clinical trial protocols specify a baseline (time 0) QoL assessment, Q_0, followed by at least one further assessment at a fixed time point following treatment (time 1) to obtain Q_1. Pre-treatment QoL may influence later values, and this study design allows an estimation of both the treatment effect upon Q_1 and the association of Q_1 with Q_0. By analogy with equation (12.14), the regression model to describe this situation for two treatment groups is

$$Q_1 = \beta_0 + \beta_{\text{Treatment}} v + \beta_{\text{QoL}} Q_0. \tag{12.18}$$

In this model, the effect of treatment on QoL can be assessed while adjusting for Q_0. This approach is also equivalent to analysis of covariance, with the baseline assessment being regarded as an explanatory covariate.

An alternative method of analysis is to first calculate for each subject the change score, $D_{\text{QoL}} = Q_1 - Q_0$. Then the following regression equation could be fitted:

$$D_{\text{QoL}} = \beta_0 + \beta_{\text{Treatment}} v. \tag{12.19}$$

This will not give the same values for β_0 and $\beta_{\text{Treatment}}$ as equation (12.18) unless $\beta_{\text{QoL}} = 1$ exactly, but the p-values are often similar. Frequently the baseline value Q_0 is added to model (12.19) as a covariate, in which case the p-values will be identical to those of equation (12.18) and the choice of method comes down to a preference in the style of reporting (European Medicines Agency, 2003).

The use of change scores provides a simple and intuitive analysis – although a number of cautions should be noted if Q_0 is not added as a covariate. First of all, it is not always advisable to make use of baseline measurements. Frequently, Q_1 and Q_0 will have similar variances, and both these variances will contribute to the overall variance of D_{QoL}. It can be shown that if the correlation of Q_1 with Q_0 is less than 0.5 (*partial correlation*, after allowing for other factors), D_{QoL} will have larger variance, and thus also larger SD, than Q_1. In effect, subtracting the baseline measurement has added noise.

In a clinical trial, the baseline characteristics will tend to be balanced across the treatment groups, the principal reason for adjusting for Q_0 is to reduce the unexplained variance, which implies that Q_0 is only useful if its correlation with Q_1 is appreciably greater than 0.5.

Another problem with change scores is that many QoL scales consist of discrete categorical data with unknown scale intervals. The validity of change scores makes a strong assumption of linearity. For example, on a typical short scale, that a change from, say, a score of 0 (representing 'not at all') to a score of 2 ('a little') is equivalent to a change from 2 ('a little') to 3 ('quite a bit'). Arguably, change scores should only be used for categorical data if IRT or similar techniques have been used to ensure linearity.

An *analysis of covariance* (ANCOVA) models the actual values of QoL at follow-up, while an analysis of D_{QoL} models the change from baseline. Clinicians instinctively tend to prefer the second approach because of its apparent simplicity and because it reflects more directly the changes in each patient. Whichever approach is used, for group comparisons, statisticians recommend regarding the baseline measurement as a covariate because (i) the regression coefficient $\beta_{Treatment}$ estimates the difference between groups, and (ii) the value of β_{QoL} is allowed to vary from 1 and is chosen so as to minimize the unexplained variance.

12.5 Analysis of variance

We have described the test for the comparison of two means in two equivalent ways: the z- or t-test (depending on the sample size), and a regression analysis approach. A third equivalent way is by means of *analysis of variance* (ANOVA). Thus calculations summarised by equations (12.9) and (12.10) can be cast into an ANOVA format as in Table 12.8. Here the variance, V, is merely the SD squared.

In this table, $g = 2$ is the number of treatment groups, T_I is the sum of all the n_I observations of treatment I, T_{II} is the sum of all the n_{II} observations of treatment II and $T = T_I + T_{II}$ is the sum of all the $N = n_I + n_{II}$ observations. It should also be noted that V_{Within} is the square of SD_{Pooled} used in equation (12.8), while $V_{Between}$ is proportional to d^2. The final column gives the value of Fisher's F-test; this requires two sets of degrees of freedom, one for the Between groups with $df_{Between} = g - 1$, and one for Within groups with $df_{Within} = N - g$. This is often expressed using the notation $F(df_{Between}, df_{Within})$. It can be shown in this situation when we are comparing two groups that $F = t^2$, the square of equation (12.10), so that the two procedures lead to exactly the same test.

The ANOVA of Table 12.8 refers only to a single QoL observation per patient, with no repeats. It can readily be extended to $g > 2$ groups. For example, if there are $g = 3$ groups, then an extra term T_{III}^2 / n_{III} will be added to $S_{Between}$, and $n_{III} - 1$ added to the degrees of freedom for S_{Within}. However, in this case F is not simply t^2 and Table T5 is required to obtain the corresponding p-value.

Table 12.8 Analysis of variance (ANOVA) table to compare $g = 2$ means

Source of variation	Sums of squares	Degrees of freedom (df)	Variances	Variance ratio
Between treatments	$S_{Between} = \dfrac{T_I^2}{n_I} + \dfrac{T_{II}^2}{n_{II}} - \dfrac{T^2}{N}$	$g - 1$	$V_{Between} = \dfrac{S_{Between}}{g-1}$	$F = \dfrac{V_{Between}}{V_{Within}}$
Within treatments	$S_{Within} = S_{Total} - S_{Between}$	$(n_I - 1) + (n_{II} - 1)$	$V_{Within} = \dfrac{S_{Within}}{(n_I - 1) + (n_{II} - 1)}$	
Total	$S_{Total} = \displaystyle\sum x_i^2 - \dfrac{T^2}{N}$	$n_I + n_{II} - 1 = N - 1$		

Example from the literature

Greimel *et al.* (1997) used ANOVA to compare comorbidity (total score) between three age groups among cancer patients who had been discharged. Table 12.9 gives the mean comorbidity score for each age group. The resulting significance test, calculated using ANOVA, gave $F = 13.7$.

Here $N = 227$ patients and there are $g = 3$ groups; thus $df_{Between} = g - 1 = 2$ and $df_{Within} = N - g = 224$. This latter figure is large and one therefore uses the entries corresponding to $df = \infty$ in Table T5. Thus, with $df_{Between} = 2$ and $df_{Within} = \infty$ in Table T5, the critical value for $\alpha = 0.05$ is $F(2, \infty) = 3.00$; for $\alpha = 0.01$ it is $F(2, \infty) = 4.61$. The observed F is considerably larger than this, giving a p-value < 0.01 (the actual value is $p = 0.0001$)

The authors conclude: "The results showed that patients older than 65 years of age have a significantly higher level of comorbidity than patients 65 years of age and younger ..."

Table 12.9 Age differences in co-morbidity in patients who have been discharged following treatment for cancer

Total comorbidity score	Age (years)			F	p-value
	<45	45–65	>65		
N	37	106	84		
Mean	3.0	4.3	5.2	13.7	< 0.0001
SD	0.9	2.2	2.1		

Source: Greimel *et al.*, 1997, Table 3. Reprinted with permission of Macmillan Publishers Ltd on behalf of Cancer Research UK.

Doubtless the results do indicate such a conclusion, but ANOVA is not the best approach for an analysis of these data. ANOVA is more appropriate when comparing three or more treatment groups, or perhaps several categorical groups, rather than groups defined arbitrarily from what is a continuous variable such as age. Thus ANOVA is may be used when comparing more than two treatment arms in a clinical trial.

Example from the literature

Sharp *et al.* (2010) randomised 183 women with early breast cancer to three groups: self-initiated support (SIS), SIS plus reflexology, or SIS plus scalp massage. The primary endpoint was the Trial Outcome Index (TOI) of the Functional Assessment of Cancer Therapy (FACT-B) – breast cancer version, at 18 weeks post surgery. ANOVA was used to compare the three groups, and paired comparisons between groups were only carried out when the three-group comparison achieved the critical *p* value of 0.05.

The TOI scores differed significantly across the three groups ($p = 0.02$). In the ensuing paired comparisons, massage patients had significantly higher scores on the TOI (indicating a better quality of life) than those receiving SIS ($p = 0.03$), but the differences between reflexology and SIS, and massage and reflexology, were not statistically significant. However, the authors noted that the mean difference between massage and self-initiated support was 4.01 points, which falls short of the suggested minimally important difference of between 5 and 6.

Grouping age as in Table 12.9 implies that there is a jump in comorbidity score at each age group boundary, whereas there is if anything more likely to be a gradual and smooth change with age. A scatter plot of comorbidity against age would reveal the shape of this change. Since age is continuous, a regression approach to the analysis would be more statistically efficient. ANOVA is more suitable for factors such as marital status, which have no natural ranking of categories.

Example from the literature

Smets *et al.* (1998, Table 3) investigated the influence of gender and educational level on levels of mental fatigue in 154 disease-free cancer patients treated with radiotherapy. The *F*-tests following ANOVA are $F(1, 150) = 8.08$ for gender differences and $F(3,148) = 2.11$ for educational level.

From Table T5, the corresponding *p*-values are < 0.01 and approximately 0.1, suggesting a gender difference in mental fatigue score, but not one by educational level.

When comparing two groups, we can use either an ANOVA or a regression approach to the analysis. However, in the case of more than two treatment groups ANOVA is easily extended, whereas some care has to be taken with equation (12.13). Thus we cannot merely regard treatment as variable v in equation (12.13) and give it values of, say, 0, 1 and 2, as this would imply that the three treatments (I, II and III) were of an ordered nature – although this is precisely what we should do if they were. Instead, when comparing three (unordered) treatments, we have to express the regression model in the following way:

$$\text{QoL} = \beta_0 + \gamma_1 v_1 + \gamma_2 v_2. \tag{12.20}$$

The variables v_1 and v_2 are termed *dummy variables*. In this model, $v_1 = 1$ if the treatment group is I but $v_1 = 0$ if the treatment group is not I, and $v_2 = 1$ if the treatment group is II but $v_2 = 0$ if the treatment group is not II. In this way, the three treatment groups correspond to different pairs of values of (v_1, v_2) in the following way. The pair $(v_1 = 1, v_2 = 0)$ defines treatment I patients. Similarly the pair $(v_1 = 0, v_2 = 1)$ defines treatment II patients. Finally, the pair $(v_1 = 0, v_2 = 0)$ defines treatment III since the values of v indicate neither a treatment I patient nor a treatment II patient.

In this model there are therefore two regression coefficients, γ_1 and γ_2, to be estimated for the treatment effects. The null hypothesis of no treatment differences corresponds to testing whether the regression coefficients are simultaneously zero, that is, if $\gamma_1 = \gamma_2 = 0$. Extending this approach, if there are g treatment groups then $g - 1$ dummy variables will need to be created.

The advantage of the regression model approach of equation (12.20) over the ANOVA of Table 12.8 is that covariates can be more readily added to the model so that the final treatment comparisons can be adjusted for the (possible) influence of these variables. In some studies ANOVA can also be adjusted for covariates (ANCOVA), but this is not as flexible as the regression approach. Therefore we recommend the use of regression techniques for QoL analysis.

Checking for Normality

When analysing data from PROs, it is often advantageous to be able to assume that they have an approximately Normal distribution shape. We have suggested that comparing the magnitudes of the mean and SD may lead one to suspect a rather skew distribution, which can be confirmed by a histogram of the data. For small samples, it may be difficult to judge the degree of non-Normality of the data, and Altman (1991) describes how a *Normal plot* aids this process. When data are clearly not from a Normal distribution, statistical procedures based on the ranks are available.

Non-Normally distributed data

Although the ANOVA described earlier relates to a PRO that can be assumed to have a Normal distribution form, the method of analysis can be extended to continuous data that are skewed. In this case, the individual values of the PRO are replaced by their ranked values. For example, if five patients recorded pain on a visual analogue scale (VAS) as 2.2, 2.3, 2.4, 3.6 and 7.8 cm, these indicate a rather skew distribution. These are then replaced by their ranks 1, 2, 3, 4 and 5 respectively. The ANOVA, termed *Kruskal–Wallis*, then proceeds as we have previously described but now utilising the rank values rather than the individual observed values. It should be emphasised that the ranking is made by first combining all the N observations from the three or more (treatment) groups. The ranks are then summed for each of the g different groups separately; the corresponding test statistic is

$$KW = \frac{12\sum n_i \left(\bar{R}_i - \frac{(N+1)}{2} \right)^2}{N(N+1)}, \tag{12.21}$$

where there are n_i observations and $\bar{R}_i$ is the mean of the ranks in the ith group. If the null hypothesis is true, the test statistic KW follows the χ^2 distribution of Table T4 with $df = (g - 1)$.

This method can also be applied to ordered categorical data, but difficulties arise if there are (and there usually will be) many tied observations – as is the case with HADS depression scores of Table 12.4.

12.6   Analysis of variance models

Relationship with regression

In equation (12.12) we described the linear regression equation of QoL on age, and we repeat this equation here with one adjustment; we add the so-called *error term*, ε:

$$Q = \left[\beta_0 + \beta_{Age} Age\right] + \varepsilon. \tag{12.22}$$

With this equation we are stating that a particular observed value of QoL for a subject with a certain age will be equal to $[\beta_0 + \beta_{Age} Age]$. However, at the same time, we recognize that there may be other factors associated with QoL, which we are not considering here. For example, there may be additional variation owing to differences between subjects, such as gender, ethnic origin or stage of disease, as well as more random differences for which there is no obvious explanation. As a consequence, the model will not be perfect and so there may be (and usually will be) some departure in the observed QoL value from that predicted by the model were we to know β_0 and β_{Age} precisely. This departure is termed the *error component* in the model that we have denoted by ε in equation (12.22). Once the model is fitted to the data, it can be estimated as:

$$e = Q - \left[b_0 + b_{Age} Age\right]. \tag{12.23}$$

Here b_0 and b_{Age} again represent the estimates of β_0 and β_{Age} respectively; and e, the estimate of ε, is often termed the *residual* (from the fitted model). The true value ε may be positive, zero or negative. It is usually taken to be random and to average out to zero over all the subjects in a particular study. It is also assumed that the particular value of ε for one subject will not be influenced by the value in any other subject, and that the ε values are therefore uncorrelated. In technical terms, ε is often assumed to have a Normal distribution with mean zero and a constant standard deviation σ across all age groups.

For notational convenience and since in general we will not be confined to age as the covariate, we rewrite equation (12.22) as

$$Q_j = \alpha + \beta x_j + \varepsilon_j, \tag{12.24}$$

where α replaces β_0, β replaces β_{Age} and x_j replaces *Age*. The *j* refers to the individual subjects in the study. If there were two treatment groups, x_j takes the value of 0 or 1 depending on which treatment the patient is given.

We have also pointed out that the approach to the analysis for comparing groups can be made either by ANOVA or by linear regression techniques. Regression methods are (statistical) model-based approaches and so, since the methods are equivalent, ANOVA too is model-based. However, the model is usually formulated in a slightly different way.

The object of the ANOVA is to ascribe some of the variation in QoL observed amongst the *N* subjects to specific factors, for example treatments. The remaining (unexplained) proportion of the variation in QoL is then described as *random variation*. The ANOVA model takes the following form:

$$Q_{ij} = (\mu + \pi_i) + \varepsilon_{ij}. \tag{12.25}$$

Here *i* corresponds to the different treatment groups and *j* to the different patients. Those of treatment 1 will take the value π_1 in the above model and those of treatment 2 take the value π_2. Thus $\mu + \pi_1$ corresponds to α of the regression model (12.24), when $x_i = 0$. Similarly, $\mu + \pi_2$ corresponds to $\alpha + \beta$ in the same model, when $x_i = 1$. If we take $\pi_1 + \pi_2 = 0$, this implies $\pi_1 = -\pi_2$, which we can label simply π. This is equivalent to stating that treatment 1 is above the mean μ by $+\pi$ and treatment 2 is below the mean by $-\pi$, implying $\beta = 2\pi$ and $\alpha = \mu - \pi$. Thus there is a direct relationship between μ and π, and between α and β. Consequently, the ANOVA model of equation (12.25) is equivalent to the linear regression equation (12.24), although it is written in a somewhat different format.

In the situation of no differences between treatments, $\pi = 0$ while μ is estimated by the overall mean of the data, $\overline{Q}$. The term in brackets on the right-hand side of equation (12.25) is that part of the variation in Q explained by the model. In contrast, ε_{ij} is the remaining, or *residual*, variation in Q that we have not been able to explain. As already noted, for the purposes of brevity we did not include this term with the corresponding regression equations, but it is there just the same. It implies that the models we are discussing are not perfect descriptors of how the PRO behaves for a patient. Here in the ANOVA model format, as well as the regression format, this residual variation is assumed to follow a Normal distribution with a mean of zero and a constant standard deviation, σ, which is estimated by $\sqrt{V_{Within}}$ of Table 12.8.

12.7   Graphical summaries

Analysis of QoL data from clinical trials and other studies can be classified into two broad categories: *confirmatory data analysis*, and descriptive or *exploratory data analysis*.

Confirmatory data analysis is used when a number of hypotheses are to be tested. These should have been formulated before the study was commenced and should be specified in the clinical trial protocol. The testing of hypotheses can be based largely upon standard statistical significance testing, although there may be practical problems arising from the multidimensional nature of QoL assessments, the 'longitudinal' nature of the repeated measurements over time and the occurrence of missing data for individual patients.

Exploratory and descriptive data analyses, as their names suggest, are used to explore, clarify, describe and interpret the QoL data. Frequently these analyses will reveal unexpected patterns in the data, for example suggesting differences in QoL with respect to treatment or other factors. However, exploratory analyses often consist of a large number of individual comparisons and significance tests, and some apparently strong effects may in fact arise out of chance fluctuations in the data. Thus exploratory analyses may result in the generation of new hypotheses that should then be explored in subsequent studies.

Because exploratory analyses are less concerned with significance testing, graphical methods may be especially suitable. These largely visual methods have a number of advantages over purely numerical techniques. In particular, a judicious use of graphics can succinctly summarise complex data that would otherwise require extensive tabulations. At the same time, graphics can be used to emphasize the high degree of variability in QoL data. Graphical techniques can highlight changes in PROs that are large and clinically significant, while making it clearer to readers which changes are unimportant even though some clinically unimportant changes may represent statistically significant departures from zero.

Histograms and bar charts

The simplest summaries are *histograms* and *bar charts*, which show the frequency distribution of the data. These are often used to establish basic characteristics of the data. For example, prior to using a *t*-test one ought to check whether the data are distributed symmetrically and whether they appear to have a Normal distribution.

Most clinical trials compare two or more treatments, and many other investigations and analyses are also of a comparative nature. Thus graphs comparing two groups are particularly common in publications. One useful way of displaying the differences between groups of patients is a bar chart.

Example

Wisløff *et al.* (1996) evaluated QoL in 524 multiple myeloma patients from a randomised clinical trial that compared the use of melphalan–prednisone alone (MP) against MP + α-interferon (MP+IFN). They report EORTC QLQ-C30 scores at baseline, and then at 1, 6, 12, 24, 36 and 48 months.

Figure 12.2 shows the histogram of baseline emotional functioning (EF) scores of patients with multiple myeloma. In this case the data are concentrated at the higher levels with a clear ceiling effect, and the shape does not conform to that of the Normal distribution.

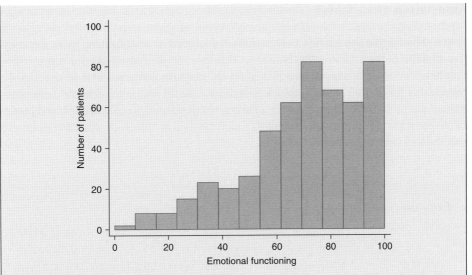

Figure 12.2   Histogram of baseline emotional functioning (EF) in patients with multiple myeloma. *Source:* Data from Wisløff *et al.,* 1996.

Example

Figure 12.3 displays the mean EF scores for males and females, according to age group. The reported EF is consistently higher (better) in males than in females, although the magnitude of the difference appears quite small. There seems to be a slight increase with age.

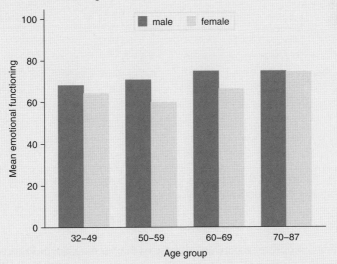

Figure 12.3   Bar chart illustrating the baseline EF scores from multiple myeloma patients, by gender and age group. *Source:* Data from Wisløff *et al.,* 1996.

Association of variables

When showing the association between two variables, the simplest and most informative graphic is the *scatter plot*. However, this may be of limited use for those PROs that have fewer than, say, 10 categorical levels, because many points will overlap. To reduce this limitation, some graphics programs have an option to increase the magnitude of the plotted symbols to reflect a number of overlapping observations, and others allow the addition of a small amount of random noise to 'jitter' overlapping points so that the individual points can be seen.

Example

Figure 12.4 shows the relationship of age with EF scores. Because the EF scale can only take 12 distinct values, a large proportion of the 524 patients have the same few values. A small amount of 'jitter' has been added to make the patterns clearer. In this example, there is only a weak relationship between age and EF – the correlation is $r = 0.14$.

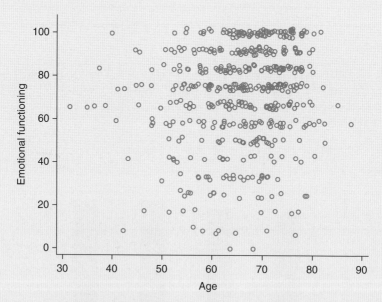

Figure 12.4 Scatter plot of the baseline EF in patients with multiple myeloma at different ages. *Source:* Data from Wisløff *et al.*, 1996.

A convenient compromise between the use of the bar diagram of Figure 12.3, which gives no indication of the variability, and the scatter diagram of Figure 12.4 is to use a series of box-and-whisker plots. A *box-and-whisker plot* indicates the median value at the centre of the box, and the 25th and 75th percentiles are indicated by the edges of the box. The *whiskers* each side of the *box* extend to the largest and smallest observed values within 1.5 box lengths. *Outliers* are indicated by open circles.

Example

Figure 12.5 shows the same data as Figure 12.3, using a series of box-and-whisker plots. From this one can see that the median EF varies little with age, except perhaps in the youngest age group (which is also the smallest group of patients). There is, however, considerable variability within each age group.

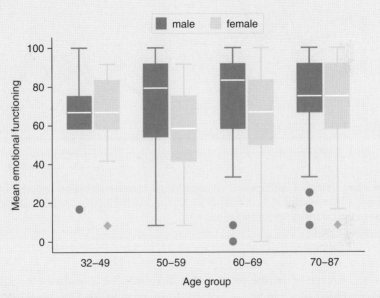

Figure 12.5 Box-and-whisker plot of the baseline EF in patients with multiple myeloma, by gender and age group. *Source:* Data from Wisløff *et al.*, 1996.

Patient profiles

One form of presentation that is particularly useful in QoL analyses is the *profile plot*. This attempts to display many dimensions simultaneously, divided on the basis of a grouping variable. Profile plots are convenient ways to summarise changes in many dimensions, but can handle only a single, grouped explanatory variable. They may be particularly useful when a consistent and unambiguous pattern is seen across successive groups.

Example

Figure 12.6 summarises the mean score profiles of patients after one month of treatment either with or without IFN. The bold line indicates the patients allocated to IFN and shows that, at one month, the IFN group tended to report worse functioning and more symptoms for nearly all scales of the EORTC QLQ-C30. Wisløff *et al.* (1996) report that many of these differences during the first year of treatment were statistically significant.

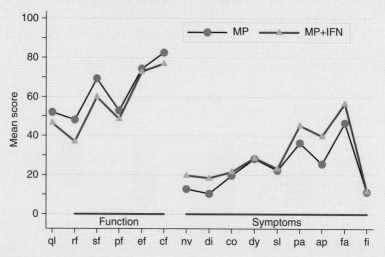

Figure 12.6   Profile of function and symptom values at one month after commencing treatment with α-interferon (bold line) or without α-interferon (thin line), in patients with myeloma. *Source:* Data from Wisløff *et al.*, 1996.

One disadvantage of profile plots is that there may be a tendency to assume that the different dimensions can be compared. However, items on QoL questionnaires are rarely scaled uniformly, and so it is usually meaningless to describe whether one item or scale takes higher (or lower) values than other items and scales.

12.8   Endpoints

In this chapter we have not taken particular note of which of the often numerous QoL items or scales we have chosen for analysis. However, in practice it is important to identify the key components of the QoL instrument that are the most relevant for the study concerned. These components should be identified clearly as the main study endpoints. Their number should be few, preferably no more than two or three. In designing a study and determining sample size it is imperative that the key endpoints are so identified. The same is true at the analysis stage. In any event, it is not usually possible to explore in great detail all QoL items or scales on an instrument. It is better to select the important ones in advance of conducting the study, and these would also shape the form of the analysis, be it cross-sectional, graphical or longitudinal in nature.

12.9   Conclusions

In any analysis attempting to summarise a QoL study there are many issues that need addressing. Fundamental to these is the choice of variables for analysis, the form the analysis will take, and whether the underlying (statistical) assumptions are satisfied by these data. It is often useful to commence with some initial graphical displays of the data. There are usually many QoL items and scales for examination, but the main focus should remain on the previously identified primary endpoints. In most circumstances, the final analysis may be best approached using regression techniques since these are generally the most flexible.

13

Exploring longitudinal data

Summary

The majority of studies involving QoL assessment include repeat assessments over time. Thus in a randomised trial and other studies there may be a baseline assessment, followed by a series of further assessments during the active treatment period, followed by (often less frequent) further assessments. QoL data are therefore longitudinal in form, the analysis and presentation of which is relatively straightforward if the number of observations per patient is equal. However, for QoL assessment this will seldom if ever be the case. The final dataset will usually be very ragged with the numbers of assessments available for analysis differing from patient to patient. In this chapter we introduce a summary of such data by means of the *area under the curve* (*AUC*). However, the main focus is on how such longitudinal data can be represented in a graphical format.

13.1   Area under the curve

In describing the cross-sectional analyses in Chapter 12, we considered a single aspect of the QoL assessment for a particular instrument, measured at one particular time. For example, if we had been describing an analysis from the HADS, we might have been referring to depression at a fixed time from the commencement of treatment, with no reference to depression levels at earlier or later assessment times. Such an analysis will rarely encapsulate all the features of the total data collected. Thus usually we will wish to examine the QoL profiles of patients over time, to summarise these for the individual patients, to describe collectively all those receiving the same treatment, and finally to compare treatments.

> ### Example
>
> Figure 13.1 shows the pain profile of two patients assessed on a daily basis during hospitalisation for severe burns. However, one missed two assessments and furthermore the duration of hospitalisation for the two patients differs. Hence the number of pain evaluations is not the same.

Quality of Life: The Assessment, Analysis and Reporting of Patient-Reported Outcomes, Third Edition.
Peter M. Fayers and David Machin.
© 2016 John Wiley & Sons, Ltd. Published 2016 by John Wiley & Sons, Ltd.

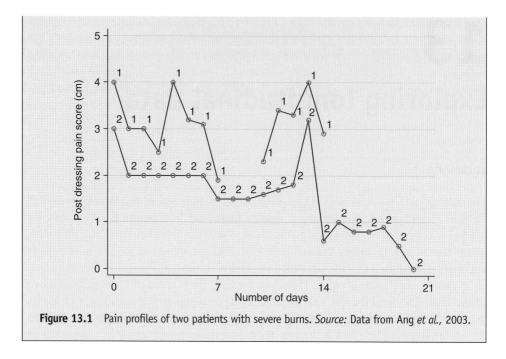

Figure 13.1 Pain profiles of two patients with severe burns. *Source:* Data from Ang *et al.,* 2003.

Even when QoL data have a longitudinal format, it is often advisable to summarise them by extracting key elements from the patient profile. Examples are the patient's QoL at a fixed time after the active treatment period has been completed or perhaps a measure such as the time from randomisation until QoL is improved by a prespecified amount. Another such measure, but one that uses all the QoL data of each available assessment, is the *AUC*. In Figure 13.1, the *AUC* is the area between the pain profile of each patient and the horizontal axis representing zero pain. Once calculated, the *AUC* for pain may be used as a summary value for each patient.

To calculate the *AUC* the data points are first joined by straight lines as in the complete profile of Figure 13.1. These then describe the shape of the 'curve'. The area is calculated by adding the areas under the curve between each pair of consecutive observations. For the first two QoL assessments, taking values QoL_0 and QoL_1 of one patient at consecutive times t_0 and t_1, the corresponding area is

$$A_1 = \frac{(QoL_1 + QoL_0)(t_1 - t_0)}{2}.$$

Similarly

$$A_2 = \frac{(QoL_2 + QoL_1)(t_2 - t_1)}{2},$$

and if there are $k + 1$ assessments in all, then

$$A_k = \frac{(QoL_k + QoL_{k-1})(t_k - t_{k-1})}{2}.$$

After calculating the corresponding areas, we have

$$AUC = (A_1 + A_2 + \ldots + A_k)/T. \tag{13.1}$$

The final divisor T is the duration of time from the first or baseline assessment (time 0) until the final assessment (assessment $k + 1$). This takes into account the possible and usual different times and periods of assessment of each patient.

The AUC is calculated individually for each patient, providing for each a single summary score. These can then be averaged across all patients within each separate treatment group. A useful property is that although the original measurements may show floor and ceiling effects, the AUC is more likely to follow a Normal distribution (see Figure 13.9 and the associated example). Thus the corresponding treatment means may be compared using the appropriate z- or t-tests, ANOVA or regression techniques, as outlined in Chapter 12.

We can calculate the AUC even when there are missing data. Thus patient 1, in Figure 13.1, does not complete assessments on days 8 and 9. The observations at days 7 and 10 have not been joined to emphasise this loss of data. However, the calculation proceeds without these, as there is no requirement in equation (13.1) that the time intervals be equal between successive observations. Therefore, in situations where despite a fixed schedule being specified, there are some deviations from the observation schedule for virtually every patient, the calculation of AUC can still be made.

This type of calculation may not be appropriate if the final observation that is anticipated is missing. However, in studies in which patients with an ultimately fatal disease are assessed until as close to death as is reasonable, the last-reported QoL observation may be assumed to be the worst possible QoL value for that item or scale. This then provides the final value and so an AUC can then be calculated using equation (13.1). In this situation T will correspond to the time from baseline assessment to patient death.

With the AUC we have summarised each patient's longitudinal experience as a single quantity, and so the analysis once more becomes cross-sectional in nature and the methods of Chapter 12 may again be applied. Lydick *et al.* (1995) discuss methodological problems associated with the use of AUC in the context of patients with episodic diseases.

Example from the literature

Kottschade *et al.* (2011) explored the use of vitamin E for the prevention of chemotherapy-induced peripheral neuropathy in a randomised phase III clinical trial with 207 patients. The values over time of patient-reported peripheral neuropathy scores on the 7-item Symptom Experience Diary and a single-item Neuropathy Specific Question were collapsed into AUC summary statistics for each patient (pro-rated for the number of time periods reported). All values for each question ranged from 0 to 10 (with 0 being no symptoms and 10 being as bad as it can be). For each of the eight outcomes, two-sample t-tests were used to compare the average AUC for each treatment arm. There were no differences in the patient-reported AUC outcomes between treatment groups (p-values ranging from 0.11 to 0.88).

13.2   Graphical presentations

A fundamental decision to be made when graphing aggregated longitudinal data from QoL instruments is what measure to plot against time. The four principal choices are: the percentage of patients with values exceeding a certain level, median scores of items and scales, mean scores of items and scales, and individual data points. Which to choose may be determined by the context.

Percentages

Example from the literature

The Medical Research Council (MRC) Lung Cancer Working Party (1992) conducted a randomised trial of palliative radiotherapy with two fractions (F2) or a single fraction (F1), in poor-performance patients with inoperable non-small-cell lung cancer. Of particular concern was the distress caused by dysphagia with this disease.

The percentage of patients reporting dysphagia 'mild soreness when swallowing' or worse on a daily basis is shown in Figure 13.2. This basic plot shows that there is a large difference in the percentage of patients reporting dysphagia between the F1 and F2 regimens. This is particularly noticeable in the second and third weeks post randomisation.

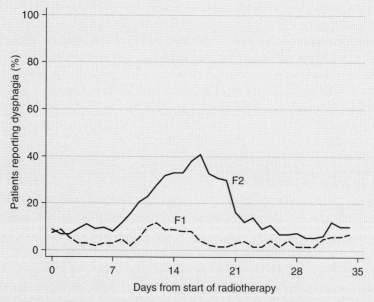

Figure 13.2   A trial comparing two radiotherapy regimens for non-small-cell lung cancer, which used a daily diary card to assess QoL. *Source:* Bllehen *et al.* 1992, Table 3. Reprinted by permission from Macmillan Publishers Ltd on behalf of Cancer Research UK.

The difficulty with this form of presentation is that it does not indicate the reducing number of patients (and hence how precisely the associated percentages are estimated) in the plot as time progresses from diagnosis. A sensible addition to this (and many plots) is to include the number at risk by treatment group at various points beneath the time axis. In this example assessments are made daily so that patient numbers would be given only at convenient intervals. If there is a less frequent or irregular schedule it is important to give numbers observed on these occasions.

There may be more than two response possibilities (that is, more than 'present' or 'absent' categories), and the concept of percentage plots can be extended to handle these. Thus, in the example of reported dysphagia levels, this might be done by superimposing plots corresponding to the cumulative percentage of patients in the successive categories. These categories could correspond to 'no soreness when swallowing', 'mild soreness when swallowing', 'quite a bit of soreness when swallowing' and 'very much soreness when swallowing'. The cumulative total of these is then 100% at each assessment time point. However, with such a plot it is not so easy to include two (or more) patient groups within the same panel as the likelihood of superimposed data points is high and any substantial overlap can obscure the underlying patterns.

Means versus medians

The EORTC QLQ-C30 and the Hospital Anxiety and Depression Scale (HADS) are typical QoL instruments that, like many others, use raw items with four-point categories, often with labels such as 'not at all', 'a little', 'quite a bit' and 'very much' for the respective categories that are then scored 1–4. Also, many QoL items have strongly skewed distributions in the associated responses. Thus for items representing rare symptoms and side effects or infrequent problems, the majority of patients may report 'not at all'; that is, the minimal response for the QoL item. In contrast, with items concerning more common problems there may be a large proportion of patients reporting 'very much'; that is, the maximum response for the item. As a consequence, it is not unusual for as many as half the patients to report the maximum for some items and the minimum for others. In these cases, the medians for the QoL items would be these *floor* or *ceiling* values of either 1 or 4. Such medians carry limited information when presented in graphical format, and it becomes better to plot mean values rather than medians.

All available data

Since QoL measurements are usually collected repeatedly over time, it is almost inevitable that there will be a lot of incomplete data. In fact, if it weren't for this the presentation and analysis of QoL data would be greatly simplified and would not differ substantially from methods used in many other applications. One can rapidly assess the magnitude of the 'missing problem' by a plot of all available data at each time point. Such a plot is useful in examining simultaneously both attrition and departures from the assessment schedule. This plot is likely to be only useful for QoL scales, as individual items will usually have too few categories for the technique to be helpful.

Example from the literature

Figure 13.3 shows a scatter diagram of Functional Assessment of Cancer – General version (FACT-G) QoL assessments completed by 375 anaemic cancer patients receiving non-platinum-based chemotherapy (Fallowfield *et al.*, 2002). The patients were included in a randomised trial comparing epoetin alfa against placebo. Because patients could be enrolled with a variable number of expected chemotherapy cycles, and because those cycles could be of varying durations, the timing of QoL assessments could not be standardised to specific days or weeks in the study. The actual timing of the QoL assessments that resulted from this study design is illustrated in Figure 13.3, where the vertical axis represents patients (sorted by days in the study) and the horizontal axis represents study duration.

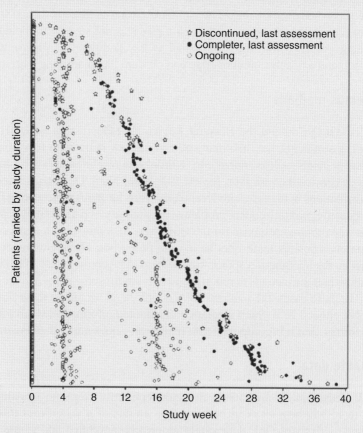

Figure 13.3 Scatter plot showing the timing of FACT QoL assessments in a group of anaemic cancer patients. Each symbol represents a QoL assessment for a patient at the specified time in the study. The last assessment for a patient who withdrew early is represented by a star, the last assessment for a completer is a closed circle, and a continuing assessment is shown by an open circle. *Source:* Fallowfield *et al.*, 2002, Figure 2. Reprinted with permission of Macmillan Publishers Ltd on behalf of Cancer Research UK.

Example from the literature

Machin and Weeden (1998) examined the adherence of patients in a lung cancer trial to a schedule of planned assessments. They provide a multi-panel plot of the data (Figure 13.4), from which it is clear that an increasing proportion of patients depart from the fixed schedule as time goes on. The increasing scatter of the QoL assessments relative to the scheduled assessment times indicates the increasing departures from the protocol schedule. Even the baseline QoL assessments were not all made immediately prior to randomisation and start of treatment (day 0).

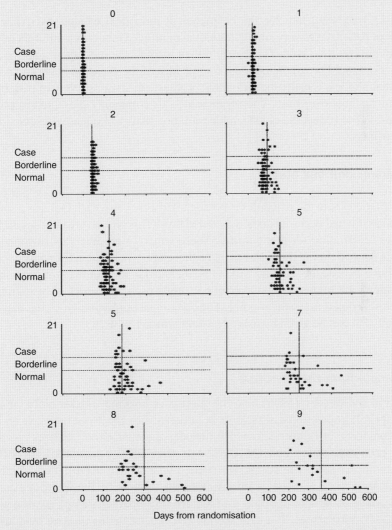

Figure 13.4 Scatter plot of the HADS depression score at each assessment against day of assessment for patients with small-cell lung cancer. *Source:* Machin and Weeden 1998. Reproduced with permission of John Wiley & Sons, Ltd.

Figure 13.4 takes up considerable space on the printed page. However, to illustrate the patterns within both treatment groups would require even more space, unless of course different plotting symbols or colour codes are used within each panel. This is not usually practicable as many points may be obscured due to coinciding values at some times. Nevertheless, the plots of Figure 13.3 and Figure 13.4 do indicate the attrition following the baseline QoL values since the number of observations in the successive clouds of points reduces as time progresses.

Individual profiles

Figure 13.3 does not indicate the behaviour of individual patients over time. If the number of patients was very small, individual plotting symbols or a different colour for each patient could be used. These would then identify the individuals and the respective patterns could be examined to give some idea of the variation between and within individual profiles. Usually the individual profiles will show a variety of patterns, with large fluctuations over time. The mean values, as commonly presented in published analyses, fail to reflect the considerable variation that is frequently observed in individual patients.

Histograms and box plots

If the variation about the schedules is not regarded as serious, each QoL assessment can be taken as if it had occurred at the scheduled time. This effectively imposes acceptable *windows* of variation for this purpose. These windows are intervals surrounding the schedule dates, defining those assessments that can be included in the analysis. Assessments lying outside the window will not be included in the summary or analysis. Once the windows are imposed, the data can be summarised as a series of histograms, one for each scheduled assessment point. Thus a compact presentation of the data shown in Figure 13.4 can be given by using box-and-whisker plots.

Example from the literature

Machin and Weeden (1998) give the successive box-and-whisker plots for each of 10 HADS depression assessments in patients with small-cell lung cancer. This is reproduced in Figure 13.5, which includes the numbers of patients completing each assessment and the thresholds that classify patients into normal, borderline or case. The successive median values have been joined to form a summary profile. However, care needs to be taken with the interpretation of this profile as patient attrition may remove those patients with, say, the worst (highest) HAD scores. The data are plotted separately for the two randomised treatment regimens, a two-drug (2D) and a four-drug (4D) regimen as described by MRC Lung Cancer Working Party (1996).

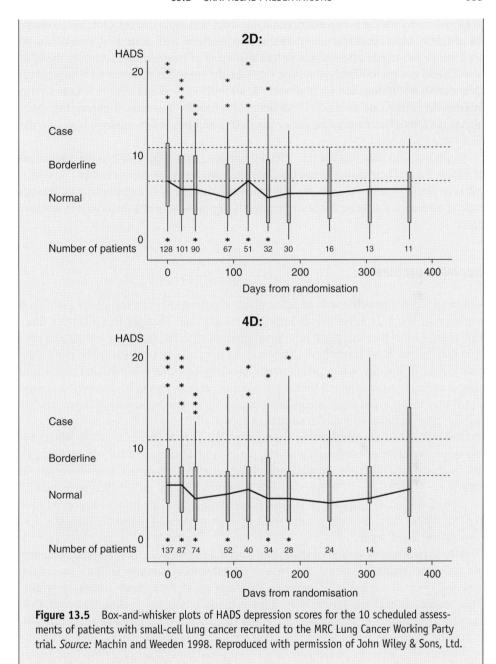

Figure 13.5 Box-and-whisker plots of HADS depression scores for the 10 scheduled assessments of patients with small-cell lung cancer recruited to the MRC Lung Cancer Working Party trial. *Source:* Machin and Weeden 1998. Reproduced with permission of John Wiley & Sons, Ltd.

In constraining the data into windows we are assuming that the variations in day-to-day values over the short spans of time are regarded as minor. Nevertheless, there may be circumstances when this is clearly not the case. In these situations the windows need to be selected with care. For example, if the study schedule defines QoL assessments immediately after receiving chemotherapy in patients with cancer, it would not be appropriate to include assessments before that cycle of treatment. In addition, the window should not go too far beyond the cycle as the immediate impact of treatment on QoL may have diminished by that time. A wide window could lead to a rather false impression of the true situation. It is better if windows are defined before the study begins, as later choices may be rather subjective and possibly introduce bias into the analytical procedures.

Any remaining data outside the selected windows could be added to the equivalent of Figure 13.5. Their clouds would occupy the gaps between the successive box-and-whisker plots. In this way, all the information collected is summarised even though little analytical use may be made of the clouds of points between the box-and-whisker plots.

Summary profiles

Although it is not possible with large numbers of patients to examine all the individual patient profiles, it is nevertheless important to evaluate changes in QoL over time. However, it must be recognised that those patients with the fewest assessments available may be the most severely ill. This may be particularly so towards the end of the time course of a study, when patients may possibly be close to death, and this would almost certainly have affected their QoL were we able to assess it. These data 'omissions' may result in the assessments that we are able to observe seriously misrepresenting the 'true' patterns of the overall patient group.

One method of examining this situation in detail is to present, group-by-group, the summary profiles comprising all the patients in 'duration of follow-up groups'. To do this, separate mean profiles are plotted for those patients who were lost to follow-up at 0, 1, 2, ..., 9 months. For example, one of these summaries would be provided by data from those patients completing baseline plus four consecutive HADS. These data are then summarised at each scheduled assessment by the corresponding mean score.

If these profiles are similar in shape and have similar mean values over the comparable assessment schedule times, it may be reasonable to summarise all the data at each schedule over all the available patients. This then provides a single summary profile. This profile, despite the absent data, may provide a reasonable description of QoL changes over time. On the other hand, if the shapes of the profiles are very different, it may be inadvisable to collapse the data further. This might also be the case if the profiles are similar in shape but parallel to each other rather than superimposed. In this case, treatment and follow-up influence QoL in a similar way but initial values are a strong indicator for prognosis.

A final step in this graphical analysis will be to divide the data into treatment groups and plot the corresponding means at each assessment point for each treatment group separately.

Example from the literature

Hopwood *et al.* (1994) utilised this approach with part of the data from the MRC Lung Cancer Working Party (1996) trial. They considered the HADS anxiety rather than depression assessments. They excluded all data from patients having gaps in their assessment profiles as they were describing a methodology rather than the actual results of the clinical trial. Figure 13.6a shows the mean HADS for each follow-up profile. Since the plots appeared fairly consistent, it was concluded that there were no major differences in these subgroups so that the combined (all-patient) profile of Figure 13.6b could be calculated. This is divided by treatment group in Figure 13.6c.

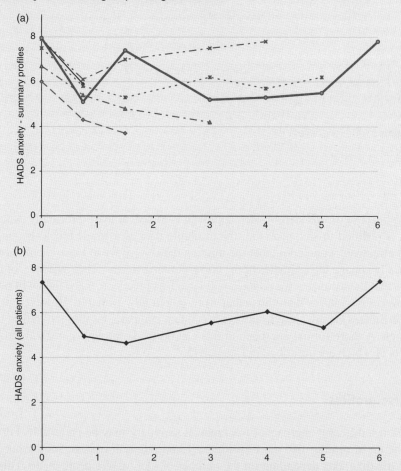

Figure 13.6   Profiles of HADS anxiety score for patients with small-cell lung cancer (a) according to number of assessments completed, (b) by all patients and (c) by treatment group. *Source:* Hopwood *et al.*, 1994, Figures 2, 3 and 4. Reproduced with permission of Springer Science and Business Media.

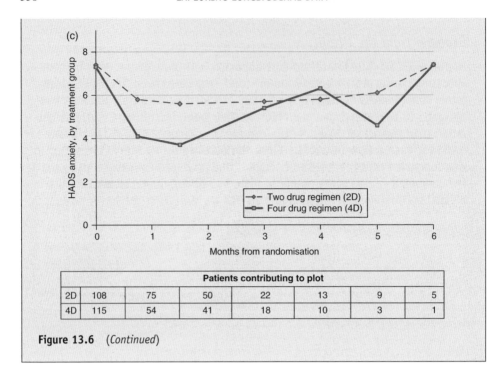

Figure 13.6 (*Continued*)

The purpose of this step-by-step approach is to see, at least informally, whether or not it is justified to summarise all the available data as a single block. If one could, this is effectively concluding that the missing data (were we to know them) would not materially change the estimates of the corresponding means. Their absence, of course, means that the estimates we do have will have less precision, since they will be based on fewer observations than those that were potentially available. However, provided these estimates are not biased, between-treatment comparisons may still reflect the true situation. A more formal approach to this can be made through statistical modelling, aspects of which are described in Chapter 15.

Reverse profiles

Sometimes different approaches to graphical summary may be preferable. For example, the mean profiles like those of Figure 13.6a might have been similar but shifted along the time axis depending on the number of QoL assessments made. This could occur if the QoL profiles of patients tended to be similar at critical stages, for example similar for all patients close to death. In this case placing the origin as the date of last assessment and plotting backwards in time, rather than forwards from baseline, may result in similar profiles that could then be averaged.

Example

Figure 13.7 shows a reverse profile plot of HADS depression scores in patients with small-cell lung cancer, calculated from date of last assessment as the reference point. In these patients, this time was usually when the patient was close to death. These data suggest that HADS depression levels rise as death approaches. The integers used as plotting symbols indicate the number of assessments completed by that particular group of patients.

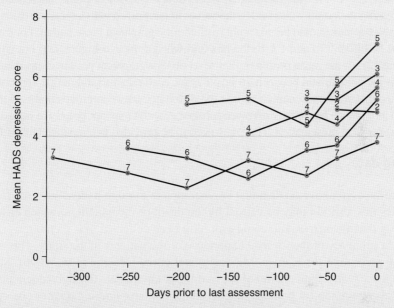

Figure 13.7 Mean HADS depression score in patients with small-cell lung cancer, reverse plotted from date of last assessment, subdivided by the number of available assessments. *Source:* Machin and Weeden, 1998. Reproduced with permission of John Wiley & Sons, Ltd.

Variability

One advantage of the repeated box-and-whisker plots in Figure 13.5 is that they not only summarise the changing median QoL levels with time but also summarise and quantify the associated variability. This variability is described by both the interquartile range and the whiskers themselves. The number of patients contributing to each point in this graph can be added beneath the time axis, displaying in a compact form all the principal features of the data.

It is unlikely that any approach to data presentation will be entirely appropriate or optimal for all situations. Indeed, what may seem the best for one QoL item or scale in a particular instrument may not be optimal for another. However, some compromise is needed. What we suggest is that the method of presentation should be that which satisfies best the needs of the most important QoL scale in the context of the particular study – once determined, this presentation would be carried throughout. It would be perplexing for the reader if each QoL variable were to be presented in its own unique way. If a comparison is to be made between the current study and work conducted previously by others, choosing the same style of presentation clearly facilitates the comparison even in situations where the method of presentation may not be optimal. However, one must avoid repeating poor methods of presentation.

For studies describing a single group of patients, it may be useful to add 95% confidence intervals (*CI*) for the mean at each scheduled assessment point. These emphasize the increasing uncertainty attached to the values at later times with increasing patient attrition. However, care should be taken not to clutter the graphical presentation. For example, it would be difficult to add *CI*s to the box-and-whisker plot of Figure 13.5 but would be quite feasible for the mean profile of Figure 13.6b. For graphical presentations intended to illustrate the comparison between groups, *CI*s for each mean would not be appropriate to add to the graphical presentation as it is the difference between groups that is if interest. Any *CI* should then be for the differences observed, and it may not be easy to include these into the graphical presentation. They may need to be provided in a separate tabular format.

Missing data

We have focused above on data that are incomplete through patient attrition. In many examples this attrition may be caused by the death of the patient, in which case there is no way that the *absent data* could ever have been collected. It is then often useful to include a summary of the survival experience of the patients in the study. This may be done by presenting the Kaplan–Meier survival curve (Machin *et al.*, 2006). Survival curves give a ready appreciation of the reason for absent data through patient attrition.

It is also common for patients in QoL studies to have *missing data* at one or more scheduled times in an otherwise complete set of QoL reports. In this case, attempts are often made to impute their value (see Chapter 15). Such imputed values should not be added to the clouds of data points, such as those of Figure 13.4, even though they may be used to estimate the mean QoL at each scheduled assessment time.

13.3 Tabular presentations

Much of the information summarised in graphical form above could have been presented in tabular format, perhaps even in a more compact way. However, in reporting longitudinal QoL studies it is important to convey the extent of attrition (and hence absent data), and this can usually be best illustrated graphically. Such detail can really only be given for a limited number of scales from each QoL instrument used in the study; the remaining variables will have to be presented in tabular format. Such tables should indicate the numbers of subjects providing information for each item or scale, the proportion of missing as opposed to absent values, a summary statistic such as the mean or percentage, and a measure of the variability. The tables should also highlight the principal endpoints of the investigation in some way.

Example from the literature

Wisløff *et al.* (1996) give a tabular summary of the symptom and toxicity aspects of their trial in the tabular format of Table 13.1, in which for each assessment the mean score is given for each treatment and this is repeated for each symptom. One way in which this table could be modified would be to rank the symptoms in terms of frequency of occurrence from month 0 onwards – starting with 'muscle pain', 'joint pain', 'night sweats' and so on until 'hair loss'. The reason that 'joint pain' precedes 'night sweats' in this ranking, although they are numerically equal at month 0, is that there is more of the former at month 1. The rows of the table would then follow this ranking. In this way it would be a little easier to follow the patterns of the major symptoms as they would be grouped close together.

Table 13.1 Means of toxicity and symptom scores for patients with myeloma, by treatment received. Symptom scores range from 0 to 100, with higher scores representing higher levels of symptoms or toxicity

| | Month after start of therapy | | | | | | | | | | | |
| | 0 | | 1 | | 6 | | 12 | | 24 | | 36 | |
Treatment	MP	MP+IFN	MP	MP+IFN	MP	MP+IFN	MP	MP+IFN	MP	MP+IFN	MP	MP+IFN
No. of patients who completed questionnaires	271	253	255	232	218	206	196	181	142	144	67	74
No. of drop-outs[a]	24	33	5	8	6	4	4	4	3	5	0	0
Symptoms												
Night sweats	21	23	19	20	15	14	14	13	15	12	17	16
Fever	5	11	6	12	3	8	4	6	3	5	5	6
Chills	6	10	11	17	8	13	8	12	8	11	9	14
Dizziness	15	14	14	18	13	17	11	16	9	17	14	15
Hair loss	4	4	6	7	11	22	10	13	8	9	12	12
Headache	12	14	12	15	13	12	13	11	12	13	14	12
Sore mouth	8	8	10	11	8	13	7	10	8	11	13	6
Muscle pain	28	31	26	31	25	27	24	26	25	24	30	29
Joint pain	21	23	21	24	21	20	23	23	25	21	26	24
Dry skin	17	20	20	27	16	28	17	23	21	22	20	22
Coughing	16	16	16	18	16	14	19	16	15	13	14	13

[a] Number of patients who are alive and who have completed all previous questionnaires, but not the one at this time point.
Source: Wisløff *et al.*, 1996. Reproduced with permission of John Wiley & Sons, Ltd.

One difficulty with a tabular format such as Table 13.1 is that the times of QoL assessment, although clearly indicated here, are often not equally spaced. As a consequence, it is often difficult to appreciate the true shape of the changes with time by scanning entries in a table. This is also a difficulty with successive bar charts that are presented equally spaced on the printed page rather than at locations determined by their relative positions in time. Although this may be easy to rectify using other forms of plot, as we do in Figure 16.2b later, unequally spaced columns would not be a practical format for tabular display.

Although we recommend that some measure of variability should be included in a tabular display, it is difficult to see how this could be added to all the entries of Table 13.1 without making it unacceptably complicated. A compromise is to identify the *major* symptoms of concern at the protocol development stage and provide the variability measure for these only. This could be done by listing these major symptoms first in Table 13.1 and in the order of importance as specified by the protocol (not by the results). The measure of variability would then be added alongside or beneath the corresponding mean. Following a break in the table, the remainder of the symptoms could then be listed in rank order of observed importance at baseline assessment in the manner that we have previously indicated.

13.4   Reporting

From the previous sections it is clear that the process of examining longitudinal QoL data in detail may be a complex and lengthy one. Seldom will the patterns revealed be simple; indeed, they may be very intricate, and so their summary will usually be daunting. However, by first focusing on the few major questions posed by the study and reporting these in careful detail, it may not be so important to report with the same level of detail the other endpoints. The guidelines for reporting outlined in Section 16.6 set out some vital aspects that we will concentrate upon. It is inevitable in reporting any study that compromises have to be made as journal editors and readers will wish for clear messages uncluttered by detail.

Compliance with schedule and attrition

As we have indicated, if the study involves repeated QoL assessments on patients whose ability to complete the questionnaire is likely to be compromised, for example by death itself, as time goes on it is useful to summarise the survival experience by a Kaplan–Meier survival curve. A single survival curve may suffice if there is no major difference in survival between the therapeutic groups, but only if there is also no major difference in compliance. If there is a marked difference in survival and/or if the pattern or rate of non-compliant patients differs substantially, treatment-specific detail should be provided.

Example

Figure 13.8 shows the survival over 48 months of patients with myeloma treated in the randomised study of the Nordic Myeloma Study Group (1996), whose QoL data are described by Wisløff *et al.* (1996).

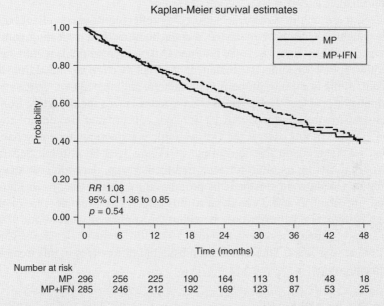

Figure 13.8 Kaplan–Meier estimates of the survival curves for patients with myeloma, by treatment received. The apparent survival advantage to MP+IFN (relative risk, RR, = 1.08) is not statistically significant. *Source:* Data from Wisløff *et al.*, 1996.

One advantage of this plot is that it also enables the QoL assessment schedule to be indicated by marking the time axis in an appropriate way. It is customary in reporting survival curves that the numbers of patients at risk be indicated at key points beneath the time axis. These numbers can be supplemented by the compliance, possibly for each group, especially at key stages such as when important patient management events take place. Examples of critical events include the time that active (protocol) therapy ceases, the time of disease response assessment, or the anticipated time of discharge to community care. When the principal QoL endpoint under consideration is one that poses personal difficulties with respect to the ability or willingness to respond for many subjects, it may sometimes be appropriate to count these patients as *non-compliant*, even though they may have completed the other assessment items. It will be a matter of judgement which figures to report.

The upper panel of Table 13.1 provides a tabular alternative to the graphical format of Figure 13.8. This shows the number of patients completing the QoL questionnaire at each scheduled assessment together with the number of patients who were alive at that time but who did not complete the questionnaire. The total of these two gives the numbers still alive at the respective assessment points and declines quite rapidly over the three years of the study. This tabular format is more compact than the corresponding graphical alternative.

However, these methods of presentation may reflect not the compliant but the *off-schedule* patients. As we have indicated, a convenient method of dealing with these is to impose acceptable windows. If the returned QoL assessment falls within the respective window for that schedule, it is included; but otherwise it is excluded from analysis. Once again, if this is a minor proportion of the total anticipated QoL assessments, this causes no major problem. However, in other circumstances the departure from schedule (being outside the windows) may be of major concern and also differ between the treatment groups. In this case, if the QoL variable is numeric with a reasonable range of values, we recommend that the format of Figure 13.3 be utilised. Separate panels may or may not be required for each treatment group, depending on the context. If keeping to schedule slips as patients progress through the trial, as in Figure 13.4, it may be important to add a comment to this effect. For example, one might state: 'Although compliance with schedule is within the stipulated window for 98% of the patients at the baseline assessment, this reduces to 50% at the one-year assessment and is only 25% at two years. There were no substantial differences in this trend between the treatment groups.'

Treatment comparisons

In randomised trials the main focus is to make comparisons between treatments, and it will often be useful to provide a graphical summary similar to Figure 13.6c (another example is given in Figure 16.2b) after going through the stages we have described. Whether such a plot provides an unbiased summary of the QoL changes over time and between treatments will depend to a large extent on the pattern and proportion of compliant patients. Again, it is a matter of judgement as to whether this is indeed the case in a particular situation. Any concerns in this respect should be included in the accompanying text. Indications of the associated variability can be added to this graph at each assessment point. If the summary measure plotted is a mean, a horizontal line spanning two standard deviations above and below the mean can be indicated. For the two treatments at each QoL assessment point, the two corresponding lines can be displaced slightly horizontally so as not to overlap directly. Judgement again will have to be made as to whether a single-panel (Figure 13.6c) or a double-panel format (Figure 13.5) is the more suitable. What is not recommended is to include the 95% *CI* for the difference between treatments at each assessment point, since these tend to encourage point-by-point comparisons that introduce problems similar to those of repeated statistical tests. However, if the protocol had stipulated that a major endpoint was the QoL at a particular time point, it would be appropriate to give an indication of the 95% *CI* for that comparison only.

On the other hand, if longitudinal data have been summarised for each patient by a single quantity, the longitudinal component of the presentation disappears and one is left with a cross-sectional analysis to report. Thus, if the *AUC* is used, each treatment group will have a corresponding mean, $\overline{AUC}$, with a standard error of *SE(AUC)*. The *AUC* data can then be presented graphically by either box-and-whisker plots or histograms, one for each treatment group. However, it is essential that the difference in means be quoted and the corresponding 95% *CI* stated. Because this measure is derived from the original and multiple QoL responses it may less easily convey its own meaning to the reader. Thus it may be best to provide the combination of a tabular format to summarise the component data for this derived measure with a graphical display of the resulting distributions, such as the distributions of the *AUC*s.

Example

Figure 13.9 shows the histograms of the *AUC*, here denoted AUC_{36}, calculated for the assessment of fatigue over the whole 36 months from the date of randomisation in the trial described by Wisløff *et al.* (1996). The corresponding numbers of patients for the melphalan-prednisone (MP) alone and with interferon (IFN) treatment groups are 238 and 213 with respective means 43.5 (*SD* = 22.3) and 47.5 (*SD* = 16.0). The difference between these means of 4.0 (95% *CI* 0.02–8.02) is suggestive of more fatigue reported by those patients receiving IFN ($p = 0.049$).

Although histograms of data at each of the assessment points showed an excess of patients with low levels of fatigue, the Normal distribution curves that are superimposed in Figure 13.9 show that the *AUC* values are approximately Normal. However, such superimposed curves would not usually be added to a figure for the published report.

Just as for any other endpoint, it should have been indicated in the protocol that AUC_{36} is an important one that will be the focus of analysis. In fact, repeating the *AUC* calculations for this trial but using only the first 24 months' data (AUC_{24}) and again using AUC_{12} produces *p*-values of 0.003 and 0.001 respectively. These indicate that the excess symptom levels reported with IFN are greater in the early part of the treatment period. Any investigator, albeit pre-specifying that AUC_{36} was the key variable, would be foolish not to explore the data in detail and, once the phenomenon is noticed, should report it as an observation requiring confirmatory study on another occasion. Thus in future trials earlier endpoints, for example AUC_6, might replace AUC_{36} as the major endpoint.

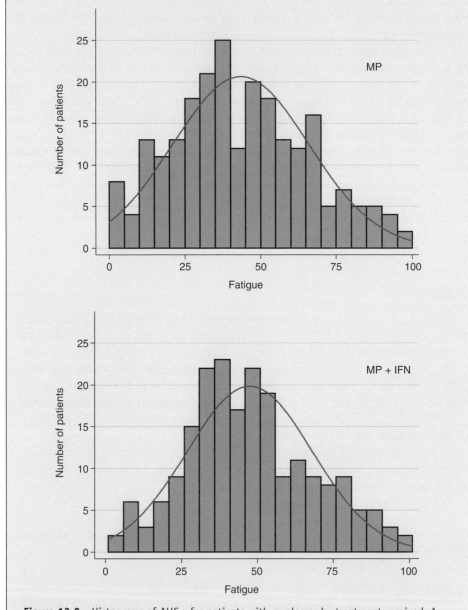

Figure 13.9 Histograms of AUC_{36} for patients with myeloma, by treatment received. A Normal distribution is superimposed. *Source:* Data from Wisløff *et al.*, 1996.

13.5 Conclusions

Longitudinal data, especially when there is attrition due to missing data and death, presents a number of problems in analysis and interpretation. These difficulties are further compounded by unequally spaced scheduled assessment times and variability in the time of the actual assessment. For these reasons, the initial exploration of the data should place emphasis upon summary tabulations and graphical methods. Summary measures, such as the *AUC* or the percentage of time that a patient has QoL levels above a specific threshold, can reduce longitudinal data to a single summary score for each patient. This has the advantage that the methods of Chapter 12 can then be applied, for example to provide significance testing of treatment differences. *AUC* is one method of combining QoL values over time. An alternative method, using *QALYs*, is described in Chapter 17; this weights different health states according to patients' values, or *utilities*. However, the modelling methods described in Chapter 14 may also be applied in order to explore the data in greater depth and in particular to estimate the magnitude of the treatment effect and test its significance.

13.5 Conclusions

14

Modelling longitudinal data

Summary

In Chapter 13, emphasis was placed on describing in graphical form changes in outcomes with time and their summary across groups of patients. However, these comparisons were not quantified to any extent. This chapter describes a modelling approach to the description of longitudinal data that permits both an estimation of effect sizes and statistical tests of hypotheses. These models are an extension of the linear regression and ANOVA techniques described in Chapter 12. In particular, they take account of the fact that successive PRO assessments by a particular patient are likely to be correlated. The alternative approaches are classified as repeated measures, general estimating equations and multilevel models. They all require the specification of an autocorrelation structure, and this is described. Some of the statistical assumptions underpinning the techniques for fitting these models to QoL data are complex; so we have focused more on interpretation than on technical aspects. Although the mathematical details of some models might appear complex, the aim is only to find a model that describes the data well and thereby enables a simple estimate of the treatment effect.

14.1 Preliminaries

In Chapter 13, we used graphical approaches for exploring PRO data to provide a visual summary that is relatively easy to interpret while taking account of the possible impact of missing data through attrition. However, such approaches do not permit formal statistical comparisons to be made. Tabular presentations, including confidence intervals (*CI*s) for between-group summary differences, can to some extent be useful for this purpose although these too may not necessarily give a complete or appropriate summary of the situation. Just as the use of a regression model was the more powerful analytic tool when investigating the role of age on PROs in Chapter 12, so modelling is also important here. However, modelling longitudinal data with missing observations is a relatively complex process, and it will usually benefit from a detailed examination of the data by the methods discussed in Chapter 13 before proceeding to this stage.

One important aspect of longitudinal data is that the observations may not be independent. This contrasts with cross-sectional data in which there is, for the particular PRO item under consideration, a single variable whose value in a subject will not depend on the magnitude of the corresponding value in other subjects. In longitudinal analysis we have repeated measures on the same subject, and so successive observations are unlikely to be independent. This is one reason why care in analysis and presentation are important.

14.2 Auto-correlation

Section 5.3 introduced the use of the correlation coefficient in several situations and defined the correlation coefficient with equation (5.1). We repeat that equation here, introducing some notational differences with x_1 and x_2 replacing the variables x and y respectively of the former equation. Thus:

$$r_T(1,2) = \frac{\sum (x_{i1} - \bar{x}_1)(x_{i2} - \bar{x}_2)}{\sqrt{\sum (x_{i1} - \bar{x}_1)^2 \sum (x_{i2} - \bar{x}_2)^2}}. \tag{14.1}$$

Here x_{i1} and x_{i2} represent the values of two successive assessments of the *same* PRO item or scale, from the *same* instrument, made by the *i*th patient. For example, these may be their emotional functioning (EF) values at the time of randomisation and one month later. Previously x and y had represented two different PROs from the same or different instruments, reported at a single time – for example, EF and performance status (PS) values immediately before treatment commences.

Equation (14.1) is termed the *auto-*, or *serial-*correlation, and measures the strength of the association between successive (longitudinal) measurements of a single PRO on the same patient.

This will be a Pearson correlation if x_1 and x_2 have the Normal distribution form, or the Spearman rank correlation if they do not. The expression is symmetric in terms of x_1 and x_2, and hence $r_T(1,2) = r_T(2,1)$. The notation for correlation coefficients such as $r_T(1,2)$ is reduced to r_T if the context is clear.

Auto-correlation matrix

Suppose QoL is assessed on numerous occasions and the values of one PRO at different times are $Q_{j0}, Q_{j1}, \ldots, Q_{jT}$ for patient j in the study. Then equation (14.1) can be utilised, one pair of these observations at a time, with the respective Q replacing the x values. The resulting correlations are the auto-correlations that we denote by, for example, $r_T(0,3)$. We use T to emphasise the time element and the 0 and 3 indicating that we are correlating the baseline and third follow-up PRO assessments. If there are assessments at $T + 1$ time points, there will be $(T + 1)T/2$ pairs of assessments leading to separate auto-correlation coefficients. For example, for $T = 5$ there are $(6 \times 5)/2 = 15$ auto-correlation coefficients that may be calculated, from $r_T(0,1)$ through to $r_T(4,5)$.

Example

Figure 14.1 shows the scatter plot of EORTC QLQ-C30 EF scores at the baseline (pre-treatment) assessment (EF_0) against the corresponding scores one month after starting treatment (EF_1), for 457 patients with multiple myeloma. The Pearson auto-correlation coefficient between these two assessments (one month apart) is 0.61. The Spearman auto-correlation coefficient with the same data gives 0.58 – a very similar figure.

In fact, QoL assessment in this example was also carried out at 6, 12, 24, 36 and 48 months during therapy. Thus Table 14.1 summarises the resulting 15 auto-correlation pairs for the assessments until month 36, while Figure 14.2 gives a panel of the corresponding scatter diagrams.

It can be seen from Table 14.1 that the auto-correlation coefficients are moderately large (between 0.39 and 0.65) and that once on-treatment (month one onwards) the auto-correlations are above 0.54 for all pairs of measurements up to two years apart.

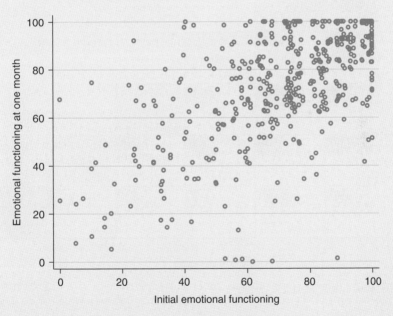

Figure 14.1 Scatter plot of emotional functioning (*EF*) for multiple myeloma patients, prior to treatment and one month after starting treatment. *Source:* Data from Wisløff *et al.*, 1996.

Table 14.1 Matrix of Pearson auto-correlation coefficients for *EF* of multiple myeloma patients immediately prior to and during the first 36 months of therapy

Emotional functioning	0	1	6	12	24	36
0	1					
1	0.61	1				
6	0.44	0.54	1			
12	0.46	0.57	0.65	1		
24	0.39	0.54	0.55	0.60	1	
36	0.47	0.47	0.49	0.57	0.54	1

Source: Data from Wisløff *et al.*, 1996.

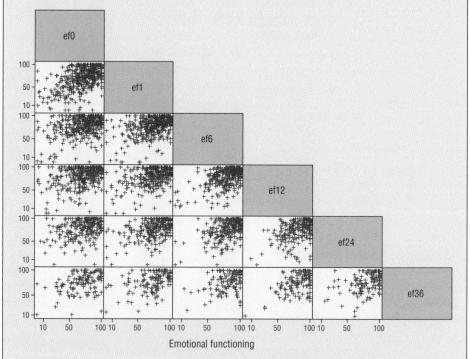

Figure 14.2 Pairwise scatter diagrams for *EF* of multiple myeloma patients immediately prior to and during the first 36 months of therapy. *Source:* Data from Wisløff *et al.*, 1996.

It should be noted from Figure 14.2 (and similarly for Table 14.1) that the scatter plots are only given beneath the leading diagonal since the plot of, for example, x_1 against x_2 provides the same information as x_2 against x_1 and so has the same value for the correlation coefficient.

Auto-correlation patterns

The pattern of an auto-correlation matrix, such as that of Table 14.1, gives a guide to the so-called *error structure* associated with the successive measurements.

Example from the literature

Cnaan *et al.* (1997, Table IV) give the correlation matrix after fitting a statistical model to patients assessed by the total score from the Brief Psychiatric Rating Scale (BPRS). One correlation matrix was calculated after fitting a statistical model that included the variables: baseline BPRS, treatment, centre and week. These correlations are given in the lower left half of Table 14.2.

Examination of these values suggests an underlying pattern of decreasing correlation as the observations become further apart. For example $r_T(2,3) = 0.76$ whereas $r_T(2,6) = 0.60$. The time difference or lag between the observations are $3 - 2 = 1$ week and $6 - 2 = 4$ weeks respectively.

Table 14.2 Auto-correlation matrices derived from patients with schizophrenia assessed with the BPRS calculated after fitting two statistical models

Week	1	2	3	4	5	6
1	1	*0.61*	*0.50*	*0.27*	–	*0.32*
2	0.63	1	*0.75*	*0.59*	–	*0.60*
3	0.52	0.76	1	*0.73*	–	*0.67*
4	0.34	0.64	0.77	1	–	*0.77*
5	–	–	–	–	1	–
6	0.35	0.60	0.72	0.85	–	1

Source: Adapted from Cnaan *et al.*, 1997, Tables IV and V. Reproduced with permission of John Wiley & Sons, Ltd.

Although in this example no assessment was made at week 5, we have included the corresponding row and column in Table 14.2 to emphasise this gap in observations. In general QoL assessments will not be evenly spaced, and this may obscure the underlying patterns somewhat. Thus it is more difficult to examine the patterns given in Table 14.1 as the time intervals between successive assessments are mostly unequal and of quite different periods. A further problem arises if patients depart from the prescribed QoL assessment schedules, although this may be partially overcome by identifying acceptable windows as outlined in Chapter 13.

Several underlying patterns of the auto-correlation matrix are used in the modelling of longitudinal PRO data. These include *independent*, *exchangeable*, *multiplicative*, *unstructured* and *user-fixed*. Burton *et al.* (1998) give a detailed description.

The error structure is *independent* (sometimes termed *random*) if the off-diagonal terms of the auto-correlation matrix are zero. The repeated observations of an outcome on the same subject are then independent of each other and can be regarded as though they were observations from different individuals.

On the other hand, if all the correlations are approximately equal the matrix of correlation coefficients is termed *exchangeable*, or *compound symmetric*. This means that we can re-order (exchange) the successive (timed) observations in any way we choose in our data file without affecting the pattern in the correlation matrix. It may be reasonable to suppose that this is the underlying pattern suggested by the correlation matrix of Table 14.1 in which the values of the auto-correlations fluctuate around approximately $r_T = 0.5$.

Frequently, as the time or lag between the successive observations increases, the auto-correlation between the observations decreases. Thus we would expect a higher auto-correlation between PRO assessments made only two days apart than between two PRO assessments made one month apart. In such a situation one may postulate that the relationship between the size of the correlation and the *lag*, that is the time between t_1 and t_2, may be of the form

$$\rho_T(t_1, t_2) = \rho^{\varphi|t_2 - t_1|}.$$

$$(14.2)$$

The $|t_2 - t_1|$ implies that if the difference between t_2 and t_1 is negative the sign should be ignored, and φ takes a constant value that is usually less than one. A correlation matrix of this form is called *multiplicative*, or *time series*.

Example

Suppose the true auto-correlation between the first two of many successive but equally spaced PRO assessments is $\rho_T(0,1) = \rho_T = 0.546$. Then, on the basis of equation (14.2) with $\varphi = 0.6$, the auto-correlation between the baseline ($t = 0$) and the second follow-up assessments ($t = 2$) is anticipated to be $\rho_T(0,2) = \rho^{0.6 \times |2-0|} = 0.546^{0.6 \times 2} = 0.484$. Further, that between baseline and third assessment, $\rho_T(0,3) = \rho^{0.6 \times |3-0|} = 0.546^{0.6 \times 3} = 0.336$ and is clearly smaller.

Finally, the *unstructured* auto-correlation matrix presumes no particular pattern or structure to the correlation matrix, while one that is *user-fixed* has, as the term indicates, values that are specified by the user.

The auto-correlation pattern materially affects the way in which the computer package estimates the regression coefficients in the corresponding statistical model, and so it should be chosen with care.

14.3   Repeated measures

ANOVA

In some situations, QoL assessment may be made over a limited period rather than over an extended time span. In this case it may be reasonable to assume that all subjects complete all the assessments. Thus instead of having a ragged data file with the number of observations for each subject varying from subject to subject, the file has a rectangular shape. This enables an ANOVA approach to be considered.

The rationale for repeated-measures ANOVA is to regard time also as a factor in addition to, for example, treatment. In a two-treatment randomised clinical trial, the treatment factor has two levels and each patient is randomised to one of the treatment options, or factor levels. However, although time may also be considered a factor with T levels it is not randomised, as successive QoL assessments necessarily follow one after the other. As a consequence, the structure of the underlying statistical model has to be modified to take account of this.

This structure is a *split-plot* design, where the term *plot* arises as the particular design was first introduced in agricultural research and the plot referred to a small piece of ground. In our situation each 'plot' is a subject and the time of the QoL assessment is a 'sub-plot'.

For the case of g treatments being compared in a clinical trial having T QoL assessments on each of m patients per treatment group, the ANOVA corresponding to Table 12.8 is extended to take the form of Table 14.3.

The sub-plot nature of this design results in two residual or error variance terms in Table 14.3. One assesses the between-patient variability within treatment groups and is used to test the hypothesis of no differences between treatments using the F-ratio of Table T5 with $(g - 1)$ and $g(m - 1)$ degrees of freedom. The second is used to test the hypothesis of no change in a PRO measure over time using the F-ratio with $(T - 1)$ and $g(m - 1)(T - 1)$ degrees of freedom. The F-ratio is used also to test for the interaction between Treatment and Time. If an interaction is present, this suggests that any differences in treatments observed do not remain constant over time. We discuss this in detail later.

Repeated-measures ANOVA is an attempt to provide a single analysis of a complete longitudinal dataset. In such studies, the patients are often termed *Level 2* units and the repeated PRO assessments the *Level 1* units. This terminology leads to the more general *multilevel* models that we return to later. The use of the repeated-measures ANOVA implies an *exchangeable* auto-correlation between any two observations on the same patient (Diggle *et al.*, 2002). This may not always be appropriate for PRO assessments.

Modelling

The main difficulty with repeated-measures ANOVA, in the context of QoL research, is that there are seldom equal numbers of QoL assessments recorded per patient or subject. Although ANOVA methodology can be extended to handle some *unbalanced* situations, in the standard format shown in Table 14.3 the number of assessments must

Table 14.3 Layout for the repeated measures ANOVA for comparing g treatments, in m subjects per treatment with an outcome observed on T successive occasions

Source of variation	Sums of squares	df	Mean squares	F
Between treatments	$S_{Treatment}$	$g-1$	$M_{Treatment} = S_{Treatment}/(g-1)$	$F_{Treatment} = M_{Treatment}/M_{Patient}$
Patient residual	$S_{Patient}$	$g(m-1)$	$M_{Patient} = S_{Patient}/g(m-1)$	
Between times	S_{Time}	$T-1$	$M_{Time} = S_{Time}/(T-1)$	$F_{Time} = M_{Time}/M_{TimeResidual}$
Interaction	$S_{Treatment*Time}$	$(g-1)(T-1)$	$M_{Treatment*Time} = S_{Treatment*Time}/(T-1)$	$F_{Treatment*Time} = M_{Treatment*Time}/M_{TimeResidual}$
Time residual	$S_{TimeResidual}$	$g(m-1)(T-1)$	$M_{TimeResidual} = S_{TimeResidual}/[(m-g)(T-1)]$	
Total	S_{Total}	$gmT-1$		

Example

Wisløff *et al.* (1996) describe a randomised clinical trial in which the fatigue (*FA*) of patients with myeloma receiving either melphalan-prednisone (MP) or melphalan–prednisone + interferon (MP+IFN) was assessed on several occasions over a four-year period. If we assume the exchangeable pattern for the correlation matrix, the bold entries of Table 14.4 give a summary of the results of fitting equation (14.3) to part of the data. The numbers in parentheses represent the respective standard errors (*SE*s).

Considering the on-treatment data from month 1 to month 36, the results of fitting this model are shown as model II of Table 14.4, in which:

$$FA = 41.41 + 5.26x_i - 0.30t.$$

Table 14.4 Analysis of fatigue (*FA*) levels in patients with myeloma receiving either MP or MP+IFN. Patients with complete information on assessments from month 1 up to and including month 36. Cells contain estimates and *SE*.

Model	Regression coefficient	Type of auto-correlation matrix			
		Exchangeable	Independent	Unstructured	Multiplicative
I	Constant, α	38.21	38.21	36.60	39.35
	Treatment, τ	5.26 (2. 40)	5.26 (1.54)	5.30 (2.40)	5.10 (2.24)
II	Constant, α	**41.41**	41.40	41.73	42.23
	Treatment, τ	**5.26 (2.40)**	5.26 (1.53)	5.18 (2.40)	5.10 (2.23)
	Time, β	**−0.30 (0.06)**	−0.30 (0.09)	−0.30 (0.07)	−0.25 (0.08)
III	Constant, α	39.02	39.02	39.32	39.85
	Treatment, τ	10.05 (2.76)	10.05 (2.45)	9.97 (2.82)	9.86 (2.92)
	Time, β	−0.07 (0.09)	−0.07 (0.13)	−0.09 (0.10)	−0.04 (0.12)
	Interaction, γ	−0.45 (0.13)	−0.45 (0.18)	−0.43 (0.13)	−0.42 (0.17)
IV	Constant, α	22.36	22.36	21.43	22.36
	Treatment, τ	9.25 (2.49)	9.25 (2.45)	9.07 (2.47)	9.05 (2.65)
	Time, β	−0.07 (0.09)	−0.07 (0.12)	−0.01 (0.12)	−0.05 (0.11)
	Interaction, γ	−0.45 (0.13)	−0.45 (0.16)	−0.43 (0.13)	−0.42 (0.16)
	Baseline FA, ϕ	0.35 (0.04)	0.35 (0.03)	0.37 (0.04)	0.37 (0.04)

Source: Data from Wisløff *et al.*, 1996.

From this model one deduces that as time goes by, that is as *t* increases, reported fatigue decreases while those patients also receiving IFN score approximately 5.3 units higher on each occasion. For example, at $t = 1$, the first assessment post-commencement of treatment, those who received MP alone had $FA_{MP} = 41.41 - 0.30 = 41.11$, while those also receiving IFN had $FA_{IFN} = 41.41 + 5.26 - 0.30 = 46.37$. The contribution due to time, −0.30, is in both expressions, as is the constant term 41.41, and so the difference $FA_{IFN} - FA_{MP} = 5.26$ remains the same at each assessment. Using equation (12.1) the ratios $z = -0.30/0.06 = -5.0$ and $z = 5.26/2.40 = 2.2$ imply, from Table T1, p-values of < 0.0001 and 0.026 for the time and treatment effects respectively. These suggest a statistically significant decline in fatigue with time, but higher levels of fatigue in those receiving IFN.

be equal for all patients. However, we mentioned in Chapter 12 that ANOVA is a model-based form of analysis and this remains so in the repeated-measures situation. It is therefore possible – and usually simpler – to use a regression-modelling approach rather than repeated-measures ANOVA. The regression model corresponding to the analysis of Table 14.3 can be written as

$$Q_{jit} = \alpha + \tau x_i + \beta t + \omega_{jit}. \tag{14.3}$$

Here Q_{jit} is the assessment of a PRO for patient j at assessment time t and who is receiving treatment i, and $x_i = 0$ corresponds to the patient receiving one of the treatments whereas $x_i = 1$ for the other treatment. The ω_{jit} is the *error* or *residual term* similar to the ε introduced in equation (12.22). However, as shown in Table 14.3, there are two residual terms corresponding to 'Patient Residual' and 'Time Residual'. This implies that each ω_{jit} really has two parts, one a between-patients component and the other a within-patient component. We have been investigating the within-patient component when examining the patterns in the auto-correlation matrices.

Use of the basic model in equation (14.3) implies that the outcome changes in a linear way with time. That is, the scatter diagrams of PRO profiles of patients against time should appear, at least approximately, as straight lines and have the same slope from patient to patient. A second assumption is that if the value if the outcome differs between patients on the two treatments, it is the same difference at each assessment time.

Once we specify the form of the model and the pattern of the auto-correlation, this model can be fitted using most standard statistical packages.

In the model indicated by bold numbers in Table 14.4, we have not considered the interaction component of Table 14.3, and so the comparison with repeated-measures ANOVA is not quite complete. However, before discussing the interaction we show the basic steps involved in constructing statistical models.

Model building

The major research question in the context of a clinical trial is the treatment effect, and so of primary interest is τ in the following model:

$$Q_{jit} = \alpha + \tau x_i + \omega_{jit}. \tag{14.4}$$

This is a simplified version of equation (14.3), setting $\beta = 0$ so that the time element is not included. Fitting this model, again using the exchangeable auto-correlation matrix, gives (model I of Table 14.4) $FA = 38.21 + 5.26x_i$. The treatment effect is significant since $z = 5.26/2.40 = 2.2, p = 0.026$. Although this is statistically significant, the model building process asks if there are other and additional variables that might also explain some of the variation in the outcome. In our context, the next model to consider is equation (14.3), which, once fitted, confirms the statistical significance of the treatment effect but also suggests that time plays a role ($z = -0.30/0.06 = -5.0, p < 0.0001$). However the view of the effect of treatment remains unchanged.

Auto-regression

Although we have already introduced an auto-regression model in equation (14.3) as a means of effecting a repeated-measures ANOVA, we now examine a rather simpler model so as to explain the role of β. Since in longitudinal studies there are not only observations

Example from the literature

Hart *et al.* (1997) investigated the value of homeopathic arnica C30 for pain in patients after total abdominal hysterectomy. They present individual plots to demonstrate the variety of pain score changes against time after operation. One of these profiles, for a patient receiving arnica as opposed to placebo, is reproduced in Figure 14.3. The profile chosen is approximately linear over the study period so that equation (14.5) may be a reasonable description in this case.

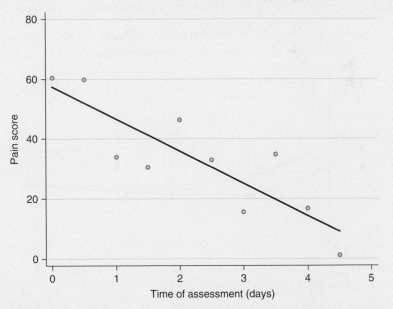

Figure 14.3   Pain score changes for a patient receiving arnica following total abdominal hysterectomy. *Source:* Adapted from Hart *et al.*, 1997. Reproduced with permission of Sage Publications, Ltd.

on many subjects but also repeating observations over time on the same subjects, we may wish to investigate changes in the outcomes over time, using a linear regression model. Thus we might propose that the outcome changes with time according to the expression

$$Q_t = \alpha + \beta t + \omega_t. \tag{14.5}$$

This has much the same form as equation (12.24) but t, denoting time, replaces x_j and we write ω_t in place of ε_j. With this expression we are saying that the outcome for *an individual patient* changes with *time* according to this linear model. Now, in contrast to equation (12.24), the observations are all made on the same subject and so the ω values cannot be assumed to be independent or uncorrelated.

In general we will have more than a single subject and so the more general form of equation (14.5) for subject j is

$$Q_{jt} = \alpha + \beta t + \omega_{jt}. \tag{14.6}$$

Interactions

A plot of the Wisløff *et al.* data is shown in Figure 14.4, and this suggests that it is unrealistic to assume that the mean difference between the values remains constant over time. The graph suggests there is a treatment difference at month 1, which has largely disappeared by month 36. This is a Treatment × Time *interaction*. The corresponding statistical test using the repeated-measures ANOVA of Table 14.3 compares $F_{Treatment*Time}$ against an F-ratio that has $(g-1)(T-1)$ and $g(m-1)(T-1)$ degrees of freedom.

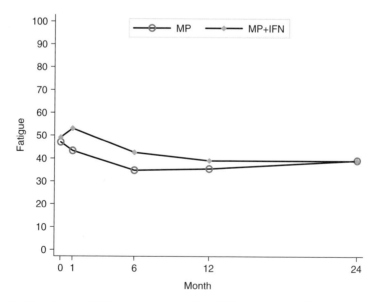

Figure 14.4 Mean levels of fatigue in patients with multiple myeloma, before and during treatment with MP or MP+IFN. *Source:* Data from Wisløff *et al.*, 1996.

To model the interaction a further regression coefficient, γ, has to be added to equation (14.3). This is attached to the product of x_i and t, giving

$$Q_{jit} = \alpha + \tau x_i + \beta t + \gamma x_i t + \omega_{jit}. \tag{14.7}$$

Using the example data, this is shown as model III in Table 14.4. The corresponding z is $-0.45/0.13 = -3.5$, which from Table T1 gives $p = 0.0023$ and is statistically significant.

It is important to note that there is a large change in the regression coefficient for treatment, from 5.26 with model II to 10.05 with model III. This arises because there is also a change in the interpretation of τ. In model II, τ represents the average treatment effect, averaged over the observations at 1, 6, 12 and 24 months. Inspecting Figure 14.4, at month one the difference is of the order of 10 units of FA, while at month 24 it is close to zero, with intermediate values at months 6 and 12. These provide an average value of approximately 5 units of FA. In contrast, the τ of 10.05 in model III is interpreted as the estimated difference between treatments were observations to be made at $t = 0$, just after treatment commenced, rather than at baseline which is just before treatment commenced. At $t = 0$ the contribution of the interaction term of equation (14.7) is zero, whereas at later assessments the interaction term enters the model given by equation (14.7) and reduces the value of the estimated treatment effect. Thus for IFN at $t = 1$ (the first post-treatment assessment), $x_i = 1$, $\gamma x_i t = -0.45 \times 1 \times 1 = -0.45$. This reduces the estimated effect of treatment to $10.05 - 0.45 = 9.60$ units of FA. By 12 months, at $t = 12$, we have $\gamma x_i t = -0.45 \times 1 \times 12 = -5.40$ and so the treatment effect is reduced to $10.05 - 5.40 = 4.65$. The estimates that are provided by model III are close to those suggested by Figure 14.4.

Paired data

We have discussed a special case of equation (14.7) in Section 12.4 when the baseline outcome measure (at $t = 0$) is compared with a later value at some fixed time (which can be arbitrarily labelled $t = 1$). Using equation (14.7) at $t = 0$ and $t = 1$ we have for subject j, $Q_{j0} = \alpha + \omega_{j0}$ and $Q_{j1} = \alpha + \beta + \omega_{j1}$ respectively. Their difference is $D_j = Q_{j1} - Q_{j0} = \alpha + \beta + \omega_{j1} - \alpha - \omega_{j0}$, giving

$$D_j = \beta + (\omega_{j1} - \omega_{j0}).$$

The null hypothesis of no difference between baseline and subsequent outcome assessments corresponds to $\beta = 0$. Each subject has his or her own error term, here $(\omega_{j1} - \omega_{j0})$, which comprises the residuals from both the time 0 (baseline) and time 1 observations. The value that this difference takes for a particular patient will be independent of the values taken by other subjects in the study. They are thus uncorrelated.

The data in this situation are termed *paired*. For a particular study with N subjects observed at baseline and at one further occasion, the estimate of β is $b = \bar{D}$ with $SE(b) = SD / \sqrt{N}$ where SD is the standard deviation obtained from the differences D_j.

This in turn leads to a paired z-test version of equation (12.1), or a paired t-test if the study is small, for testing the differences in an outcome on these two occasions. Thus, if there are only two assessment times, longitudinal data can be reduced to single measurements per patient (change in outcome), and so no new principles are involved and the analysis has become cross-sectional in nature.

Between- and within-subject variation

Earlier we examined the possible forms of the error term in the regression model of equation (14.3), and there were several options available. The model described a particular subject, j, but we may wish to extend this to a group of N subjects. In doing this, there are several further choices to make. One possibility is to assume that all subjects have the same PRO profile with respect to time, apart from random variation. In this case, the model remains as equation (14.7) but the error must now contain components that include random fluctuations accounting for both within- and between-subject variation. We shall explore this using generalised estimating equations.

Generalised estimating equations

Repeated-measures ANOVA is a form of *fixed effects model*, and it also implies that the auto-correlation structure is of the exchangeable form. Applying this methodology to some of the data of Wisløff *et al.* (1996) gave the model introduced in bold in Table 14.4. However, models using the other forms of auto-correlation matrix, independent, unstructured or multiplicative, can be fitted using so-called generalised estimating equations (GEE). This methodology is implemented in many statistical packages.

Example

Applying the GEE methodology to the fatigue data of Wisløff *et al.* (1996), assuming independent, unstructured and multiplicative forms of the auto-correlation matrix, gives the results summarised in Table 14.4. Focusing on model III as this seems most appropriate for these data, the estimated regression provided by the exchangeable and independent models are the same, but the *SE* associated with the treatment effect is smaller, while the *SE* for time and the interaction *SE* are somewhat larger. Both the corresponding estimates of the regression coefficients and their *SE*s of the unstructured and multiplicative auto-correlation models differ from one another and from both the exchangeable and independent models. Thus the results change with the underlying auto-correlation structure assumed. Nevertheless, the models are in broad agreement, suggesting a statistically significant Treatment effect and evidence of a Treatment × Time interaction.

In practice it is often difficult to choose whether an exchangeable, unstructured or multiplicative auto-correlation structure is appropriate. Sometimes the choice remains unclear despite examining the initial and subsequent (after model fitting) correlation matrices. In this case, models may be developed using each of the alternatives and these are then compared. If the models are all similar both with respect to the variables included and the corresponding regression coefficients, there is little difficulty about which to choose for interpretation. Conversely, if there are major differences, this is an indication for further investigation.

The general methodology of GEE is very flexible and in principle can deal with all the observed data from a QoL study. The subjects are not required to have exactly the same numbers of assessments, and the assessments can be made at variable times. The latter allows the modelling to proceed even if a subject misses an assessment. This assumes that the probability of being missing is independent of any of the random terms (the residuals) in the model. However, care is still needed here, as this assumption may not hold. The very fact that the data are 'missing' may itself be informative (see Section 15.5). In this circumstance, taking no particular note of its absence may result in incorrect conclusions being drawn from the data.

Although the detail need not concern us too much, the process of fitting GEE models begins by assuming the independence form of the auto-correlation matrix. Thus it begins by fitting the model as if each assessment were from a different patient. Once this model is obtained, the corresponding residuals – see equation (12.23) – are calculated and these are then used to estimate the auto-correlation matrix assuming it is the exchangeable type. This matrix is then used to fit the model again and the residual once more calculated and the auto-correlation matrix obtained. This process is repeated until the corresponding regression coefficients that are obtained in the successive models differ little on successive occasions, that is, they converge. This process is termed *iteration*.

Example

The lower diagonal of Table 14.5 shows the independence form of the auto-correlation matrix of the Wisløff *et al.* (1996) data prior to fitting a GEE model of treatment, time and their interaction.

Thus while the model-fitting values of r_T average approximately 0.5, the final exchangeable value is lower at 0.4. It will usually be the case that after model fitting the auto-correlations will appear to have been reduced.

Table 14.5 Matrices of auto-correlation coefficients for *FA* of multiple myeloma patients during the first 24 months of therapy. The lower diagonal gives the independence matrix before model-fitting, while the upper gives the exchangeable form after model-fitting

Fatigue	1	6	12	24
1	1	0.40	0.40	0.40
6	0.62	1	0.40	0.40
12	0.48	0.61	1	0.40
24	0.39	0.47	0.56	1

Source: Data from Wisløff *et al.*, 1996.

Fixed and random effects

Although we may postulate that the slope of the regression line β can be assumed the same for all subjects, each may have a different starting point. This can be expressed by modifying α of equation (14.6) to α_j to give

$$Q_{jt} = \alpha_j + \beta t + \omega_{jt}. \tag{14.8}$$

Again there are options here. One is to assume that α_j (the intercept) is unique for each of the N subjects and so there are N of these to estimate. This model is termed a *fixed-effects model*, since a different effect is estimated (or fixed) for each subject. An alternative is to assume that the subjects chosen for study are a random sample of subjects from a population that has mean α and a standard deviation σ_α. In fitting this latter model we estimate for the first term of equation (14.8) with only the two parameters, α and σ_α, rather than N individual values for α_j. This second approach is termed a *random-effects model*.

It is important to note that a possible confusion of terms arises, as 'random' is used in two contexts. Here, it describes a property of the α_j regression coefficients in the model of equation (14.8). In descriptions of auto-correlation matrices (see Table 14.2), it is commonly applied to the ω_{jt} error part of the model, when *random* is an alternative term for the *independent* error structure.

In the random-effects model, one is effectively modelling α by means of the following equation:

$$\alpha_j = \alpha + v_j, \tag{14.9}$$

where α is the fixed part of this model and v_j is the residual, error or random part, which is assumed to have a mean of zero and standard deviation σ_α. In this case, the format of equation (14.8) changes to

$$Q_{jt} = \alpha + \beta t + v_j + \omega_{jt}. \tag{14.10}$$

Thus we are introducing a second component to the residual variation, which now comprises both v_j and ω_{jt}.

One can go a step further than having a random-effects model for the intercept α alone by also postulating that the slope β can be dealt with in a similar way, so that different patients can have different slopes. This leads from equation (14.8) to

$$Q_{jt} = \alpha_j + \beta_j t + \omega_{jt}. \tag{14.11}$$

In this situation, the β_j can either be estimated from a fixed-effects model or regarded as having mean β and a standard deviation σ_β in a random-effects model. The latter can be expressed as $\beta_j = \beta + \eta_j$, where η_j is the corresponding residual that is assumed to have a mean of zero and standard deviation σ_β.

Finally, in order to make use of regression techniques to compare two treatments with respect to longitudinal outcomes, we have to extend the above models to include a regression coefficient for treatment. Thus we write, for example:

$$Q_{jit} = \alpha_j + \tau x_i + \beta_j t + \omega_{jit}, \qquad (14.12)$$

This model can specify either fixed- or random-effects for either or both of α and β. Models that contain both fixed and random effects are termed *mixed*.

The advantage of the random-effects model is that there are fewer regression parameters to estimate. It is based upon the assumption that the subjects in the study are chosen at

---

Example from the literature

A mixed-effects repeated measures model was used by Homs *et al.* (2004) in reporting a multicentre randomised trial that compared brachytherapy versus stent placement for the palliation of dysphagia from oesophageal cancer. Day of assessment and treatment group were fixed effects. Baseline scores were used as covariates. A day by treatment group interaction term allowed for differing curves. Brachytherapy was beneficial over time on most of the QoL endpoints, including dysphagia. There was a significant time-treatment interaction. The authors also fit so-called cubic spline functions, to obtain smooth-curve esti-mates of the degree of dysphagia over time for each treatment with 95% CIs (Figure 14.5). This plot confirmed the presence of a treatment-time interaction, with brachytherapy being beneficial after about six months, and a suggestion that stents might be more effective during the first four months.

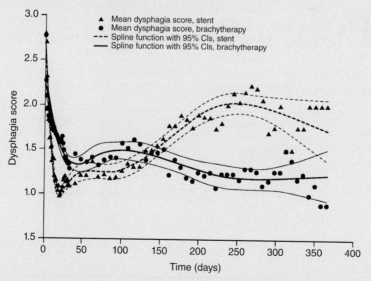

Figure 14.5 Brachytherapy or metal stent for palliation of dysphagia from oesophageal cancer. *Source:* Homs *et al.*, 2004. Reproduced with permission of Elsevier.

random from some wider patient population. This will seldom be true, at least in the context of a clinical trial for which trial patients are screened for eligibility and entered only after giving informed consent. Thus although the treatment assigned is 'at random', this is a very different use of the word random, and does not imply that random-effects models are necessarily appropriate; once again, there is multiple use of the same word describing different situations. However, it is usually reasonable to assume that the trial patients have been chosen at random from a large number of potentially eligible patients, and that they represent a random selection from this artificial population. Thus a random-effects model is frequently applied whenever a study includes large numbers of patients.

In clinical trials it is common for the randomisation to be stratified by centre. In this case centre should be one of the covariates, but should it be regarded as a fixed or a random effect? Some authors suggest that random is preferable (Kahan and Morris, 2013).

Multilevel models

If we assume a random-effects model is appropriate, models can be fitted using *multilevel modelling*. This is available both in many standard statistical packages or in

---

Example

Applying the multilevel methodology to the selected *FA* data from Wisløff *et al.* (1996) gives the results summarised in model III of Table 14.6. Here the mixed model includes the treatment (τ) as a *fixed effect*, and the intercept (α) and time (β) are *random effects*. This can be compared with the model III results summarised in Table 14.4. The model suggests a statistically significant treatment effect and a strong Treatment × Time interaction as we had observed before. The regression coefficients and *SEs* do not differ materially from those of Table 14.4.

Table 14.6 Multilevel modelling analysis of *FA* levels in patients with myeloma receiving either MP or MP+IFN. Patients with complete information on assessments up to and including month 24 only

Regression coefficient	Model III		Model IV	
	Estimate (*SE*)	*p*-value	Estimate (*SE*)	*p*-value
Constant, α	39.01		21.56	
Treatment, τ 95% *CI*	10.06 (2.87) 4.43 to 15.69	0.0004	9.22 (2.44) 4.43 to 14.00	0.0002
Time, β	−0.08 (0.10)	0.47	−0.08 (0.10)	0.47
Interaction, γ	−0.45 (0.15)	0.002	−0.45 (0.13)	0.002
Baseline, ϕ	–	–	0.37 (0.04)	< 0.0001

Source: Data from Wisløff *et al.*, 1996.

specialised statistical software such as MLwiN (Rasbash *et al.*, 2009). In multilevel models, the repeated assessments within a patient are the 'Level 1' units and the patients themselves are the 'Level 2' units. Use of multilevel modelling as opposed to GEE allows a more detailed examination of the sources of variance ('errors') in the model.

It should be noted that the analysis was from 1 to 36 months with the baseline value as a covariate. Thus, because of the presence of a strong Treatment × Time interaction, the estimated effect of 10.06 and the associated 95% *CI* of 4.43–15.69 are estimates of the treatment effect at month one.

Covariates

All the models can be extended further to include covariates, in a similar way to that which we have described in equation (12.15), as it is recognised that patient-specific details may influence subsequent patient outcome measures. In the context of QoL studies, the pre-treatment values, or *baseline assessment*, may be particularly critical. For example, this is likely to be the case in circumstances where these baseline levels determine to some extent the pattern of subsequent missing data.

Example

Adding the baseline *FA* measure to the random-effects model previously discussed for the data of Wisløff *et al.* (1996) gives the model IV summarised both in Table 14.4 and the final columns of Table 14.6. The regression coefficient of baseline fatigue (FA_0) is statistically significant, suggesting its major influence on subsequent reported levels.

If baseline variables or other prognostic indicators are important predictors of outcome, they may be expected to account for some of the otherwise unexplained variability in the data. As a consequence, some of the *SE*s for other coefficients may become smaller when these strong predictors are included. This means both that we have better estimates of the coefficients – including those for the treatment effect – and that their *p*-values may become more highly significant. However, if we include unnecessary variables in the model, such as those baseline characteristics that are irrelevant to subsequent outcome, we are in effect adding more noise, which will weaken the estimation of treatment effect. One should resist the temptation to add a large number of covariates just because 'they may be important'.

In a randomised trial, the baseline (pre-randomisation) characteristics may be anticipated to be broadly similar in the different groups of patients because of the randomisation procedure itself, and so the estimate of the treatment effect is unlikely to be biased. However, as in this example, including covariates can alter the estimate of the treatment effect. Thus there is a suggestion that perhaps the true difference between the treatments may be a little bit smaller than when we ignored the baseline *FA* score (for example 9.25 instead of 10.05 if we assume exchangeable or independent auto-correlations).

Example from the literature

Cnaan *et al.* (1997) describe the application of general linear mixed models to a randomised clinical trial of patients with schizophrenia assessed by the total score from the BPRS. There were four treatments: three doses (low, medium and high) of an experimental drug and a control drug. Patients were evaluated at baseline, one, two, three, four and six weeks. However, of 245 patients randomised only 60% completed the six-week assessment. The results of part of their analysis using the random-effects model is summarised in Table 14.7.

The corresponding algebraic model, for a patient receiving low-dose treatment, at week W is

$$BPRS = \alpha + \tau_L + \beta_{\text{Linear}}(W-3) + \beta_{\text{Quadratic}}(W-3)^2 + \varphi BPRS_0, \qquad (14.13)$$

where τ_L indicates an offset for the low-dose group, W is the week number and $BPRS_0$ is the baseline value. The corresponding fitted equation is

$$BPRS = 1.90 + 2.04 - 1.52(W-3) + 0.37(W-3)^2 + 0.65BPRS_0.$$

At week 3, this reduces to $BPRS = 3.94 + 0.65\ BPRS_0$. Thus for patients with $BPRS_0 = 40$, the predicted score at week 3 with low-dose treatment is $3.94 + (0.65 \times 40) = 29.94$ or approximately 30.

Table 14.7   Random-effects model for changes in BPRS in patients with schizophrenia

Variable name	Parameter	Estimate	SE
Intercept	α	1.90	2.51
Low dose	τ_L	2.04	1.06
Medium dose	τ_M	−1.64	1.03
High dose	τ_H	−0.13	1.05
Week	β_{Linear}	−1.52	0.25
Week*Week	$\beta_{\text{Quadratic}}$	0.37	0.09
Baseline BPRS	φ	0.65	0.07

Source: Cnaan *et al.*, 1997, Table VI. Reproduced with permission of John Wiley & Sons, Ltd.

There are several details in this last example that require further explanation. The first is that there are four treatments involved (doses, in this example), rather than the two different treatments of equation (14.3). This implies that the τx_i part of that equation has to be expanded to $\tau_L x_{Lj} + \tau_M x_{2j} + \tau_H x_{3j}$. A patient j receiving the control treatment is indicated by $x_{Lj} = x_{Mj} = x_{Hj} = 0$. For a patient receiving a low dose, $x_{Lj} = 1$,

$x_{Mj} = x_{Hj} = 0$; for one receiving a moderate dose, $x_{Lj} = 0$, $x_{Mj} = 1$, $x_{Hj} = 0$; and for one receiving a high dose, $x_{Lj} = x_{Mj} = 0$, $x_{Hj} = 1$. The variables x_{Lj}, x_{Mj}, and x_{Hj} are called *dummy variables*.

Secondly, time in weeks occurs twice in equation (14.13). The first term with regression coefficient, β_{Linear}, is the linear and the second, $\beta_{\text{Quadratic}}$, the time-squared or quadratic part (written as Week*Week in Table 14.7). Together they express the fact that, in contrast to the example of Figure 14.3, the change in the PRO score over time may not be linear but may be somewhat curved. This can be interpreted as a decrease in BPRS scores with time, but the decrease is larger initially and then levels off; the quadratic model is analogous to an interaction in this context. Further, the equation includes $(W - 3)$ rather than W, but subtracting the 3 is merely a convenience device to ease the computational problems as squared terms tend to get large and this makes the fitting process less stable.

Finally, there is a covariate term with regression coefficient φ. This is included here since it is well known that the initial BPRS is an important predictor of future values irrespective of the treatment given. Thus any treatment comparisons need to be adjusted for variation in the baseline values for the patients.

Choosing the auto-correlation structure

Although we have illustrated this chapter with the auto-correlation matrix calculated from successive observations of *FA* in patients with myeloma, the actual matrix we really wish to examine is that obtained from the residuals. As we have noted, the residual is the difference between the observed outcome measure and the one predicted from the fitted model; this is a quantity w, which estimates the respective ω. However, we cannot determine this without first fitting the model, leading to a circular process. To avoid this, the usual procedure is to make an initial assumption about the auto-correlation structure, often as in our example based upon the auto-correlations of the observed values. Then we can fit the model, and examine whether the residuals have the form that we assumed in the first place. If so, we may accept the assumption as reasonable; if not, we may try an alternative.

Example from the literature

The model of equation (14.13) led to the lower diagonal auto-correlation matrix of Table 14.2 (Cnaan *et al.*, 1997). The upper and italicised corner was calculated using the same model but with a further covariate (patient status) added. It can be seen that the values of the auto-correlation coefficients are smaller in the upper corner than the corresponding values in the lower corner. For example, the first model gives $r_T(1, 6) = r_T(6, 1) = 0.35$ and the second model 0.32. This will generally be the case if one model contains one or more extra variables over and above those already contained in the first model. The extra variables reduce the amount of otherwise unexplained residual variation, and so the size of the ω values will in general be smaller leading to smaller correlation coefficients.

14.4   Other situations

Logistic models

So far we have assumed that the outcome under study is a continuous or scale variable that can be assumed to have a Normal distribution. However, the methodology is not confined to this situation. For example, the outcome could be an item with binary responses, in which case allowance would be made in the model-fitting process. This is done by specifying a *link function*. If the basic distribution is Normal the link is known as an *identity link*, which means the outcome is not changed for the fitting process. On the other hand, if the PRO item is binary, the basic distribution is often taken as binomial and the corresponding link is the *logit* (logistic) transformation. The left-hand side of the above equations now becomes of the form $\log_e[Q/(1-Q)]$, with equation (14.14) corresponding to equation (14.3), giving

$$\log_e\left[Q_{ji} \,/\, (1-Q_{ji})\right] = \alpha + \tau x_i + \beta t + \omega_{jit}. \tag{14.14}$$

The technical details of the methods for fitting the above models become complex, but the processes are implemented in most statistical packages that provide GEE or multilevel models. The theoretical approach is a very general one, and other distributions can be accommodated by specifying suitable link functions. Statistical packages incorporating these methods usually provide a number of choices.

MANOVA

In the previous sections we have assumed that we are dealing with a single scale or item from a QoL instrument. However, most instruments comprise several items and scales that are assessed concurrently, ranging, for example, from two for HADS (anxiety and depression) to 15 with the EORTC QLQ-C30 (five functional scales, one global health status, three symptom scales and six items). Thus the complete analysis of QoL data from a clinical study may seek to summarise multiple features, even though sensible study design should have specified in advance the one or two aspects of QoL that are of principal interest. The 'all features' analysis poses major problems for the investigator in terms of the magnitude of the task and of the complexity of the eventual summary. In principle at least, such a multivariable analysis can be drawn into a single one by extending the repeated-measures ANOVA to *multivariate analysis of variance*, or MANOVA.

MANOVA leaves unchanged the right-hand side of equations such as (14.5), which contain the *independent* or *explanatory* variables. However, the left-hand side now reflects all the PRO measures and not just the single *dependent* variable that we have so far included. This poses some immediate problems as the variables may not all be of the same type. That is, some may be binary, some ordered categorical and others continuous with a Normal distribution. However, MANOVA is not applicable unless all of the outcome variables can be assumed to have the same form, or all are reduced to, say, binary form despite the resultant loss of information. This makes the methodology less attractive. Another major difficulty is that some but not all of the responses at a particular assessment may be missing; that is, some of the items within an otherwise complete QoL assessment are not available, as opposed to the whole form being missing. The resulting patterns of items missing from forms and whole forms missing can be very complex.

In theory, a single MANOVA, perhaps focusing on a between-treatments comparison, reduces the number of statistical significance tests conducted on the data and so avoids some of the difficulties associated with multiple testing (see Section 11.9). Rasbash *et al.* (2015, Chapter 4) describe how the multilevel modelling approach can be extended to include this multivariate situation, which then removes the constraints of equal numbers of observations per subject but does not necessarily overcome difficulties associated with the pattern of missing values.

Perhaps the single greatest difficulty with the use of MANOVA arises when summarising what has taken place. This approach is not easy to explain and the results are difficult to interpret, which detracts from its routine use.

Missing data

For reasons of clarity, when describing the techniques included in this chapter we have purposely omitted detailed reference to missing data but have recognised that the numbers of observations per subject may not be equal owing to attrition. For example, in a trial with patients in advanced cancer the attrition may be caused by the death of the patient. We have assumed that prior to this the QoL assessments are all complete although not necessarily on schedule. In practice, there will be missing data and, depending on their type and volume, this may have a serious impact on the analysis and interpretation. The GEE and multilevel methodologies can be applied when some data are absent, but for every missing observation there is a reduction in the statistical power of the analysis and, perhaps more importantly, the possibility of bias leading to incorrect conclusions.

14.5   Modelling versus area under the curve

Modelling fits an overall (average) model to all patients, while allowing for random variability. Thus it implicitly assumes that all patients have broadly similar-shaped curves describing their experience. In contrast, *area under the curve (AUC)* condenses each individual patient's measurements into a summary score, and thus the shape for each patient's experience can be completely different. To that extent, *AUC* is the more robust of the two procedures. On the other hand, *AUC* loses the richness of the patterns over time, although this may to some extent be compensated by judicious accompaniment of graphical displays. Both *AUC* and modelling make a number of assumptions about linearity of responses, for example if a 100-point scale is being analysed that a shift in score from 0 to 10 is as important as a shift from 50 to 60. Both methods work best if the outcome variable has many states and can therefore be assumed to be continuous, but are generally quite robust down to seven or even fewer categories. To some extent, increasing the number/frequency of assessments over time can compensate for loss of precision due to using scales with few categories – and it is clearly of advantage to ensure that multiple assessments are made over the periods of greatest interest and/or largest variation in the patient's state. *AUC* makes explicit assumption about the equivalence of time-severity states, for example that six months with a score of 50 is equivalent to three months at 100 followed by three months at 0. However, equivalent – and equally dubious – assumptions are implicit in most modelling approaches.

Most modelling methods additionally assume that the residual unexplained variability follows a Normal distribution. Therefore floor or ceiling effects can present a serious threat to the validity of many models. *AUC*, by contrast, tends to follow a Normal distribution closely even when the original data are distinctly non-Normal; this facilitates the subsequent application of regression or other models on *AUC* scores.

The study protocol should specify the primary method analysis that will be used for hypothesis testing and claims concerning efficacy. It may well propose the use of additional methods for further exploration of the data and to support the primary analysis. Thus one pragmatic approach is to take advantage of the simplicity and robustness of *AUC* for the basic significance testing, and present this alongside a more detailed explanatory analysis that uses modelling, graphical displays and descriptive cross-sectional estimates at critical time points.

14.6   Conclusions

It should be mentioned that a wide variety of names are used in the statistical literature to describe versions of the same model, or closely similar models. These names include mixed linear; two-stage random-effects; multilevel linear; hierarchical linear and random regression coefficient models. Some of these differ only by the technical way in which the standard errors are estimated.

One difficulty associated with powerful statistical packages, which can fit numerous and complex statistical models almost instantly, is that they may be used as a black box by the unwary. All of the models used in these procedures make assumptions about the nature of the data, and these assumptions are then reflected in the resulting output. In some situations, any visual inspection of the data will indicate what is and what is not sensible in relation to the non-error part of the model. For example, Figure 13.6c would suggest that baseline values are very similar across the treatment groups, but it may not be sensible to assume that PROs change linearly with time. An appropriate model would attempt to describe the early advantage in the reduction of HADS anxiety of the four-drug regimen. In addition, there is the problem of specifying the appropriate auto-correlation structure.

There is a further difficulty. We have stated repeatedly that the major endpoint measures for any study of PROs must be pre-specified in the protocol, and this should also be true of the models proposed to describe these data. Our experience is that this is rarely done, one reason being the unfamiliarity of many investigators with the longitudinal values, in the context of any particular study, of the outcomes being assessed. When there is a lack of experience, simple cross-sectional analyses may be appropriate, with the more complex statistical models being regarded as tentative and exploratory. These models can then form the basis for a better understanding of the processes in future studies.

15
Missing data

Summary

This chapter describes problems that arise through missing QoL assessment data. Situations are outlined where values are missing from otherwise complete questionnaires or where entire forms are missing. The main difficulty with either type of missing data is the bias they may introduce at the analysis stage. We distinguish QoL data that are 'missing' through *attrition* because the patient has died, from that which is *missing* in the sense that the patient was alive and could have completed a questionnaire although one was not returned.

We describe how missing values may be estimated, often termed as *imputed*, to ease the statistical analysis, but stress that imputing values is no substitute for collecting real data.

15.1   Introduction

Difficulties with data collection and compliance are major barriers to the successful implementation of QoL assessments in clinical trials. The principal problem is that bias may be introduced through data that are missing because patients either drop out of the trial completely or do not participate comprehensively in the QoL assessment. The issue is then whether the data actually collected are representative of the QoL of all study patients, including those without data, in such a way that the analysis can be taken as a reliable reflection of the study outcome. If the missing data can be regarded as absent at random, they will on average be similar to the available data. If not, the summary derived only from those who provide data may no longer be representative. In this case, the available patient data will give a biased view that will not reflect the true situation.

Considerations of potential bias raise questions of whether the missing data are missing at random or not at random, and what proportion of missing data is acceptable in a trial or study. In the context of a randomised trial, there is the question of the

Quality of Life: The Assessment, Analysis and Reporting of Patient-Reported Outcomes, Third Edition.
Peter M. Fayers and David Machin.
© 2016 John Wiley & Sons, Ltd. Published 2016 by John Wiley & Sons, Ltd.

impact of ignoring missing data. For example, what are the implications of assuming that if the patterns of missing data are similar in all treatment groups, treatment comparisons will be unbiased? If the impact of missing data cannot be ignored, how can one estimate or allow for the missing data when analysing the trial?

In some situations, the fact that data are absent may be *informative*, in that this tells us something about the patient from whom they are missing. We need to take note of this information. For example, suppose the likelihood of a missing assessment is high when a patient's health deteriorates just prior to death. Then any analysis of QoL should take account of this pattern, and should recognise that missing values immediately prior to death are more likely to be associated with poor QoL. These values are likely to be different from those that are missing at times distant from death, when patients are expected to be healthier and when the reason for their being missing is more likely to be accidental.

QoL data are usually collected using a self-assessment questionnaire containing a series of questions. Critically, once a patient has missed a QoL assessment, the retrospective collection of the patient response is rarely possible although some other types of clinical data may often be collected from the patient's routine medical charts.

There is a clear distinction between data that was anticipated but are missing, and data that are absent because they cannot be collected. In the context of a clinical trial for a life-threatening disease, QoL may be assessed at monthly intervals. However, data can be expected – and hence have the potential to be missing – only for the period while the patient is alive. Attrition due to death is covered in Chapter 17. In that situation, we do not anticipate equal numbers of observations per patient. Nor is it sensible to impute values of PROs in the period after death.

Complete-case analysis

The simplest approach to analysis when some data are missing is to remove all patients with incomplete data from the analysis. Then standard complete-data methods can be used. However, this leaves only those patients for whom the relevant QoL information is entirely complete. In studies of advanced disease, where the assessment just prior to death may be difficult, this generally means deleting an unacceptable number of patients. In addition, during follow-up of patients, those who are in a good condition might be expected to have less missing information than those who are not so well. Consequently, QoL as summarised from solely those patients who complete all questionnaires (*complete-case analysis*) may be overestimated, particularly at later time points. Therefore complete-case analysis has two distinct disadvantages: it reduces the sample size by excluding patients with incomplete data and may produce misleading results. Complete-case analysis is usually equivalent to assuming that, if we had been able to retrieve the data, the patients with missing information would have had the same values as the mean of the observed patients; this implies that the data are *missing completely at random*. This can be extremely bias-prone. We do not recommend it unless the proportion with missing data is very small, perhaps in less than 5% of patients.

Available-case analysis

Suppose we wish to compare two treatments with respect to QoL at specific time points, using standard statistical tests such as the *t*-test or the Mann–Whitney test. One possibility is to include in the comparison all the QoL information available at that assessment time point and carry out a series of cross-sectional comparisons. Although the sample size may then vary at each assessment time point, this method makes use of all available data.

The main disadvantage of this method is that different sets of patients contribute information at different time points depending on the pattern of missing data, and this makes comparisons unclear. Additionally, an overall comparison of treatments is usually preferable to simple cross-sectional comparisons at specific time points because longitudinal analyses (as described in Chapter 14) allow general statements about treatment effects, are statistically more powerful and safeguard against multiple testing.

Summary measures

As discussed in Chapter 13, a widely used method for an analysis of data collected serially over time is to reduce the data on each patient to a single summary statistic, such as the area under the curve (*AUC*). In trials where a treatment is provided with the intent of palliating a certain symptom, another useful summary statistic may be the patient's worst QoL score for that symptom. Alternatively, a certain change score from baseline may be defined as clinically or subjectively important, and the time taken to reach this change score may be calculated. The summary for all patients is then analysed using an appropriate univariate test.

However, such an approach does not necessarily circumvent the occurrence of missing values as the key response, perhaps the worst QoL score for that symptom, may be the very item that was missing. Thus this approach may also be prone to bias.

Imputing missing data

To avoid the problems with respect to complete-case and available-case analyses, an option frequently used is to replace the missing values by imputed values, estimated using the data that has been observed. Imputation can make use of available assessments and other details about the patients whose values are missing, as well as information from comparable patients who did not have missing data. This can include:

- from the patient with missing data:
  a. baseline characteristics, especially factors known to be of prognostic value
  b. any available previous PRO measurements
  c. any PRO measurements that became available at later assessments

- from other patients:
  a. patterns of change over time
  b. information from a subset of patients that has similar characteristics to the patient with missing data

The aim of imputation is to make full use of all available information, both from the patients with missing data and from other similar patients. Thus the imputed values may be regarded as the *best estimate* of what the missing values would have been, and these estimates are inserted into the data file to make a now augmented (and complete) file on which the analysis can then be undertaken.

In theory, carefully imputed values should be close to the presumed 'true' values that might have been observed, and therefore the biases should be less than when using a naïve analysis that ignores the missing data – such as the complete-case analysis as described above. However, as we shall discuss, imputation carries a number of disadvantages, one of which is that it is easy to fall into the trap of thinking one has observed more data than was really collected; clearly it is not possible to increase the sample size by 'creating' new data, and so care must be taken to ensure that the appropriate degrees of freedom (*df*) are used throughout the analyses. Another danger is that many forms of imputation result in the underestimation of the sample standard deviation (*SD*); again, care must be taken to ensure a suitable correction factor is used.

The attraction of imputation is that, compared to the model-based approaches, it can be fairly simple to implement, the assumptions are explicit and the results are relatively easy to interpret. Therefore, despite its serious shortcomings, we present a detailed description of the major imputation methods.

15.2   Why do missing data matter?

Bias

The main cause for concern is that missing data may result in bias, and that the apparent results of a clinical trial will not reflect the true situation. That is, we will not know if the difference we observe between treatments is a truly reliable estimate of the real difference. If the proportion of anticipated data missing is small, then, provided the data are analysed appropriately, we can be confident that little bias will result. However, if the proportion of data that is missing is not small, then a key question is: 'Are the characteristics of patients with missing data different from those for whom complete data are available?' For example, it may be that the more-ill patients, or patients with more problems, are less willing or less able to complete the questionnaires satisfactorily. Then the missing QoL assessments (had we been able to receive them) might have indicated a poor outcome whereas those that were completed may reflect a better QoL.

Alternatively, perhaps patients without problems are less convinced about the need to return comprehensive information. In that case, the questionnaires that have been completed may reflect a worse QoL. In practice, there may be a mixture of these two possibilities within a particular trial. There may also be different patterns among patients receiving the different protocol treatments within one trial. Any analysis that ignores the presence of missing data may result in biased conclusions about both the changing QoL profiles over time and the between-treatment differences.

Consider a randomised clinical trial where we wish to estimate the overall QoL scores of patients at one time point and compare these between treatments. If we first consider one of the treatment groups, suppose that of the N patients recruited to that treatment M ($<N$) fail to complete the key QoL assessment. The proportion of missing data is $P = M/N$, and the proportion of patients with complete data is therefore $1 - P$. We assume that the responding and the non-responding patients do have different mean QoL values and these are $\mu_{Responding}$ and $\mu_{NotResponding}$ respectively. The patients recruited to the trial comprise of a mixture of those who ultimately do respond and those who do not. The combined mean for all patients, were we able to observe it, is

$$\mu = (1 - P)\mu_{Responding} + P\mu_{NotResponding}. \tag{15.1}$$

But here we are assuming that we do have responses from the non-responders. However, since one clearly cannot observe the non-responders, we cannot estimate μ with the QoL data recorded but only $\mu_{Responding}$. Thus the bias, B, will be

$$\begin{aligned} B &= \mu - \mu_{Responding} \\ &= (1 - P)\mu_{Responding} + P\mu_{NotResponding} - \mu_{Responding} \\ &= P(\mu_{NotResponding} - \mu_{Responding}). \end{aligned} \tag{15.2}$$

The bias will be zero if the mean scores of responders and non-responders are in fact equal, that is, $\mu_{NotResponding} = \mu_{Responding}$. However, since the non-responders do not record their QoL, we have no means of knowing if this is indeed the case. If there is no missing data, $P = 0$ and there will be no bias.

In a clinical trial comparing two treatments there will be a potential bias of the form of equation (15.2) for each treatment. The aim of a clinical trial is to estimate the difference in QoL between treatments. Thus the bias of this difference, for a trial comparing a test and control therapy, will therefore be

$$B_{Difference} = B_{Test} - B_{Control}. \tag{15.3}$$

The treatment comparison will be unbiased only if the bias happens to be the same (or absent) in both treatment arms, but again we have no means of knowing this.

There can be considerable bias in the estimated treatment difference if the proportion of missing assessments differs substantially between the treatment arms. Information regarding the reason for non-response, if known, may be useful in determining whether the analysis is biased or not. Additionally, if the probability of completing the QoL assessment is associated with patient characteristics measured at entry into the trial, such as their age, performance status or clinical stage of disease, it may be possible to reduce the bias by adjusting for these factors. It is important to note that the bias of equation (15.2), and hence (15.3) depends upon the proportion of missing data

---

Example from the literature

Curran *et al.* (1998b) describe a sample of metastatic breast cancer patients who completed the EORTC QLQ-C30. Physical functioning (PF) was assessed using items Q_1 to Q_5. In this study the QLQ-C30 (version 2) was used, and these items were scored 1 (No) or 2 (Yes). Thus the minimum sum-score is 5 and the maximum 10, which is then scaled to range from 0 to 100. There were 86 patients completing the first, or baseline, assessment. However, following recruitment, some patients dropped out before the next QoL assessment was made while the remainder carried on until the next monthly assessment, following which others dropped out.

Figure 15.1 presents the mean PF score by time of dropout either by death or failure to complete the QoL assessment. Each profile is calculated from those patients completing all QoL assessments up to the specified number of months. As may be seen, those patients who provide information on all five PF assessments tend to have a higher baseline mean PF score than the other groups of patients. Thus there is an intrinsic bias that tends to include only the better patients into the QoL analysis at later time points. Care should therefore be taken in interpreting any graphs or tabular displays that include mean scores calculated from all the data available being regarded as if they were all from one homogeneous group albeit comprising subjects for whom differing numbers of QoL assessments are available. The overall mean PF score, the bold broken line of Figure 15.1, rises steadily from 55.4 at baseline to 70.8 at the last assessment, suggesting an overall improvement in PF. This contrasts with the decline in PF that has occurred in, for example, those patient groups with three and four assessments in which the last observed mean PF dropped below previous levels. Since only a few patients dropped out at each month, the overall mean score is dominated by the patients who completed all five assessments.

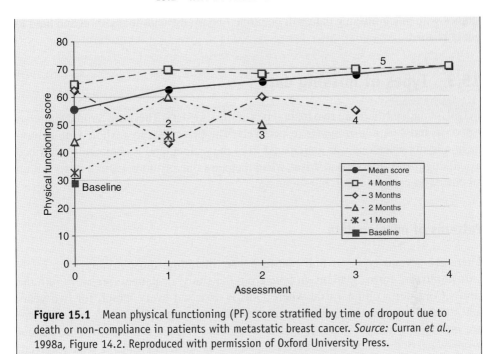

Figure 15.1 Mean physical functioning (PF) score stratified by time of dropout due to death or non-compliance in patients with metastatic breast cancer. *Source:* Curran *et al.,* 1998a, Figure 14.2. Reproduced with permission of Oxford University Press.

and not the number of observations. Bias cannot be reduced by increasing the total sample size.

Sample size

The other problem of missing data is more obvious: fewer data are available for analysis, resulting in a loss of power to detect differences in a clinical trial or other study. Loss of power also means that confidence intervals about the parameter estimates will be wider. However, unlike bias, we can compensate for loss of power by increasing the sample size. This will ideally have been done at the time of preparing the protocol, when a realistic estimate of the amount of missing data should have been made, and the planned sample size increased accordingly.

Compliance

It cannot be emphasised too strongly, the best solution is to take every possible measure to improve compliance and to avoid, or at least minimise, missing data. In the chapter on planning clinical trials we describe methods for achieving this, and also caution that studies with much missing data will be prone to bias, difficult to interpret and hard to get published.

15.3   Types of missing data

In QoL situations there are two main types of missing data. These are termed *unit non-response* and *item non-response* respectively. The first refers to a whole QoL assessment missing when one was anticipated from the patient, and is commonly described as *missing forms*; the second arises when there are one or more *missing items* within an otherwise complete QoL questionnaire.

Patterns of missing data

There are several types of unit non-response, including those arising from *intermittent missing* forms, patient *dropout* from the study, or patient *late entry* into the study. Consider a clinical trial where QoL is assessed every month for two years but a patient completed QoL assessments only at months 0, 2, 3, 5 and 6. There are *intermittent* missing questionnaires at months 1 and 4. At month 7 the patient *dropped out* of the study and therefore no additional QoL assessments were received; this is sometimes described as *terminal missing*. In contrast, suppose a patient was randomised into this trial in, say, September 2013 and an interim analysis of the ongoing trial was performed at the beginning of December 2013. In this case, the patient would have completed QoL assessments only at months 0, 1 and 2. This is a case of *late entry* into the trial since one could not expect more questionnaires for this patient at this time.

In some clinical trials of chronic diseases QoL assessments continue for the remaining life of the patient. However, especially in advanced disease, it is evident that not all patients will complete the same number of assessments, sometimes for medical reasons but ultimately because of death.

Example

Curran *et al.* (1998b) give the Kaplan–Meier plot (Figure 15.2) of time on protocol treatment for breast cancer patients with newly diagnosed bone metastases. The median time on treatment was 6.4 months. The patients were requested to complete a QoL questionnaire pre-treatment, monthly for the first seven months and three-monthly thereafter until progression.

As may be seen, there is substantial attrition of patients, mainly due to progression of their disease. By month 13 only about 12 patients were still on protocol treatment.

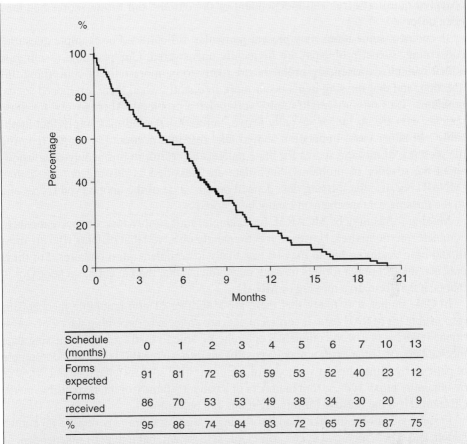

Schedule (months)	0	1	2	3	4	5	6	7	10	13
Forms expected	91	81	72	63	59	53	52	40	23	12
Forms received	86	70	53	53	49	38	34	30	20	9
%		95	86	74	84	83	72	65	75	87	75

Figure 15.2   Kaplan–Meier estimate of the time to progression for patients with metastatic breast cancer. *Source:* Curran *et al.*, 1998a, Figure 14.1. Reproduced with permission of Oxford University Press.

Mechanisms of missing data: MCAR, MAR, MNAR

Analysis of the patterns of missing PROs suggests that they do often occur at random. Thus, although those patients who, perhaps through carelessness, omit answers to one question are more likely to omit answers to other questions, the reason for their so doing may be unrelated to the (unrecorded) level of the particular PRO. Also, although missing items within forms may take the pattern of a run of adjacent questions, often the questions are unrelated, implying oversight rather than intentional omission. In both these circumstances, it is reasonable to assume the data are *missing completely at random* (MCAR). In formal terms, an item is MCAR if the probability of having a missing item is independent of that item's scores on previous observed questionnaires and independent of the current and future scores had they been observed.

In contrast, some items may present particular difficulties. For example questions concerning 'sexual problems' are frequently unanswered. One plausible assumption is that patients experiencing problems are likely to be more reticent concerning this question, and that missing items occur more frequently when there are indeed sexual problems. Thus missing might imply 'very much a problem'. Alternatively, for those patients who are no longer sexually active, failure to respond may imply 'not applicable'. In either case, imputation should take this into account, as simply ignoring the presence of missing scores for these patients can result in misleading conclusions about the severity of problems. Such data are classified as *missing not at random* (MNAR) because the missing data depend on the value of the unobserved scores and so the missing data mechanism cannot be ignored.

Missing forms may be MCAR if, for example, staff simply forget to ask patients to complete questionnaires. However, it is frequently observed that patients who are most ill and have declining health may be less likely to complete questionnaires. For these patients, the fact that a form is missing may indicate that the patient has a poor QoL – that is, it is informative missing or MNAR.

In QoL studies it is likely that there are a number of non-ignorable mechanisms responsible for MNAR data. If sufficient data are collected concerning why QoL questionnaires have not been completed, one may be able to distinguish the missing data mechanisms. In some cases it may be possible to retrieve the PROs of a random sample of patients by using alternative modes of administration such as telephone interview or by obtaining proxy scores from members of a patient's family or the responsible medical team. Then the reasons for missing items can be explored.

In some situations, the likelihood of having a missing score may depend on known factors and scores recorded at an earlier QoL assessment, but it may be independent of the current (not recorded) score. Such data are termed *missing at random* (MAR). An example might be age group: older people are more likely to have a higher rate of missing items and are also likely to have poorer physical functioning scores. Within any particular age group the data are MCAR, but when considering all patients together the data are MAR because those with missing values are likely to have lower true levels of PF than those with complete data.

When it comes to analysis, MCAR is frequently described as ignorable missing, because it is unlikely to result in biased analyses (although it will still cause loss of power). At the other extreme, MNAR is non-ignorable and may well bias any comparison. For the analyst, MNAR is the most challenging. In between, MAR is the focus of most analytical approaches because, firstly, MCAR is usually unrealistic, and secondly, MNAR is so problematic. Provided we can identify a sufficient number of explanatory factors, and provided the assumption of MAR is valid, we can use robust methods to impute estimated values for the missing items and missing forms.

Statistical tests are available to evaluate whether missing data are MCAR or MAR; it is not possible to test for MNAR as, by definition, the data that are needed to determine this are themselves missing. Fielding *et al.* (2009) describe four methods for distinguishing MCAR from MAR and apply them to five clinical trials. They also emphasise the importance of minimising the amount of missing data by use of reminders, and illustrate how the data recovered following a reminder may be utilised to further test the nature of the missingness pattern.

15.4 Missing items

The problem

Experience reported for a variety of clinical trials suggests that, for most single items, between 0.5% and 2% of values will be missing from returned questionnaires. Thus, overall, the problem of missing items might seem relatively unimportant. However, for a questionnaire that contains about 30 questions, a one per cent missing rate for items would, if it occurred at random, imply that about a quarter of patients could have a missing item on their initial QoL assessment. A missing rate as low as 0.5% could result in 14% of patients with at least one item missing. Furthermore, at each subsequent assessment there may be additional missing data and many patients are likely to have some degree of missing QoL data.

Examples from the literature

Reports of clinical trials describe compliance in terms of missing forms, but rarely provide the corresponding information about missing items within forms. Other studies provide estimates of typical proportions of missing items. It is frequently observed that there can be high proportions of missing values for embarrassing questions, including items about sexual function and sexual activity. One might speculate that that those with sexual problems would be the most likely to choose not to respond, leading to potential bias in the analyses.

In two large prospective observational studies of male adult patients receiving haemodialysis for chronic kidney disease (Veteran End-Stage Renal Disease Study, 314 patients, and the DOPPS Dialysis Outcomes and Practice Patterns Study, 3,300 patients), QoL was measured with the KDQOL-SF. This consists of the SF-36 and 11 multi-item scales specific to patients with kidney disease (Saban *et al.*, 2010). There were between 1% and 10% missing values for all items except for sexual function which was missing for greater than 50% of data. Between 0 and 5% of items were missing in the Veterans study, versus 6% and 10% for the DOPPS study. This difference may have been attributed to the Veteran data being collected over the telephone whereas DOPPS data were collected via written questionnaire. Because of the large amounts of missing data from both the VETERANS and DOPPS samples for the sexual function subscale, sexual function was not included in the calculation of the KDCS.

> Two thousand Dutch households were surveyed by van de Poll-Franse *et al.* (2011), to determine normative values for the EORTC QLQ-C30 and the EORTC sexuality items. The authors found that 197 respondents (11%) chose not to respond to the questions on sexual interest and activity. These individuals were more often female (14% versus 9% male; $p = 0.002$) and, on average, younger ($p < 0.0001$), less well educated ($p < 0.0001$), and reported a lower net family-income ($p < 0.0001$) than those who completed these questions. This study investigated Dutch patients; it is likely that the percentages could be very different in other countries or cultures.

Thus, even when there is only a small proportion of missing values for each item, a substantial proportion of patients may have at least one or more missing items during their follow-up period. Analyses based solely upon those patients for whom complete data are available may find that the cumulative exclusion of patients results in too few patients remaining in the final analyses, and hence a severe loss of statistical power. In addition, there is a process of selection of patients into the analysis since only those with complete data are retained. The subsequent subset of patients who have complete data may not be representative of all the patients in the trial.

15.5   Methods for missing items within a form

When individual items from a multi-item scale are missing, there are problems in calculating scores for the summated scale. In such cases, methods have been developed to impute the most likely values for these items. Such methods are no substitute for real observations but merely a device to facilitate analysis. The objective of imputation is to replace the missing data by estimated values that preserve the relationships between items, and which reflect as far as possible the most likely true value. If properly carried out, imputation should reduce the bias that can arise by ignoring non-response. By filling in the gaps in the data, it also restores balance to the data and permits simpler analyses. There are several approaches that can be used for imputation but the final choice is likely to depend on the particular context.

Treat the score for the scale as missing

If any of the constituent items are missing, the scale score for that patient is excluded from all statistical analysis. When data are MCAR, this reduced dataset represents a randomly drawn sub-sample of the full dataset and inferences drawn can be considered reasonable. This exclusion method is the simplest approach to the analysis, but results in overall loss of data (and so loss of statistical power in the analysis) because the scores based upon several items are excluded whenever even a single item is missing.

Far more important, however, is that it may lead to serious bias when there is an informative reason for the item being missing.

Simple mean imputation

For those QoL instruments that use unweighted sum-scores, the missing scale score can be estimated from the mean of those items that are available. This process is usually restricted to cases where the respondent has completed at least half of the items in the scale.

If no items are missing, the *raw score (RS)* is calculated as the average of the items:

$$RS = \frac{\sum_{i=1}^{L} Q_i}{L},$$

(15.4)

where the Q_i are the individual response to the L items in the domain. This is then transformed to the *standardised score (SS)* over the range 0 to 100 by

$$SS = \left\{ 1 - \frac{(RS - minimum)}{range} \right\} \times 100,$$

(15.5)

where the *range* is the difference between the largest (*maximum*) and smallest (*minimum*) scores possible.

Example

The emotional functioning (EF) scale of the EORTC QLQ-C30 is formed by summing responses to the $L = 4$ items of Figure 15.3. These items are all on four-point scales scored from 1 to 4, and hence the *range* is $4 - 1 = 3$. One patient indicated $Q_{21} = 1$, $Q_{23} = 2$ and $Q_{24} = 2$ but left Q_{22} as missing. Taking account of the missing response,

$$RS = (Q_{21} + Q_{21} + Q_{21})/3 = (1 + 2 + 2)/3 = 1.6677,$$

and

$$SS = \{1 - (1.6667 - 1)/3\} \times 100 = 77.8$$

	Not at all	A little	Quite a bit	Very much
21. Did you feel tense?	1✓	2	3	4
22. Did you worry?	1	2	3	4
23. Did you feel irritable?	1	2✓	3	4
24. Did you feel depressed?	1	2✓	3	4

Figure 15.3   The emotional functioning (EF) scale of the EORTC QLQ-C30.

If no more than half the items are missing, the *RS* is still calculated from equation (15.4) but with *L* replaced by the number of items available, and only the corresponding PRO values actually observed in the numerator. The corresponding value of *RS* is then substituted directly into equation (15.5) to obtain the *SS*.

One disadvantage of simple mean imputation is that, as in this example, it can result in some strange scores, such as 77.8, that are intermediate between the scale scores calculated for patients with complete data. This can be inconvenient when tabulating summary scores against treatment or other factors.

Hierarchical scales

Simple mean imputation is a very easy method to implement. However, there are a number of situations in which this may result in misleading values of the resulting QoL scores. For example, the EORTC QLQ-C30 scale for PF is *hierarchical* in that it contains an implicit ordering of responses. Thus if a patient replies 'Yes' to Q_3 about difficulties with a short walk but does not answer Q_2 about taking a long walk, it would not be sensible to base an imputed value for this missing response on the average of all the answered items. Clearly, those who have difficulty with short walks would have even greater problems with a long walk. In this case, the structure of the QoL questionnaire may imply that the replies to some questions will restrict the range of plausible answers to other questions. Thus if we assume the response to 'long walk' is missing but the patient responds as having difficulty with short walks, it would seem reasonable to assume that long walks would also cause difficulty and so we would accordingly impute a value of 2. On the other hand, if the response to 'short walk' is missing but the subject responds indicating no difficulty with long walks, we may assume there is unlikely to be difficulty with short walks and would impute a value of 1.

In contrast, simple mean imputation may still be more appropriate for the other two possible situations, that is, no difficulty with short walks but 'long walk' is missing, and difficulty with long walks but 'short walk' is missing.

Regression imputation

Regression imputation replaces missing values by predicted values obtained from a regression of the missing item variable, Q_{Miss}, on the remaining items of the scale. The data used for this calculation are from all those subjects in the study with complete information on all variables within the scale. More generally, regression imputation is a modelling technique. First the relationship of the missing item to the other items in the subscale is estimated using regression and the data from other subjects. Then the values of the non-missing items within the scale for the subjects with the missing response are substituted in this regression equation, to predict the value of the missing item.

Example

Suppose the missing item is Q_{22} from the EF scale of Figure 15.4, but the patient completed questions Q_{21}, Q_{23} and Q_{24}. Then the corresponding multiple regression equation required is

$$Q_{22} = \beta_0 + \beta_1 Q_{21} + \beta_3 Q_{23} + \beta_4 Q_{24}, \tag{15.6}$$

where the β_0, β_1, β_3 and β_4 are the regression coefficients. This equation is then fitted to the data obtained from those patients who have complete data on all items.

Suppose equation (15.6) has been estimated using data from the other patients, giving $Q_{22} = 0.3 + 0.5Q_{21} + 0.4Q_{23} + 0.6Q_{24}$, and that the current patient had responded with $Q_{21} = 1$, $Q_{23} = 2$ and $Q_{24} = 2$. Substituting in these values, we have the imputed value for $Q_{22} = 0.3 + (0.5 \times 1) + (0.4 \times 2) + (0.6 \times 2) = 2.8$. In practice, this imputed value will be rounded to **3**, the nearest integer, so that finally the scale score for this patient is imputed as $1 + 3 + 2 + 2 = 8$.

Mean imputation of equation (15.4) can be regarded as a special case of regression imputation in which $\beta_0 = 0$ and, for the above example, $\beta_1 = \beta_3 = \beta_4 = 1/3$. In general, if L items in a scale are all scored with the same range and one item is missing then, apart from $\beta_0 = 0$, the remaining βs will all equal $1/(L-1)$.

Regression imputation has the advantage that it can easily be extended to allow other predictive factors to be added to the equation, for example age, gender or stage of disease.

Score depends upon external variables

The value of an item may be more strongly associated with variables external to the scale – for example clinical or demographic variables of the patient – than with other items within the scale. In this case, rather than use the associated QoL variables on the right-hand side of regression equation (15.6), it may be more appropriate to predict the missing item by using only the clinical or demographic variables.

Informative censoring

In situations where the fact that the item is missing may be informative, it would not be appropriate to assume that the average value (or a regression model) of the other items should be used to impute the missing score. If 'missing' tends to imply that the patient has problems, the estimated score should in some way reflect this. The term *censoring* here indicates that the item is missing, albeit in circumstances when it was anticipated since the QoL assessment was essentially complete except for this item. The presumption of *informative* implies that this item was deliberately skipped rather than merely overlooked. If those who have sexual problems were embarrassed and likely to skip questions about decreased interest, missing would be informative and might imply likely problems.

Item 'not applicable'

It is questionable how to estimate scale scores when some constituent items are missing through not being applicable. For example, patients may return missing for Q_1 in the EORTC QLQ-C30 PF scale because they never try to perform strenuous activities. It is debatable as to how best to allow for these non-applicable items, and the decision will partly depend upon the scientific question being posed. However, in the example cited, it might be argued that if 'not applicable' implies limitations in terms of PF it would be reflected by the other items in the scale, in which case regression imputation could still be appropriate.

15.6   Missing forms

The problem

Missing forms tend to be a far more serious problem than missing items. Forms are more frequently missing, and if a form is missing so are all constituent items on it. Forms may be essentially MCAR if, for example, the patient was inadvertently not asked to complete the QoL assessment for a reason unrelated to his or her health status. On the other hand, they may be missing at critical stages depending on the relative health of the patient at the scheduled assessment time. For example, they may be missing just before death. Intermittent forms may also be missing because the patient feels too ill and so unable to complete the questionnaire, or perhaps feels so well that the assessment no longer seems relevant. Hospital staff may also avoid giving the form during a period of severe illness of the patient. Such patients may, however, complete the succeeding form as their relative health state may have changed by that time. These types of missing form will usually not be MCAR or MAR, but are more likely to be MNAR.

Example from the literature

Curran *et al.* (2009) explored the nature of missing data in a clinical trial of palliative chemotherapy for gastric cancer. A dichotomous indicator variable was used to represent dropout (no more forms returned). Table 15.1 shows logistic regression used to explore the effect of QoL scores on dropout.

The authors comment that the two QoL terms in the model, 'difference in QL' and 'sum of QL', were significant indicating that if the sum of the two previous QoL scores were low then the probability of dropout was high and if there was a decrease in QoL score from the previous assessment then the probability of dropout was also high. They concluded that the missing data are not MCAR and "caution needs to be taken when analysing the QoL data".

Table 15.1 Logistic regression to explore the nature of missing data in a trial of palliative chemotherapy for gastric cancer

Parameter	Estimate	Standard error	Chi-squared	*p*-value
Intercept	0.015	1.006		
Time	−0.235	0.254	0.854	0.356
Treatment	−0.086	0.368	0.054	0.816
Time × treatment	0.160	0.110	2.124	0.145
Difference in QoL	−0.018	0.006	8.231	0.004
Sum of QoL	−0.008	0.003	7.156	0.008

Source: Curran *et al.*, 2009, Table 4.CC NC 4.0 (<http://creativecommons.org/licenses/by/4.0/>). Reproduced commercially with kind permission from Springer Science and Business Media.

Examples from the literature

Missing data has long been recognised as a major problem. Ganz *et al.* (1988), using the FLIC scale in a study of patients with lung cancer, report that while 87% of patients returned a baseline questionnaire, overall only 58% of expected forms were completed. Hürny *et al.* (1992), with similar patients, report a compliance rate of about 50% when using the EORTC QLQ-C30 with a linear analogue scale (LASA) and a mood-adjective checklist (BF-S). They note that the institution, not the patients, appeared to be the major variable contributing to high or low compliance rates.

Geddes *et al.* (1990), on behalf of the UK Cancer Research Campaign, report 68% compliance again in patients with lung cancer. They opine that patients find it difficult to continue completing the assessment when they become ill with progressive disease, "and this poses a methodological problem for investigators who wish to assess effects throughout an entire treatment programme".

Randomised phase III trials in cancer patients normally require several hundreds of patients to be recruited, and thus such trials are frequently organised on a multicentre basis. Whereas a single-centre trial may be able to assemble an enthusiastic team that is committed to assessing QoL, there may be severe problems in motivating some participants of larger multicentre trials. This can lead to major problems in compliance. In general, multicentre trials are the most demanding environment for conducting QoL assessments.

15.7 Methods for missing forms

Statistical methods have been developed to impute the most likely values for missing data when whole QoL assessments are missing. We have shown how values may be calculated for missing items within a form, and how these methods may or may not make use of other information collected on the same form. In contrast, when a whole QoL assessment is missing, the imputation procedure must use information from other similar patients, values from previous and/or later assessments by the same patient, or a mixture of both. We note that, if items are used only as components of a scale, it may not be necessary to impute values for those items, only for the scale score itself. As with missing items, once values have been imputed for the particular missing assessments they may then be stored with the remaining data to give the appearance of a full dataset.

15.8 Simple methods for missing forms

Last value carried forward

One straightforward imputation technique is the *last value carried forward* (LVCF) method. The values that were recorded by a patient at the last previously completed QoL assessment are used for items on the current (missing) QoL assessment. Thus, for example, if a patient completes the first assessment but fails to complete the second one, the patient's score from the first assessment would be used as the imputed value for the second (missing) assessment.

A key disadvantage of the LVCF method is that it assumes the patient's score remains essentially constant over time. In the above example, we may be reasonably confident of the imputed value for the first missing state but perhaps not so certain of the second imputation, as that (missing) assessment was followed by a worsening state 2. An imputation method that took account of what follows might have imputed 2 here rather than 1.

It should be noted that had the second instance of state 3 been missing in the above sequence, then, if the patient were known to be alive at that time, the only possible option for the LVCF or any other method would be 3. Rarely will such certainty regarding the true value be justified.

Example from the literature

Curran *et al.* (1998a) describe an example in which the EORTC QLQ-C30 PF scale was used to assess QoL in post-orchidectomy patients with poor-prognosis metastatic prostate cancer. The individual items were summed and then transformed to range from 0 to 100. These scores were then used to define four categories, or states, coded as 1 = Good PF (score ≥ 60), 2 = Poor PF (score < 60), 3 = Progression and 4 = Death.

A typical patient might therefore have a sequence of states as shown here:

$$1 \quad 1 \quad 2 \quad 1 \quad - \quad - \quad 2 \quad 2 \quad 3 \quad 3 \quad 4$$

This patient initially has Good PF (state 1), drops temporarily to Poor (state 2) and then improves. There are then two missing QoL assessments, after which the patient is in state 2, has disease progression (state 3) and eventually dies (state 4). Note that once a patient enters state 3 (progression) or state 4 (death) the patient cannot return to one of the previous states.

Using LVCF, the first missing value would be replaced by a state 1. This gives a still incomplete sequence, and so the LVCF method can be applied a second time to obtain:

$$1 \quad 1 \quad 2 \quad 1 \quad \mathit{1} \quad \mathit{1} \quad 2 \quad 2 \quad 3 \quad 3 \quad 4$$

If an assessment is missing after a patient has commenced a treatment that is known to have major side effects, it would seem silly to impute an LVCF value based on the previous pre-treatment assessment. More generally, it is apparent that LVCF is likely to be biased whenever there are known to be consistent changes over time that may affect the items of interest. An example is progressive chronic diseases, where patents may be expected to deteriorate over time.

In summary, LVCF is one of the simplest approaches, but in many situations it will be inappropriate and cannot in general be recommended. When it is used, care should be taken to evaluate and justify the inherent assumptions regarding the validity of LVCF.

Sample-mean imputation

In the context of a missing form, *sample-mean imputation* is usually the replacement of missing QoL scores by the mean score calculated from those patients who did complete the QoL assessment. That is, if there are N patients for QoL assessment of whom M have missing values, the mean $\bar{Q}_{N-M}$ from the $N - M$ patients with QoL observations is used for imputation. This procedure is also called mean value substitution, or simply *mean imputation*.

Example

At a particular assessment time, the mean QoL score (on a scale 0–100) was $\bar{Q} = 20$ for those patients who were assessed. Thus, for those patients for whom the assessment is missing, the corresponding score will be imputed as $Q = \bar{Q} = 20$.

A feature of mean imputation is that the estimate of the mean of the augmented dataset remains the same as the mean $\bar{Q}$ that was calculated for the original non-missing data. In contrast, the estimate of the *SD* will be reduced artificially as the imputed values are all placed at the centre (mean) of the distribution. This can lead to distorted significance tests and falsely narrow confidence intervals (*CIs*).

However, the *SD* can be corrected by two equivalent methods. Thus (i) either the *SD* of the $N - M$ non-missing values (denoted SD_{N-M}) is retained and used, or (ii) the *SD* of the now complete set of N augmented observations (which includes the missing M) is corrected by multiplying by f, from equation (15.7), to give SD_{N-M} once more.

$$f = \sqrt{\frac{N-1}{N-M-1}}. \tag{15.7}$$

Example

At the time of a particular QoL assessment there were $N = 10$ patients, but $M = 2$ of these failed to complete the assessment. The eight observed and ordered QoL values were 1, 1, 2, 2, 2, 2, 3 and 3, with mean = 2.0 and $SD_8 = 0.7559$.

The $M = 2$ missing values are both imputed as $\bar{Q} = 2.0$, giving the full augmented ordered dataset of 1, 1, 2, 2, **2, 2**, 2, 2, 3, 3. The mean of the resulting ten values remains as 2, but the corresponding *SD* is reduced to 0.6667. However, $f = \sqrt{(10-1)/(10-2-1)} = 1.1339$ and the adjusted $SD = 1.1339 \times 0.6667 = 0.7560$. This also equals the SD_8 of the eight values actually observed.

As we have indicated, the two methods are equivalent. In some situations, particularly if the dataset is large, it is easiest to add the imputed values to the data file merely to facilitate analysis by standard computer packages. In this case, the adjustment method may be the most convenient, as it can be applied to all variables including those that have no missing values, since when $M = 0$ we have $f = 1$, and the calculated *SD* remains unchanged.

It is also important to note that the correlation between different scores (or items) may be affected by the imputation. Imputing a missing value by the corresponding mean value of the remainder of the data will tend to reduce the size of the observed correlation coefficient if the calculation is carried out on the augmented dataset.

The sample-mean imputation method that we have described here uses the full dataset from all available patients, but a modification is to take only the mean score of a subset of patients. Patients with similar characteristics to the patient with the missing data would be chosen. The presumption here is that matched patients will behave in a similar way; a generalised version of this approach is discussed under pattern mixture models.

Horizontal mean imputation

Unlike the LVCF method, sample-mean imputation takes no account of the longitudinal nature of an individual's QoL data. Thus an alternative to sample-mean imputation is to impute the missing value from the mean of the patient's own previous scores. This method is sometimes termed *horizontal* as it takes into account the longitudinal nature of the QoL data. It reduces to the LVCF method if there is only one previous assessment available or if there has been no change in PROs over the assessments to date.

Example

For the sequence 1, 1, 2, 1, −, −, 2, 2, 3, 3, 4 discussed previously, horizontal mean imputation would give 1, 1, 2, 1, *1.25*, *1.25*, 2, 2, 3, 3. Here 1.25 is the mean of the first four item values in the sequence. In practice, these values could be rounded to the nearest integer before being added to the augmented dataset.

The same reservations as for LVCF apply here. Thus horizontal mean imputation is not recommended if there is evidence of a systematic decline or fall in PROs over time.

Example

For the sequence 1, 1, 1, 1, 2, 2, 2, 2, 3, −, 4, horizontal mean imputation would result in 1, 1, 1, 1, 2, 2, 2, 2, 3, *1.67*, 4. Here, *1.67* (rounded to 2 before addition to the dataset) is the mean of the first nine item values in the sequence. This is clearly not a good estimate in this situation.

When imputing *intermittent* missing items, this (and other) approaches may readily be extended to make use of information from later assessments in addition to the previous ones.

Regression models

Regression models provide a wide range of methods for improving imputation. The method most frequently entails using those patients for whom the value of the item in question is known at the time point of interest, and developing a regression model for 'predicting' this value. The regression equation is then applied to the patients with missing values of the item, to obtain an estimate of the unknown value. In its simplest form, regression could be used as a substitute for LVCF. Then we would use the patients with complete data at the time point of interest, calculate the regression equation based on the previous assessment, and apply this equation to impute values for patients with missing forms. This adjusts for any shift or trend in the general levels of QoL in the patient population over time and overcomes that major disadvantage of LVCF. It also makes use of knowledge about each patient's previous score.

This simple form of regression imputation can be extended, by exploring and testing for other predictive indicators. The regression models may contain baseline characteristics or other prognostic factors as covariates, and may include other previous or later assessments in addition to the previous value. If the sample size is sufficiently large, separate equations may be developed for the randomised treatment arms; failing this, creating *dummy variables* for the treatment effects enables the exploration of interactions between the treatments and the covariates.

By including the relevant factors, regression modelling can be efficient if the pattern of missing is MAR. One major disadvantage is that, as with sample-mean imputation, the *SD* will be artificially reduced; however, it is now less clear what correction factor to use. It is even less clear how to correct the standard errors (*SEs*) of estimated parameters, and thus how to calculate *p*-values. Despite this, regression modelling provides a useful stage in the analysis of data when there are missing values.

Example

Figure 15.4 illustrates the different methods of imputation *for a single patient*. The upper trace shows the mean values for patients with complete data. Beneath is a patient who completed two assessments, but with a missing form at month 6. It can be seen that the method of imputation makes a huge impact on the value that is generated. Imputation is clearly dubious for predicting values of a single patient, as the implicit assumptions markedly affect the outcomes.

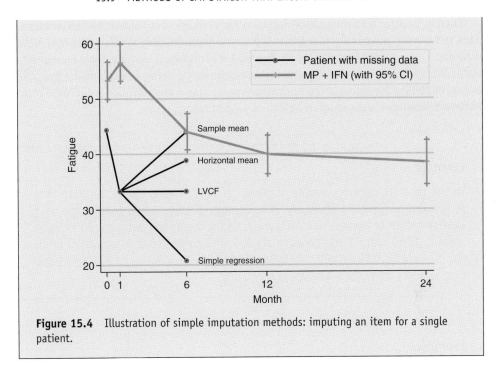

Figure 15.4   Illustration of simple imputation methods: imputing an item for a single patient.

Although one might hope that imputation would perform more satisfactorily when applied to the whole sample, a few points should be noted.

1. If the patients with the poorest QoL tend to have missing forms, the sample mean will consistently overestimate the missing values.

2. If patients fail to return forms when their health is declining, both horizontal mean and LVCF will overestimate the true values.

3. If QoL for the whole sample is declining over time, simple regression will tend to result in lower estimates than the other methods.

15.9   Methods of imputation that incorporate variability

Markov chain imputation

In the methods described so far, the imputed values will be the same for any two patients with the same profile of successive non-missing values. Such methods are termed *deterministic*. A major disadvantage of all these simple methods is that the variance of the observations is underestimated. This can result in a falsely reduced *SD*, artificially narrow *CI*s and misleading significance.

Another approach to imputation is to use the concept of a so-called Markov chain. This reflects the possibility that the two patients with missing assessments may have differing QoL profiles had they been recorded. This method assigns, for a patient in a particular QoL state at one assessment, probabilities of being in each of the possible states, including the same, at the next assessment. These probabilities are termed *transition probabilities* and are often described in percentage terms.

Example

In the prostate cancer example of Curran *et al.* (1998a), above, suppose that at one QoL assessment there are 100 patients in state 1 and that at the next assessment 65 of these remain in state 1. Of the remaining patients, 20 move to state 2, 12 to state 3 and three to state 4. The corresponding transition probabilities are $65/100 = 0.65$, $20/100 = 0.20$, $12/100 = 0.12$ and $3/100 = 0.03$, that is, 65%, 20%, 12% and 3% respectively.

Example

In fact, the observed transition probabilities for the prostate cancer trial are shown in Table 15.2. These were constructed from all the data available from QoL assessments four, five and six combined together. This table is referred to as a *matrix of transition probabilities*. Thus at this stage of the trial a patient with Good PF has a transition probability of 76.0% for remaining in the same state, whereas the transition probability for Progression is 12.6%. For a patient already in Progression, the probability of remaining in that state is 91.4% and the transition probability of Death of 8.6%. These probabilities can be used to impute missing QoL data.

Table 15.2 Transition probabilities between states, expressed as percentages, for a prostate cancer trial

	Resultant state			
	1 = Good PF	2 = Bad PF	3 = Progression	4 = Death
Initial state:				
1 = Good PF	76.0	11.4	12.6	0.0
2 = Bad PF	11.1	75.0	13.9	0.0
3 = Progression			91.4	8.6
4 = Death				100.0

Source: Curran *et al.*, 1998a, Table 14.1. Reproduced with permission of Oxford University Press.

Example

In the missing pattern above, the fifth and sixth QoL assessments were missing, but we know the patient is alive and without progression. Therefore we know that the missing states must be replaced by either a 1 or a 2 since a patient cannot return to state 2 from either Progression or Death.

1   1   2   1   –   –

The state observed immediately before the first missing QoL value was 1. Thus the only possible transitions from the fourth to the fifth QoL assessment are, from Table 15.2, 1→1 (76.0%) and 1→2 (11.4%). However, these transition probabilities total 87.4% rather than 100%. Therefore we divide each of the two possible transition probabilities by 87.4 to obtain: 76.0/87.4 = 0.87 or 87% and 11.4/87.4 = 0.13 or 13%.

To impute the missing values, we make use of these transition probabilities together with a table of random numbers or a computer random number generator, giving random numbers from 0 to 100. If the random number so generated is less than or equal to 87, we impute for the missing QoL state as state 1; otherwise we impute state 2.

Example

Suppose the first random number is 10, which is ≤ 87. Then state 1 is imputed, giving:

1   1   2   1   1   –

Since the fifth assessment was imputed as state 1, the transition probabilities for the sixth assessment remain as 87% and 13%. Thus to complete the sequence the same procedure is followed. If the second random number is 68 and is thus ≤ 87, state 1 is again imputed and we have:

1   1   2   1   1   1

This is the same sequence that was generated using the LVCF method. However, this need not necessarily have been the case had other random numbers been drawn. Thus all the alternatives to *1 1* are possible; that is, *1 2, 2 1* and *2 2*. As a consequence, a second patient with exactly the same QoL profile may have a randomly different missing sequence imputed.

In the method just described, we used the knowledge that the missing values could not have been either state 3 or state 4. Thus we restricted and simplified our transition matrix accordingly. However, we ignored the fact that we have additional information about the next (seventh) state, which had been reported to be 2. More comprehensive calculations are shown in the next table, improving the imputation process by taking into account the known value of the observation following the missing values.

Example

In the incomplete patient sequence given previously 1 1 2 1 − − 2 2 3 3 4, the last value before the missing value was state 1 and the first value after the missing sequence was state 2. The four possible intermittent sequences of 1 1, 1 2, 2 1 and 2 2 for the missing values are given in Table 15.3, with the associated transition probabilities. The probability of each sequence occurring is then calculated by multiplying the corresponding transition probabilities. Thus for the first sequence, that is *1 1* (moving from state 1 to 1, then 1 again, and ending in 2), the probability is: $0.870 \times 0.870 \times 0.130 = 0.098$. Once the probabilities for all possible sequences are calculated, they are adjusted to ensure that they sum to 1 or 100%. Thus the adjusted probability for the first sequence is $0.098/(0.098 + 0.099 + 0.002 + 0.099) = 0.329$. Finally, to facilitate the choice of sequence using random numbers, the cumulative probability is then calculated by adding the probabilities of the individual sequences.

Using random number tables, we select a number randomly between 000 to 999. If this number is in the range from 001 to 329, sequence 1 1 is imputed. Similarly, if from 330 to 661, the sequence is 1 2; if from 662 to 668, the sequence is 2 1; and, if from 669 to 999 or equal to 000, the sequence 2 2 is chosen.

Suppose the random number generator gave 831. This is in the range 669 to 999 and so 2 2 is chosen for the imputation, giving the complete sequence of states for the patient as:

$$1 \quad 1 \quad 2 \quad 1 \quad \mathbf{2} \quad \mathbf{2} \quad 2 \quad 2 \quad 3 \quad 3 \quad 4$$

Table 15.3 Probabilities of sequences for imputing values for missing data in the prostate cancer trial

Possible sequence	All possible sequences with associated transition probabilities							Probability	Adjusted probability	Cumulative probability (%)
1 1	1	0.870*	1	0.870	1	0.130*	2	0.098	0.329	32.9
1 2	1	0.870	1	0.130	2	0.871	2	0.099	0.332	66.1
2 1	1	0.130	2	0.129	1	0.130	2	0.002	0.007	66.8
2 1	1	0.130	2	0.871	2	0.871	2	0.099	0.332	100.0

*From Table 15.2: $76.0/(76.0 + 11.4) = 0.870$ and $11.4/(76.0 + 11.3) = 0.130$.
Source: Curran *et al.*, 1998a, Table 14.3. Reproduced with permission of Oxford University Press.

If there are more than one successive missing items, an alternative method of imputation is to calculate probabilities for the possible sequences that may be imputed for the missing sequence. The sequence chosen to impute the missing sequence is itself chosen at random in proportion to the corresponding probability.

There are several difficulties with this approach. One is its complexity compared with methods such as LVCF. A second difficulty is the assumption about the relative stability of transition probabilities over time. In our example, Table 15.2 was calculated using only information from QoL assessments four, five and six. It was judged that the transition probabilities would be stable over this period. However, perhaps probabilities are different for the first three assessments or from the seventh assessment onwards. It is difficult to make decisions about the stability of the transition probabilities over time. Another problem is that scales often have larger numbers of categories, leading to many cells in the corresponding table of transition probabilities. Consequently, these probabilities may be based upon relatively few observed patients and may be unreliable, making their use for imputation problematic.

However, an important advantage of this method over the deterministic LVCF or mean imputation methods is that the variability of the data is preserved in the augmented dataset, and hence the value of the *SD* is maintained.

Hot deck imputation

Hot deck (a pack of playing cards) imputation selects at random, from patients with observed QoL data, the QoL score from one of these and substitutes this as the imputed value for the patient with the missing QoL assessment. The hot deck literally refers to the deck (here computer file) of responses of patients with observed data from which the missing QoL score is selected. The particular deck chosen may be restricted to those patients that, in some way, are similar to the patient with the missing QoL score.

Curran *et al.* (1998a) describe how this method can be extended to more-complex situations with differing imputation probabilities assigned taking into account WHO performance status, treatment group and initial pain levels. This basic form of hot deck imputation has been largely superseded by more sophisticated computer-intensive variants.

Example from the literature

Curran *et al.* (1998a) indicate that in patients with prostate cancer the baseline WHO performance status (PS) affects the probability of being in a subsequent QoL state. Thus in Table 15.4, 73.3% of patients with PS = 0 at baseline were state 1 (Good PF), but this was so for only 20.0% for those with PS = 2.

To impute a missing value using information about the baseline PS, we first identify the corresponding 'deck' of patients. Thus if a patient with a missing baseline QoL value has PS = 0, the deck consists of patients with this PS. Table 15.4 shows that, for this deck, state 1 (Good PF) would be imputed with probability 0.733 and state 2 (Bad PF) with probability 0.267. On the other hand, if the deck were PS = 1, states 1 and 2 would be imputed with probabilities 0.476 and 0.524 respectively. Finally, if the deck is PS = 2, states 1 and 2 would be imputed with probabilities 0.200 and 0.800 respectively. Although the possible imputed values (states 1 or 2) remain the same for all patients with missing assessments, the probabilities attached to the (two) alternatives within the deck are varied according to baseline PS values. Thus the three PS decks considered here all consist of two types of 'cards', Good or Bad PF, but these are present in the three decks in differing proportions.

Table 15.4 Percentages of patients with good or bad physical functioning (PF), by WHO performance status. These percentages are used for the hot deck imputation

WHO Performance Status	1 = Good PF	2 = Bad PF
0	73.3	26.7
1	47.6	52.4
2	20.0	80.0

Source: Curran *et al.*, 1998a, Table 14.4. Reproduced with permission of Oxford University Press.

EM algorithm

When the missing values arise through a known censoring mechanism, the so-called *EM algorithm* can be used to impute missing values. (The E stands for expectation and M for maximum likelihood, but these details need not concern us.) The EM algorithm is particularly useful when many patients have missing forms at different assessment points, because then there may be few patients with complete data from whom we are able derive hot decks or transition probabilities.

To apply the EM algorithm, we first need to decide upon an imputation method for estimating the missing items. This could be one of the methods described above, or could be multiple regression as described for missing items. If using regression models, we can of course include various factors that are expected to be predictive of the PROs, for example age, gender, stage of disease. Let us assume we decide to use regression and have developed a regression model. The procedure of the EM algorithm is:

1. Replace all missing values with the estimates that are predicted from the regression.

2. With the new dataset, recalculate the parameters of the regression equation.

3. Now repeat from (1), using the revised regression equation as just calculated in (2).

This iterative procedure is continued until the values put back do not differ from those just taken out. The process is then deemed to have converged.

When using regression methods, the EM algorithm will usually converge after only a few cycles. When there is much missing data, the resultant estimates will be far more reliable than if a simple (non-iterative) regression approach were used.

15.10 Multiple imputation

It is clear that there are several options for the methods of imputation chosen. If deterministic methods such as LVCF are used, the augmented dataset will be unique. In contrast, if a random element is included in the imputation of missing values, the resultant augmented dataset will be equivalent to a single random one chosen from many potential datasets. We can then use this dataset for analysis. For example, we might perhaps carry out a *t*-test or estimate *CI*s for a treatment comparison.

The idea of multiple imputation is that many alternative 'complete' datasets can be created instead of just one. The analysis (*t*-tests, or whatever) can be repeated for each dataset and then combined in some way. Common practice suggests that five repetitions should suffice. Rubin (1987) gives some rules for combining these separate analyses into a final summary analysis. Kenward and Carpenter (2007) provide a review of multiple imputation procedures, with full details of how it may be implemented.

Multiple imputation is a powerful technique, and overcomes the disadvantages associated with both deterministic methods (such as underestimated *SD*s, *CI*s and correlations) and Markov or hot deck models (the randomly chosen values may be randomly atypical). Although it was initially developed for use in large population surveys and tends to require large samples, multiple imputation has been repeatedly shown to be superior to simpler methods and is becoming increasingly used with PROs. Sterne *et al.* (2009) found 59 examples of multiple imputation in four leading medical journals over a five-year period to 2007, reviewed its use, commented on pitfalls, and proposed reporting guidelines. They concluded: "We are enthusiastic about the potential for multiple imputation and other methods to improve the validity of medical research results and to reduce the waste of resources caused by missing data. The cost of multiple imputation analyses is small compared with the cost of collecting the data. It would be a pity if the avoidable pitfalls of multiple imputation slowed progress towards the wider use of these methods. It is no longer excusable for missing values and the reason they arose to be swept under the carpet, nor for potentially misleading and inefficient analyses of complete cases to be considered adequate."

15.11 Pattern mixture models

Frequently, missing PRO data might be expected to be MNAR, or non-ignorable missing. This is particularly likely to be the case when the presence of missing data is associated with, for example, severe toxicity or disease progression. Studies with MNAR data are difficult to analyse satisfactorily because the very data needed to evaluate or explore models for imputation are, by definition, missing. One approach that attempts to overcome this is to use *pattern mixture models*.

In a pattern mixture approach, patients are divided into subgroups according to the pattern of missingness. For example, patients might be classified as early dropouts, later dropouts during therapy, dropouts during post-treatment follow-up, and those with intermittent missing data; this would result in four subgroups or *patterns*. Alternatively, data might be stratified by reason for dropout or missing values (for example, side effects, lack of efficacy, deteriorating health or "unexplained, presumed random"). Patterns may also be formed by subdividing these strata according to additional prognostic factors, as in the example below.

Choice of patterns is one of the most critical – and difficult – aspects of the pattern mixture approach. Pattern groups should be chosen on the basis of best reflecting the suspected mechanism of missingness, such that patients within each group may plausibly be thought to be homogeneous. This decision may be partly founded on clinical perspectives, and partly by exploring and contrasting data from

---

Example from the literature

Curran *et al.* (2009) rejected the assumption of MCAR in their trial of palliative chemotherapy for gastric cancer, and used a pattern mixture model to evaluate the PRO measures. This allowed modelling of the repeated measures structure of the data, taking into account the dropout pattern. Terms in the model included treatment, time, dropout pattern and their interactions. Thus they were able to allow the fixed effects as well as the covariance parameters to vary according to the dropout pattern. In addition, several baseline clinical variables (age, gender, WHO performance status, pain assessed by the clinician, prior surgery and weight loss) were considered as covariates in the model.

patients with missing values against those with complete data. However, the sample size of the study will also restrict the number of pattern groups that are feasible for analysis.

Having selected the pattern groups to be used, data are then analysed separately for each of these groups and values can be imputed for the missing data. Analysis of the study is completed by combining the stratum-specific results.

Multiple imputation and pattern mixture models are frequently used together, with the overall estimates and significance tests being derived by combining the multiple repeated imputations as described in the previous section (also see Figure 15.5). Pauler *et al.* (2003) provide a detailed example of how pattern mixture models may be used when analysing QoL results in a clinical trial. The choice of pattern groups is clearly to a large extent arbitrary, and consequences of alternative groupings should be explored in a sensitivity analysis (see Section 15.14).

Another alternative is a *selection model*, which provides a two-stage approach for handling missing data that cannot be ignored. First, a model is developed to predict whether or not a patient is likely to drop out. This predicted dropout probability can then be used in the longitudinal model as a covariate. A criticism of selection models is that their validity cannot be tested because the model includes the missing values as an explanatory variable.

1. Identify potential missing data patterns, based on exploratory analyses and clinical or other experience. Choose groups of respondents who share similar missingness characteristics (pattern groups). Respondents with complete data (no missing values) are often divided into subgroups by treatment arm.

2. For each pattern,

   a) specify an imputation model to be used.

   b) estimate the parameters of the imputation model from the observed data.

3. Apply the models and parameter estimates from step 2, so as to impute missing data in each pattern group.

4. Combine the groups to form a dataset with "complete" data.

5. Repeat the imputation process of steps 3 and 4 multiple (typically five or more) times, resulting in multiple datasets with "complete" data.

6. Analyse each of the multiple datasets separately.

7. Combine the results for the multiple datasets, using standard multiple-imputation methods of stratified analysis.

Figure 15.5   Pattern mixture model with multiple imputation.

Example from the literature

Post *et al.* (2010) describe a trial comparing standard-dose and high-dose chemotherapy for patients with breast cancer. The authors used a pattern mixture approach because they suspected informative drop-out. The physical functioning (PF) scale of the SF-36 was analysed. Patterns were based on the state of the patient at the end of the study period: deceased, alive with relapse, and disease free. Within each pattern the drop-out was assumed to be MAR, so that the missing PF values could be predicted from the observed measurements of patients within the pattern group. The model included terms for time, treatment and time by treatment interaction. From this, the course of PF was estimated for each state and treatment combination. Finally, the stratified analysis provided overall estimates of PF by time for each treatment group (Figure 15.6). For a sensitivity analysis, models were also explored using only patients with complete five-year follow up, and similar results were obtained.

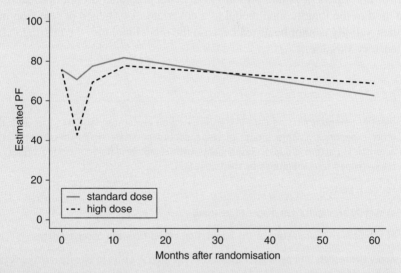

Figure 15.6   The course of PF over time by treatment, estimated using pattern mixture models. *Source:* Post *et al.*, 2010, Figure 5.CC NC 4.0 (<http://creativecommons.org/licenses/by/4.0/>). Reproduced commercially with permission of Springer Science+Business Media.

15.12   Comments

One possibility is not to impute any values at all and resort to either complete-case or available-case analysis. There are clearly difficulties associated with such an approach. For example, in the analysis of the breast cancer data of Figure 15.1, if we include only the 52 patients for whom up to five assessments are available, we may be seriously misled. We might incorrectly conclude that the overall mean was 64.6 at baseline and that by the assessment at four months the mean QoL score has risen by 6.2 to 70.8. As can be seen from Figure 15.1, this method of analysis considerably overestimates the mean QoL score at all but the final assessment time points. Case-wise deletion can result in significant bias.

An alternative to imputation is to make use of complex analytical models offering facilities for handling non-ignorable missing data. These include random-effects mixture models, shared-parameter models and selection models. Although such models may appear attractive, Fairclough (2010) notes that all these models make strong assumptions that cannot be formally tested and the estimates 'are not robust to model misspecification'. Complex statistical models do not offer a panacea, but those who wish to explore them are referred to the further reading list (Section 15.16).

15.13   Degrees of freedom

A major advantage of imputing missing values is that, once the values have been filled in, standard methods of analysis can be used – with some provisos. The augmented dataset comprising the observed values and the imputed values cannot be regarded as the same as one consisting of complete real data; obviously it is not possible to create data that do not exist. This can cause problems since, although summary statistics such as the mean and median may not be distorted, the corresponding SDs may be affected with consequences for the associated CIs and any significance tests. Even if the SD remains unaffected or is adjusted as we have described earlier, the degrees of freedom (df) must be reduced to reflect the availability of less information. Thus calculated CIs and p-values have to take account of the corresponding (reduced) df. A cautious approach to calculating the df when there are missing data is to reduce the df by 1 for every patient with missing values for the variable under consideration. Thus suppose that there are N patients recruited to each of two treatment groups in a clinical trial and QoL information is available from all but M patients. Then if the CI of the difference in mean QoL between treatments is required, the df will be reduced from $2N - 1$ to $(2N - 1) - M$; that is, $df = 2N - M - 1$ will be used to obtain the value of t from statistical tables, which will be then used in the calculation of the correct CI.

However, if this method is applied when there are single items missing within a scale and the scale score has been imputed, the final df may be too small as it is reduced by 1 for every such item. A possible compromise in this situation is to reduce the df by a fraction for every observation missing. For example, if an L-item scale is calculated for a particular patient but one item is missing, df can be reduced by $1/L$. These fractions are then summed over all the M patients who have only one missing data item, to obtain

$$df = (2N - 1) - \frac{M}{L},$$
(15.8)

and this is rounded down to the nearest integer.

15.14 Sensitivity analysis

Imputation is never an ideal solution; it is a salvage job. A major aim is to reduce bias by making full use of additional known information about the patients with missing data, and information about the patients with complete data. Thus the analyst is making many assumptions about the relationship of the observed data to the unobserved missing values. An essential aspect of making the conclusions of a trial more convincing is to show readers the consequences of the various assumptions. This leads to what is termed a *sensitivity analysis*, in which the stability of the imputation methods is examined against their impact upon the analyses. An extreme case of this would be to replace the missing data first with extremely low QoL values and then with extremely high values. If the results from both these analyses are consistent with those obtained using more formal imputation, the conclusions gain credence. If, on the other hand, the results disagree, it is necessary to explore and explain the possible reasons for the discrepancy. This may involve using a variety of imputation methods to explore which assumptions are most critical for influencing the study conclusions.

15.15 Conclusions

Many investigators are suspicious about using imputation techniques, because of the assumptions that are overtly involved. However, it should be remembered that *not* imputing missing data also involves making assumptions – namely, that the patients failing to respond are similar to those study patients for whom data have been recorded. One difference between imputing or not imputing is simply that the assumptions are explicit for the former and implicit for the latter. Thus, for example, if patients with poor baseline performance status tend to have follow-up QoL assessments missing, it is presumably better to make use of this baseline characteristic by imputing values rather than (implicitly) assuming that these patients are likely to be similar on average to the other patients in the study, many of whom are known to have a high performance status. Imputation tries to use the available information, so as to make better allowance for patients with missing data.

   Of the imputation techniques described, the multiple imputation and pattern mixture approaches seem the most efficient, as they take additional patient information into account in the imputation process, and they preserve the magnitude of the *SD*s, ensuring that the *CI*s can be correctly estimated. They also allow the user's prior knowledge and experience to be incorporated into the imputation process.

   The simplest of the methods described are based on MCAR; this is usually unlikely to be realistic. The recommended methods assume MAR, which is more plausible than MCAR. Even so, MAR is only a justifiable assumption for this purpose if there are enough explanatory variables to predict the missing values and their pattern. In the absence of sufficient predictive variables, MAR ceases to be applicable and the missing data must be regarded as MNAR. In this case, the presence of the missing measurement is in itself informative, and we cannot predict the missing value without making further untestable assumptions. Then, any imputation becomes suspect and bias cannot be ruled out. Of the methods described in this chapter, only the pattern mixture approach is suitable when the missing data are MNAR.

An intrinsic difficulty, especially when there is a large amount of missing data, whether missing forms or items, is the final choice of imputation method. The best method may be specific to the individual missing items or scales concerned as well as the particular assessment sequence. In many QoL questionnaires there are so many items that to tailor the imputation for each component may not be practical. In any event it is probably important, at least in most circumstances, to decide the method of imputation in advance of examining the data. Previous experience with similar data will often guide the choice of method. Of particular concern are those few PROs and scales that have been selected as the major endpoints for the study concerned. These should be the major focus for determining the imputation process. Secondary QoL endpoints may perhaps be imputed using the less sophisticated approaches.

It is important to emphasise that estimating missing values is an extra burden on the analyst and therefore consumes resources, some of which would be better deployed by giving greater attention to patient compliance at an earlier stage in the study process. Sophisticated imputation methods are merely devices for facilitating the final analysis. They are no substitute for the real data. It is a fallacy to think that one can create new data by analyses and imputation. The *only* way to be confident of avoiding bias is to have high compliance rates. Studies with poor compliance will remain unconvincing and unpublishable, no matter how carefully the data are analysed. Always aim for 100% compliance.

15.16   Further reading

Most texts on analysis of longitudinal studies with missing data assume a deep understanding of statistical modelling. The classic text on this subject is Little and Rubin (2002) *Statistical Analysis with Missing Data*. For a modern and simpler approach, focusing on QoL data, Fairclough (2010) *Design and Analysis of Quality of Life Studies in Clinical Trials* is highly recommended and contains many worked examples of analyses with accompanying code in the statistical computer package SAS (SAS Inst. Inc., 2008). Sterne *et al.* (2009) provide accessible advice regarding multiple imputation for clinical research. The European Medicines Agency (2010) provides general advice on all aspects of handling missing data in trials.

16

Practical and reporting issues

Summary

At various stages in the book, we have indicated issues on which decisions have to be made when analysing, presenting and reporting QoL studies. With the wealth of data that is usually generated, it is clear that compromises have to be made, and these mean that the major focus will need to be placed on relatively few aspects. Choices made will have implications ranging from the way compliance is summarised to which particular comparisons will be presented with the associated confidence intervals (*CI*s). Although QoL data pose unique difficulties, there are general aspects of presenting and reporting the results of clinical studies that should always be adhered to. We assume that good reporting standards are indeed followed, and our focus will be on those aspects that relate to QoL studies in particular.

16.1   Introduction

Guidelines to assist investigators on reporting QoL studies have been suggested by a number of authors (e.g. Revicki, 2005). These guidelines addressed aspects of QoL as well as more general recommendations for all types of clinical studies. Meanwhile, standards of reporting for clinical trials were set by the CONSORT statement (Schulz *et al.*, 2010), which initially arose as a direct consequence of poor reporting standards for randomised clinical trials. The CONSORT Quality of Life Extension (Calvert *et al.*, 2013) sets a similar standard for reporting QoL and PROs.

Prior to these guidelines, weaknesses of the published reports of QoL in clinical trials have ranged from the lack of information on specific items, such as the psychometric properties of the instruments, to the handling of missing data caused especially through patient attrition (Brundage *et al.*, 2011).

Quality of Life: The Assessment, Analysis and Reporting of Patient-Reported Outcomes, Third Edition.
Peter M. Fayers and David Machin.
© 2016 John Wiley & Sons, Ltd. Published 2016 by John Wiley & Sons, Ltd.

16.2   The reporting of design issues

Instruments

The justification for the selection of a health profile (descriptive) and/or a patient pref-erence (utility) approach for the QoL assessment as well as of a particular question-naire should be given. If a QoL instrument is not well known or is new, it must be described in detail and the psychometric properties should be summarised. The ration-ale for creating a new instrument and the method by which the items were created is indispensable. For disease-specific instruments, an indication as to whether or not the psychometric properties were established in the same type of population as the study subjects is essential.

Of particular importance are the time frame over which the subject has to assess their responses to the items of the questionnaire (e.g. the past week) and the method by which the instrument was administered (e.g. by face-to-face interview). If appropri-ate, information on the process by which the measure was adapted for cross-cultural administration must be detailed.

Sources relevant to the development and format of the chosen QoL instruments should be referenced. When an instrument, item or scale is being used in a new popu-lation or disease from that in which it was originally developed, the psychometric properties of the instrument in the new context must be reported.

The choice of instrument will often be specific to the type of patients involved, for example children (Solans *et al.*, 2008), or disease, for example osteoarthritis (Veenhof *et al.*, 2006).

Sample size

In a comparative study, and particularly a randomised trial, the anticipated effect size that it was planned to detect should be specified. As indicated in Chapter 11, an esti-mate of the required sample size calculated on the basis of the endpoints of the study should be provided. The test size (α) and power ($1 - \beta$) must be specified. If (unusu-ally) a one-sided test is used, it needs to be justified.

As noted in Chapter 11, sample size and power estimation must always be made during the design stage, and these pre-study estimates should be reported. There is no value in reporting calculations carried out retrospectively, after completing the study.

16.3   Data analysis

When describing the choice of instrument, it is important to give details of how the responses are scored, preferably by reference to a published scoring manual or other available source document. Any departure from such procedures should be detailed and justified. Information on how to interpret the scores is necessary; for example, do higher scores indicate better or worse functioning or symptoms?

Ideally, only those QoL endpoints that were defined before the trial commenced should be used for the formal analysis. For these endpoints, *CI*s and *p*-values should be quoted. Other variables will be used only for descriptive purposes and to generate hypotheses for testing in later studies.

The statistical methods of analysis must be described in sufficient detail for other researchers to be able to repeat the analysis if the full data were made available. When appropriate, assumptions about the distribution of the data should be indicated. It should be indicated whether the analysis is by 'intention to treat' or otherwise. In case of multiple comparisons, attention must be paid to the total number of comparisons, to the need for any adjustment of the significance level, and to the interpretation of the results. If applicable, the definition of a clinically important difference should be given.

Missing items

It is imperative to document the causes of all missing data. Several types of missing data are possible and should be identified and documented separately in the publication. If patients or subjects fail to complete all items on a QoL instrument, possibly accidentally, the corresponding scoring manual for the instrument will usually describe methods of calculating scale scores when there are a few missing values for some items. Particular note should be taken if missing data tend to concern particular items on the QoL instrument or occur with a certain type of patient.

In the study report, the percentages of missing data for each item in the questionnaire should be compared, always focusing on the pre-specified major endpoints. Any difference in the percentages by patient group should be commented upon.

Missing forms

It should be specified whether missing data are due to informative (non-random) censoring – that is, due to the patient's health state or particular treatment – or to non-informative (essentially random) censoring mechanisms. The methods by which missing data were defined and analysed, including any imputation methods, must be clearly stated. In appropriate contexts, it is important to specify how data from patients who die before attaining the study endpoints are dealt with in the analysis.

As described in Chapter 15, missing the whole of a QoL form, and not just some items, poses a particular problem as their absence may lead to serious bias and hence incorrect conclusions. When forms are missing, there is no easy solution for eliminating this potential bias. Therefore, emphasis must always be placed upon avoiding the problem by ensuring optimal compliance with assessment. Any form of correction to the analysis is second best and the study results will be convincing only if compliance is high and missing data are kept to a minimum. Data forms may be missing for a variety of reasons, ranging from death of the patient to refusal to comply for no given reason.

Compliance with completion of the questionnaires can be defined as the percentage of completed forms received by the investigator from the number anticipated by the study design, taking due account of factors that would make completion impossible, such as the death of the patient. Thus the number of expected forms is based on the number of people alive. A special issue of the journal *Statistics in Medicine* is devoted to this topic alone (Bernhard and Gelber, 1998).

Choice of summary statistics

In certain cases – for example if a PRO follows an approximately Normal distribution shape (it need not be continuous for this) – the mean and *SD* encapsulate the essential features of the data. As we have discussed, the Normal distribution form may require a transformation from the original scale of measurement. If the underlying PRO variable is of an ordered categorical form, we would not recommend such an approach; rather we would use the median as the measure of location and the range as the measure of spread as are used in the box-and-whisker plot of Figure 12.5. In some situations, especially if the number of categories is small, there may be a tendency for the observations to cluster towards one or other end of the scale; that is, to take the minimum or maximum values, sometimes termed the floor and ceiling values. In this situation, the median and minimum (or maximum) may coincide. In such cases, there is no entirely satisfactory summary that can be used. We suggest that for these variables the simple proportion falling in the first (or last) category be quoted, thus converting the ordered categorical variable to a binary one.

Choice of analysis

PROs are mostly either continuous or of an ordered categorical form (a binary variable is a special case of the latter), and standard statistical methods as described in Chapter 12 can be used for between-group comparisons of two groups. These methods can be extended to the comparison of three or more groups and can be adjusted to take account of patient characteristics (e.g. age), which might also be influencing QoL apart from group membership itself. This leads us, in the case of a variable that has a Normal distribution, from the comparison of two means via the z- or t-tests, to ANOVA for three or more groups and the F-test, to multiple regression to adjust for patient characteristics. Similarly, we are led from the comparison of two proportions using the z- or χ^2-tests, to logistic regression with between-group differences expressed in terms of the odds ratio (*OR*), to the extension to an ordered categorical variable and finally to multiple logistic regression.

All the methods described are interconnected and are examples of multiple regression analysis with either continuous or categorical variables. As a consequence, it is usually best to approach analysis in this way. It should be noted, however, that the computer programs for multiple regression and multiple logistic regression are not the same.

Simple comparisons

Many of the complications in analysis arise because studies that assess PROs usually assess each patient at multiple time points. When cross-sectional analyses are carried out, many of the problems disappear. Sometimes straightforward comparison of two means is required so that *t*-tests may be appropriate with associated *CI*s. Some of these comparisons may need to be adjusted by multiple regression techniques to examine the effect of prognostic variables upon PROs. Non-parametric tests, such as the Wilcoxon or Mann–Whitney, may often be better because many of the PRO single items and some of the functioning scales can have asymmetric (non-Normal) distributions. Where single items are, for example, four-point scales, ordered logistic regression might be appropriate if one wants to examine the effect of prognostic variables.

For single items, a percentage rather than a mean may be a better summary of the corresponding variable. When percentages are used, the analyses often reduce to comparisons of binomial proportions by use of simple logistic regression.

Multiplicity of outcomes

A typical QoL instrument contains many questions often with supplementary modules containing additional items and scales. Thus there are potentially many pairwise statistical comparisons that might be made in any clinical study with two – or more – groups. Even if no treatment effect is truly present, some of these comparisons would be spuriously statistically significant, and hence be *false positives*. Specifically, if a single comparison is evaluated and *p* is found to be less than 0.05, it indicates that there is a less than 5% chance that this is a false positive. If we assume for convenience that the comparisons are independent (that is, the outcomes are uncorrelated) and that all are tested against an alpha of $p < 0.05$, the overall probability that at least one of the outcomes is deemed 'statistically significant, $p < 0.05$' rapidly increases. With two outcomes the chance of at least one false positive is no longer 5%, but becomes 10%; for three, 14%; five, 23% … ten, 40% and so on. For *k* comparisons, the equation is $1 - (1 - p)^k$. Of course PROs are unlikely to be uncorrelated, but the risk of at least one false positive will nonetheless rapidly become unacceptable as the number of comparisons increases, and individual *p*-values will fail to capture the overall risk.

One way of avoiding this problem is to identify in the protocol itself one or two PROs as being the ones of principal interest. These few outcomes will then be the main focus of the analysis, and therefore there will be no problem of multiple testing. We recommend (with caution) that the *p*-values for these should not be corrected but perhaps a comment be made concerning the problem of multiple testing in the discussion of the results. This approach is recommended by Perneger (1998), who concludes that: "Simply describing what tests of significance have been performed, and why, is generally the best way of dealing with multiple comparisons." For these comparisons, we suggest a corresponding confidence interval be reported (Altman *et al.*, 2000). A precautionary recommendation here may be to have in mind a 99% *CI* as an aid to interpretation.

The alternative, especially if, despite the above recommendations, many PROs are being investigated with a large number of statistical hypothesis tests, is to use the Bonferroni correction as mentioned in Chapter 11. For k hypothesis tests, the Bonferroni-corrected p-values are the observed p-values multiplied by k. This correction assumes that the comparisons are independent of each other (which for PROs is unlikely to be true), and becomes progressively conservative (that is, over corrects) as the outcomes become more highly correlated. Although the Bonferroni procedure is widely used, there exist alternative procedures that are more efficient, such as the Holm step-down procedure (Holm, 1979). In this, the p-values calculated by the significance tests are ranked in order, from most to least significant. The first (most highly significant) value is multiplied by k (as for the Bonferroni correction). If this is significant (e.g. $p < 0.05$ if 5% has been specified as the target denoting 'significance'), the next p-value is multiplied by $(k - 1)$. If this is significant, the next is multiplied by $(k - 2)$, and so on. The process terminates as soon as a comparison is not significant, whereupon all subsequent values are deemed not significant. A variety of more efficient procedures, of varying complexity, is reviewed by Dmitrienko *et al.* (2013).

For the remaining PROs, we recommend a less exhaustive analysis. All these analyses may then be regarded as primarily hypothesis generating and the associated p-values merely indicative of possible differences to be explored at a later stage in further study. Even here it may be sensible to adopt 'conservative' p-values, either by using

---

Example

Suppose $k = 5$ outcomes were pre-specified for hypothesis testing, and the corresponding p-values calculated using a statistical test such as the t-test; statistical significance was denoted by $p < 0.05$. The observed p-values were 0.046, 0.032, 0.136, 0.011 and 0.006. Four values are less than 0.05, but (conservatively assuming independence) there is overall a 23% chance of at least one false positive. Applying the Bonferroni correction, only $0.006 \times 5 = 0.03$ meets the criterion of $p < 0.05$ and all other values are not significant.

If it had been pre-specified in the protocol that the Holm procedure was to be used, the p-values would have been sorted to give 0.006, 0.011, 0.032, 0.046 and 0.136. The corresponding correction factors are 5, 4, 3, 2, 1. Then both 0.006×5 and 0.011×4 are less than 0.05 and thus significant. Since 0.032×3 is not significant, testing ceases and the remaining two comparisons are also not significant.

the more stringent $p \leq 0.01$ (or even $p \leq 0.001$) or, as discussed in the chapter on sample size estimation, by applying the Bonferroni correction. If a large number of outcomes are considered in an exploratory analysis, the Benyamini–Hochberg (1995) false discovery rate might be considered instead of p-values.

In the case of multiple comparisons, attention must be paid to the total number of comparisons, to the adjustment, if any, of the significance level, and to the interpretation of the results. Seldom will a global multivariate test producing a single (or composite) p-value be of use. Best is to circumvent the problems of multiple testing by defining a single outcome, or possibly a couple of outcomes, as the primary hypothesis to be tested, with other outcomes and hypothesis tests being regarded as exploratory.

Repeated measurements

This raises similar issues to those just preceding, but rather than the numerous items on a QoL instrument leading to many comparisons, it is the longitudinal nature of the patient follow-up that can lead to repeat statistical testing of the difference between treatments at successive time points. Thus, of the various methods available, one of the simplest and yet most informative approaches is to use graphical displays (Chapter 13) and accompany these by cross-sectional analyses (Chapter 12) at a few specific time points. Ideally, the study protocol will have pre-specified that the analysis will focus both upon the aspect of QoL concerned and the particular time points. Nevertheless, the difficulty remains, there are still repeated tests and the problems associated with false positives remains.

A more satisfactory alternative is to encapsulate these repeated measurements into a single summary for each patient. Examples are: the overall mean QoL, the worst QoL experienced during therapy or the area under the curve (AUC) (Chapter 13). The choice of which to use will depend on the study objectives. The analyses can then compare and test using these summaries as the basic data for each patient in an appropriate cross-sectional manner.

Modelling

For the truly primary endpoints, more sophisticated methods are available and these allow for the auto-correlation between QoL values at successive time points. The main methods include the hierarchical or multilevel models and the generalised estimating equations (Chapter 14), as well as methods to cope with missing values (Chapter 15). Some of these methods do ideally require specialist statistical software to implement, such as MLwiN (Rasbash *et al.*, 2015) or HLM (Raudenbush *et al.*, 2004) for multilevel models and BUGS (Lunn *et al.*, 2009) for Bayesian modelling; for that reason, in this book we do not describe the application of these methods. However, many of the methods are also becoming more widely available in standard statistical packages; for example, GEE is available in widely used statistical computer packages such as SAS and STATA.

In general, we would not recommend use of multivariate analysis of variance (MANOVA) for repeated measures because the conclusions to be drawn from, for example, a statistically significant result are in many instances far from clear.

A sensible precaution before embarking on the modelling process (or for that matter using repeated measures ANOVA and related techniques) is first to plot the data. This will give a general idea of models that may or may not be appropriate. For example, there is unlikely to be a linear trend in values of, say, nausea and vomiting when assessed before active treatment commences, several times during chemotherapy and then several times during post-treatment follow-up in cancer patients. However, an indiscriminate use of statistical packages leads some analysts to simply read off the significant *p*-values giving little thought to the appropriateness or otherwise of the underlying statistical procedure.

Clinical significance

Although it is not possible to give a clear definition of clinical significance, nevertheless specific examples are given in Chapter 18. It is clear that statistical and clinical significance should not be confused. Statistical significance tells us whether the observed differences can be explained by chance fluctuations alone, but says nothing about clinical significance. Despite the difficulty of determining what is *clinically significant*, an idea of its magnitude has to be elicited for trial planning purposes.

16.4   Elements of good graphics

Exploratory and descriptive data analyses explore, clarify, describe and help to interpret the QoL data. These less formal analyses may reveal unexpected patterns in the data. Because these analyses are less concerned with significance testing, graphical methods are especially suitable. A judicious use of graphics can succinctly summarise complex data that would otherwise require extensive tabulations, and can clarify and display the complex inter-relationships of QoL data. At the same time, graphics help to emphasise the high degree of variability in QoL data. Current computing facilities offer unrivalled facilities for the production of extensive and high-quality graphics.

Simple graphical summaries

Perhaps the simplest summaries of all are histogram and bar charts, which show the frequency distribution of the data. These are often used for the initial inspection of data and to establish basic characteristics of the data. For example, prior to using a *t*-test one ought to check whether the data are distributed symmetrically and whether they appear to follow a Normal distribution. Thus Figure 12.2 illustrates a histogram of baseline emotional functioning (EF) in patients with multiple myeloma. This is a common method of displaying information.

Although this is a simple graphical display, there are a number of variations that may improve the presentation. Thus Figure 16.1 shows the same information, adding 'blank lines' to make it visually easier to assess the height of the histogram bars, and using light shading of the blocks.

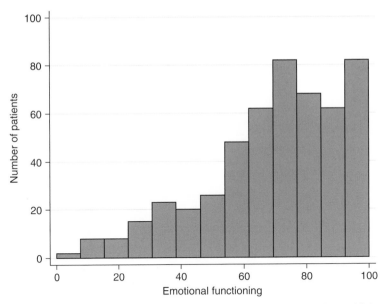

Figure 16.1 Histogram of baseline emotional functioning (EF) in patients with multiple myeloma. *Source:* Data from Wisløff *et al.,* 1996.

Comparison of two groups

One common way of displaying the differences between two treatments or two groups of patients is a bar chart. An example is shown in Figure 16.2a, which displays the mean fatigue levels for males and females at various times over the duration of the study.

However, the format of Figure 16.2b is preferable since it more readily conveys the shape of the relationship with time and helps quantify more readily the gender differences. Also, in contrast to Figure 16.2a, the unequal time intervals between assessments are correctly represented along the horizontal axis. This figure could be further enhanced to provide *CI*s.

Association of variables

When showing the association between two variables, the simplest graphic is perhaps the scatter plot, as shown for anxiety versus age in Figure 16.3a. One of the difficulties with such a plot is that two or more patients may supply the same pair of values, leading to plotting symbols being overprinted and their true impact lost. One device to expose this overlap is to 'jitter' these multiple observation points about the true plotting position. Thus Figure 16.3b represents exactly the same data as Figure 16.3a, but there now appears to be more data points. The second figure gives a more complete picture of the true situation. In the latter figure, the marginal box-and-whisker plots for EF and age are added above and to the right-hand side of the main panel to assist interpretation further.

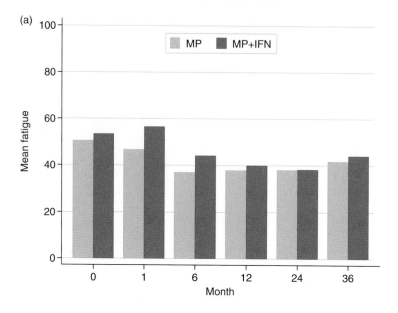

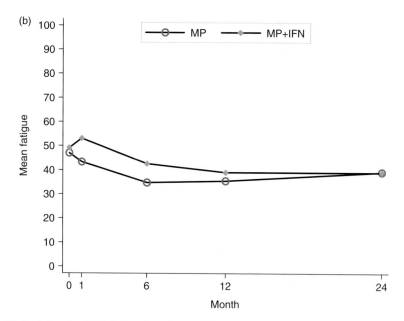

Figure 16.2 Mean levels of fatigue in patients with multiple myeloma, before and during treatment with MP or MP+IFN: (a) bar chart; (b) line plot. *Source:* Data from Wisløff *et al.*, 1996.

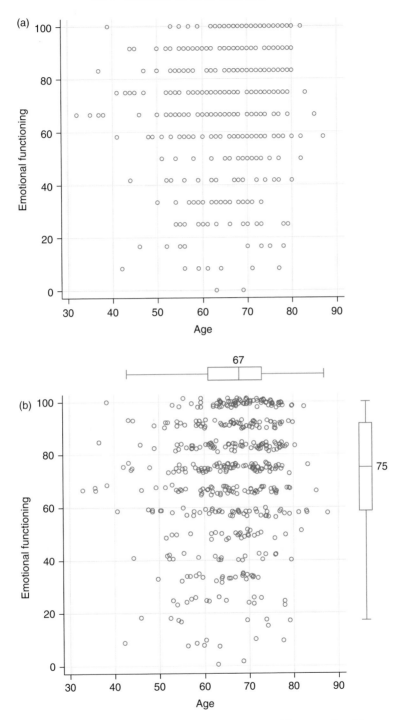

Figure 16.3   Baseline EF by age, in patients with multiple myeloma: (a) scatter plot; (b) scatter plot with 'jitter' and marginal box plots. In the box plots, the box shows the 25% and 75% quartiles and the median, and the 'whiskers' indicate the so-called 'adjacent values'. *Source:* Data from Wisløff *et al.*, 1996.

16.5   Some errors

Baseline variables

In the reporting of any study, presentation of, for example, basic demographic and other baseline data in tabular format by patient group is always valuable. In this respect, QoL studies are no different. However, these tables are usually for descriptive purposes only and so would usually contain, for example, means (or medians) and SDs, and possibly minimum and maximum values, rather than means and CIs.

In randomised clinical trials, statistical tests of significance between baseline characteristics of the groups are rarely pertinent. If the group membership was determined at random, as is the case of allocation to treatment groups in a randomised trial, any statistically significant difference in baseline characteristics will either be solely due to chance or be an indication of violation of the randomisation procedure (Fayers and King, 2008a,b). Provided one is confident that the randomisation methods are reliable, there is no point in carrying out a significance test. Statistical tests and CIs should be confined to the endpoint variables alone, although these comparisons may be adjusted for baseline variables that were included in the tabulation just referred to. It should be noted that the decision to adjust for baseline variables should depend primarily on their prognostic or predictive relevance. It is particularly important to allow for prognostic factors that are imbalanced at the baseline assessment, irrespective of whether that imbalance is statistically significant.

A common mistake is to calculate and quote CIs of, say, the mean of each group separately, whereas in any comparative study it is the CI of the difference between groups that is relevant. As already indicated, such problems are not confined to QoL studies alone, but they are compounded in such studies as the number of baseline and endpoint measures may be very large.

Confidence intervals

In published QoL research, some investigators summarise differences between subject groups for each of the QoL items or scales under study by merely reporting in a tabular format the corresponding p-value. Often they fail to quote the precise p-value unless it is less than 0.05, instead using the notation NS (not statistically significant). This is very bad practice and is now actively discouraged by the leading medical journals since NS covers a range of p-values from a little over 0.05 to 1. The conclusions drawn from a result with $p = 0.06$ are quite different from one for which it is 0.6. It is important, even when there is no statistically significant difference, to provide not just the p-values but also an estimate of the magnitude of the difference between groups together with the associated CI. This is emphasised by Altman et al. (2000), with clear recommendations.

Graphical

One disadvantage to profile plots is that there may be a tendency for naïve readers of such plots to assume that the different dimensions may be compared – for example in Figure 12.6, to think that overall quality of life (ql) is slightly greater than or 'better' than role functioning (rf), and that social functioning (sf) is much 'better' than both ql and rf. However, responses to items on QoL questionnaires are not calibrated uniformly across dimensions, and it is meaningless to describe whether one scale takes higher (or lower) values than other scales.

A common and, at first sight, apparently reasonable form of analysis is to compare change in QoL scores for patients against their baseline values. Thus one might seek to determine whether patients who start with a poor QoL are likely to have an even poorer QoL after treatment, or whether they tend to improve. Hence one might plot the baseline score (QoL_0) against the change between baseline and, say, month-1 (QoL_1) values. Thus Figure 16.4a, for EF, shows a moderate degree of correlation between the change ($QoL_1 - QoL_0$) and the baseline measurement.

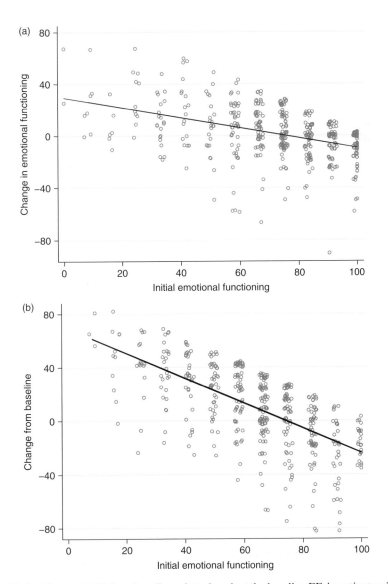

Figure 16.4   Change in EF from baseline, plotted against the baseline EF, in patients with multiple myeloma: (a) plotting ($EF_1 - EF_0$) against EF_0; (b) substituting random numbers in place of EF_0, the initial measurement. *Source:* Data from Wisløff *et al.*, 1996.

However, this plot cannot be interpreted. This is because a similar plot can be obtained by replacing the initial EF observations by random numbers over the same range of possible values and using these in the calculation of the change from baseline! Such a 'random numbers' plot against initial EF is shown in Figure 16.4b. The reason for the association in Figure 16.4a is that the vertical axis measure $y = (QoL_1 - QoL_0)$ and the horizontal axis measure $x = QoL_0$ both contain the same quantity QoL_0. Thus, in part, one is correlating $-QoL_0$ with $+QoL_0$ itself, and this correlation is perfect but negative (-1). This correlation then dominates both panels of Figure 16.4, creating the illusion of an association.

A comparison of change against initial value may be of clinical importance, and more rigorous methods of analysis are available. These issues are discussed by Bland and Altman (1986), who suggest plots corresponding to change in score $(QoL_1 - QoL_0)$ against the average score $(QoL_1 + QoL_0)/2$.

16.6   Guidelines for reporting

In recent years, the number of clinical trials incorporating measurement of health-related QoL has substantially increased. We introduce here general guidelines for the reporting of clinical trials that include a QoL measurement. These proposals are intended for researchers reporting a new study as well as for those who are asked to evaluate critically the published reports.

Checklist

Some of the headings in this section repeat those already mentioned above, but the topics are collected here as a checklist. The associated comments add some detail not included previously.

- **Abstract**
  Describe the purpose of the study, the methods, the key results and the principal conclusions.

- **Introduction**

  a. Describe the objective of the study in detail. Its rationale must be supported with a comprehensive review of the literature relevant to the disease or the treatment of interest.

  b. The natural history of the disease and its treatment should be described succinctly so that it is clear why QoL is being assessed.

  c. The pre-study hypotheses for QoL assessment must be stated, indicating the domains or scales that were expected to show a difference between treatment arms. The definition of QoL should be presented.

- **Materials and methods**

- **Population and sample**

    a. A description of the patient population, including the study inclusion and exclusion criteria, is mandatory. The population sample must be described with appropriate demographic data, for example age, gender and ethnicity, depending on the context. Other variables, such as the clinical and mental status, should also be included if they were likely to alter the ability of the patient to answer a questionnaire.

    b. It is important to indicate how and from where the patients were recruited to the study. For instance, indicate whether the sample was random or one of convenience, and the number of centres involved. If a subset of the total sample size is deemed to be sufficient for the QoL part of the trial, the method used to select the patients in the subset must be explained.

- **QoL instrument selection**

    a. Rationale for the choice of instrument, including where appropriate references to previous validation, or details of the validation and the psychometric properties.

    b. Justify the suitability of the instrument – are *all* the relevant domains covered?

- **Trial size**
  Definition of the target difference to be detected, and details of the pre-study sample size calculations.

- **Endpoints**
  State the dimension(s) or the item(s) of the instrument that were selected as endpoint(s) before subject accrual. When overall QoL is not the primary endpoint, the major endpoints of the trial should have been specified in the protocol. Endpoints not chosen before the start of the trial are to be avoided.

- **Timing and administration of assessments**

    a. The scheduled times of instrument completion must be given (for example every four weeks), as should the timing of the follow-up assessment. For instance, at the completion of treatment or discontinuation of treatment, every three months, or at the end of the study, and so on.

    b. Describe the method of administration. For example by self-completion, interview or proxy-assessment; at home or at hospital; by post or administered in the clinic.

- **Data**
  The means by which the data were collected and the procedure for evaluating their quality should be described. The criteria for what is to be considered adequate/inadequate must be specified.

- **Method of analysis**
  Definition of *p*-value level for statistical significance. If there will be multiple significance tests, what allowance will be made for multiplicity?

- **Results**

- **Presentation of data**

  a. The results of planned primary and secondary analyses should be presented along with the results of appropriate tests of statistical significance, such as *p*-value, effect size and *CI*s.

  b. The report should include reference to all the other items or scales from each instrument used in the study. In particular, it is important not to pick and choose which scales to report from an instrument without indicating very clearly why this has been done.

- **Patient data**

  a. All patients entered in the study must be accounted for and their characteristics presented. For example, how many centres were involved, how many eligible patients were approached, how many were accrued, how many refused to participate, how many were unable to complete the questionnaires, and so on.

  b. In the context of a clinical trial or comparative study, numbers of patients should be given for each group. Thus details are required on the numbers: eligible and entered; excluded from the analysis (with inadequate data, with missing data); losses to follow-up and death; adequately treated according to protocol; failed to complete the treatment according to protocol and received treatments not specified in the protocol.

- **Scheduling of instrument administration**
  Descriptive information is required that contributes to an understanding of treatment schedules, patient compliance, time windows, median follow-up times, and other practical aspects of QoL data collection and follow-up.

- **Missing data and compliance**
  Details of compliance/completion rates of the QoL questionnaires, divided by date of assessment (visit number), presented for each randomisation group. Report the methods of handling missing data, including specification of any imputation methods or adjustments to the analyses. Assess the potential bias that might arise from incomplete QoL data.

- **Statistical analysis**

  a. The main analysis should address the hypothesis identified in the introduction. Although it is recognised that there are often large numbers of items on a QoL questionnaire, the particular and few dimensions which were selected as design endpoint(s) should be the most relevant part of the report.

b. Analysis of other variables as well as any subgroup analysis not pre-specified should be reported only as *exploratory* or tentative.

c. If appropriate, the reasons for not adhering to the pre-trial sample size should be discussed.

d. In the case of a graphical presentation, it is important to specify the number at risk by treatment group beneath the time axis in the plot.

- **Discussion and conclusions**

  a. The findings should be discussed in the context of results of previous studies and research.

  b. Some particular issues in the interpretation of QoL data should be addressed here, including (as appropriate) the clinical interpretation of score change.

  c. A summary of the therapeutic results should be reported alongside the QoL results so that a balanced interpretation of the trial results can be made.

- **Appendices**
  In addition to describing the instruments that were used, as part of the Methods of the report, it may be appropriate to provide a copy if the instrument or measure is not well known. For a copyright instrument, information should be provided about the source of the instrument. If the instrument has been modified, any changes must be justified and fully documented.

16.7 Further reading

The main CONSORT statement includes a list of 25 items that should be reported for all clinical trials. There is also a flow chart describing patient progress through the trial, which should be included in the trial report. In addition, a few specific subheadings are suggested within the 'Methods and Results' sections of the paper. In the spirit of the times, the recommendations are evidence-based where possible, with common sense dictating the remainder. The CONSORT Quality of Life Extension lists the additional issues that must be addressed when using PROs.

In essence, the requirement is that authors should provide enough information for readers to know how the trial was performed and analysed, so that they can judge whether the findings are likely to be reliable. The CONSORT suggestions mean that authors will no longer be able to hide study inadequacies by omission of important information. Full details of the CONSORT statement (2011) and QoL Extension (Calvert *et al.*, 2013) are available at the CONSORT website (http://www.consort-statement.org). CONSORT guidelines are published in and endorsed by the many of leading medical journals, for example Schulz *et al.* (2010), and are further explained and elaborated by Moher *et al.* (2010).

17

Death, and quality-adjusted survival

Summary

Attrition due to death can complicate the analysis of clinical trials, especially if there are different death rates in the treatment arms. One approach is to explore the trade-off involved in choosing an aggressive therapy, with serious side effects, in the hope of improved survival versus a milder therapy that offers poorer survival prospects.

The overall survival time in a patient newly diagnosed with a life-threatening disease may be considered as being partitioned into distinct periods during which the QoL levels of the patient may expect to differ. These states may include, for example, the active treatment period. Once the time in each of these states is determined, they can be used to calculate the *time without symptoms and toxicity* (*TWiST*), the time actually experiencing symptoms and/or toxicity (*TOX*), and the time in relapse following progression of the disease (*PROG*).

Utility coefficients corresponding to each of these states can be evaluated and used as multipliers of *TOX*, *TWiST* and *PROG* to obtain a weighted *quality-adjusted time without symptoms and toxicity* (*Q-TWiST*). These are then averaged over all patients receiving a particular treatment and so can be used to compare treatments.

Threshold analysis enables an investigation into how sensitive this quantified difference in treatments is to the values of the utility coefficients for each state. The way in which *Q-TWiST* may be compared between different prognostic groups, and changes over successive time intervals from diagnosis, are described.

17.1 Introduction

The measures described so far in this book are sometimes called *profile instruments* because they provide a descriptive profile as to how each patient is feeling. This information may be used to describe groups of patients, as we have seen, or may be

Quality of Life: The Assessment, Analysis and Reporting of Patient-Reported Outcomes, Third Edition.
Peter M. Fayers and David Machin.
© 2016 John Wiley & Sons, Ltd. Published 2016 by John Wiley & Sons, Ltd.

used for comparative purposes in a clinical trial. Thus it can be used by clinicians when deciding whether one treatment results in, on average, better or worse QoL and whether this should result in a wider use of that treatment or even preclude its use altogether. Although the summary scores may seem at first sight difficult to interpret, Chapter 18 examines ways in which these scores may be interpreted clinically. The QoL profiles also provide a source of information about the possible consequences of therapy, and this information can be discussed with patients when deciding which treatment may be the most suitable. Thus clinicians can contrast the potential therapeutic benefits against possible impact upon QoL, and this can be used as the basis for patient decisions when choosing between alternative treatments.

However, for some decision purposes it is desirable to weigh up the therapeutic benefits and contrast them more formally against the changes in QoL. Specifically, if the more efficacious therapy is associated with poorer PROs, is it worthwhile?

Just as QoL can be assessed only by the patients themselves, so for clinical decisions the value judgement of treatment preference should similarly be determined by asking the patients. Various methods are available for determining patient preference ratings, some of which aim to combine QoL and survival duration into a single summary score that may be broadly summarized as equating actual years of survival to the (smaller) number of equivalent healthy years. The aim of this is to enable overall benefits of various treatment or management policies to be contrasted.

An alternative approach to combining QoL and survival duration is used for health economic studies. In this setting, cost is also considered and in contrast to the clinical approach it is usual to base utility values on the opinions of a sample of the general population. Although this book does not attempt to address health economics, the techniques developed for that purpose can be of value when analysing PROs in trials in which the survival rates differ across the randomisation groups.

17.2   Attrition due to death

In some diseases, such as cancer, more aggressive therapy may be associated with improved survival but at the expense of greater incidence of severe side effects. In some clinical trials this can result in the randomised groups having different survival durations, and indeed in such trials survival is frequently the primary outcome of interest. However, this leads to greater amounts of PRO or QoL data being available in one arm of the trial than the other. Although, superficially, this may seem analogous to missing data – with one treatment arm having more missing data than the other – it is rarely sensible to impute expected values for the 'missing' assessments that occur after death. Thus we use the term *attrition*, instead of *missing*, to encompass the additional loss of data due to death. One important distinction is that high rates of missing data indicate a poorly designed or poorly executed trial, in which there is a strong risk of biased results. In contrast, high levels of attrition due to deaths may sometimes be anticipated yet unavoidable, and do not imply that the trial is biased. However, a naïve analysis that ignores the consequences of attrition, especially when the rates of attrition due to death differ across randomisation arms of the study, may lead to misleading results.

A *landmark analysis* is a simple cross-sectional analysis at a prespecified time. This can provide a non-controversial and clinically relevant comparison of the patients who remain alive at that time. However, problems arise when carrying out analyses of the repeated measurements. Repeated cross-sectional analyses will be based on declining numbers of patients, making it difficult to compare the results at the various time points. Some authors attempt to address this by using a *complete case* analysis, in which analyses are restricted to patients alive at, for example, one year and carrying out a longitudinal analysis from baseline up to that time point. Quite apart from the wasteful loss of data, such an analysis provides results that are only applicable to similar patients surviving to that time and tells us nothing about patients who die earlier, nor does it inform what happens at later times.

An alternative approach, which is the topic of this chapter, is to evaluate patients' preferences. Specifically, suppose a patient is given the choice between two treatments, where one increases their probability of living slightly longer relative to the other treatment but at the expense of serious toxicity. Which treatment option would they prefer?

17.3 Preferences and utilities

When the outcomes are known in advance, patients can express a *preference* for one treatment or another. For example, if it can be stated that treatment will result in cure but at the cost of specified QoL disadvantages, patients can decide whether or not to accept the treatment. However, in most clinical situations there will be uncertainty regarding both the cure and the QoL outcomes. Usually, we can state only that there is a certain probability of cure and that this may be gained at possible QoL disadvantages. When preferences are assessed in the face of uncertainty, they are called *utilities*, because a patient might make one selection under uncertainty but might express a different preference if it were known what outcome would ensue.

Visual analogue scales (VAS)

The simplest way of establishing preference ratings is by means of a *visual analogue scale*, in which the extreme anchors are usually 'best possible QoL' and 'worst possible QoL', or some equivalent wording. The patient is then asked to indicate on the 10-cm line the position of their current state, and also to mark positions corresponding to various scenarios, such as their likely condition during or following therapy. For the least favourable state, 'death' is often avoided because some patients may declare particular states of health to be worse than death; thus for alternative wording one might consider 'worst imaginable state of health'.

This method has been found to be efficient and easy to use, and appears to provide meaningful values for relative preferences of various states of health and treatment. It can be extended to include the concept of uncertainty, thereby providing utilities, if the scenarios include suitably phrased descriptions that indicate a risk of side effects or disease progression; in this case, extra care is needed in choosing appropriately worded endpoints for the scale.

Time trade-off (TTO)

Time trade-off involves comparing QoL against length of survival. A typical strategy for evaluating TTO is to present a scenario under which health is impaired by specific disabilities or symptoms, and to ask the patient whether he or she would choose one year in perfect health or one year with impaired health; presumably, the healthy year would be selected. Then the duration of the healthy period is gradually reduced: 'Would you choose 11 months in perfect health, or one year with impaired health?' and so on. At some stage, equilibrium should be reached, and it may then be concluded that the value of impaired life is equivalent to a certain percentage of time relative to healthy life.

As we shall see, TTO is conceptually equivalent to the *QALY* approach (Section 17.6), and might therefore seem attractive. Since it does not involve uncertainty, it is a method for eliciting patient *preferences*. However, many patients find the concepts difficult to apply.

Standard gamble (SG)

The *standard gamble* method involves decisions in the face of uncertainty, where the uncertainty involves a risk of death or some other outcome. Thus SG attempts to estimate patient *utilities*.

For example, SG might be used to establish the value of anti-hypertensive therapy by offering the following alternatives to patients: 'Suppose there is a P percent chance

---

Example from the literature

De Haes and Stiggelbout (1996) compare VAS, TTO and SG methods in 30 testicular cancer patients. In line with other reports, the VAS method yielded the lowest scores and TTO was slightly lower than SG. The authors note that since many patients are reluctant to trade survival for QoL, and are willing to accept high levels of toxicity for a relatively modest increase in survival time, it is perhaps not unexpected that TTO results in higher scores than VAS. Similarly, SG patients are asked to consider the possibility of immediate death, which is even less acceptable to many. The authors suggest that the choice between the three methods might be made according to the disease and the intended application of the ratings; for example, in a surgical trial that involves a risk of early death, the SG approach might be preferred.

of death within the following year if you do not take anti-hypertensive therapy, but on the other hand you would have to take therapy for the rest of your life and it has these side effects …' By varying the percentage, P, the point of indifference can be established. The value $(1 - P)$ then provides the utility value for impairment due to this form of therapy.

As with TTO, many patients find the concepts of SG unrealistic and have difficulty in making consistent responses. One particular problem is that it is frequently difficult to provide realistic scenarios for some of the medical conditions and therapies that are under consideration.

Willingness to pay (WTP)

Whereas SG involves a gamble and the element of risk when comparing the value of different health states, and TTO uses varying time periods, *willingness to pay* introduces the concept of monetary value. The foundation for this is that people are accustomed to making decisions about how much they are willing to spend upon most things relating to life – from small items such as food and clothing, and medium-cost decisions such as annual holidays, through to major expenses including car and house. The amount that an individual is willing to pay is an indicator of the utility or satisfaction that they expect to gain from the particular commodity.

Various methods have been used to elicit WTP values, including basic questions such as 'What is the most that you would be willing to pay for … ?'. A variation on this is to present a list of options or a set of cards containing 'bids' of increasing amounts, from which the respondent selects the amount they would be willing to pay.

WTP has rarely been used in QoL research.

Discrete choice experiments (DCE)

Another technique for assessing preferences of health states is a *discrete choice experiment*, also known as *conjoint analysis*. This has been used extensively in market research and transport economics, and is increasingly used in health economics. DCEs involve constructing a number of realistic scenarios that represent combinations of different health states (item levels). Obviously, there are too many possible states to be able to present them all (see Section 17.4), and so particular scenarios must be selected. The patient is then presented with two or more of the scenarios and asked to rank them, rate them or indicate their preferred option. Since the majority of people are accustomed to making what are effectively pairwise comparisons and decisions on a daily basis, a single binary choice may be the preferred approach for DCEs (Ryan, 1999).

DCEs offer an alternative to SG, TTO and VAS. It has been found that many people find SG difficult, and make inconsistent choices; DCEs appear to be easier to apply. TTO has the disadvantage of being less rooted in economic theory. Although DCEs do not need to incorporate risk assessment, this can be included as part of the scenarios if so desired. If single binary choices are used, the resultant data consist of binary preferences that can be analysed using logistic (or the related probit) regression models; some of the models are complex, requiring specialised software for their fitting (Ryan and Gerard, 2005).

Example from the literature

Ryan *et al.* (2006) illustrate the use of DCEs to estimate a preference-based measure of outcome for social care of older people. Five core domains were identified: Food/nutrition, Personal care, Safety, Social participation and Control over daily living. Within each domain, three levels of need were defined: no unmet needs, low needs and high needs. Thus there were 243 (3^5) possible outcomes. Using experimental design techniques, 14 'choice sets' or pairs of scenarios were identified, enabling the fit of a linear additive model. To reduce respondent burden, each person was only asked to rate 7 choice sets and for each of these the respondent was asked to identify which scenario they least preferred. An example is shown in Figure 17.1.

There were 326 individuals over the age of 60, drawn from 14 day-centres, completing the evaluation exercise. A regression model revealed problems with the assessment of Safety and so a reduced model was explored, provisionally excluding Safety and retaining four domains. Quality weights were estimated, with high unmet needs anchored as zero for each domain. The quality weights for unmet needs were: Food, no or low = 0.141; Personal care, no = 0.353, low = 0.176; Social, no = 0.293, low = 0.193; and Control, no or low = 0.213.

Thus for someone who had no unmet needs on all four domains,

$$\text{Utility score} = 0.141 + 0.353 + 0.293 + 0.213 = 1.0.$$

Similarly, another person with low needs on all domains would have

$$\text{Utility score} = 0.141 + 0.176 + 0.193 + 0.213 = 0.723.$$

Which of these two situations do you think is worse?

SITUATION 1	SITUATION 2
You have as much control over daily living as possible.	You have sufficient, varied, timely meals and you are always clean and appropriately dressed.
But, you have an inadequate diet potentially resulting in a health risk. You are occasionally unwashed or not properly dressed and you have some worries about safety. You are also socially isolated with little or no contact from others.	But you have some worries about safety and you feel lonely and socially isolated with little or no contact from others. You have some control over daily living but could have more.

Figure 17.1 Example of a choice in the DCE. *Source:* Ryan *et al.*, 2006. Reproduced with permission of Elsevier.

A number of more complex DCE methods have been proposed. *Best attribute scaling* additionally asks respondents to indicate the attributes of the scenarios that they most and least prefer. Multiple-choice options can be used to allow individuals to choose from a number of scenarios. Respondents can also be asked to rate the strength of their preferences. Bridges *et al.* (2011) discuss the role of DCEs in healthcare and offer a checklist of good practice.

17.4 Multi-attribute utility (MAU) measures

Having assessed patient preferences or utilities for individual items, for example by using VAS, SG or TTO, there remains the issue of how to combine them. Some schemes use utilities as a form of item weighting for forming a summary index. However, there are few grounds for assuming that, for example, a patient with vomiting, pain and headaches should score the same as the sum of the three individual utility scores. *Multi-attribute utility theory* (MAUT) is a method for investigating the utilities associated with health states represented by a combination of item scores.

If an instrument has, say, three 5-point scales, there are a total of $5^3 = 125$ possible combinations of scores. Each such combination is called a *state*, and for example a score of 4 on the first scale, 3 on the second, 4 on the third could be written as the state (4,3,4). Ideally, preferences or utilities should be established for each of these states, but for many instruments this would not be feasible – an instrument with as few as six 5-point dimensions would result in 15,625 states and, for example, the SF-36 has millions of possible combinations. This has led to some utility-based instruments being deliberately brief; the EuroQol EQ-5D-3L has five dimensions that result in a total of 243 states. Of course, it is also possible to base the assessment of patients upon a single global item, in which case all that is required are the utilities corresponding to each level of the global item.

For longer instruments, there are a number of possible strategies. If it is thought reasonable to regard the dimensions as independent, only the *marginal* utilities are required and so each dimension can be studied separately when investigating the utilities. A multiplicative model is frequently used to combine *disutility* dimensions, where disutility is (1 – utility). The rationale for this is that symptoms or other deteriorations are likely to have the greatest impact if they are the first and only problem, and will reduce overall QoL to a lesser degree if they are but one of many problems. Equally, an improvement in a single area will not be sufficient to restore good QoL if there are many other problems. For example, with a three-dimension instrument, if a score of, say, 4 on the first dimension d_1 has utility $U_{d1}(4)$, a score 3 on dimension d_2 has utility $U_{d2}(3)$, and 4 on dimension d_3 has utility $U_{d3}(4)$, then

$$\text{Utility of } (d_1 = 4, d_2 = 3, d_3 = 4)$$
$$= U(4,3,4)$$
$$= 1 - [1 - U_{d1}(4)] \times [1 - U_{d2}(3)] \times [1 - U_{d3}(4)].$$

Other, more complex, schemes are available for rendering manageable the task of assessing multi-state utilities. One alternative is to evaluate the *corner* state utilities, such as, for example, the corner states of $U(1,1,1)$, $U(1,1,4)$, $U(1,4,1)$ etc. for a three-dimension instrument that has 4-point scales. Other schemes involve a combination of the marginal and corner states.

17.5 Utility-based instruments

Some QoL instruments have been designed explicitly with preference- or utility-based methods in mind, and can be described as MAU instruments. The Quality of Well-Being scale (QWB) of Kaplan *et al.* (1979) combines preference values with scale scores for mobility, physical activity, social activity and symptoms. The preference values were obtained by using rating scales to assess each possible state on a VAS scale from 0 to 1, and were obtained from the general community. The resultant scores range from 0, death, to 1, full functioning without adverse symptoms. It has been suggested that, since this instrument is sometimes used for resource allocation, the preferences of the payers – the community – are more relevant than those of the patient; in the UK, the National Institute for Health and Care Excellence declares that "Economic evaluations should quantify how the technologies under comparison affect disease progression and patients' health-related quality of life, and value those effects to reflect the preferences of the general population" (NICE, 2013). In any event, it is also often claimed that community-expressed preferences are usually not too dissimilar from patient opinions. The QWB was used extensively by the Oregon Health Services Commission in the USA, and in 1990 a priority list was produced based upon the rank ordering of services according to cost-utility.

The Health Utilities Index (HUI-3) as described by Feeny *et al.* (1995, 2002), used patient-generated utilities derived from TTO and SG methods. The HUI-3 evaluates eight attributes (emotion, cognition, pain, dexterity, vision, speech, hearing and ambulation), each on five- or six-category scales. An earlier version, HUI-2, used seven attributes and therefore provided less discriminative power.

Example from the literature

The HUI-3 was used in the 1991 population health survey in Canada. Feeny *et al.* (1995) report that 75% of the 11,567 participants were in the 12 most common states, with 30% reporting 'perfect health'.

Preference scores are available for the HUI-3, and it has been used to develop a population health index, comparing the health of different subgroups and monitoring changes over time.

The EuroQol EQ-5D, with five dimensions each originally having three categorical levels, is a brief instrument intended for use in economic evaluation. However, this still results in a total of 243 health states, and so the designers decided to focus on 13 of the most commonly occurring states, covering a broad range of health conditions. The revised version, the EQ-5D-5L extends the number of levels to five and potentially offers improved discrimination with fewer floor and ceiling effects, although the number of states is increased to 3125 (Herdman *et al.*, 2011). The SF-6D is a six-dimensional instrument derived from the SF-36 and is described in the Example in Section 17.6 (Brazier *et al.*, 2002). The EQ-5D, HUI-2 and HUI-3, SF-6D and QWB all focus on the same three underlying dimensions of QoL: physical, psychosocial and pain (Cherepanov *et al.*, 2010). However, these measures generate different health state values, even on the same populations (Tsuchiya *et al.*, 2006), so comparisons using different instruments should be interpreted with caution, especially when instruments use different valuation methods (SG, TTO, VAS).

Examples from the literature

Brooks *et al.* (1996) report the valuations for the 13 'common core' states of the EuroQol EQ-5D, using VAS, TTO and SG. Although the three methods resulted in very different scores, the ranking of the health states was broadly similar.

Example

Different methods (SG, TTO, WTP, DCE) result in different utility values, as does the choice of whose values should be solicited (patients or national populations); similarly, different instruments also produce results that are difficult to compare. This leads national health technology organisations to declare standards that should be used for cost effectiveness studies in their country. In the UK, the National Institute for Health and Clinical Excellence states that "For the cost-effectiveness analyses health effects should be expressed in QALYs. For the reference case, the measurement of changes in health-related quality of life should be reported directly from patients and the utility of these changes should be based on public preferences using a choice-based method. The EQ-5D is the preferred measure of health-related quality of life in adults." Further, "A set of preference values elicited from a large UK population study using a choice-based method of valuation (the time trade-off method) is available for the EQ-5D health state descriptions. This set of values should be applied to measurements of health-related quality of life to generate health-related utility values." (NICE, 2013).

17.6   Quality-adjusted life years (QALYs)

Having established values for preference ratings or utilities, the next stage is to attempt to combine them with the patient's likely duration in each condition. *Quality-adjusted life years* (*QALYs*) allow for varying times spent in different states by calculating an overall score for each patient. In broad terms, if the state of health during disease or treatment has been assigned a utility of 60%, then one year spent in this state is considered equivalent to 0.6 of a year in perfect health. Thus, if a patient progresses through four states that have estimated utilities of U_1, U_2, U_3, U_4, spending time T in each state, we have

$$QALY = U_1 T_1 + U_2 T_2 + U_3 T_3 + U_4 T_4. \tag{17.1}$$

This is analogous to the area under the curve (*AUC*) discussed in Chapter 13, but using utility values instead of scale scores. *QALYs* can be calculated for various medical conditions, and although the scores may be difficult to interpret in absolute terms, they provide relative rankings for alternative states and treatments in different disease areas.

Since *QALYs* explicitly make use of utilities when combining scales and when incorporating survival, it is arguable that they are a more realistic method for deriving summary indexes of QoL than the more naïve summation across dimensions and *AUC* calculations. *QALYs* have become widely used in health-economic analysis, and used to provide a summary index that enables the comparison of different policies of treatment or management, and which is consistent across various disease areas. However, whether or not it is meaningful to combine such disparate dimensions as QoL and survival into a single number must remain debatable, although this is clearly a convenient procedure for policy-making. Thus Fayers and Hand (1997b) point to the logical difficulties of declaring one treatment to be 'better' than another when there are gains in some dimensions that are offset by losses in others; the comparison depends heavily upon the trade-off across dimensions, and different people will have different opinions about the relative values – and these opinions will change over time, according to circumstances, contexts and experiences. Patients have different priorities from others, and community-averaged opinions may reflect only the views of a few central individuals. All the implicit assumptions regarding value judgements can too easily become obscured, or conveniently disguised, when only a single summary index such as cost per *QALY* is cited and presented in a league table.

As mentioned, *QALYs* are commonly used for health economic comparisons, when it is desirable to have an index that can be applied across a variety of disease areas. Consequently, generic instruments are most commonly used. Furthermore, the use of brief instruments (or a small subset of items/scales from a longer instrument) simplifies the evaluation of utilities for the many combinations of health states. Widely used MAU instruments for health economics include the EuroQol EQ-5D, SF-6D, HUI-2 or HUI-3 and QWB. To facilitate general applicability of the *QALY* scores and comparability across disease areas, the utilities may be based on the preferences of general population groups. Since health economic decisions are made at national level, the utilities are frequently evaluated from national population samples. However, values may be stable over comparable populations and so, for example, Greiner *et al.* (2003) suggest that for the EQ-5D a single European value set may suffice.

17.7   Utilities for traditional instruments

Preference-based indexes have also been developed for some of the widely used traditional health status instruments such as the SF-36. This has led to the SF-6D, a preference-based measure of health derived from the SF-36 and intended for use in economic evaluation. In creating the SF-6D, the SF-36 was revised into a six-dimensional health state classification. This offers a method for analysing existing SF-36 data from trials and other sources of evidence where there is no other means of estimating the preference-based health values for generating *QALY*s. Thus it provides an alternative to existing preference-based measures of health for use in cost utility analysis.

Example from the literature

Brazier *et al.* (2002) report the estimation of utilities for the SF-6D in a sample of 611 people from the UK general population. SG was used to evaluate a sample of 249 different health states, and from this models were used to predict the health state valuations of all 18,000 possible states defined by the SF-6D.

An example of a 'health state' is the following (abbreviated from the original):

Your health limits you *a little* in vigorous activities; You are *limited in the kind of work or other activities* as a result of your physical health; Your health limits you in your social activities *some of the times*; You have pain but it does *not* interfere with your normal work; You feel tense or downhearted and low *a little of the time*; You have a lot of energy *most of the time*.

This covers the six dimensions of physical functioning, role limitations, social functioning, pain, mental health and vitality. In this example, the level of the first dimension (physical functioning) is 2, corresponding to 'a little', and so on, resulting in a SF-6D health state categorised as 223222.

Respondents were asked to choose between living in one such hypothetical health state for the rest of their life, and living with the uncertain prospect of either the worst possible or best possible health state. Using the SG approach, the chance of living in the best state was varied until the respondent was indifferent to the certain and uncertain scenarios. The results from various models were used to derive health state utility values. These values can be used for weighting data in future clinical trials and other studies. Kharroubi *et al.* (2007) update this approach using a nonparametric Bayesian approach to provide revised values for the SF-6D.

Mapping across instruments

Health economic analyses have mostly been calculated using generic preference-based instruments such as the EuroQol EQ-5D, HUI-3 or SF-6D, and it is generally thought that these measures are applicable to all patients and all treatments. However, the generality of such brief generic instruments comes at the expense of not including disease- or treatment-specific items. Therefore, many clinicians and other investigators prefer to use targeted, condition-specific instruments; these can be more relevant, sensitive and informative regarding both group differences and within-patient changes over time. If health-economic analyses have been planned, generic utility-based instruments may be used alongside the disease-specific instruments. Frequently, however, data from generic utility instruments is not available.

These considerations have led a number of authors to report *mapping* studies that provide algorithms for predicting utility values from the scores of the disease-specific instruments. To that end, patients are asked to complete both the preference-based and the condition-specific instrument, enabling cross-calibration and a mapping function to be derived. This then enables the calculation of *QALY*s in clinical studies that have not used a preference-based instrument.

Example from the literature

McKenzie and van der Pol (2009) use two approaches to model the EQ-5D data. First, the EQ-5D values were modelled as a function of the EORTC QLQ-C30 data, using ordinary least squares regressions. Second, the five EQ-5D dimensions were modelled using ordered probit regression. The mapping equations were tested on a separate dataset, for which the QLQ-C30 data were used to predict EQ-5D values and estimate *QALY*s; these results were compared against the observed EQ-5D values and the corresponding *QALY*s. The authors found that the simpler first method was best, although they also suggest this may be because they ignored correlations and did not explore multivariate probit analysis.

The development data was from a clinical trial of palliative therapies for inoperable oesophageal cancer, and the validation data from a trial of radiotherapy after breast cancer surgery for low-risk elderly women. Table 17.1 shows that although there were some differences between the estimated and predicted EQ-5D values and the *QALY*s, the difference in *QALY*s were small (−0.019 and −0.017).

However, in this confirmatory trial the randomised groups did not differ significantly; it would have be interesting if the authors had also been able to evaluate the results in a trial for which there was a significant treatment effect. Crott and Briggs (2010) also describe mapping the EORTC QLQ-C30 to the EQ-5D, and summarise the results of a number of other studies.

Table 17.1 Actual and predicted EQ-5D values and *QALYs* by treatment arm, for 254 elderly women with low-risk breast cancer in a trial of post-operative radiotherapy

	Radiotherapy	No radiotherapy	Difference	*t*-value
EQ-5D mean value				
Actual	0.765	0.755	-0.010	0.77
Predicted from QLQ-C30	0.779	0.769	-0.009	0.70
QALYs				
Actual	0.954	0.935	-0.019	0.69
Predicted from QLQ-C30	0.972	0.955	-0.017	0.54

Source: McKenzie and van der Pol, 2009, Table 5. Reproduced with permission of Elsevier.

Brazier *et al.* (2010) review 30 studies that report a total of 119 different methods and models for mapping. They found that prediction of values for individual patients is generally relatively inaccurate, especially for patients with severe problems in who the gains may be underestimated. However, for health economics the aim of mapping functions is to estimate differences across groups of patients in clinical trials, and not to predict individual-level index values. Fayers and Hays (2014b) show regression to the mean results in attenuated estimates of SD, and that mapping studies should not use linear regression unless compensatory adjustments are made; alternative methods are preferable for linking measurement scales. The use of mapping functions is always a second-best solution to using a preference-based generic measure in the first place (or arguably using a preference-weighted condition-specific measure), but it is often necessary for pragmatic reasons.

Deriving a mapping function is a relatively simple approach. To derive a preference-based measure, it is necessary to use a full psychometric approach with preference elicitation methods. Examples of this are Rowen *et al.* (2011) for the EORTC QLQ-C30 and Dobrez *et al.* (2007) for the FACT-G.

Assumptions of *QALYs*

The value of *QALYs* is that they provide a common unit that can be compared across different disease areas and treatment groups. However, this is at the expense of a number of assumptions.

Utility independence is the assumption that individuals value length of life in a health state independently of the value of that health state. For example, if one were indifferent to the choice between two years with severe pain and one year's survival that is pain-free, one should also be indifferent to the choice between two weeks with severe pain and one week of pain-free survival.

Risk neutrality assumes a linear function for utility of life years. Thus, suppose one is willing to gamble on a 50–50 chance of either dying in one year or living for four years, versus the certainty of living for two years. Then, under risk neutrality, one should also be willing to gamble similarly in the future between a 50–50 chance of either dying in 21 years or living to 24 years versus the certainty of living 22 years.

Constant proportional trade-off is the assumption that the proportion of remaining life that one is willing to give up for a specified improvement in quality of life is independent of the number of remaining years of life.

QALY maximisation is the assumption that the objective of health care is to maximise the number of *QALYs* gained, irrespective of whom those *QALYs* go to and how they are distributed across society.

These are strong assumptions, and there is some evidence that none of them is realistic. For example, Brazier *et al.* (1999) provide a general review, while Dolan *et al.* (2005) comment on problems of *QALY* maximisation and constant proportional trade-off.

Discounting of *QALYs*

Most people place a greater value upon benefits that are immediate rather than those that may arise many years later. Thus it may be relevant to discount distant gains by proportionally reducing that component of the *QALYs* that relate to distant benefits. This concept of discounting is widely applied in economic analyses and appears equally important in the context of *QALYs*, especially when the utilities are derived from TTO evaluations.

Cost-utility ratios

One application for *QALYs* is to provide a single summary statistic for the economic evaluation of the cost-utility of interventions. This, coupled with the possibility of calculating *QALYs* in order to compare the impact of treatment across different diseases, has led to their widespread use by economists. The cost of each intervention is determined, and the cost-utility per expected number *QALYs* is estimated as

$$\text{Cost-utility per } QALY = \text{Cost}/QALY. \tag{17.2}$$

When comparing a new treatment A versus a standard (control) B, for example, we have

$$\text{Cost-utility per } QALY \text{ gained} = (\text{Cost}_A - \text{Cost}_B)/(QALY_A - QALY_B). \tag{17.3}$$

This ratio, also called the *incremental cost-effectiveness ratio* (*ICER*), can then be used as a measure to guide efficient use of healthcare funds.

Example from the literature

Grant *et al.* (2008) evaluated the relative benefits and risks of laparoscopic fundoplication surgery as an alternative to long-term drug treatment for chronic gastro-oesophageal reflux disease (GORD), in a multicentre randomised trial. They randomised 357 participants to either surgery (178) or medicine (179), and additionally recruited 453 participants who chose surgery (261) or medicine (192). Participants completed a set of questionnaires, including EQ-5D as well as other health status questionnaires. After one year there were substantial differences (one-third to one-half standard deviation) favouring the randomised surgical group across the health status measures.

Baseline and follow-up EQ-5D scores and *QALYs* are shown in Table 17.2a. A within-trial cost-effectiveness analysis suggested that the surgery policy was more costly (mean £2,049) but also more effective (+0.088 *QALYs*), as detailed in Table 17.2b. The estimated incremental cost per *QALY* was £19,000–£23,000, with a probability between 46% (when 62% received surgery) and 19% (when all received surgery) of cost-effectiveness at a threshold of £20,000 per *QALY*. Modelling plausible longer-term scenarios (such as lifetime benefit after surgery) indicated a greater likelihood (74%) of cost-effectiveness at a threshold of £20,000, but applying a range of alternative scenarios indicated wide uncertainty. The authors concluded that amongst patients requiring long-term medication to control symptoms of GORD, surgical management significantly increases general and reflux-specific health-related quality of life measures, at least up to 12 months after surgery. Complications of surgery were rare. A surgical policy is, however, more costly than continued medical management. At a threshold of £20,000 per *QALY* it may well be cost-effective, especially when putative longer-term benefits are taken into account, but this is uncertain.

Table 17.2a   Predicted unadjusted HRQoL and *QALY*, and *QALY* adjusted for baseline differences in HRQoL for patients receiving randomised treatment per protocol and followed up for one year

	Medical (*n* = 155)		Surgical (*n* = 104)	
	Mean	SE	Mean	SE
Baseline EQ-5D index	0.736	0.020	0.722	0.023
First follow-up EQ-5D	0.700	0.024	0.800	0.024
Second follow-up EQ-5D	0.710	0.022	0.777	0.023
Unadjusted QALY	0.710	0.019	0.786	0.020
QALY adjusted for baseline differences in EQ-5D	0.706	0.014	0.793	0.017

Source: Grant *et al.*, 2008, Table 36. Reproduced commercially with permission of the National Institute for Health Research (NIHR).

Table 17.2b Cost-effectiveness results for patients receiving randomised treatment per protocol and followed up for one year

	Mean	95% *CI*
Difference in mean costs (£)	2,049	1,907–2,198
Difference in mean QALYs	0.088	0.046–0.130
ICER (£/QALY)	23,284	
Probability surgery is cost-effective when threshold = £20,000	19%	
Probability surgery is cost-effective when threshold = £30,000	80%	

Source: Grant *et al.*, 2008, Table 37. Reproduced commercially with permission of the National Institute for Health Research (NIHR).

17.8   *Q-TWiST*

The *quality-adjusted time without symptoms and toxicity* (*Q-TWiST*) approach is similar in concept to *QALYs*, in that it uses utility scores to reduce the importance of years survived when health is impaired. Unlike *QALYs*, however, *Q-TWiST* can be applied to censored survival data and is therefore particularly appropriate for use in clinical trials. The principle is to partition the overall treatment-related survival curves into a few – typically three – regions that define the time spent in particular clinical states. The areas of the regions are then used to provide scores for these states, and the scores are weighted according to utilities that have been derived as for the *QALY* method.

Q-TWiST versus *QALY*

QALYs aim to provide health-economic comparisons, frequently across different disease areas. The instruments used are therefore usually generic ones, such as the EQ-5D, HUI-2 and HUI-3, SF-6D and QWB (or disease-specific instruments for which a mapping onto a generic instrument is available). Comparisons usually aim to inform decisions about resource allocation or management policies at the national level, and so utility values are likely to be derived from random samples of the national population, or based on existing utility estimates available for countries thought to be in some sense similar. In contrast, *Q-TWiST* utilities are patient orientated. Therefore, disease-specific instruments are more commonly used, with patient-derived utility weights. *Q-TWiST* is appropriate for use in clinical trials, and aims to inform clinical decisions.

Choice of health states

The initial task in calculating *Q-TWiST* is to define the health states. The overall survival time (*OS*) of each patient may include a time without symptoms or toxicity (*TWiST*). This will usually represent the optimal state, or the best possible QoL that is realistic and attainable for patients with chronic diseases such as cancer, and is therefore usually one of the health states included in a *Q-TWiST* analysis. This state has by definition a utility of 1. In contrast, death has a utility of 0. The other states are chosen according to clinical relevance, but two states might be, for example, the period with symptoms and toxicity (state 1 = *TOX*), and when in relapse (state 2 = *REL*). In this case, *OS* = *TOX* + *TWiST* + *REL* with progression-free survival (*PFS*) = *TOX* + *TWiST*; but other states might be more suitable for partitioning survival in other contexts.

Example

Suppose a patient with operable lung cancer has the tumour surgically removed so that in practical terms the patient is (almost) free of disease and hence symptom-free. However, post-operative chemotherapy of three cycles is given in the hope of eliminating any potential metastases. Following each cycle of chemotherapy, the patient experiences severe toxicity for five, three and seven days. Thereafter the patient remains without either symptoms or toxicity until the disease recurs at 250 days after surgery when symptoms also reoccur and he dies 50 days later. Here *TOX* = 5 + 3 + 7 = 15, *TWiST* = 235, *REL* = 50 and *OS* = 15 + 235 + 50 = 300 days.

Survival curves

A standard survival analysis is based upon *OS* for each patient, and the treatment-specific groups can be compared using the Kaplan–Meier method as described by Machin *et al.* (2006). This form of analysis also takes into account survival times of patients who have not yet died at the time of analysis. In very broad terms, the treatment that is most effective corresponds to the upper of these two survival curves, and the magnitude of the area between them represents the size of their difference.

To partition the survival curves, the time in each of the *Q-TWiST* states is quantified for each patient and summarised using the corresponding Kaplan–Meier estimates to graph the curves for the different states. The area beneath the corresponding Kaplan–Meier curve provides an estimate of the mean duration of time spent in each particular health state. The areas between the curves for *TOX*, *PFS* and *OS* are estimates of the respective mean health state durations. Thus the area between the *PFS* and *TOX* survival curves is an estimate of the mean duration of *TWiST*, while the area between the *OS* and *TWiST* survival curves is an estimate of the mean duration of *REL*.

Example from the literature

Wang *et al.* (2011) use *Q-TWiST* analysis to evaluate the benefit of adding panitumumab to best supportive care for patients with metastatic colorectal cancer. The partitioned survival curves are shown in Figure 17.2. Toxicity was defined as the time spent with grade 3 or 4 adverse events, during the period from randomisation until disease progression.

The panitumumab patients spent on average 3.5 weeks in *TOX*, 13.3 weeks in *TWiST* and 9.4 weeks in *REL*; the corresponding periods for the control group were 1.1, 8.0 and 16.1 weeks.

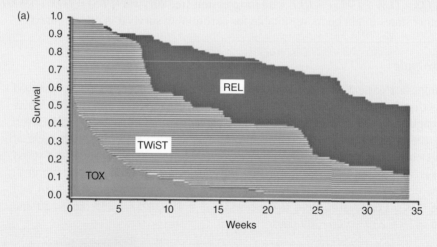

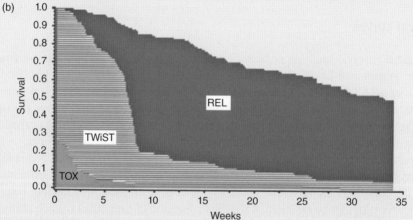

Figure 17.2 Partitioned survival curves for the two treatment arms of the metastatic colorectal cancer trial. (a) panitumumab+BSC and (b) BSC alone, where BSC=best supportive care. REL is the relapse period until death or end of follow up; TOX represents days with grade 3 or worse adverse events; TWiST is the time without symptoms or toxicity. *Source:* Wang *et al.*, 2011, Figure 1. Reprinted with permission of Macmillan Publishers Ltd on behalf of Cancer Research UK.

Calculating *Q-TWiST*

The period in *TWiST* is regarded as optimal, with a utility of 1, but we need utilities u_{TOX} for *TOX*, and u_{REL} for *REL*. These presumably have utilities between 0 and 1, and could be determined using the methods of VAS, SG or TTO, or could be chosen arbitrarily on the basis of experience of clinicians or other staff. The utilities might be specified as part of the protocol documentation, or could be collected during the trial itself. *Q-TWiST* is then calculated by summing the utility-weighted values for *TOX*, *TWiST* and *REL*. Thus,

$$Q\text{-}TWiST = (u_{TOX} \times TOX) + (u_{TWiST} \times TWiST) + (u_{REL} \times REL). \qquad (17.4)$$

Since *TOX*, *TWiST* and *REL* are measured in units of time, such as months, *Q-TWiST* too is measured in the same time units.

Example from the literature

Gelber *et al.* (1995) calculate the survival curves for *OS*, *PFS* and *TOX* for the individual treatments of the International Breast Cancer Study Group (IBCSG) Trial V. This trial tested the benefits of Long versus Short chemotherapy. The estimated mean times for their three states are *TOX* = 1, *TWiST* = 47 and *REL* = 16 months for the Short chemotherapy arm in the IBCSG Trial V. They also define $u_{TWiST} = 1.0$, $u_{TOX} = 0.5$ and $u_{REL} = 0.5$. Thus,

$$Q\text{-}TWiST = (0.5 \times 1) + (1.0 \times 47) + (0.5 \times 16) = 55.5 \text{ months.}$$

If the utilities used were different, a different value of *Q-TWiST* would be obtained. For example, suppose relapse were followed by a period of much lower QoL than when *TOX* was being experienced. In such a case perhaps $u_{TWiST} = 1.0$ and $u_{TOX} = 0.5$ as previously, but $u_{REL} = 0.25$. Then

$$Q\text{-}TWiST = (0.5 \times 1) + (1.0 \times 47) + (0.25 \times 16) = 51.5 \text{ months.}$$

Here the value of one month spent during the relapse period is one-quarter that spent with the better QoL of the *TWiST* interval, and one half of that during the period of symptoms and/or toxicity.

The utility model of equation (17.4) makes the assumption that the quality-adjusted time spent in a health state is directly proportional to the actual time spent in the health state. It also assumes that the value of the utility coefficient for a health state is independent of the time the health state is entered. This implies, for example, that if toxicity is experienced on three separate occasions then the associated u_{TOX} will be the same for each occasion.

Example from the literature

In the study of Wang *et al.* (2011), the EQ-5D was also used. This permits an alternative approach to determining the values of u_{TOX} and u_{REL}. Utility values for u_{TWiST}, u_{TOX} and u_{REL} were obtained from the observed EQ-5D utility data for the *TOX* and *REL* periods. Since *Q-TWiST* compares *TOX* and *REL* relative to *TWiST*, all three utility values are scaled through division by the patient-estimated u_{TWiST}, following the example of Bernhard *et al.* (2004).

The authors note that EQ-5D scores were higher for patients on panitumumab compared to the control group during periods of both *TOX* and *TWiST*. They also comment that in these patients skin rash was a common side effect of treatment and has a detrimental effect on HRQoL.

Comparing treatments

In a randomised trial to compare treatments, *Q-TWiST* itself becomes the variable for analysis. In theory, the value of *Q-TWiST* for each patient could be calculated, which would then enable the Mann–Whitney test described in Section 12.2 to be used for testing significance. However, the methods described above based upon partitioned survival curves are advocated for use with censored data or when there are missing values, and these result in a single summary statistic for each treatment group. One way of testing the statistical significance of this observed treatment difference is to use computer-based *bootstrap* methods to calculate confidence intervals (*CIs*) and *p*-values, as described in Altman *et al.* (2000). Revicki *et al.* (2006) reviewed published studies in oncology that used *Q-TWiST* and suggest that a clinically important difference is 10% of the overall survival in a study, and that differences of 15% are clearly clinically important. For planning studies, if little is known about the treatment and/or disease area, they recommend using an effect size of 5% to 10% for sample size estimation.

Example from the literature

Gelber *et al.* (1995) describe the steps taken in the calculation of *Q-TWiST* using data from the IBCSG Trial V. These calculations are summarised in Table 17.3. In broad terms, they conclude that the advantages for long-term chemotherapy in terms of *OS* and *PFS* over the short-term chemotherapy are not offset by the disadvantages associated with the greater toxicity. Thus the *Q-TWiST* difference of five months favours the use of long-term therapy for these patients. *CIs* were calculated using bootstrap methods.

Table 17.3 Calculation of *Q-TWiST* from International Breast Cancer Study Group Trial V

Endpoint	Utility coefficient	Mean time (months)		Difference	95% *CI*
		Long	Short		
Survival (*OS*)	—	69	64	5	2 to 8
Disease-free survival (*DFS*)	—	59	48	11	8 to 15
Time with toxicity (*TOX*)	0.5	6	1	5	—
TWiST	1.0	54	47	7	—
Time in relapse (*REL*)	0.5	9	16	−7	—
Q-TWiST	—	61.5	55.5	6	3 to 8

Source: Gelber *et al.,* 1995, Table 2.

17.9 Sensitivity analysis

The final value of *Q-TWiST* depends critically on the values assigned to the utility coefficients. Thus, in Table 17.4, had the utilities $u_{TWiST} = 1.0$, $u_{TOX} = 0.75$ and $u_{REL} = 0.25$ been used in place of 1.0, 0.5 and 0.5, we would have $Q\text{-}TWiST_{\text{Long}} = 60.75$ and $Q\text{-}TWiST_{\text{Short}} = 51.75$ months. Then the advantage of the Long regimen is extended to the equivalent of $60.75 - 51.75 = 9.00$ disease-free months. Thus there is value in exploring how robust the conclusion is to changes from the utility coefficients specified. If this exploration concludes that whatever the values of the utilities provided there always remains an advantage to one particular treatment, the message is clear. However, if there are conflicting suggestions depending on the choices made, the situation may become ambiguous. Or at least, the choice of best treatment option should be based on individual (patient-specific) values.

Such a *sensitivity analysis*, or *threshold utility analysis*, begins by comparing equation (17.4) calculated for each of the two treatment options. For brevity, we term these treatments A and B. For a particular clinical trial, we will have calculated TOX_A, $TWiST_A$, REL_A and TOX_B, $TWiST_B$, REL_B and hence $Q\text{-}TWiST_A$ and $Q\text{-}TWiST_B$. The difference between these two values of *Q-TWiST* is termed the *gain*, *G*:

$$G = Q\text{-}TWiST_A - Q\text{-}TWiST_B. \tag{17.5}$$

This equals

$$G = u_{TOX} \times (TOX_A - TOX_B) + u_{TWiST}(TWiST_A - TWiST_B) + u_{REL} \times (REL_A - REL_B).$$

Further, if we assume $u_{TWiST} = 1$, as will be the case in most applications, then *G* simplifies to

$$G = u_{TOX} \times (TOX_A - TOX_B) + (TWiST_A - TWiST_B) + u_{REL} \times (REL_A - REL_B). \tag{17.6}$$

From equation (17.5) the gain will be zero, that is $G = 0$, if Q-$TWiST$ for the two treatments is the same. To achieve this, one can search for values of the pair (u_{TOX}, u_{REL}) that, once substituted in equation (17.6), make this true. The values of both u_{TOX} and u_{REL} are confined to the range between 0 and 1. We can also search for values of (u_{TOX}, u_{REL}) that have $G > 0$. In this case, treatment A would be preferred to B. Similarly, we can search for values that have $G < 0$, in which case treatment B is preferred to A.

This sensitivity analysis can be presented as a two-dimensional plot of u_{TOX} against u_{REL}. The straight line obtained by setting $G = 0$ is the *threshold line* that indicates all pairs of utility coefficients (u_{TOX}, u_{REL}) for which the two treatments have equal Q-$TWiST$. The threshold line is determined by setting $G = 0$ in equation (17.5). In effect, we rewrite that equation in the following way:

$$u_{TOX} = \frac{(TWiST_A - TWiST_B)}{(TOX_A - TOX_B)} - u_{REL}\frac{(REL_A - REL_B)}{(TOX_A - TOX_B)}. \tag{17.7}$$

This is in the form of the equation of a straight line $y = \alpha + \beta x$, where

$$y = u_{TOX}, \; x = u_{REL}, \; \alpha = -\frac{(TWiST_A - TWiST_B)}{(TOX_A - TOX_B)} \text{ and } \beta = -\frac{(REL_A - REL_B)}{(TOX_A - TOX_B)}.$$

Example from the literature

For the IBCSG Trial V comparing Long and Short chemotherapy, Gelber *et al.* (1995) use the data of Table 17.4 to specify equation (17.7). This gives

$$G = u_{TOX} \times (6 - 1) + (54 - 47) + u_{REL} \times (9 - 16)$$
$$= 5u_{TOX} + 7 - 7u_{REL}.$$

Setting $G = 0$ we have, from equation (17.7):

$$u_{TOX} = -\frac{7}{5} + \frac{7 \times u_{REL}}{5} = -1.4 + 1.4u_{REL}.$$

This implies that the threshold line has intercept $\alpha = -1.4$ and slope $\beta = 1.4$. In fact, the authors quote $u_{TOX} = -1.2 + 1.4u_{REL}$ but the difference between the two expressions is due to rounding to whole numbers when presenting the summary calculations.

Example from the literature

Wang *et al.* (2011) apply this approach and summarise their threshold sensitivity analysis as shown in Figure 17.3. The threshold line for which the two treatments have equal *Q-TWiST* (that is, $G = 0$) is shown by the second line from the bottom right corner in Figure 17.3. The other lines show the differences in *Q-TWiST* (weeks) corresponding to varying values of u_{TOX} and u_{REL}.

Results were statistically significant ($p < 0.05$) for all *TOX* utility levels when $u_{REL} \leq 0.4$, and when $u_{REL} = 0.6$ results were still significant for all values of $u_{TOX} \geq 0.5$. The authors concluded that the addition of panitumumab to best supportive care provided significant improvements in quality-adjusted *PFS* and quality-adjusted *OS* and, that the toxicities associated with panitumumab are more than offset by the associated increase in time without severe toxicity.

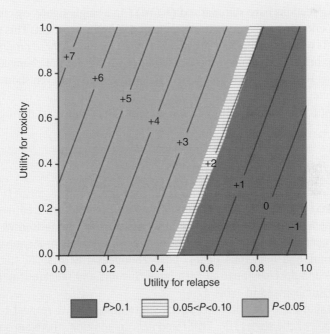

Figure 17.3   Threshold utility analysis, showing differences in *Q-TWiST* (number of weeks) for varying toxicity and relapse utility levels. Positive numbers indicate a benefit in favour of the panitumumab arm. *Source:* Wang *et al.,* 2011, Figure 3. Reprinted with permission of Macmillan Publishers Ltd., on behalf of Cancer Research UK.

17.10   Prognosis and variation with time

Prognostic factors

In many clinical situations, the appropriate treatments and the patient's final choice of therapeutic option may differ depending on circumstances. Nevertheless there may be groups of patients, perhaps pre-menopausal women with breast cancer, who might choose a different approach from that chosen by post-menopausal women with the same disease. The *Q-TWiST* methodology extends to this situation and can also be used for comparing patient groups receiving the same treatment. From such studies one may conclude, for example, that pre-menopausal women gain additional disease-free equivalent days by use of a particular therapy when compared with the post-menopausal women receiving the same treatment. More generally, one can make comparisons between treatments within each of these patient groups.

Variation of *Q-TWiST* with time

The preceding sections have summarised *Q-TWiST* in a single figure, essentially encapsulating the period from diagnosis to subsequent death of the patient. This may be relevant to patients with relatively poor prognosis, but not for those whose prognosis is good. However, the principles involved in calculating *Q-TWiST* are not changed if the time from diagnosis is divided into segments – perhaps into yearly or even shorter intervals.

Thus in some situations patients diagnosed with a certain disease receive an aggressive treatment for a relatively short period (say less than one year) during which they

---

Example from the literature

In describing a *Q-TWiST* analysis, Cole *et al.* (1994) present the mean times spent in *TOX*, *TWiST* and *REL* for four groups of women according to treatment (Short or Long chemotherapy) received. The prognostic groups comprised women who were pre-menopausal with small tumours and few nodes, pre-menopausal with large tumours and numerous nodes, post-menopausal with small tumours and few nodes, and post-menopausal with large tumours and numerous nodes. Their results are summarised in Table 17.4.

In this table there are differences between treatments with respect to the time spent in each of the states *TOX*, *TWiST* and *REL*. In addition, there are some major differences between patient groups. For example, for the pre-menopausal women with small tumours receiving Short chemotherapy, $Q\text{-}TWiST = 0.8u_{TOX} + 74.5 + 19.0u_{REL}$, whereas for those who are pre-menopausal but have large tumours it is $0.8u_{TOX} + 38.1 + 23.5u_{REL}$. Thus whatever the values given to u_{TOX} and u_{REL} by these two groups of women, those with the smaller tumours will have the greater *Q-TWiST* with short-duration therapy. The *TWiST* values of 74.5 and 38.1 months, respectively, dominate the corresponding *Q-TWiST* values.

Table 17.4 Average number of months in each of three health states for four groups of patients with breast cancer receiving one of two chemotherapy regimens

	Chemotherapy	
	Short	Long
Tumours <2 cm and <4 nodes		
Pre-menopausal		
TOX	0.8	5.8
TWiST	74.5	83.5
REL	19.0	7.7
Post-menopausal		
TOX	0.8	5.8
TWiST	80.1	87.9
REL	16.8	6.7
Tumours ≥2 cm and ≥4 nodes		
Pre-menopausal		
TOX	0.8	5.8
TWiST	38.1	50.1
REL	23.5	9.9
Post-menopausal		
TOX	0.8	5.8
TWiST	43.9	55.8
REL	22.1	9.4

Source: Adapted from Cole *et al.*, 1994.

experience both treatment-related toxicity and symptoms of their disease. Thereafter they may have an extensive period in which they are disease-free, followed by the remote possibility of relapse and the emergence of long-term side effects of treatment. In this example, for all patients on therapy, the first post-diagnosis year may be dominated by *TOX*, and the remaining parts with *TWiST* and *REL* within this year may be of relatively short duration. Whereas in the second post-diagnosis year a few patients may be still experiencing toxicity, the majority are disease-free, while a few may relapse. Thus the balance between *TOX*, *TWiST* and *REL* may change. This implies that the gain, *G*, of equation (17.6) may well vary from period to period following diagnosis.

Example from the literature

Gelber *et al.* (1995) show, with their example of Short and Long chemotherapy regimens of the IBCSG Trial V, how the gain changes with time during the first seven years post-diagnosis. In Figure 17.4, the bold central horizontal line shows the relative gain when $u_{TOX} = 0.5$ and $u_{REL} = 0.5$, and the shaded region denotes the range of Q-TWiST gains as the utility coefficients vary between zero and one.

Thus Figure 17.4 illustrates how the balance in the first year after diagnosis favours the Short regimen. This is clearly because all the active treatment occurs in this period and the *TOX* component of Short is much less than that of Long. As a consequence *Q-TWiST*, when confined to this period, will be dominated by *TOX* unless the associated utility coefficient, u_{TOX}, is very small. However, in later years the contribution of *TOX* to *Q-TWiST* is less, and so the balance between the two options shifts in favour of the Long regimen.

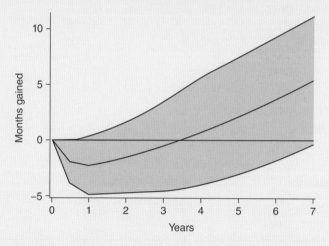

Figure 17.4 Change in *Q-TWiST* gain (months) over time for women with breast cancer receiving Short or Long duration chemotherapy; 'gain' indicates the advantage of Long over Short. *Source:* Gelber *et al.*, 1995, Figure 4.

Thus with *Q-TWiST* potentially varying with time following diagnosis, the attending physician may discuss with the patient with breast cancer the pattern of possible gain over the coming years. This in turn may then influence the patient's choice of treatment.

17.11   Alternatives to *QALY*

Various alternatives to *QALY*s and *Q-TWiST* have been proposed, but none have gained matching popularity. *Healthy-years equivalent* (*HYE*) and *Disability-adjusted life years* (*DALY*) are two of the principal alternatives.

HYE is claimed by its advocates to be superior to *QALY* because it avoids some of the assumptions (Gafni *et al.*, 1993). The principle of *HYE* is to avoid the need for expressing the preferences of patients in terms of utilities, which are an abstract concept, but instead to obtain an estimate of the equivalent number of years in full health that the patients would trade for their health-state profile.

The original procedure involved a two-stage estimation to obtain patients' *HYE* values, but it has been shown that *HYE* is very closely related to *QALYs* calculated using TTO. The difference is as follows. For *QALYs*, we need to know the utility of each health state, and the overall *QALY* score is calculated by assuming that this utility then applies uniformly to the time in that particular health state, as in equation (17.1). In the *HYE* formulation, the number of *HYEs* has to be measured for every possible duration of time in each possible health state. Thus *HYE* avoids the 'risk-neutrality over time' assumption of *QALY*, but at the major expense of having to evaluate *HYEs* for every possible state duration.

The *DALY* is a measure of disease burden, with disability weights for loss of functioning. One *DALY* represents the loss of one year of equivalent full health, whereas one *QALY* corresponds to the gain of an extra year of full health. The weighting function assigns different weights to life years lived at different ages, and the method of estimating *DALY* and *QALY* weights differs (Murray, 1997). Detailed examples of calculating *DALYs* are provided by Fox-Rushby and Hansen (2001) and Sassi (2006).

Whether or not *HYE* or *DALY* have benefits over *QALY* and *Q-TWiST* remains controversial. In any event, in clinical trial settings *HYE* or *DALY* will rarely be feasible unless utility values have been evaluated and are available.

17.12 Conclusions

Utility approaches attempt to combine QoL with survival, enabling a comparison of different policies of management when both QoL and survival vary simultaneously. They do this by equating a year of survival with good QoL as being equivalent to a longer period with poor QoL. However, there are clearly some difficulties with assessing this quality-adjusted survival. These include the determination of the utilities themselves and the rather simplified concept of health states during which QoL remains essentially constant. Although cost utility may remain constant, a patient's attitude and hence QoL with respect to successive cycles of chemotherapy may well be very variable and far from even approximately constant. Thus although the threshold analysis examines the robustness of this approach to some extent, it does not challenge some basic assumptions.

Another problem is that different patients may have very different sets of utilities. The concept of asking patients to assess their utilities for themselves is likely to be feasible only in relatively small groups of patients. Furthermore, an individual patient's utilities need not remain constant but may change over time or according to experience and circumstances. Thus, unless a threshold analysis confirms that conclusions regarding treatment superiority hold for a very wide range of utilities, it would be difficult to maintain that the results have general applicability.

Although this chapter has touched on heath economics, the main focus of this book remains clinical trials and clinical interpretation of the results; anyone interested in health economic studies are advised to read specialist texts on that subject. In many clinical trial situations it would seem preferable to report the observed QoL and the overall survival differences and let the individual – whether patient, clinician or health-care planner – decide what relative importance to attach to the separate dimensions. That is, one possibility is to aim to present sufficient information to let the individual apply their own set of utilities.

17.13   Further reading

This chapter has touched upon health economic analyses, mainly with respect to *QALYs* as a means of integrating QoL and survival. However, health economics is a subject in its own right, and anyone embarking on such studies is recommended to seek specialist advice. Books on this topic include Drummond *et al.* (2005), Brazier *et al.* (2007) and Glick *et al.* (2007). Ramsey *et al.* (2005) propose standards for good cost-effectiveness research alongside clinical trials.

18

Clinical interpretation

Summary

The interpretation of QoL scores raises many issues. The scales and instruments used may be unfamiliar to many clinicians and patients, who may be uncertain of the meaning of the scale values and summary scores. We describe various methods aimed at providing familiarity of scale scores and understanding the meaning of changes in scores. We describe the use of *population-based* reference values from healthy individuals and from groups of patients with known health status and various illnesses. We also discuss *patient-orientated* methods. These include the identification of the minimal changes in PROs that are discernible by patients or are important to patients, the impact of QoL states upon behaviour, and the changes in QoL which are caused by major life events. Data-derived *effect sizes*, which consider the random variability of the observed data, provide yet another method and can be particularly useful when reference values and patient-orientated information are not available. Threshold values used for interpretation are also useful for determining suitable targets to be used when calculating the sample size for a study.

18.1 Introduction

Previous chapters have described methods of collecting, analysing and summarising PROs. What do the results mean? What is the clinical relevance of a particular score for QoL, and how important are the changes in patients' PROs?

Sometimes results for single items are reported. For example, when a seven-point global question about overall QoL has been used, the results might indicate that treatment improves overall QoL by, say, on average 0.8 points. A clinician (or a patient) might quite reasonably demand to know how to interpret such a change. If QoL for an individual patient changes by that amount, would it be a noticeable change? Would it be an important change? Similarly, when scores are calculated for multi-item scales, what do they mean? What are the clinically important differences between groups of patients?

Quality of Life: The Assessment, Analysis and Reporting of Patient-Reported Outcomes, Third Edition.
Peter M. Fayers and David Machin.
© 2016 John Wiley & Sons, Ltd. Published 2016 by John Wiley & Sons, Ltd.

Although some clinicians may hope to identify a single value that will serve as a clinically significant difference in QoL, it can be argued that this is a demand that is unfairly imposed more frequently upon QoL scales than other clinical scales. Suppose we consider blood pressure (BP) measurement. Systolic and diastolic BP are two of the most widely used medical measurements, and the association between elevated BP and increased mortality is well recognised. The epidemiology of BP and its relationship with age and gender are also well established. Yet there is little consensus as to what critical levels should be taken as indications of hypertension demanding treatment. Most clinicians would probably consider initiating therapy if repeated diastolic BP measurements exceed 100 mmHg, but some might start at 95 mmHg. Some would use diastolic BP in conjunction with systolic BP. Some would make allowance for age when setting the threshold for commencing therapy. Given this divergence of agreement about thresholds, it is not surprising to find that there is even less agreement as to what *differences* are clinically worthwhile. If beta-blockers lower diastolic BP by 20 mm, from 120 mmHg to 100 mmHg, is it worth continuing long-term therapy? Many might say yes. But what if the change is 10 mm? Or even as little as 5 mm? Despite international guidelines, national practices vary.

One could level similar arguments against other simple measurements. If a course of cytotoxic drugs prolongs survival by an average of 50% in small-cell lung cancer patients, is it worth giving routinely? Most would agree that it is worthwhile for good-prognosis patients, but how about patients with advanced disease who are expected to have very short survival and for whom a 50% increase results in a gain of only a few weeks? Would therapy still be worthwhile if it prolongs average survival by less than 10%? Clearly there is little consensus about survival, either. It appears to be recognised and accepted that clinically important survival benefits are very much a matter of personal value judgements, on the part of both the patient and the treating clinician.

One obvious distinction is familiarity with the scales. Most people can understand the concept of survival, and thus many patients justly demand to be involved in decisions about their survival. Patients have less feeling for the meaning of BP measurement, but realise that their clinicians have a better understanding of it than they do. Therefore they expect the clinician to help assess the value of treatment. Unfortunately, with PRO scales, both patients and clinicians may feel uncertain what a score change of, say, 10% means. Hence the need for information about the levels of QoL that are to be expected for ill patients and guidelines to help decide what magnitude change in QoL is worthwhile.

No single approach is likely to provide a complete feel for the meaning of PROs, and thus it is important to use a variety of methods for obtaining familiarity and understanding of QoL scores.

18.2   Statistical significance

The meaning of statistical significance and the power of tests was covered in Chapter 11. Here, we merely emphasise that statistical significance does not imply clinical significance. Statistical significance tests are concerned solely with examining the observed data values, to determine whether differences or changes can be attributed to chance and patient variability, or whether there is sufficient weight of evidence to claim that there is almost certainly a pattern in the data. Highly statistically significant p-values indicate little about the magnitude of the differences, and tell us only that the differences are probably real as opposed to chance events. They tell us even less about the *clinical significance* of the observed changes.

It is particularly important to bear this in mind when reading reports of survival studies. Many of these enrol large numbers of patients in order to be certain of detecting small, yet clinically important, differences in survival. Sample sizes of several hundred are not uncommon in multicentre randomised trials, and some recruit thousands of patients. PROs are often secondary endpoints in those clinical trials that aim to compare two treatments for survival differences. This large sample size means that if there is even a very small difference in QoL it will be detected and found to be statistically highly significant. A p-value of, say, $p < 0.01$ tells us that, because of the large sample size, it is unlikely (a chance of less than 1 in 100) that we would have observed such extreme data purely by chance. Therefore we are reasonably confident that there is likely to be a difference in QoL. However, despite being 'highly significant' in statistical terms, the observed difference in a PRO (which is our best estimate of the true difference between patients taking these treatments) might in fact be very small. It might be clinically unimportant.

Conversely, in a small study a difference might be found to be barely significant at the 5% level (say, $p = 0.049$). Yet the observed difference in QoL could be substantial and, if confirmed to be true, might be exceedingly important in clinical terms.

In summary, statistical significance does not necessarily indicate clinical relevance of the findings. Statistical significance tests are concerned solely with evaluating the probability that the observed patterns in the data could have arisen purely by chance.

18.3 Absolute levels and changes over time

The interpretation of scores will take different forms according to the purpose for which the outcome is being assessed.

- *Cross-sectional studies* may collect data representing the levels of an outcome in a group of patients, and often it will be appropriate to contrast the observed average values against reference data from other groups, such as the general population.

- *Follow-up studies* that collect repeated measurements for each patient may be interested in the same issues as cross-sectional studies, but in addition they are likely to place greater emphasis upon changes over time rather than absolute levels. Large follow-up studies have the power to detect small variations in the mean level of an outcome, and some of these changes may be so small that they are of little consequence to individual patients.

- *Sample size estimation* requires specification of a target difference. Although the emphasis of this chapter is on interpretation of results, there is a close relationship between interpretation and the definition of the effect size to be used as the target when estimating the number of patients required for a study. Generally, at the study design stage, the investigator wishes to ensure that the sample size is large enough to have a reasonable probability of detecting relevant differences, where relevance is typically either differences that are large enough to influence the management of patients, or differences that patients notice and are considered by them to be important.

- *Clinical trials* place the focus upon differences between the randomised groups. Usually the investigators will carry out a significance test to determine whether there is evidence that the observed differences are larger than can be attributed to chance alone. If statistical significance is established, they will next want to know whether the between-group differences are large enough to be clinically important. They may also want to know whether one or both groups of patients in the trial have lower or higher scores than reference groups such as the general population. Also, in clinical trials, assessments are usually made at baseline, during treatment and during follow-up. Investigators may be interested in differences between groups of people or within-person changes over time.

    a. If one group has worse (or better) outcomes than another group, are the differences large enough to be important?

    b. If PROs change over time, how large do the changes need to be before they are noticed?

    c. What magnitude of change in scores is big enough to be important?

    d. Do differences between the groups diminish over time? If so, when do they cease to become clinically important?

    e. Do some individuals have such a large reduction in QoL that psychosocial intervention is necessary?

Many forms of information are necessary to answer the above questions. The interpretation of QoL data may often be based upon a consideration of absolute levels relative to a reference population, combined with a judgement concerning the magnitude and clinical importance of observed differences between groups of patients and changes over time. We need to define a reference population. Often this will consist of healthy people or the general population. We need to know what levels of QoL are present in the reference population and how much variability there is in the data. This variability is often summarised by the *SD* calculated from the reference population. We need to know what magnitude of differences or changes are perceived by patients or others as being noticeable, important and worthwhile.

18.4 Threshold values: percentages

One of the simplest forms of presentation – and therefore one of the simplest for interpretation – is to show the percentage of patients above some specific value. For example, when comparing treatment groups one might tabulate the percentage of patients that report 'good' QoL. For a few instruments, such as the Hospital Anxiety and Depression Scale (HADS), there are guidelines for values that denote 'cases' and 'doubtful cases' requiring treatment. Even without such guideline levels, many readers seem to find it intuitively easier to visualise a comparison based upon the percentage of patients above and below some arbitrary cut-point rather than a difference in group means.

In some situations, such as when many patients rate themselves at the maximum (ceiling) value, it may be helpful to compare the proportion of patients at this maximum.

Similarly, when using odds ratios (OR) it is also in principle possible to choose a critical value and compare the proportion of patients lying above and below that threshold. This approach has not been widely used and so for most instruments it is less clear what critical values might be appropriate.

18.5   Population norms

Interpretation of PROs may use population-based *reference values*, which provide expected or typical scores that are called *norms*. Tables of normative data, taken from surveys of randomly selected subjects from the general population, provide a useful guide for interpretation. Norms can consist of values for the general population as a whole or for various subgroups, such as healthy people or those with particular disease conditions. Norm-based interpretation of PROs consists of defining one (or more) reference groups for whom norms are available, and treating these scores as target values against which the scores observed in an individual patient, or the average for a group of patients, can be compared. For comparative purposes, the average patient values and the norms can be listed side by side. A possibly better method is to regard the norms as anticipated values; these can be subtracted from the patient averages to give the difference-scores of observed-minus-expected values. These differences can be standardised, to allow for differences in variability of the measurements and scales. Usually, if a measurement scale has a small *SD* in the general population (indicating that most people have very similar values to each other), even a small difference from the norm will be noticeable and important. Conversely, if the population *SD* is large, there will be a large amount of variation from one person to another and only large differences between the observed patient values and the norms will be clinically important. Therefore the standardised differences, in which the differences are divided by the *SD*, may be easier to interpret than plain observed-minus-expected differences. Standardisation is also related to the concept of effect sizes, as described in Section 18.12.

What reference population should be chosen? The two obvious choices are the general population, which includes both the healthy and those with chronic or acute illness, or the healthy population after excluding those with illnesses. Random samples from the general population may find that more than half of the subjects report chronic illnesses of varying severity, although the proportions will vary according to the composition of the sample (e.g. age range and distribution) and the definition of 'chronic illness'. Often the optimal choice of reference population will be debatable. In some studies, patients who are recruited into the study will be as likely as the general population to have concomitant diseases. For example, a study of QoL in patients with cardiovascular diseases may find that many patients have chronic lung disease too. In such cases, the general population would seem the most suitable choice. This is the reference population that is most frequently used. However, the healthy population could be used to provide an indication of the 'ideal' target value. Sometimes the healthy population may be more appropriate as the reference group. For example, some clinical trials may have eligibility criteria that exclude patients with serious comorbid conditions. In such trials, contrast with values from the healthy population is preferable. In other circumstances, neither reference population is ideal. For example, when considering the meaning of QoL states in patients who are receiving active therapy or recovering from side effects, sometimes the target and potentially achievable QoL might be defined as that obtained by long-term survivors or cured patients. These data are less frequently available for QoL instruments, and most investigators make use of the general population or, less commonly, the healthy population.

Normative data, also called reference values, are available for many QoL instruments. Mostly, these are based upon cross-sectional surveys of the general population and are presented as values tabulated by age and gender. Norms are also sometimes available for different disease groups. Less common, although important, are norms from longitudinal studies, showing the changes over time that may be expected for healthy or ill subjects. For example, it could be important for the interpretation of results to know the anticipated rate of change in palliative care patients, or in those responding to therapy.

Example from the literature

Hjermstad *et al.* (1998a) report normative data for the EORTC QLQ-C30 in a randomly selected sample of 3,000 people from the Norwegian population, aged between 18 and 93. Data were available for 1,965 individuals. Table 18.1 summarises their results, by age and gender, for the functioning and global health/QoL scales of the QLQ-C30 (version 2.0).

Apart from emotional functioning, all functioning scales and the global score show a decline with age. The fall is particularly marked for physical functioning above the age of 50. Men tend to have markedly higher levels than women. These patterns are clearly shown in Figure 18.1. The authors also present bar charts of the data, showing that there is a large amount of variability in the data; the distributions are inevitably asymmetric since the mean values are close to the ceiling of 100.

Table 18.1 Mean scores for EORTC QLQ-C30 (version 2.0) functioning scales and global health/QoL, by age and gender, from a sample of the general Norwegian population

	Male							Female							Total
	All	18–29	30–39	40–49	50–59	60–69	≥ 70	All	18–29	30–39	40–49	50–59	60–69	≥ 70	
Number	(1016)	(205)	(228)	(182)	(153)	(114)	(134)	(949)	(185)	(159)	(147)	(145)	(142)	(171)	(1965)
Functioning scales															
Cognitive	87.1	91.6	88.9	89.5	86.5	82.7	77.6	85.8	89.5	87.3	86.9	86.1	86.4	77.9	86.5
Emotional	85.4	87.8	83.7	84.6	83.9	84.8	87.7	79.9	78.7	77.2	76.8	83.2	79.4	84.4	82.8
Physical	93.2	98.0	97.3	91.1	92.9	89.1	77.7	86.4	97.6	93.6	89.9	87.6	78.2	67.7	89.9
Role	85.7	92.4	91.0	85.5	84.4	79.0	73.3	80.6	88.4	85.9	82.6	81.3	75.5	68.1	83.3
Social	87.7	94.5	89.4	89.0	84.4	80.9	81.6	83.6	88.9	84.0	80.0	83.9	83.4	80.1	85.8
Global Health/QOL	77.3	80.1	78.8	79.0	75.9	75.2	71.4	73.2	77.9	75.7	72.7	74.1	70.2	67.6	75.3

Source: Adapted from Hjermstad *et al.,* 1998a.

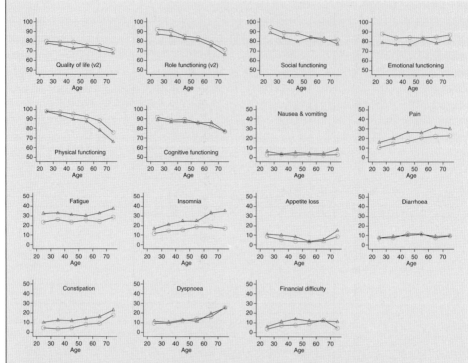

Figure 18.1 Age-distribution of the mean scores for the subscales of the EORTC QLQ-C30 (version 2.0), for males (0) and females (Δ) from a sample of the general Norwegian population. *Source:* Adapted from Hjermstad *et al.,* 1998a. Reproduced with permission from the American Society of Clinical Oncology.

One way of using normative data for interpreting values observed in individual patients is to note the decrease in levels with increasing age. Physical functioning declines by nearly 5 units per decade of life, both for men and for women. This may help give a feeling for what an average change of 5 units might mean to patients. Similarly, global health/QoL declines by approximately 2 units per decade, role functioning by 3.5, cognitive functioning and social functioning by 2, and emotional functioning by 0.5.

Anchor methods

Approaches such as the above are sometimes described as *anchor methods*. The outcome of interest is *anchored* by using either a patient's or health professional's judgement to define a (clinically) important difference. Other examples are anchoring against patients' global rating of change (Section 18.6); comparing before and after treatment and then linking the observed change to participants who had a clinical improvement as defined by other criteria; anchoring contrasts between groups of patients to determine an important difference; and comparisons with other life-affecting events (Section 18.11).

Adjusting for age and gender

The patterns in Figure 18.1 emphasise the need to allow for age and gender when contrasting normative data against groups of patients who may have very different age–gender profiles. People with chronic health problems may tend to be older than those who are healthy, and for many disease areas the patients in clinical trials may be older than people in normative samples. Thus an adjustment should be made for differing age and gender distributions.

There are two principal approaches to this problem. First, it is possible to regard the age distribution of the reference population as being the standard to which all other datasets should be adjusted. The age-specific scores for the patients are calculated, and the age distribution of the reference population is used with these scores so as to estimate the mean level of QoL that would be expected for the reference age-structure. This leads to adjusted, or standardised, mean scores for each of the disease groups. This procedure is equivalent to *direct standardisation* as used in epidemiology. This method is not often used because, unless the disease group is large, age-specific mean scores cannot be estimated very accurately.

The second approach, illustrated in Table 18.2, is based upon the concept of calculating *expected mean scores* for the disease group. The population reference values are used to calculate the expected scores that would be observed for subjects of the same age and gender distribution as in the disease group. Since each disease group will have a different age–gender distribution, separate expected values are calculated for each group. The calculations use basic reference data, such as those in Table 18.1. Similar *indirect standardisation* is used in epidemiology when comparing incidence or prevalence rates amongst different subgroups.

Although we illustrate the calculations using the age-grouped data presented in Table 18.1, a variation on this approach is to use the individual-patient raw data and apply regression modelling to fit an equation that includes age and gender. This can be used to generate expected (predicted) values for each individual. In principle this should be a more accurate method since it makes full use of the individual values and involves fitting a smooth curve. In practice, however, it usually makes negligible difference to the estimates and has two disadvantages: it requires access to the individual-patient data, and the regression models will often involve different non-linear functions of age for each gender.

Age- and gender-adjusted normative reference values are frequently compared against the observed results of studies, often as a simple table. Alternatively, profile plots as shown in Figure 12.6 may be used.

As noted for Figure 12.6, the mean scores for different dimensions, whether symptom or functioning scales, should not be contrasted against each other as PROs are rarely scaled uniformly. For example, when describing it would be incorrect to suggest that pain in the LRRC group, with a mean value just over 40, is worse than fatigue or other symptoms. This would be an unfounded statement as there is no evidence that a particular score on one scale is equivalent to the same score on other scales. We can only say that pain in the LRRC group is worse than in the other groups. Consequently, some authors prefer to use bar charts to compare PROs for groups of patients and the corresponding normative values. However, we find that the underlying patterns are easier to discern in profile plots.

Example from the literature

Hjermstad *et al.* (1998b) illustrate how to allow for age and gender when using normative reference data. They compared the cognitive functioning of 265 patients with cardiac problems, as given in Table 18.2, against the reference data of Table 18.1. There are 17 females aged 18–29 years and, if we examine the comparable age–gender group in the normative data of Table 18.1, we see that the expected value of their cognitive functioning is 89.5. Therefore the expected total score for these females is $17 \times 89.5 = 1,521.5$. Similarly, we can estimate the expected total score for the remaining female groups. Combining these gives an expected total score of

$$(17 \times 89.5) + (8 \times 87.3) + (14 \times 86.9) + (14 \times 86.1) + (23 \times 86.4) +$$
$$(48 \times 77.9) = 103,68.3.$$

Similarly, for the 141 males:

$$(9 \times 91.6) + (21 \times 88.9) + (15 \times 89.5) + (16 \times 86.5) + (26 \times 82.7) +$$
$$(54 \times 77.6) = 11,758.4.$$

The expected total score for all 265 cardiac-problem patients is therefore 10,368.3 + 11,758.4 = 22,126.7, giving an expected mean score 22,126.7/265 = 83.5. The observed mean score for cognitive functioning of the 265 patients with cardiac problems was 75.9 which, even after allowing for age and gender, is lower than that of the general population by $83.5 - 75.9 = 7.6$.

Note that, if we had not allowed for age and gender but used the mean score for the total normative sample directly, the difference ($86.5 - 75.9 = 10.6$) would be more than three points larger ($10.6 - 7.6 = 3.7$).

Table 18.2   Age and gender distribution of a group of 265 patients with cardiac problems

Age group	Female	Male	Total
18–29	17	9	26
30–39	8	21	29
40–49	14	15	29
50–59	14	16	30
60–69	23	26	49
≥ 70	48	54	102
Total	124	141	265

Source: Hjermstad *et al.*, 1998b. Reproduced with permission of Elsevier.

Example from the literature

Traa *et al.* (2014) report the HRQoL of patents who received treatment for rectal cancer at a tertiary referral centre in The Netherlands. Treatment for rectal cancer is based on clinical T-stage, pathological lymph nodes and distant metastasis. The standard treatment for non-advanced rectal cancer in The Netherlands is neo-adjuvant radiotherapy followed by a total mesorectal excision with autonomous nerve preservation, except for cT1N0 patients where radiotherapy is not indicated. Patients with locally advanced rectal cancer (LARC) or locally recurrent rectal cancer (LRRC) are treated with neo-adjuvant radio-chemotherapy often followed by more extensive extra-anatomical surgery in order to achieve a curative resection.

Table 18.3 EORTC QLQ-C30 scale scores, for 439 patients with rectal cancer divided into non-advanced disease (NAD), locally advanced rectal cancer (LARC) and locally recurrent rectal cancer (LRRC). The normative group consists of age- and gender-matched reference values in a sample of the general population in the Netherlands

	NAD (*N*=80)		LARC (*N*=292)		LRRC (*N*=67)		Normative (Reference values)	
	Mean	*SD*	*Mean*	*SD*	*Mean*	*SD*	*Mean*	*SD*
ql	70.5	22.1	68.1	23.4	64.0	24.0	77.2	17.4
pf	80.3	19.1	79.5	20.4	71.9	22.8	86.0	17.1
rf	75.0	28.4	75.3	28.1	69.6	31.6	86.4	21.6
ef	84.8	18.8	82.6	20.7	81.1	22.6	90.3	15.0
cf	84.4	20.9	83.7	21.1	80.9	22.1	90.8	14.1
sf	82.7	22.4	79.2	25.2	69.6	29.2	93.1	16.8
fa	23.1	22.3	26.8	23.9	26.2	22.1	17.8	20.5
nv	3.0	8.3	4.4	11.8	4.0	11.6	3.0	11.8
pa	14.8	21.3	15.8	22.8	41.9	22.3	17.8	23.0
dy	16.0	24.4	13.8	22.5	12.4	19.3	9.4	19.6
sl	19.4	27.5	18.7	26.5	21.3	30.4	14.9	22.0
ap	3.8	10.7	6.7	17.7	3.2	9.9	3.3	12.0
co	8.4	16.4	9.1	20.5	9.3	23.7	5.6	15.3
di	21.5	27.8	18.7	25.3	19.4	26.0	4.5	15.1
fi	5.6	17.3	11.9	23.3	8.2	19.9	3.0	12.0

ql, global quality of life; pf, physical functioning; rf, role functioning; ef, emotional functioning; cf, cognitive functioning; sf, social functioning; fa, fatigue; nv, nausea and vomiting; pa, pain; dy, dyspnoea; sl, insomnia; ap, appetite loss; co, constipation; di, diarrhoea; fi, financial difficulties.

All patients who were still alive in 2010 were contacted to ask them if they were willing to participate in this study. In total, 80 patients with NAD (median years since surgery = 4.5), 292 patients with LARC (median years = 2.3) and 67 patients (median years = 3.3) with LRRC returned completed EORTC QLQ-C30 questionnaires (as well as the EORTC QLQ-CR38 colorectal module) and were included in the current study. This reflected an 85% response rate. The authors compared the three groups of patients with the age- and gender-matched normative sample, presenting a table showing the means, standard deviations and *p*-values; Table 18.3 summarises the means and *SD*s for the EORTC QLQ-C30 outcomes. Figure 18.2 shows the corresponding profile plot, and in our opinion this visual display makes the patterns in the outcomes much easier to discern.

The authors observed that, compared to the other two rectal groups, LRRC patients reported lower functioning scores and more pain. Compared with the normative population, rectal cancer patients had lower scores on Global Quality of Life, all five functioning scales and more constipation and diarrhoea, regardless of treatment ($p < 0.05$). In addition, LARC and LRRC patients experienced a lower PF, but more fatigue than the normative population ($p < 0.05$). Finally, LRRC patients reported more pain ($p < 0.0001$) than the normative population, while the LARC group reported more appetite Loss ($p = 0.017$) and dyspnoea ($p = 0.026$) compared with the normative population.

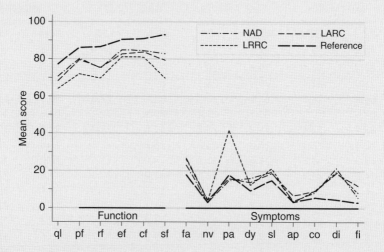

Figure 18.2   EORTC QLQ-C30 *scale scores* for 439 patients with rectal cancer, divided into non-advanced disease (NAD), locally advanced rectal cancer (LARC) and locally recurrent rectal cancer (LRRC). The bold line shows age- and gender-matched reference values in a sample of the general population in the Netherlands. The reference group had highest QoL, best functioning and least symptoms (based on the data shown in Table 18.3).

In this observational (non-randomised) study the three rectal cancer groups differed in age (medians 70.4, 65.6 and 63.7 respectively), but the normative values presented by the authors are based age and gender averaged across all three groups.

Example

Figure 18.3 shows the bar plot corresponding to Figure 18.2. Arguably, the visual benefits of the profile plot have been forfeited and it is now more difficult to discern the underlying patterns. However, this presentation makes it less likely that naïve readers will assume that values on different dimensions are directly comparable.

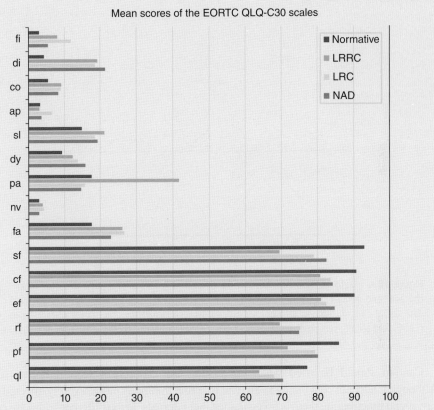

Figure 18.3 *Bar chart* of the mean EORTC QLQ-C30 scale scores shown in Figure 18.2, for 439 patients with rectal cancer, divided into non-advanced disease (NAD), locally advanced rectal cancer (LARC) and locally recurrent rectal cancer (LRRC) (based on the data shown in Table 18.3).

Although the format of is widely used, many people find it easier to see patterns in data if the reference group is drawn as the baseline, or target, level of QoL and the patient means are plotted as differences about this baseline. This format is shown in Figure 18.4. An additional advantage is that, like the bar-chart of Figure 18.3, it discourages casual readers from comparing absolute values of the different scales with each other.

Example

In Figure 18.4 it is easy to see that Global QoL and all functioning scales have lower values for patients than for the general population. Also, all three patient groups have more diarrhoea that the normative sample, by between 15 and 20 units. For LRRC patients, pain is worse by about 25 units. It is visually more difficult to read these values from Figure 18.2, and involves subtraction to obtain the differences.

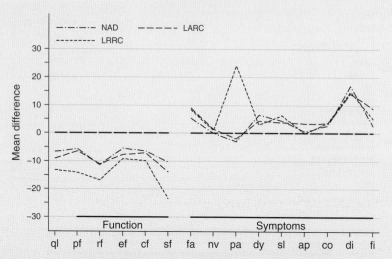

Figure 18.4 Data of Figure 18.2, showing *mean differences* of the patient scores from the age- and gender-matched reference values of the general population for 439 patients with rectal cancer, divided into non-advanced disease (NAD), locally advanced rectal cancer (LARC) and locally recurrent rectal cancer (LRRC). See footnote to Table 18.3 for scale names.

Caution should be used when contrasting the differences from different scales. Although it appears convincing from that role functioning is more severely affected than, say, social functioning, there is no guarantee that intervals on the different scales are equivalent. It is possible that a change of 5 units may be important on one scale, while changes of less than 10 may be unimportant on another. An alternative method, which may be preferable when comparing scales, is to plot effect sizes, as described in Section 18.12.

18.6   Minimal important difference

Whereas norms are based upon surveys of the prevailing QoL states in reference populations, the minimal important difference (*MID*) takes into account the opinions and values of patients. Also sometimes called the minimal *clinically* important difference or *MCID*, the *MID* is the smallest difference in score in the domain of interest that patients perceive as beneficial and which would cause clinicians to consider a change in the patient's management (assuming no side effects or major cost considerations).

In order to determine the size of this difference, patients can be asked whether they have noticed a change in their condition and how important they regard that change. Most QoL questionnaires relate to present or recent QoL status; for example: 'During the past week, did you feel depressed?' Therefore, the strategy is to ask the patient to complete a questionnaire at their first visit and then again at the second visit. Immediately following this second assessment, they are asked whether they perceived any change between the two visits and whether this has been an important change. Questions regarding the change in level are sometimes called *transition questions*, or *global ratings of change*. The number of categories in the transition questions, and their descriptive wording, may influence the value obtained for the minimal clinically important difference. Most investigators have used at least seven categories, with the central one being 'no change' and the extreme categories being something like 'very much better' (or worse) or 'a great deal better' (or worse).

Example from the literature

The first published example of using a global rating of change was for the Chronic Respiratory Questionnaire and Chronic Heart Failure Questionnaire, investigated by Jaeschke *et al.* (1989) to determine the *MIDs*. Initial discussion with staff experienced in administering the questionnaires suggested that a mean change of 0.5 on the seven-point scales represents a change that a patient would feel was important to their daily life. In a subsequent study, 75 patients completed QoL questionnaires at baseline and at 2, 6, 12 and 24 weeks. After completing the second and subsequent assessments, they also scored themselves on 15-point global rating scales according to whether their condition was 'a very great deal worse' (−7) through to 'a very great deal better' (+7).

Small changes of 'somewhat worse' were defined as those between −3 and −1, moderate changes were −5 and −4 ('moderately or a good deal worse'), and large were −7 and −6 ('a great deal or a very great deal worse'). Corresponding positive values were defined for getting better. Table 18.4 shows the mean

Table 18.4 Mean change scores for dyspnoea, fatigue and emotional function,by size of global rating of the change

	Global rating of change			
	None	Small	Moderate	Large
Dyspnoea	0.10	0.43	0.96	1.47
Fatigue	0.12	0.64	0.87	0.94
Emotion	0.02	0.49	0.81	0.86

Source: Jaeschke *et al.*, 1989. Reproduced with permission of Elsevier.

change in reported levels of dyspnoea, fatigue and emotional function, divided according to whether patients thought that the overall change was none, small, moderate or large. In this table, positive and negative changes have been combined. For example, the recorded levels of dyspnoea changed by an average of 0.96 in those patients who reported a moderate overall change, with a decrease in dyspnoea for those reporting benefit and a corresponding increase for those improving.

Thus Jaeschke *et al.* (1989) confirmed their preliminary estimates that a small change on the seven-point scales would correspond to a change in score of approximately 0.5, since the mean of the observed values 0.43, 0.64 and 0.49 is 0.52.

A 15-point global rating of change scale can place a cognitive challenge to patients and demands a large sample size to ensure that sufficient numbers of patients are available to enable precise estimates for all categories; indeed, as in the example above, it is frequently necessary to reduce the data from 15-point scales by merging adjacent categories. This has led some investigators to use other formats, such as seven-point scales (e.g. Osoba *et al.*, 1998). Whereas the analysis reported by Jaeschke *et al.* (1989) referred to 'changes' and did not distinguish improvement from deterioration, it has since been found in some studies that there may be a difference; for example, in the study of Cella *et al.* (2002) it was observed that *MID*s for improvement tended to be larger than those for deterioration. Recognising the similarities with diagnosis, many authors have adapted receiver operating characteristic (ROC) curves to the estimation of *MID* values; these have the advantage of making greater use of the distribution of the full sample for estimating individual values (Turner *et al.*, 2009b).

Example from the literature

Kvam *et al.* (2010) evaluated *MID* values using EORTC QLQ-C30 scores from 239 multiple myeloma patients. Seven-category scales were used for the transition questions, with response options ranging from 'very much worse' through 'no change' to 'very much better'. Figure 18.5 shows results for the four dimensions pain, fatigue, physical function and global QoL. Mean scores and confidence intervals are displayed, corresponding to each of the seven transition ratings. From the figure, *MID* values for a little better and worse were pain −14.2, 12.9; fatigue −5.0, 4.5; physical function 4.4, −4.4; global QoL 1.4, −10.7. The values for moderate changes ranged from 6 to 17. Kvam *et al.* kept deteriorations separate from improvements, and confirmed the findings of Cella *et al.* (2002) that *MID*s for improvement tended to be larger than those for deterioration.

Figure 18.6 shows a ROC curve for pain deterioration, with the suggested cut point based on a compromise between sensitivity and specificity; at this cut-point, the pain score was 16.7.

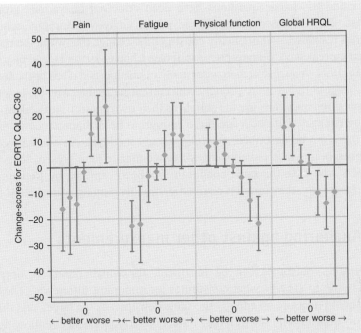

Figure 18.5 Each graph shows the mean score change and 95% *CI* for 239 patients with multiple myeloma who stated that they had become much better, moderately better, a little better, unchanged (0), a little worse, moderately worse, or much worse from time 1 (baseline) to time 2 (three months). High scores indicate more symptoms (pain and fatigue) or better functioning (physical function and global HRQL). *Source:* Kvam *et al.*, 2010. Reproduced with permission of John Wiley & Sons, Ltd.

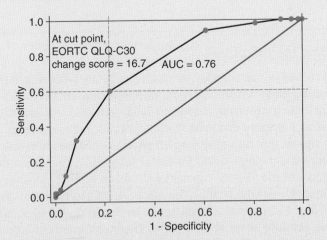

Figure 18.6 Receiver-operating characteristic (ROC) curve of the European Organization for Research and Treatment of Cancer (EORTC) QLQ-C30 change score in patients who stated that their pain had deteriorated. AUC, area under the curve. *Source:* Kvam *et al.*, 2010. Reproduced with permission of John Wiley & Sons, Ltd.

Global rating of change questions have been criticised on various grounds (e.g. Terwee *et al.*, 2010). To assess their change, patients may with varying accuracy recall their previous responses and implicitly construct the change that would be necessary to explain their current state. Both response shift (see Chapter 19) and recall bias (Schwartz and Sudman, 1994) may distort their assessment of change, and it has been observed that ratings of change correlate more strongly with current status than with the baseline score.

These transition questions use the patient as their own control, and seek to determine whether any changes that occur are large enough to be of importance to the patient. They can therefore be described as *within-person* methods. An alternative *between-person* approach, in which patients are asked to compare their present state relative to that of others who have the same condition, has been explored by Redelmeier *et al.* (1996). Reassuringly, they found it resulted in broadly similar estimates for the *MID*.

18.7   Anchoring against other measurements

Sometimes other outcomes can be identified, for which observers or preferably patients are able to specify what constitutes an important difference. These *anchor* outcomes should measure essentially the same construct as the target, and the value of these anchors depends on how well they reflect underlying change. Following Cohen's (1988) rules of thumb, Hays *et al.* (2005) recommend 0.371 as a correlation threshold to define a noteworthy (large effect) association; they also recommend that there should be multiple anchors and that the correlations should be reported. Then patients can be classified into groups according the anchor, and the corresponding values of the target measure are used to determine the *MID*.

Example from the literature

Suñer *et al.* (2009) used changes in visual acuity to propose a MID for the National Eye Institute Visual Function Questionnaire-25 (NEI VFQ-25). The authors note that a 15-letter change in best corrected visual acuity is frequently used as a primary endpoint in clinical trials and is generally accepted as clinically significant. Thus they used 15-character changes in visual acuity as the anchor for determining the *MID* for the corresponding changes in the overall composite score of the VFQ-25, formed by the mean of 24 items after omitting the single item for general health. The mean visual acuity (letter count) was 53.5, with $SD = 13.2$, and the mean score for the VFQ was 69.3, $SD = 19.2$. Patients were assessed again at 12 months. The investigators grouped patients into those who gained at least 15 letters, had fewer than 15 letter change, or lost at least 15 letters. Fitting linear regression models, they estimated a *MID* of 4.34 based on a clinically significant change of 15 letters in visual acuity.

In this example the authors, following conventional practice, analysed group mean scores and used linear regression models. However, correlations between the anchoring variable and the target score (the authors reported r to be less than 0.3) affect the slope of the regression line, and cause the slope to be shallow: in regression, slope $b = r \times (SD_{Target} / SD_{Anchor})$. This in turn will result in an attenuated estimate of the *MID*. Why does this happen? Regression aims to predict expected scores for individual patients, which is not the same as cross-calibration of scales. Instead, we are concerned with estimating the equivalent value on the target scale that corresponds to an observed change on the anchoring outcome. We suggest that an alternative approach is to apply a simple linear linking function (Fayers & Hays, 2014a). This is unaffected by r and leads to:

$$MID = AnchorChange \times (SD_{Target} / SD_{Anchor}). \tag{18.1}$$

This is equivalent to applying the effect-size ratio of the anchor to the target. A possible advantage of this approach is that it can be applied either to change-scores or to cross-sectional data, as it simply scales the anchor change by the respective *SD*s. For the above example, this would result in $MID = 15 \times 19.2/13.2 = 21.8$, which is very different from the attenuated value proposed by Suñer *et al.* (2009). However, empirical studies evaluating the merits of linking scores instead of regression models are required.

18.8   Minimum detectable change

Minimum detectable change (*MDC*), or minimal detectable difference, is the smallest change in score that can be detected after allowing for 'measurement errors' or random errors such as test-retest and patient-to-patient variability. There are several methods for estimating the *MDC*, typically involving the standard error of measurement (*SEM*) or reliability coefficients such as the test–retest correlation and Cronbach's α. Clearly, both *MDC* and *MID* are important, but they measure different things. For an instrument to be useful, it ought to be capable of detecting changes that are important to patients or are deemed clinically relevant; that is, it should be suitably sensitive and should be responsive to changes, two characteristics that are assessed as part of the validation of all new instruments. For a sensitive and reliable instrument, *MDC* should smaller than *MID*. Further, *MDC* is a statistical property of the measurement, and is sometimes described as a distribution-based approach, whereas *MID* is the value of concern for interpretation and is based on the value judgement of patients or less frequently other observers. Thus *MDC* is of little relevance for interpretation. The relationship between *MID* and *MDC* is discussed by Turner *et al.* (2010) and de Vet *et al.* (2010). Effect size statistics, based on *SD* rather than *SEM*, are sometimes also described as a distribution-based approach, but it is less confusing to term them as being a standardised-differences approach (see Section 18.9).

18.9   Expert judgement for evidence-based guidelines

Early attempts at specifying *MID* for sample size determination and interpreting results relied on expert judgement. Later studies attempted to formalise this process, using rigorous qualitative studies and Delphi methods to obtain consensus values. King *et al.* (2010) used expert judgement in another way, combining it with clinical anchors and systematic review. Three clinicians with many years of experience managing cancer patients and using PROs in clinical research each reviewed 71 publications that reported mean scores of the FACT-G. The clinicians were blinded to the FACT-G results of the individual studies, and were asked to consider the various clinical anchors that they believed might be associated with FACT-G mean differences, using these to predict which dimensions of QoL would be affected and whether the size-class of effects would be trivial, small, moderate or large. For example, if the study was a clinical trial that reported patients in one treatment arm had cancer that progressed and led to shortened survival, the experts might anticipate that there would be moderate or large deterioration of QoL accompanied with moderate increase in levels of pain. Similarly, knowledge of treatment received might lead experts to infer levels of particular toxicities. The size-classes were defined explicitly in terms of clinical relevance, for example 'Small: subtle but nevertheless clinically relevant'. The experts' judgements were then linked with the observed FACT-G mean differences and inverse-variance weighted mean differences and values were calculated for each size-class.

Example from the literature

Cocks *et al.* (2011) extended the method of King *et al.* (2010), and applied it to the QLQ-C30. They identified 152 publications of randomised clinical trials and cohort/descriptive studies. These reported QoL comparisons for 2,217 'contrasts' that could act as anchors, such as patients with early versus advanced disease, or good versus poor performance status, different treatment modalities, etc. A team of 34 experts reviewed from one to 98 articles each, according to their areas of expertise and their availability. Reviewers were mainly oncologists but the panel also possessed nursing, psychosocial, surgical, psychology, and radiotherapy expertise. For the review, the actual study results in the publications were masked, and the reviewers described what results, based on their experience, they anticipated would have been reported in the publications. Based on the meta-analysis of the results, recommendations were made for each of the multi- and single-item scales of the QLQ-C30. The results are summarised in Table 18.5. The authors suggest the threshold between trivial/small should be the smallest estimate on which to base a sample size. Depending on the individual study/interventions, larger differences may be of interest and the range of small/medium estimates could be used. This table is for cross-sectional comparisons, and Cocks *et al.* (2012) extend the analyses to include guidelines for interpreting change in scores over time.

Table 18.5 Guidelines for the size of cross-sectional differences when comparing groups of patients. Scales have been ordered according to the size of the medium differences

Lower estimate of medium differences	Scale	Mean difference			
		Trivial	Small	Medium	Large
< 10 points	DI	< 3	3–	> 7	—
	NV	< 3	3–	8–	> 15
	CF	< 3	3–	9–	> 14
	DY	< 4	4–	9–	> 15
10–15 points	FI	< 3	3–	> 10	–
	QL	< 4	4–	10–	> 15
	SF	< 5	5–	11–	> 15
	SL	< 4	4–	13–	> 24
	FA	< 5	5–	13–	> 19
	CO	< 5	5–	13–	> 19
	PA	< 6	6–	13–	> 19
	PF	< 5	5–	14–	> 22
	AP	< 5	5–	14–	> 23
> 15 points	RF	< 6	6–	19–	> 29

DI, diarrhea; NV, nausea and vomiting; CF, cognitive functioning; DY, dyspnoea; FI, financial difficulties; QL, global quality of life; SF, social functioning; SL, insomnia; FA, fatigue; CO, constipation; PA, pain; PF, physical functioning; AP, appetite loss; RF, role functioning.
Source: Adapted from Cocks *et al.* (2011). Reproduced with permission from the American Society of Clinical Oncology.

18.10   Impact of the state of quality of life

The extent to which reduced QoL affects daily living may sometimes serve as an indicator of its importance. This is likely to be particularly true for causal scales. An example is pain: patients can be asked about both *levels* of pain and its *impact* upon various activities; thus impact ratings are used to 'anchor' the pain ratings.

Thus the Brief Pain Inventory (BPI) asks patients to rate their pain at the time of completing the questionnaire (pain now) and also its worst, least and average over the previous week. One form of scoring the BPI is to use the 'pain-worst' scale as the primary response variable. To calibrate the pain-worst scale in terms of the impact of pain, patients can additionally be asked to rate how much their pain interferes with various activities and states.

Example from the literature

Table 18.6, from Cleeland (1991), shows the levels at which specific functions begin to be impaired by 'pain worst' recorded on the BPI. For example, patients were asked to rate how much pain interferes with their 'enjoyment of life', with 0 being 'no interference' and 10 being 'interferes completely'. Using an interference rating of 4 to mean 'impaired function', Table 18.6 shows that enjoyment of life becomes impaired when pain worst reaches a level of 3. Most of the items became impaired when pain reached a level of 5. This is consistent with other studies, where the midpoint of pain rating scales has been found to represent a critical value beyond which patients report disproportionate impairment of functional status. Because of these findings, Cleeland suggests, it is possible to define 'significant pain' as pain that is rated at the midpoint or higher on pain-intensity scales.

Table 18.6 Levels of pain severity that were reported as impairing function

Impaired function	Rating of worst pain
Enjoyment of life	3
Work	4
Mood	5
Sleep	5
General activity	5
Walking	7
Relations with others	8

Source: Cleeland, 1991. Reproduced with permission of Taylor and Francis Group LLC Books.

18.11   Changes in relation to life events

Since QoL scales involve unfamiliar measures, studies that relate the observed changes to changes in more familiar or objective measures can be easier to interpret. One such method is to compare (or 'anchor') changes in QoL in patients with the size of change that is expected to occur in persons who experience various major life events such as family illness, loss of a job or bereavement.

Example from the literature

Table 18.7 shows 12 items from the Social Readjustment Rating Scale (SRRS) of Holmes and Rahe (1967) that form a Life Events Index of undesirable stressful life events. The full SRRS consists of 43 scales for major life events rated from 0 to 100 according to their level of stress. For example, a minor violation of the law was associated with a change score of 11 points. Columns one and two of Table 18.7 summarise the changes relating to various life events.

Testa *et al.* (1993), in a randomised clinical trial of antihypertensive therapy, used a Life Events Index (LEI) adapted from the SRRS, the General Perceived Health (GPH) scale and several other QoL scales. The GPH scale contains 11 items relating to vitality, general health status including bodily disorders, and sleep disturbance. The changes from baseline were expressed using standardised response means as in equation (18.6), with the change scores being divided by the *SD* of the changes observed during a period while the patients were stable. The authors then used linear regression to calibrate the GPH scale in terms of the LEI (final column in Table 18.7).

They found that a change of 0.1 *SD* in the GPH scale was equivalent to approximately 37 points on the LEI, and thus corresponds to the impact that might be expected from the death of a close friend (37 points) or from sexual

Table 18.7 Undesirable life events and their corresponding weights, from the Social Readjustment Rating Scale, and four examples of change-scores from the General Perceived Health (GPH) questionnaire that correspond to a change in stressful life events

Stressful life event (undesirable events)	Life Events Index: weights	General Perceived Health (GPH) Change scores (*SD* units)
1. Minor violation of the law	−11	
2. Major change in sleeping habits	−16	
3. Major change in working conditions	−20	0.05
4. Change in residence	−20	
5. Trouble with boss	−23	
6. Death of a close friend	−37	0.10
7. Sexual difficulties	−39	
8. Being fired from work	−47	
9. Major personal injury or illness	−53	0.15
10. Death of a close family member	−63	
11. Divorce	−73	0.20
12. Death of a spouse	−100	

Source: Holmes and Rahe, 1967, reproduced with permission from Elsevier, with additional data from Testa *et al.*, 1993.

difficulties (39 points). A change of 0.15 *SD* in GPH similarly corresponds to a 55-point life-events change, and this is equivalent to the impact on QoL that a major personal illness (53 points) might have. Testa *et al.* conclude that although there was broad variability in responses from person to person, values between 0.1 and 0.2 *SD* units can be considered clinically meaningful and represent the lower bound of what constitutes a minimally important response to treatment.

In this study, overall QoL scores shifted positively by 0.11 for treatment with captopril, and negatively by 0.11 for enalapril, an overall difference of 0.22. Testa *et al.* comment: "Our findings indicate that drug-induced changes in the QoL can be substantial and clinically meaningful even when they involve drugs in the same pharmacological class."

18.12   Effect size statistics

The methods discussed so far to estimate the magnitude of important changes make use of information collected from surveys of the population or from studies that investigate QoL changes in patients. When such information is unavailable, *effect size statistics* may be useful. These are based on standardised differences, in which the variability of the measurements is accounted for by scaling the target effect through division by the standard deviation of the measurements. Some authors group effect-size statistics with other distribution-based methods, because they depend on an estimate of the *SD*. However, as mentioned in Section 18.7, this can be misleading as the objective of standardisation is very different. Standardisation is a scaling of the target values according to the variability of the data (i.e. the *SD*), whereas *MDC* statistics typically make use of the standard error instead of the *SD*, where the standard error is a function of not only the *SD* but also the sample size and is used for significance testing. Effect size measures were initially proposed for use in sample size estimation, and have been mentioned in that context in Section 11.3. Methods based upon effect size statistics have the advantage of simplicity. Their limitation is that they do not consider the values and opinions of patients. Despite this, many investigators have found that effect size statistics often seem to produce values that correspond very roughly to those obtained using patient-orientated methods.

Suppose changes in a patient's QoL are assessed using several different instruments. Some instruments may use a scale that is scored, say, from 1 to 7, while others might score the patient from 0 to 100. Thus changes will appear to be larger on some instruments than others. One way to standardise the measurements is to divide the observed changes by the *SD*. A particular change is likely to be of greater clinical significance and of more importance to patients if it occurs on a scale that has a narrow range of values and therefore shows little variation as indicated by a small *SD*.

Having scaled for the variability in this way, the standardised changes should then be of comparable magnitude to each other, despite the scales having different ranges of values.

Considering the patient's perspective, too, it can be sensible to allow for SDs. The level of QoL will vary within a patient from day-to-day. If there is a high degree of variability in QoL levels, implying a large SD, a small improvement due to therapy may not even be noticed by the patient and would not be considered useful.

Cohen (1988) proposed this form of standardisation in order to simplify the estimation of sample sizes. He noted that to calculate a sample size one must first specify the size of the effect that it is wished to detect. Sometimes the investigator will have knowledge or beliefs about likely, important, treatment effects, and will be able to base estimates upon that. Frequently, there will be no such prior information upon which to base decisions. Thus Cohen proposed that the mean change divided by the SD would serve as an *effect-size index* that is suitable for sample size estimation. Based upon his experience in the social sciences, he suggested that effect sizes of 0.2–0.5 have generally been regarded by investigators as being 'small', 0.5–0.8 are 'moderate', and those of 0.8 or above are 'large'.

These apparently arbitrary thresholds have stood the test of time very well. Perhaps surprisingly, the values 0.2, 0.5 and 0.8 have since been found to be broadly applicable in many fields of research as well as in social sciences from where Cohen had drawn his experience.

Examples from the literature

Osoba *et al.* (1998) contrasted the approach of minimal clinically important difference with the values for ES, and the two methods were broadly consistent. In most cases, the ES was 0.5 or greater ('moderate to large') when the transition questions indicated moderate or greater change. The ES was mostly between 0.2 and 0.5 ('small') when the transition question indicated little change, and was mostly less than 0.2 when no change was reported.

Norman *et al.* (2003) carried out a systematic review, identifying 38 studies (62 outcomes) that reported a minimal clinically important difference and also provided information sufficient for calculation of an effect size. They conclude that in most circumstances the threshold of discrimination for changes in health-related QoL for chronic diseases appeared to be approximately half a SD. It is noted as an explanation for this consistency that research in psychology has shown that the limit of people's ability to discriminate over a wide range of tasks is approximately one part in seven, which is very close to half a SD. However, many authors regard the use of distribution-based effect sizes as simplistic and it remains controversial.

The label *effect size* is used as a generic term to cover a wide range of standardised measures of change, and so there is some confusion sometimes over what is intended. Two in particular stand out in QoL research. The first, often simply called the 'effect size', is described next. The second method, the *standardised response mean*, is suitable for paired data and uses a different *SD*.

Effect size for two independent groups

One statistic frequently used for determining effect sizes is the *ES* statistic, called simply and confusingly *effect size*. *ES* is defined as the mean change in scores, divided by the *SD*. This can be used to compare two independent groups of patients, as in a clinical trial. If the mean values of the two groups are $\bar{x}_{Treatment}$ and $\bar{x}_{Control}$, the *SD* used for standardising the treatment difference can be calculated from the control group, giving:

$$ES = \frac{\bar{x}_{Treatment} - \bar{x}_{Control}}{SD_{Control}}. \tag{18.2}$$

Although the *SD* of one group (usually the control group, $SD_{Control}$) is frequently used for the divisor, in practice, the pooled *SD* from the two treatment groups is more commonly used:

$$ES = \frac{\bar{x}_{Group1} - \bar{x}_{Group2}}{SD_{Pooled}}, \tag{18.3}$$

where, if groups are of equal size,

$$SD_{Pooled} = \sqrt{\left[\left(SD_{Group1}^2 + SD_{Group2}^2 \right) / 2 \right]}. \tag{18.4}$$

Examples from the literature

Table 12.3, based on Islam *et al.* (2010), can be readily extended to include the effect size by calculating the mean difference divided by SD_{Pooled}, as shown in Table 18.8. The *ES* of 0.39 for HADS anxiety is small, but 0.68 for depression can be regarded as moderate.

Another example is provided by Temel *et al.* (2010), who randomised 151 patients with metastatic lung cancer to standard care alone or early palliative care integrated with standard care. QoL at baseline and at 12 weeks was assessed with three scales: the Functional Assessment of Cancer Therapy–Lung (FACT-L) scale (values can range from 0 to 136); the lung-cancer subscale (LCS) of the FACT-L scale (range 0 to 28); and the Trial Outcome Index (TOI), which is the sum of the LCS, physical well-being and functional well-being scores (range 0–84). Thus each scale had a different range of values and a different high (best) score, making the change scores difficult to interpret. Temel *et al.* used the *SD* of the pooled data to calculate the *Effect Size* for each scale, thus providing comparable standardised outcome measures. The values were 0.42, 0.41 and 0.52 respectively. The authors commented that "A comparison of measures of quality of life at 12 weeks showed that the patients assigned to early palliative care had significantly higher scores than did those assigned to standard care, for the total FACT-L scale, the LCS, and the TOI, with effect sizes in the medium range." (Although by some conventions an *ES* between 0.20 and 0.50 is classified as small.)

Table 18.8 Comparison of mean HADS scores in 50 patients with facial trauma and 50 matched controls. The addition of effect sizes may guide the interpretation of observed differences. (Adapted from Islam et al., 2010. Reproduced with permission of Elsevier).

Variable	Facial trauma group (N = 50) Mean (SD)	Control group (N = 50) Mean (SD)	Mean difference (95% CI)	p-value	Effect size*
HADS Depression	5.94 (3.1)	3.92 (2.8)	−2.0 (−3.4 to −0.6)	0.006	0.68
HADS Anxiety	5.91 (4.5)	4.33 (3.5)	−1.6 (−3.5 to 0.2)	0.07	0.39

*According to the conventional classification, an effect size of 0.20 is small, 0.50 moderate, and 0.80 large.
Source: Adapted from Islam *et al.,* 2010. Reproduced with permission of Elsevier.

Example

Figure 18.4 can be redrawn using the principle of effect sizes. The differences between the values of patients and the reference population have been divided by the between-patient *SD*s, leading to the *ES* values in Figure 18.7. The dotted lines correspond to small, moderate and large *ES* of 0.2, 0.5 and 0.8. Since many of the scales had approximately similar *SD*s of around 20 points, the plot is superficially similar to that of Figure 18.4 apart from a scaling factor. The effect sizes are in the region between small to moderate for most of the scales, but patient symptom-scores for pain (LRRC) and diarrhoea are large or moderate compared to the reference values, and the functioning scales and overall QoL show small to moderate reductions, with a large impact on social functioning for the LRRC patients.

(Continued)

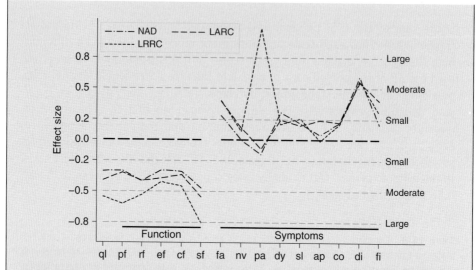

Figure 18.7 Data of Figure 18.4, showing *effect sizes* instead of absolute mean differences. For 439 patients with rectal cancer, divided into non-advanced disease (NAD), locally advanced rectal cancer (LARC) and locally recurrent rectal cancer (LRRC), compared to age- and gender-matched reference values of the general population. See footnote to Table 18.3 for scale names.

Effect size (*ES*) for paired data

The *ES* statistic can also be used for paired, or within-patient, data. It is then defined as the mean change in scores divided by the *SD* of the QoL scores. Usually the *baseline* measurement, at *Time* 1, is chosen to be either immediately prior to starting active treatment or pre-randomisation in a clinical trial, and this can be used for the calculation of the *SD*:

$$ES = \frac{\overline{x}_{Time2} - \overline{x}_{Time1}}{SD_{Time1}}. \qquad (18.5)$$

Standardised response mean (*SRM*)

The standardised response mean (*SRM*) is the mean change in a PRO from two assessments in each subject, divided by the *SD* of these changes in scores. Most commonly the paired assessments are made at two different times in each patient, for example at baseline and after treatment, and thus the *SRM* describes the course of the illness. Another example of within-patient paired observations is self-assessment compared to proxy assessment. The formula for *SRM* is:

$$SRM = \frac{\overline{x}_{Time2} - \overline{x}_{Time1}}{SD_{Difference}}. \qquad (18.6)$$

A large *SRM* indicates that the change is large relative to the background variability in the measurements. Thus the *SRM* is a form of *Cohen's effect-size* index. It is a widely used measure of the size of effects for paired data. The $SD_{Difference}$ should in principle be estimated from stable patients whose overall level of QoL is not expected to be changing. For example, if untreated patients under observation are expected to have a stable QoL, they might provide an estimate of the background variability. Sometimes $SD_{Difference}$ may be available from previous test–retest reliability studies conducted when developing the QoL instrument itself, since those studies also require stable patients. In practice, data on stable patients are often unavailable and the $SD_{Difference}$ of the study patients themselves is most frequently used.

Whereas the *ES* used the *SD* of the between-patient baseline scores, *SRM* uses the $SD_{Difference}$. An advantage of the *SRM* is that is corresponds most closely to the method of calculating a paired *t*-test, which is most sensitive for detecting differences between the two measurements. However, the *ES* is commonly considered more appropriate for assessing an effect size because it can be argued that we should use patient baseline values and variability in order to decide what magnitude of QoL change would be important.

If the correlation between X_{Time1} and X_{Time2} is ρ, and if we assume that the *SDs* at times 1 and 2 are approximately equal, there is a direct relationship between *ES* and *SRM*:

$$ES = SRM \times \sqrt{2(1-\rho)}. \qquad (18.7)$$

Thus, if the correlation ρ is 0.5, *ES* and *SRM* will be similar; if there is a high correlation, which implies that $SD_{Difference}$ will be smaller than the *SD* of the baseline scores, *ES* will be smaller than *SRM*. Despite this, the same thresholds of 0.2, 0.5 and 0.8 are commonly interpreted as indicating small, moderate and large effect sizes for both *ES* and *SRM*; this is clearly not very logical.

Table 20.1 provides the standard errors (*SEs*) for paired and unpaired *SRMs*, enabling calculation of confidence intervals.

Example from the literature

Self- and proxy-reports were compared for the Stroke Impact Scale (SIS) using data from 180 patients in Brazil (Carod-Artal *et al.*, 2009). The SIS 3.0 is a 59-item self-report assessment of stroke outcome, and has eight domains: Strength, Hand function, Mobility, Physical and instrumental activities of daily living (ADL/IADL), Memory and thinking, Communication, Emotion, and Social participation. Scores for each domain range from 0 to 100, and higher scores indicate better QoL. Four of the subscales (Strength, Hand function, ADL/IADL, and Mobility) are combined into a Composite Physical Domain (CPD).

Table 18.9 shows the comparison of SIS patient and proxy mean scores. For six of the eight domains there were no significant differences between proxy and patient scores, but proxies scored significantly lower (worse) for Strength (41.7 vs. 36.6; $p < 0.0001$) and ADL/IADL (46.2 vs. 43.1; $p < 0.01$), as well as for the composite CPD (39.7 vs. 34.9; $p < 0.0001$). The authors commented that "Nevertheless, the estimated *ES* was small (0.21 for the Strength domain)", and "The *SRM* for the CPD was 0.37 (small/moderate effect)".

Since the authors had indicated that "An *ES* or a *SRM* of 0.2 was considered a small bias, and a value between 0.20 and 0.5 a moderate bias", it seems inconsistent to use *ES* for the strength domain. Nor is it entirely clear why they reported *ES* in addition to *SRM*. They did not comment on the effect size of ADL/IADL.

Table 18.9 Self- and proxy-report assessments of the Stroke Impact Scale (SIS): *ES* and *SRM* of the differences, for 180 Brazilian patients

SIS domains	Patients N=180 Mean (SD)	Proxies N=180 Mean (SD)	Patient-Proxy difference Mean (SD)	t	P	ES	SRM
Strength	41.7 (25.8)	36.6 (23.7)	5.3 (21.4)	3.3	<0.001	0.21	0.25
Hand function	20.2 (30.9)	20.5 (30.1)	−0.5 (18.1)	−0.4	0.7	0.02	0.03
Mobility	42.2 (26.9)	40.7 (26.7)	1.5 (16.8)	1.2	0.22	0.06	0.09
ADL/IADL*	46.2 (23.7)	43.1 (22.5)	3.2 (16.6)	2.6	0.01	0.13	0.19
Memory and thinking	71.6 (22.8)	68.2 (24.5)	3.4 (25.3)	1.8	0.07	0.15	0.13
Communication	77.1 (20.2)	76.9 (20.1)	0.1 (22.3)	0.1	0.93	0.01	0.01
Emotion	52.2 (12.3)	53.7 (13.1)	−1.2 (16.3)	−0.9	0.33	0.09	0.07
Social participation	46.9 (22.8)	49.1 (23.7)	−2.3 (27.6)	−1.1	0.2	0.10	0.08
Composite Physical Domain	39.7 (22.7)	34.9 (21.6)	4.7 (12.9)	4.9	<0.001	0.21	0.37

*ADL/IADL: activities of daily living/instrumental activities of daily living.
Source: Carod-Artal *et al.*, 2009, Table 4. Reproduced with permission of Wolters Kluwer Health.

Carod-Artal *et al.* observed that proxy raters tended to report more HRQoL problems than patients themselves on the SIS physical domains. They concluded that patient and proxy ratings are valid, and that agreement between stroke patients and proxies was adequate for most SIS domains. However they also assessed agreement and warned that proxy assessment of SIS subjective domains should be evaluated with caution because the strength of the agreement was low.

Effect sizes and meta-analysis

Effect sizes are a form of standardisation, and provide a *dimensionless* number that summarises the results. For example, if a mean treatment difference were measured in millimetres, dividing by a *SD* that is also expressed in millimetres would result in a number that has no measurement units. Thus the *ES* provides a useful method for comparing results across a number of clinical trials, even when several different instruments have been used. It therefore enables *meta-analyses* to be carried out with QoL data. This is discussed in more detail in Chapter 20.

18.13 Patient variability

Most of the methods described make use of comparisons of means, and therefore inherently assume that all patients will derive the same benefit or deterioration in QoL according to their treatment. That is, all patients are assumed to change by the same average amount. It is also assumed that PRO scores may be sensibly aggregated by averaging – and that, for example, two patients scoring 50% of maximum are equivalent to one patient scoring 75% and another scoring 25%.

Clearly, there is variability in patient-to-patient responses. If QoL improves, on average, by 15%, most patients will experience changes that are either smaller or larger than this value and few if any will experience exactly this change. Thus even a small average benefit might allow some patients to obtain a major and very worthwhile improvement. Although it is important to know the overall mean changes, it is also important to consider the potential advantage (or disadvantage) to those patients who benefit (or suffer) most from the treatment. The *normal range* is the estimated range of values that includes a specified percentage of the observations. For example, the 95% normal range for the change in QoL would be the range of values that is expected to include 95% of patients from the relevant patient population. The limits of the normal range would indicate the magnitude of the likely benefit to those patients with the best 2.5% (upper limit of range) and worst 2.5% (lower limit of range) of responses, and also show the degree of variability in the observations. If the observations have a Normal distribution, the following formula estimates the normal range (for further details, see Campbell *et al.*, 2007). From Appendix Table T1, z_α is the value that corresponds to the proportion of patients outside the normal range (e.g. $1 - \alpha/2 = 0.975$ for 95% normal range, in which case $z_{1-\alpha/2} = 1.96$), $\bar{x}$ is the mean value and *SD* is the standard deviation:

$$Normal\ range = \bar{x} - z_{1-\alpha/2} \times SD \text{ to } \bar{x} + z_{1-\alpha/2} \times SD. \tag{18.8}$$

Example

Pain is frequently measured on a 0 to 10 scale. Suppose treatment causes a small reduction in average pain, with a mean change of 0.96 and corresponding $SD_{Difference}$ of 2.49. Assuming a Normal distribution for mean change, the 95% normal range would be $0.96 - (1.96 \times 2.49)$ to $0.96 + (1.96 \times 2.49)$, or -3.9 to $+5.8$. Therefore, we expect 95% of patients to lie within this range, but 2.5% are expected to have more extreme deterioration and 2.5% a more marked improvement. This is a range of 9.7 (-3.9 to 5.8) or nearly 10 points on the pain scale, and is approximately half the total range (-10 to $+10$) possible for the scale. Thus, although the mean change in pain score was 0.96, which corresponds to a small effect size, many patients could experience large and clinically important increases or decreases in pain.

18.14   Number needed to treat

An alternative way to allow for the variation in treatment effect upon QoL is known as the *number needed to treat (NNT)*. This is an estimate of the number of patients who need to be treated with the new treatment in order for one additional patient to benefit. The *NNT* can be estimated whenever a clinical trial has a binary outcome. When evaluating QoL, one possible binary outcome might be the proportion of patients with a 'moderate improvement' in QoL, where moderate improvement could be defined as an improvement greater than some specified value. Similarly, the number of psychiatric 'cases', such as cases of depression, could be used.

The proportion of patients with 'moderate deterioration' or 'cases' can be estimated for each treatment group. If the proportions *deteriorating* are p_T and p_C for the test and control treatments, the difference $p_T - p_C$ is called the *absolute risk reduction (ARR)*. The *NNT* is simply:

$$NNT = \frac{1}{ARR} = \frac{1}{p_T - p_C}. \tag{18.9}$$

When p_T and p_C are the proportions *improving*, $p_T - p_C$ is called the *absolute benefit increase (ABI)*, and $NNT = 1 / ABI$.

Example from the literature

Guyatt *et al.* (1998) describe a cross-over trial of treatment for asthma. The multicentre double-blind randomised trial recruited 140 patients. During the three periods in this cross-over study, each patient received salmeterol, salbutamol or placebo in random sequence. Patients completed the asthma-specific AQLQ.

Two AQLQ scales were examined: asthma symptoms and activity limitations. Table 18.10 shows that the mean differences between salmeterol and the other two treatments were all statistically highly significant, but are 'small' for AQLQ scores according to the classification of minimal clinically important difference in Section 18.6. The *NNT* is calculated from the proportion of patients who had obtained benefit from salmeterol, where 'better' was defined as an improvement of 0.5, minus the proportion of patients who obtained a similar sized benefit from the alternative treatment. Thus in the first row of Table 18.10, these proportions are 0.42 and 0.12 for salmeterol versus salbutamol, giving $ABI = 0.30$, and hence $NNT = 1/0.30 = 3.3$. Therefore 33 patients would need to be treated for 10 to gain an important benefit in symptom reduction.

Table 18.10   Differences between groups given different treatments for asthma, showing the number needed to treat for a single patient to benefit from salmeterol

AQLQ domains	Difference between treatments		Proportion better on salmeterol	Proportion better on salbutamol or placebo	Proportion who benefited	NNT
	Mean	*p*-value				
Salmeterol vs. salbutamol						
Asthma symptoms	0.5	< 0.0001	0.42	0.12	0.30	3.3
Activity limitations	0.3	< 0.0001	0.32	0.10	0.22	4.5
Salmeterol vs. placebo						
Asthma symptoms	0.7	< 0.0001	0.50	0.09	0.41	2.4
Activity limitations	0.4	< 0.0001	0.42	0.08	0.34	2.9

Source: Guyatt *et al.*, 1998, Table 1. Reproduced with permission of BMJ Publishing Group Ltd.

This example relates to a cross-over trial in which patients received all three treatments. Consequently, the proportion of patients better on one treatment or the other could be estimated directly. In a majority of randomised trials, each patient only receives one of the treatments, say C or T. Therefore we must estimate how many patients benefit from C and how many from T. Let us suppose that for the N_C controls the proportions improved, unchanged and deteriorated are i_C, u_C and d_C respectively. Although i_T of the N_T patients in the T-group improved, we might expect that some of these patients would have improved even if they had received the C instead. Assuming independence between the two groups, we can estimate that i_C of the i_T patients would have improved anyway. Therefore, of the improved patients in the T-group, we estimate the proportion who truly benefited from T as $i_T - (i_C \times i_T) = (u_C + d_C) \times i_T$. In addition, d_C of the T-group patients who were unchanged might have been expected to have deteriorated if they were in the C-group, giving another $d_C \times u_T$ that benefited from T. Hence, after allowing for those patients expected to benefit from C, the total proportion of the N_T patients who really benefited from T is estimated as:

$$\left[\left(u_c + d_c\right) \times i_T\right] + \left(d_c \times u_T\right).$$

Similar calculations for the C-group give the proportion of the C patients who might be expected to have benefited from C, and as before $ARR = p_C - p_T$.

Example from the literature

Guyatt *et al.* (1998) describe a parallel group trial involving 78 patients with chronic airflow limitation. In the control group, the proportions of patients whose dyspnoea was improved, unchanged and deteriorated were $i_C = 0.28$, $u_C = 0.49$ and $d_C = 0.23$. The comparable proportions for the treatment group were $i_T = 0.48$, $u_T = 0.42$ and $d_T = 0.10$. Therefore the estimated proportion that were better in the treatment group is $(0.49 + 0.23) \times 0.48 + (0.23 \times 0.42) = 0.44$. Similar calculation for the estimated proportion who are better in the control group gives $0.28 \times (0.42 + 0.10) + (0.49 \times 0.10) = 0.20$. Hence $ARR = 0.44 - 0.20 = 0.24$, and $NNT = 1/0.24 = 4.2$.

Thus for every 42 patients treated it may be expected that 10 patients would have an important improvement in dyspnoea reduction as a consequence of therapy.

Example from the literature

Many QoL instruments are multidimensional, and some authors therefore define a composite endpoint. Klinkhammer-Schalke *et al.* (2012) reported a randomised trial in 200 women with newly diagnosed breast cancer, who completed the EORTC QLQ-C30 and the supplementary breast cancer module, QLQ-BR23. 'Diseased QoL' was defined as a drop below 50 points in any of the 10 major QoL dimensions on a scale from 100 to 0 points (worst QoL). 'Healed QoL' was a shift to 50 points or more. The primary end point used meaningful changes in QoL in each patient as an immediate, personally relevant treatment goal, not mean values in the overall patient group. The effect size was calculated as the number needed to treat (*NNT*) to raise all QoL subscales above 49 in one patient at six months.

The authors report that at six months 60/85 patients in the control group or $p_C = 71\%$ (95% *CI* 51–68) showed diseased QoL in at least one dimension. In the treatment group, this occurred in 47/84 patients or $p_T = 56\%$ (95% *CI* 38–56). A χ^2-test of the difference gives $p = 0.048$. This corresponds to a relative risk reduction of $(71-56)/71 = 21\%$ (95% *CI* 0–37), an $ARR = 15\%$ (95% *CI* 0.3–29) and an *NNT* of 7 (95% *CI* 3–37). The confidence limits for *NNT* were calculated by a computer bootstrapping algorithm.

18.15   Conclusions

This chapter has described a variety of ways of approaching clinical significance and the interpretation of results. Some methods aim to provide a better feel for the interpretation and meaning of scale scores, for example by estimating the values that may be expected in patients and in other groups such as healthy people. Other methods place greater emphasis upon the patient's perspective and clinical significance. Reviews have concluded that "While no single method for determining clinical significance is unilaterally endorsed, the investigation and full reporting of multiple methods for establishing clinically significant change levels for a QOL measure, and greater direct involvement of clinicians in clinical significance studies are strongly encouraged" (Wyrwich *et al.*, 2005). Thus many authors recommend using a combination of approaches, including in particular anchor- and distribution-based methods (Revicki *et al.*, 2008; Sloan *et al.*, 2006)

The interpretation of QoL results remains essentially qualitative. Clinical significance is subjective, and therefore a matter of opinion. The values and opinions of individual patients will differ, as will the opinions of the treating clinician and those of society in general. Thus, for a QoL measurement scale, it is unlikely that a single threshold value will be universally accepted as a cut-point that separates clinically important changes from trivial and unimportant ones. It is also likely that patients may consider changes in some PROs to be more important than others, and a change of, say, 5 points on one scale may be as clinically important as a change of 20 on another. However, many investigators are finding that, for a variety of scales assessing overall QoL and some of its dimensions, changes of between 5% and 10% (or 5 to 10 points on a 100-point scale) are noticed by patients and are regarded by them as meaningful changes.

18.16   Further reading

There is extensive literature about how to interpret QoL measures and PROs. Revicki *et al.* (2008) review literature on this topic and set standards. The interpretation of changes over time is reviewed by Wyrwich *et al.* (2013), who also describe the use of "cumulative distribution function" plots. For an example of a comprehensive assessment of a particular domain, Dworkin *et al.* (2008) review research into pain and offer consensus recommendations. However, methods for establishing *MID* values remain controversial (King, 2011). Communication of results to patients presents additional challenges, and some approaches are considered by Guyatt and Schunemann (2007).

19

Biased reporting and response shift

Summary

It is well established that patients adapt to their illness, learning to accommodate and cope with their altered conditions. Thus they may change their internal standards, their values and/or their conceptualisation of QoL. Such changes are an example of *response shift*, in which a patient's responses to PRO items may vary in a manner that seems discordant with their changing health status. We discuss when and how response shift and other forms of bias, such as recall bias and selective reporting, might affect the analyses or distort the interpretation of results.

19.1   Bias

An estimate is said to be *biased* if it differs *systematically* from the true value of the parameter being estimated. An estimator with zero bias is called unbiased. Otherwise the estimator is said to be biased. There are many causes and forms of bias. This chapter examines biases that affect questionnaire assessments and, in particular response shift. Response shift occurs when a subject's views, values or expectations change over time, and especially when the changes occur during the period of observation. Thus a patient's health might be seen to be deteriorating, and yet the patient may assert that their QoL has not changed, or even that it has improved. Alternatively, a patient's health status may appear to be unchanging even though that same patient may report substantial changes in their QoL. In both cases, the patient's responses over time do not seem to agree with their corresponding health status. Of course there could be non-systematic, or random, measurement errors due to poor test–retest reliability; these do not constitute response shift, and do not result in consistent or repeatable responses from patients. Similarly, an instrument with poor sensitivity may fail to detect a change in QoL, but that does not enable a claim that a patient's QoL has not changed despite

Quality of Life: The Assessment, Analysis and Reporting of Patient-Reported Outcomes, Third Edition.
Peter M. Fayers and David Machin.
© 2016 John Wiley & Sons, Ltd. Published 2016 by John Wiley & Sons, Ltd.

their health status having deteriorated – in the latter case the implication is that, for example, the patient has adapted and is coping with their changing circumstances.

19.2   Recall bias

An important but sometimes neglected aspect of quality of life instruments is the specification of the recall period. A few instruments focus on current health status, and ask the respondent about how they feel 'Right now'. Many more, however, refer to 'How you have been in the past week', and some specify the past month or some other period. Another form of recall is to ask the patients to compare themselves against how they were when they previously attended hospital, reporting how much their condition has changed. It is clearly important that instruments pay attention to the precise specification of recall period. Caution must be exercised if this recall period is altered from that advocated by the instrument's developers, as any change is likely to violate the previous reports of validation.

The United States Food and Drug Administration (FDA, 2009) notes that it is important to consider patient ability to validly recall the information requested. They comment that the choice of recall period that is most suitable depends on the instrument's purpose and intended use; the variability, duration, frequency and intensity of the concept measured; and the disease or condition's characteristics; and the tested treatment and, in reference to clinical trials, "we intend to review the clinical trial protocols to determine what steps were taken to ensure that patients understood the instruments recall period … note also that any problems created by differential recall are likely to noise and obscure treatment effect." PRO instruments that call for patients to rely on memory, especially if they must recall over a long period of time, compare their current state with an earlier period, or average their response over a period of time, are likely to undermine content validity. Response is likely to be influenced by the patient's state at the time of recall. For these reasons, items with short recall periods or items that ask patients to describe their current or recent state are usually preferable.

Recall bias occurs when the respondent's answer to a question is affected not just by the correct answer and also by the respondent's memory. People tend to forget how extreme the past was. A patient with dental pain might say that their current pain is unbearable, but a few months later they are likely to have forgotten just how bad it was and might report that it was 'not that bad'. On the other hand, positive events they also become blurred towards neutrality: if someone has just come back from a successful holiday, it is well known that they will give enthusiastic descriptions of their experience; but if they are asked about that same holiday after a few weeks, the response is likely to be considerably weaker. Assessment of HRQoL is frequently concerned with symptoms and other problems, and patients may tend towards under-reporting the severity of past problems. If patients do, as we suggest, tend to report problems differently according to their distance from the time of the event, their responses will have systematically changed and this may be regarded as a form of *response shift*.

Example from the literature

Stone *et al.* (2004) show that pain recall may be complex: although we suggested that recall may lead to understatement of actual pain in the past, the opposite may also occur. Chronic-pain patients ($N = 121$) were asked to rate their current pain several times a day, and at the end of the week were also asked to "Place a mark on the following line to indicate the level of your USUAL PAIN over the last 7 days". An additional item asked participants about the change in pain from week to week. The question "Think about your pain over the last 7 days and compare it to the week before. How has it changed?" was answered with a five-point scale from much worse to much better.

On a scale of 0 (no pain) to 100 (worst possible pain), average momentary pain ratings were much lower (mean = 44) than recalled levels (58). The authors suggest that when subjects have to recall their average pain, they might only consider (or give greatest weight to) occasions when they are actually in pain, because those episodes are more prominent and salient, and thus more available to memory. Thus, recalled pain levels correspond more closely to the average levels experienced during episodes of pain, rather than to overall average levels.

When assessing change using momentary and recalled data there was low level of consistency and agreement. The authors suggest various reasons for this. One explanation hinges on the idea that change scores are inherently unreliable.

As Albert Schweitzer, the philosopher and physician, is reputed to have said, "Happiness is nothing more than good health and a bad memory".

19.3 Selective reporting bias

Patients may tend to ignore or discount those problems they believe to be unrelated to their illness. For example, a patient with bladder cancer who has also previously been incontinent for many years might respond to a question on this topic by reporting that it causes no problem – in effect, the patient has adapted to the illness and learnt to cope with the symptoms. However, patients who have experienced a recent change or who believe they have illness-related problems are more likely to make accurate responses. This *selective reporting bias* can distort the analyses and interpretation of results. To some extent it can be controlled by suitable *framing* of the questionnaire, which consists of instructions telling the patient whether to report *all* symptoms and problems, irrespective of origin or cause. Furthermore, many instruments ask about severity, as opposed to impact, of symptoms.

When a questionnaire is given to the general population, however, one might expect no such discounting of problems. As a consequence, QoL levels for patients may appear to be more favourable than those expected from population-based reference values. Sometimes this effect can be quite marked, even to the extent of making patients appear to have better QoL than the general population.

Example from the literature

Selective reporting may affect proxies as well as patients. Fayers *et al.* (1991) report QoL assessments in a randomised trial comparing maintenance versus no maintenance chemotherapy for small-cell lung cancer patients. Because this chemotherapy was likely to induce vomiting, the patient questionnaire asked about nausea and vomiting. These symptoms were also recorded by the clinicians.

In a total of 956 patient visits (Table 19.1), patients reported 626 (65%) episodes of vomiting, compared with 245 (26%) reports by physicians. Patients reported 371 episodes of vomiting where physicians recorded no problems with nausea and vomiting. Curiously, in 49 instances physicians reported vomiting when patients indicated no problems.

The authors suggest that if patients reported vomiting it was likely to be true. Thus there was a high degree of selective reporting by clinicians, who perhaps ignored and under-reported mild vomiting because they expected this to occur in nearly all patients.

Table 19.1　Small-cell lung cancer patients' and their physicians' assessments of nausea and vomiting

Physicians' assessments	Patients' assessments			
	None	Nausea	Vomiting	Total
Not reported	125	78	371	574
Nausea	27	31	79	137
Vomiting	49	20	176	245
Total	201	129	626	956

Source: Fayers *et al.*, 1991, Table V. Reproduced with permission of Macmillan Publishers Ltd on behalf of Cancer Research UK.

19.4　Other biases affecting PROs

Many forms of bias can affect questionnaires (Streiner and Norman, 2008), among which are the following. Responses to items on a PRO questionnaire can be influenced by a patient's current *mood*: depressed patients tend to rate themselves poorly, while happy patients are more positive. *Response acquiescence*, also described as *'yea-saying'* or acquiescence bias, is the tendency of respondents to give positive responses such as 'yes', 'true' or 'often'. Mood may be particularly important in younger females, while response acquiescence may be a source of systematic bias that can lead to underestimation of PROs among the well-educated and overestimation among older respondents. (Moum, 1988). *Framing effects* occur when responses are affected by how the question is phrased or by the preceding questions (Kahneman and Tversky, 1984); this is why most developers of QoL questionnaires specify that the sequence of items on their questionnaire must not be changed – so that any framing effects will at least remain constant. It is also the reason why some questionnaires place questions about 'your overall quality of life' at the end, so that the preceding items indicate (frame) the range of issues that should be considered in answering the global item (or, conversely, some questionnaires deliberately position the global item first, so that it remains unaffected by later items). *Halo effects* can cause ratings of specific characteristics to be influenced by the overall impression of health, and provide reason *not* to place the global item first. Proxy assessments may also be influenced by halo effects, with the rater's overall impression influencing ratings of specific characteristics.

Social desirability, or *'faking good'*, is the tendency for respondents to give what they consider to be the most socially desirable answer (Edwards, 1957). This is sometimes manifested by under-reporting side effects of treatment or over-reporting the reduction of symptoms, so as to 'please the doctor'. In social desirability the respondent is usually unaware of the bias, whereas faking good is done deliberately; an example of faking good is the cancer patient who understates side-effects of treatment so as to ensure the dose is not reduced. *'Faking bad'* is the opposite of faking good: an example is the patient who overstates the severity of their pain so as to obtain analgesics. *End aversion*, or *central tendency* bias, is the tendency for respondents to avoid the extremes of the response scale – perhaps avoiding the rating of symptoms as 10 on a scale from 0 to 10 because that would preclude the ability to indicate a worse response in future. Many forms of bias may be susceptible to cultural, gender, age or education differences (Johnson *et al.*, 2005).

When patients rate their overall QoL, an ill-defined construct, they may reasonably ask, 'Compared to what?' *Social comparison* is the process by which people compare themselves with others. *Downward comparisons* consist in comparing oneself to others whose state is worse, and tend to generate feelings of satisfaction (Wills, 1981), while the corresponding *upward comparisons* are associated with dissatisfaction. Wood *et al.* (1985) reported that breast cancer patients make the majority of comparisons with patients less fortunate than themselves. Stanton *et al.* (1999) later showed that while breast cancer patients made more downward comparisons, they preferred information and support from more fortunate others. We illustrate social comparisons as an example of response shift and reference frames (see Figure 19.2).

Example from the literature

The effects described can be substantial. A sample of 60 university students completed a survey on student issues that included two questions: 'How happy are you with life in general?' and 'How many dates did you have last month?' (Strack *et al.*, 1988). There was little correlation ($r = -0.12$) between the responses to these questions, suggesting that dating is not a major factor determining happiness. But in a second sample of 60 students the order of questions was switched, asking about frequency of dating first; now the correlation was strong ($r = 0.66$). When respondents hear 'How happy are you these days?' their answer is affected by current mood. If asked about dating first, that determines their current mood – sad or happy – and they answer the next question accordingly.

19.5 Response shift

Many patients adapt over time, and their perceptions of QoL may change. Learning to cope with problems is a well-recognised feature in the chronically ill, and frequently an important aspect of clinical therapy is to help patients to adapt to their illness. Thus, patients who experience a constant level of pain for a long period may come to cope with it, and hence report diminishing levels over time. Also, patients may meet others whose condition is better or worse than their own, and this can also lead to a recalibration of their own internal standards and values. Such subjective changes in patients' perceptions are an example of what is known as *response shift* (Schwartz and Sprangers, 1999).

Under the theoretical model proposed by Sprangers and Schwartz (1999), *response shift* is a change in the meaning of one's self-evaluation of QoL as a result of changes in internal standards, values and the conceptualisation of QoL (Figure 19.1). Rapkin and Schwartz (2004) later extended this model to include changing frame of reference. This model therefore describes four forms of response shift:

1. Recalibration – for example, someone with extreme pain might rate their pain as being 9 on a scale from no pain (0) to worst imaginable pain (10). However, when assessed again after their condition has deteriorated and the pain has become much worse, they might realise that their earlier pain should have been described as nearer 5 out of 10.

2. Reprioritisation – typified by someone who values physical function and health as the most important factors for good HRQoL until, when they become seriously and terminally ill, they find that family relationships are far more important determinants.

3. Re-conceptualisation – in addition to reprioritisation, people can redefine what they mean by HRQoL. For example, a healthy person may be unlikely to mention absence of fatigue as a major factor for good HRQoL, whereas patients with serious chronic disease might describe fatigue as one of the most important domain affecting HRQoL.

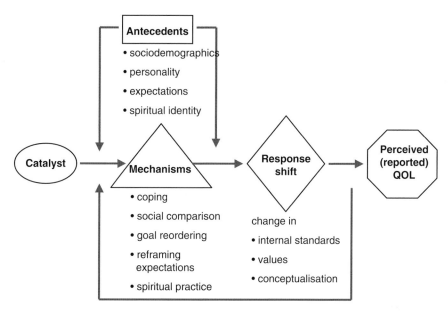

Figure 19.1   Sprangers and Schwartz (1999) theoretical model of response shift and quality of life. *Source:* Sprangers and Schwarz, 1999, Figure 1. Reproduced with permission of Elsevier.

4. Changing frame of reference – when a hospital inpatient is surrounded by others who are more severely ill than themselves, they might revise their self-assessment by making the social comparison 'I'm not so badly off as most of the others on this ward'.

These response-shift changes may be consequences of various *mechanisms*, such as coping and adaptation to illness, reframing of expectations, effects of spiritual practices, changing social comparisons, goal reordering and recalibration of responses. The impact of the mechanisms will be affected by *antecedents*, such as the patient's personality or other characteristics, their expectations and spiritual identity. We illustrate some forms of response shift by the following examples.

Example from the literature

An example of response shift was provided by Albrecht and Devlieger (1999), who posed the disability paradox: "Why do many people with serious and persistent disabilities report that they experience a good or excellent quality of life when to most external observers these individuals seem to live an undesirable daily existence?" Based on the results of interviews, they suggested that the high quality of life reported by many respondents could be a 'secondary gain' that occurs when individuals with impairments adapt to their new conditions and make sense of them. Individuals who experience disability can find an enriched meaning in their lives secondary to the disability condition. The results of this study suggest that secondary gains occurred when individuals used their disability condition and subsequent outcomes to reinterpret their lives and reconstitute personal meaning in their social roles. Thus the respondents changed their values and conceptualisation of QoL.

The implications of the study by Albrecht and Devlieger are firstly that healthy people are poor judges of the QoL and values of patients, and secondly that people change when they become ill – this latter implication being an example of response shift. Others have noted similar response shifts: as we mentioned in Chapter 1 of Part 1, there are major and consistent differences between the opinions of patients and the others, and also between the different healthcare staff. Thus Slevin (1990) observed that, contrary to the expectations of doctors or others, "(cancer) patients appear to regard a minute chance of possible benefit as worthwhile, whatever the cost" and willingly tolerate horrendously toxic cancer therapy for little improvement in chance of survival. Again, patients have changed their priorities and values after becoming ill, and their responses to questionnaires have altered as a consequence.

Example from the literature

Groenvold *et al.* (1999) investigated anxiety and depression in newly diagnosed breast cancer patients, using the HADS. A sample of 466 Danish breast cancer patients at low risk of recurrence was recruited within seven weeks following their surgery. Their level of anxiety and depression was compared with that of 609 women randomly selected from the Danish general population.

Contrary to expectations, the HADS scores of breast cancer patients were significantly lower than those of the general population sample, indicating less anxiety and depression. The respective patient and population mean scores were 5.3 and 6.0 ($p = 0.02$) for anxiety, and 2.8 and 3.4 ($p = 0.001$) for depression. The differences were consistent across all five age groups examined.

The authors were sceptical regarding the results, and questioned the validity of comparing HADS scores of breast cancer patients against those obtained from the general population. Firstly, the HADS was developed and validated in hospital patients, and had not been validated in the general population. Secondly, there might be selective reporting. Since the patients knew they were in a cancer study, they might have excluded complaints that they attributed to non-cancer causes (selective reporting bias). This might lead to an underestimate of anxiety and depression for the breast cancer patients. Thirdly, there may have been response shift. The cancer patients may have changed their internal standards as a result of their experiences – for example, some patients might now place greater value on family relationships. The authors conclude: "The results of the HADS applied in the general population are probably not directly comparable with the results from the breast cancer patients."

Example from the literature

The SEIQoL is an individualised quality of life measure that allows respondents to nominate the five most important issues that affect them. This makes it ideally suited for detecting response shift. Re-conceptualisation corresponds to changes in nomination of cues (life areas), while reprioritisation is reflected by changes in cue weights. Ring *et al.* (2005) explored the impact of denture treatment on 117 edentulous patients, with assessments pre-treatment and at three months. There was evidence of re-conceptualisation, with 81% of patients nominating at least one different cue at three months compared to baseline. There was also evidence of reprioritisation, with patients significantly changing their weightings for the cues that they rated most and least important.

In the above examples of response shift we have postulated that there is re-conceptualisation or reprioritisation, although patients may be affected by more than one type of shift as in the preceding example. Adapting to illness, learning to cope and changing of values and priorities can represent mental changes that reflect real modifications as to how patients feel. Of course, centuries ago Aristotle realised that such internal changes occur, and the quotation deserves repeating: "what constitutes happiness is a matter of dispute … some say one thing and some another, indeed very often the same man says different things different times: when he falls sick he thinks health is happiness, when he is poor, wealth" (Aristotle, 384–322 BCE). Recalibration is different, in that the patients' feelings and values may remain unchanged, but the patients are expressing themselves on a revised scale; recalibration is predominantly a measurement problem.

Example from the literature

Sprangers *et al.* (1999) describe a qualitative study in which 99 patients with newly diagnosed cancer were assessed for fatigue, before and after radiotherapy. Patients were also interviewed using non-judgemental probes. An example of the reported responses was a patient who said: "During the radiotherapy I became more tired. At that time, I may have thought that I was tired. But now I say no I was not tired at all. Now I am tired. ...So, now I may look differently upon that week, while at that time I may have thought that I was dead tired." Thus this patient recognised that she had experienced a recalibration response shift, and that by her revised standards she had overstated the level of fatigue at the pre-treatment assessment. A number of patients considered their revised values of the baseline assessment to be more valid than the responses made at the time.

Pain is another symptom that, like fatigue, may be prone to recalibration if patients experience increasingly severe pain as their illness progresses. Visser *et al.* (2013) studied 202 cancer patients and reported that that 35% experienced recalibration response shifts in the anticipated direction, while 20% showed recalibration shift in the opposite direction.

Patients may be asked the seemingly simple question 'What is your overall quality of life during the past week?', but this begs the query 'Compared to what?' Even if such a query is not made explicit, some patients may contrast their health against that of another peer group such as friends of similar age, other patients with similar condition, or even themselves before becoming ill. The need to specify a reference frame has been recognised by social scientists in the population survey context, where the concern has been to remove inherent ambiguities by directing respondents to use age-standardised comparisons. Investigators have used questions such as 'Compared to others of your age, how would you rate your health status?', commonly specifying relative response options (better/worse) and not absolute values (such as very bad to very good). Better average health status is reported by elderly people when an age comparison is explicitly invoked (e.g. Baron-Epel and Kaplan, 2001). Although it is rare for reference frames to be specified in healthcare research, there is evidence that the measurement of QoL is affected.

Example from the literature

Fayers *et al.* (2007) asked 1,325 patients with Paget's disease, who were completing the SF36 in a clinical trial, "How would you rate your overall quality of life during the past week?" The patients were then told that we realise different people have different things in mind when they answer questions about their quality of life, and asked "When you rated your overall quality of life, were you mainly comparing yourself against one or more of the following?" The options included 'before you became ill', 'how you felt a year ago', 'other people with Paget's disease', 'healthy people that you know (such as family or friends)' and 'something else (please specify)'. Patients could tick one or more response options.

The majority of patients ticked a single option. At all time points, about 20% of patients said they had in mind how they were before they became ill, nearly a third were considering themselves a year or more previously, and about 20% were comparing themselves with healthy peers. As had been hypothesised, mean HRQL scores varied substantially according to the declared frame of reference; differences were as big as 19% of the scale score, or a standardised mean effect size of 0.74 standard deviations (Figure 19.2).

Thus, reported reference frames were associated with effects of similar magnitude to the differences in HRQoL that are regarded as clinically important. This may be of particular concern in trials that randomise patients to management in different settings, such as treatment at home/in hospital, or surgery/chemotherapy and might bias or obscure HRQL differences.

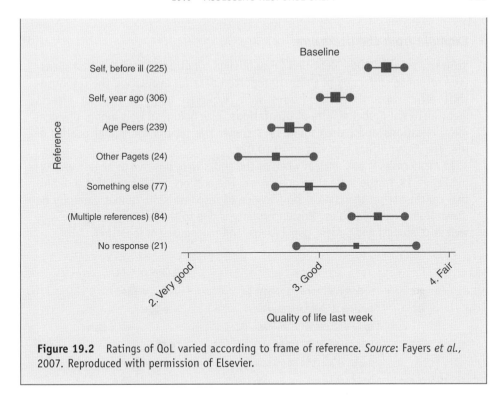

Figure 19.2 Ratings of QoL varied according to frame of reference. *Source*: Fayers *et al.*, 2007. Reproduced with permission of Elsevier.

19.6 Assessing response shift

Early attempts at assessing response shift in HRQoL mainly focused on the 'then-test'. Patients are assessed on two occasions, such as pre-treatment and post treatment. After completing the second assessment, they are given the then-test, with a question such as: 'We would like you to think back to the time of your first assessment, immediately prior to the start of your treatment. With hindsight, how would you now rate the way you felt then?' The difference between the values of the pre-treatment assessment and the then-test provides an estimate of recalibration response shift. Arguably, when estimating the change in a PRO due to treatment, the then-test value should be used in preference to the pre-treatment value.

The then-test approach is easy to understand, simple to apply and straightforward to analyse; it has been used extensively. However, it can be criticised as making unsupported assumptions about absence of recall bias, ability to recall previous states, a shared internal standard for current and previous conditions, and potential contamination because of respondent's feelings of social desirability or other concerns. A review of publications reporting then-test results also found that the then-test lacks standardised and transparent interpretation, with ambiguity in the claims of negative and positive response shifts. Schwartz and Sprangers (2010) subsequently produced guidelines for the optimal use and reporting of the then-test.

Example from the literature

Schwartz *et al.* (2006) identified 26 published longitudinal studies that measured response shift, and of these 19 reported data for evaluating the response-shift effect size. Five dimensions were explored using a random effects meta-analysis: global quality of life, fatigue, psychological well-being, physical role limitations and pain. Figure 19.3 shows the results for global quality of life. The mean effect size was small (0.02).

In many cases it was unclear whether the shifts were positive or negative, making Figure 19.3 little more than guesswork. The authors commented that a definitive conclusion on the clinical significance of response shift cannot currently be drawn from existing studies. This uncertainty is due to the heterogeneity of ESs as well as of studies and patient populations, and inadequacy of reporting.

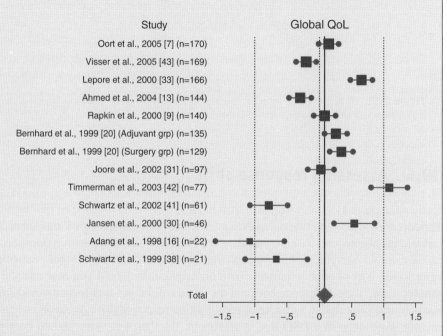

Figure 19.3 Meta-analysis of response shift affecting assessment of global QoL. (see Chapter 20 for explanation of the 'Forest plot'). Note: See Schwartz *et al.*, 2006 for detailed references of studies cited. *Source:* Schwartz *et al. 2006*, Figure 3. Reproduced with permission of Springer Science and Business Media.

While the then-test is most suitable for detecting recalibration, a variety of multivariate methods have been proposed for identifying and measuring reprioritisation and re-conceptualisation response shifts. A review by Schwartz *et al.* (2013) describes the range of statistical techniques that have been used and offer guidelines for exploring response shift in clinical studies.

19.7   Impact of response shift

It might be argued that, when assessing QoL, all that matters is the patient's current perception. Hence, if pain is perceived and reported as diminishing, we can regard it as becoming less important to the patient even though the pain stimulus may be unchanged. However, many clinicians would argue that it remains just as important to address the pain, despite claims by the patient that they can cope and that it is becoming less of a problem. Response shift might equally work in the other direction. Patients can find that persistent symptoms cause increasing distress, and may therefore report the symptoms as becoming more severe even though they do not appear to be changing in any objective physical sense. A nagging pain may not be intense, but can become extremely distressing.

There seems little doubt that response shift can occur; much of clinical practice is concerned with helping patients to adapt to their illness, or to learn how to cope with their symptoms. That is, positive response shifts are actively encouraged, and may sometimes be substantial.

Selective reporting, recall and other biases, and response shift can all be forms of measurement bias, and may all result in misleading reports of PROs. Both subjective and supposedly objective symptoms can be reported differently by patients and the general population. Selective reporting can clearly present a serious bias problem when using normative data, although response shift is arguably less important if perceptions are considered to matter more than reality. In QoL studies it is rarely possible to quantify the overall bias, and these various causes of bias can rarely be separated.

Many forms of assessment bias may be of less importance for treatment comparisons in a clinical trial, provided they apply equally to all treatment arms. However, it is important to bear in mind their potential impact on particular studies. We have already seen that clinicians may under-report symptoms such as vomiting, which they regard as the inevitable consequence of chemotherapy for cancer. Similarly, selective reporting bias could occur in a trial of long-term chemotherapy versus 'no treatment' if the treatment group gradually regarded some symptoms as inevitable and stopped reporting them; selective reporting might lead to serious underestimation of QoL differences between the chemotherapy and control groups.

19.8   Clinical trials

Can response shift affect the results of clinical trials? In many situations there may be no reason to suspect that response shifts will differ between the randomised groups. Then one might hope that there are no grounds to believe there could be a systematic bias to the treatment comparisons. Despite this, response shift may add extra noise to the comparisons, and by increasing the variability it can blur the estimates of treatment effect and reduce the power of the comparison. Thus it should not be ignored.

As we have observed, helping patients to cope and adapt to illness is a major component in many interventions – especially when there is limited choice of active treatments. Clinicians and other staff actively promote and encourage adaptation as a positive part of the patient experience, and many believe it has profound impact on patients. Thus it can be argued that coping and related adaptations are part of the overall policy of management: provided one regards the trial as comparing *policies of management*, as opposed to comparing individual treatments, there is no need to make any correction or other allowance for adaptation. Thus if one arm of the study involves more frequent hospital attendances for administration of the treatment than the other, and if patients benefit by the additional contact with hospital staff, that is all part of the policy of management and would apply just as much to future patients outside the trial as to those within it. Adopting a pragmatic perspective, we know that adaptation occurs, it is encouraged, and it is a normal part of overall patient management. But it can obscure the explanatory assessment of treatment efficacy.

Sometimes there may be unanticipated differences in the degree of response shift in the study arms, even in randomised clinical trials.

Example from the literature

The trial of Jordhøy *et al.* (2001) compared the QoL of palliative care patients who were managed in a specialist hospital unit against those who were offered a comprehensive support package that allowed them to stay at home until the end of their lives. The authors report that "The present intervention enabled more patients to stay at home to die, and according to published reports on patients' wishes, this is a favorable outcome. Several others have reported improved family and patient satisfaction". However, contrary to all expectations, there was no difference in QoL between the two groups (Jordhøy *et al.*, 2003).

One might speculate that the hospital-based patients were surrounded by others in a comparable state or, sometimes, in an even worse health state than themselves. These patients might therefore adjust their expectations accordingly, and may feel that, compared to those around them, their QoL is not so bad. In contrast, the home-care patients would be among healthy people and might use a very different yardstick when responding to QoL questionnaires. However, the trial of Jordhøy *et al.* was not designed with response shift in mind. The authors could only conclude that there was no evidence of a difference in QoL (and discussed a number of potential explanations).

In this example, response shift may have played a role because the two randomised groups were being assessed in completely different settings, and it is plausible that the settings might influence the responses in divergent ways.

> **Example from the literature**
>
> In the study of Ring *et al.* (2005), exploring the impact of implant-supported dentures compared with high-quality conventional dentures, recalibration response shift was identified in addition to the reprioritisation and re-conceptualisation that we described above. Unadjusted QoL scores revealed no significant impact of treatment at three months (baseline: 75.0; three months: 73.2, $p = 0.33$). However, after allowing for response shift there was a significant treatment effect (revised baseline: 69.2; three months: 73.2, $p = 0.016$). The authors conclude that positive impact of denture treatment for edentulous patients was seen only when response shifts were taken into consideration: "The nature of the response shifts was highly complex but the data indicated a degree of re-conceptualisation and reprioritisation. Assessment of the impact of treatments using patient-generated reports must take account of the adaptive nature of patients."

19.9 Non-randomised studies

Response shift can be a far more serious issue for non-randomised studies, because it can no longer be argued that response shift may occur equally across the randomised groups. As an example of the problems, we have already mentioned the survey of Groenvold *et al.* (1999). A more serious and far-reaching example is that of Spitzer (2012).

> **Example from the literature**
>
> In 2001, Robert Spitzer announced the first results of an influential and notorious study that evaluated the feelings of gay people who were receiving 'reparative' therapy (also known as 'sexual reorientation' or 'conversion' therapy), and which concluded that many of them reported changes in their sexual desires from homosexual to heterosexual (Spitzer, 2003). Eleven years later he recanted, acknowledging that "There was no way to judge the credibility of subject reports of change in sexual orientation. I offered several (unconvincing) reasons why it was reasonable to assume that the subject's reports of change were credible and not self-deception or outright lying. But the simple fact is that there was no way to determine if the subject's accounts of change were valid" (Spitzer, 2012). One of the flaws was that the assessment was based on what people remembered feeling years before. Thus response shift, for example in the form of self-deception or misrepresentation of their feelings, might have biased the results and may well have led to erroneous conclusion.

19.10 Conclusions

Most clinical trials and surveys either ignore response shift or assume it is negligible. In randomised trials this may sometimes be reasonable, for example when comparing two forms of pharmaceutical therapy in a double-blind trial. But response shift becomes more of a threat when trials are unblinded, although even then there is the temptation to take the pragmatic view that many forms of response shift, such as adaptation to illness, are consequences of the overall policy of management. However, the magnitude of the response shifts is usually not established and if substantial may obscure treatment effects or distort the estimates of effect size. The greatest threat is to non-randomised studies, when the interpretation of the results may become compromised. Throughout this chapter we have illustrated examples in which response-shift effects appear to have played an important role.

20

Meta-analysis

Summary

Systematic overviews and meta-analyses have become an important aspect of clinical research. In particular, they are routinely applied *before* launching new clinical trials as a means of confirming the need to carry out a clinical trial, or *after* completing trials as a means of synthesising and summarising the current knowledge on the topic of interest. In this chapter, we focus on issues that are of specific relevance to meta-analyses of QoL and PROs.

20.1 Introduction

Meta-analysis is the quantitative review and synthesis of the results from studies that have independently evaluated similar or equivalent interventions and outcomes. Thus the principal stages of meta-analysis are (i) the systematic identification of all studies that addressed the outcome of interest, (ii) the evaluation of the quality of these studies, (iii) the extraction of the relevant quantitative data and (iv) the statistical combining and analysing of the collective results.

Many books have been written about meta-analysis, and it is the focal interest of the Cochrane Collaboration. The aim of this chapter is to introduce the principles of meta-analysis, together with examples from the literature. We shall in particular focus on the two special challenges posed by QoL studies: firstly, in many disease areas there are a number of potential questionnaires, and for meta-analysis it will be necessary to combine the seemingly disparate outcome measures and, secondly, the quality of studies may vary considerably, in particular because some studies may experience poor compliance with consequent high levels of missing data. This chapter is primarily concerned with data extracted from published reports, as opposed to the more labour-intensive meta-analyses that involve obtaining individual patient data from each separate study.

It is strongly recommended that the Cochrane Handbook for Systematic Reviews of Interventions (Higgins and Green, 2011) be consulted – see the section on Further Reading.

Quality of Life: The Assessment, Analysis and Reporting of Patient-Reported Outcomes, Third Edition.
Peter M. Fayers and David Machin.
© 2016 John Wiley & Sons, Ltd. Published 2016 by John Wiley & Sons, Ltd.

20.2   Defining objectives

The first stage is to define the study objectives in a formal written protocol. Is the review examining results relating to a particular class of drugs? – If so, there must be a precise definition of what pharmaceutical compounds will be included. What patient groups will be eligible for inclusion – for example, will studies of children and adults both be relevant? Will only randomised studies be included, or are other experimental designs permitted – for treatment efficacy comparisons, many researchers only accept evidence from randomised controlled trials. Will studies be excluded if compliance is below a specified threshold? Will studies be excluded if they used instruments that are unvalidated or inadequately validated? Will foreign language publications be accepted? If at all possible, they should be; but there may be practical constraints that make it unfeasible to obtain all translations. At this stage, it is also useful to search the Cochrane Library – maybe someone else has already carried out a similar systematic review!

20.3   Defining outcomes

It is necessary to define the outcome that is to be compared across studies. For some dimensions this is easier than others, and for some PROs it may be tricky. For example, when reviewing 'quality of life' in a meta-analysis, should studies that present data on self-reported 'overall health' but not 'overall quality of life' be accepted? If pain is the main outcome, are studies useful if they only report the percentage of patients with pain, or should an eligibility criterion be that a valid score be available for severity of pain? Formal definitions and rules should be recorded in the meta-analysis protocol, defining the outcomes that must be available for the analyses.

   Another aspect needing definition is the specification of the assessment time points. Individual trials may report the PROs at different time points, or may provide only summary measures such as AUC or scores from longitudinal analysis. It is unlikely that there will be consistency of reporting across trials. It is necessary to define the target time point – such as at the end of treatment or a specified time after randomisation. It is also necessary to define the maximum eligible window. For example, if the target time point is two months after randomisation, will trials be accepted if they provide only a six-week assessment – or a six-month assessment?

   Some reviews focus on change from baseline; that is, whether patients have improved or deteriorated from the intervention. In this case, how many studies present the mean change scores or provide information enabling the calculation of change scores?

20.4   Literature searching

A major part of any systematic review or meta-analysis is the literature search, to make sure that all available studies have been identified and included. It is the literature search that takes the greatest time when carrying out a meta-analysis. The Cochrane

Collaboration offers workshops and training sessions on this topic. The quality of the literature search is largely what distinguishes a strong meta-analysis from one that is weak and unpublishable. Searching should address published and unpublished literature, uncompleted studies and studies still in progress.

A starting point is to search bibliographic databases such as Medline and Embase, and obtain abstracts of all potentially relevant articles. A key point at this stage is to ensure that a full range of relevant terms is included in the searching strategy; bibliographic searching is a science in itself.

Citations are another source of published reports. After a relevant publication has been found, its list of references may be scrutinised for *backward citations*. In most publications, clues about the value of the citations may be obtained from the introduction and the discussion sections. More recent papers that refer back to publications already found may also provide useful information, either in the form of data or references to yet other studies. These *forward citations* may be identified using citation indexes, such as the Social Sciences Citation Index.

The above searching process addresses completed, published studies. Ongoing studies can often be identified by accessing registers of clinical trials. These registers may be maintained nationally or internationally, and many of them cover trials run by the pharmaceutical industry as well as publicly funded ones. Example registers are the International Standard Randomized Controlled Trial Number Register (<http://www.controlled-trials.com/isrctn/> and the US National Institutes of Health register (<http://www.clinicaltrials.gov/>); many of the national registers are amalgamated into a central database at the World Health Organization (<http://apps.who.int/trialsearch/>). Some registries are maintained by funding institutions or by groups with interest in particular disease areas, such as the US National Cancer Institute register of clinical trials. In 2004, the International Committee of Medical Journal Editors (ICMJE) gave notice that it will consider a clinical trial for publication only if it has been registered in an appropriate registry.

Usually, multiple sources will be searched, and records should be kept of the number of new studies identified from each additional database. It can be anticipated that fewer and fewer new studies will be retrieved from successive searches, and this may be used in reports as part of the evidence regarding the thoroughness of the searching process.

In summary, searching (and the subsequent extraction of data) is a complex and time-consuming task.

20.5 Assessing quality

Full information, such as copies of publications, should be obtained for each potentially usable study. These can be graded for eligibility and overall quality. It is usually recommended that there should be multiple reviewers, with each study being reviewed by more than one person. This is partly to spread the workload, but mainly to ensure that the ratings are consistent and of a reliable standard. It is therefore important that there should be a formal pre-specified procedure both for making the ratings and for resolving rater disagreements.

The principal concern is that the reviewed studies should be free from any plausible bias that might weaken confidence in the results. The Cochrane Collaboration suggests that the simplest approach is a three-level grading into:

- Low risk of bias   All quality criteria met,
- Moderate risk of bias   One or more quality criteria only partly met,
- High risk of bias   One or more quality criteria not met.

After assessing the quality of the studies, a numeric rating can be assigned. This can later be used when calculating the mean effect across studies, such that the poorer quality studies will have lower *weight* and contribute less to the calculated mean effect.

The main sources of bias that apply to studies of interventions are described individually. The Cochrane Handbook for Systematic Reviews (Higgins and Green, 2011) covers these issues in greater depth, and discusses additional sources of bias; reporting bias, for example, includes not only outcome reporting bias but several other subheadings, too.

Selection bias

This is one of the most important factors affecting study quality. The prevention of *selection bias* is the main objective of randomisation in clinical trials. When assessing a potential participant's eligibility for a trial, both those who are recruiting the participants and the participants themselves should remain unaware of the intervention that will be assigned; the assignment is only disclosed after the eligibility has been confirmed and the participant recruited to the trial. Once revealed, neither the assignment nor the eligibility decision can be altered. It has been shown repeatedly for example by Schulz *et al.*, 1995) that *allocation concealment* of the randomised allocation is an essential component of quality, and that trials with poor concealment tend to show larger – and biased – treatment effects. The CONSORT statement (Schulz *et al.*, 2010), adopted by many medical journals, ensures that all publications about clinical trials now record full details of the randomisation procedure. This information is less frequently available for earlier publications, and one must assume that a lack of published information implies that randomisation was not used, or that it may have been of a poor standard. For example, in some early trials the randomisation may have been effected by a list of successive allocations that was printed pre-study, with the clinicians recruiting patients to the trial possibly knowing in advance what the next 'random' allocation would be. This practice, formerly common, means that the allocation was not concealed and that the randomisation is fundamentally flawed. Randomisation should ideally be by an independent central office that registers the patients' eligibility details and then provides the allocation through an automated process.

In general, non-randomised studies provide substantially weaker evidence than randomised clinical trials.

Performance bias

Performance bias refers to systematic differences in the care provided to the participants in the comparison groups. In a clinical trial the only systematic difference should be the intervention under investigation. To protect against unintended differences, those providing and receiving care can be *blinded* so that they do not know the group to which the recipients of care have been allocated. As part of the blinding process, placebos should be used whenever appropriate. Schulz *et al.* (1995) show that a lack of blinding is a major source of bias.

Of course, not all interventions can be blinded. Some treatments have such obvious side effects that it immediately becomes apparent which has been applied to which patient. But on the other hand, even some surgical trials have used 'mock surgery' for the control group: the patient responses to physically ineffective mock surgery can be so strongly positive that these trials have been deemed ethical. This highlights the importance of including assessment of blinding as a part of quality. Lack of blinding is also associated with detection bias.

Detection bias

Detection bias refers to systematic differences between the comparison groups in outcome assessment. Trials that blind the people who will assess outcomes to the intervention allocation should logically be less likely to be biased than trials that do not. *Blinding of outcome assessment* may be particularly important in research with subjective outcome measures, such as pain (for example Schulz *et al.*, 1995) or other PROs.

Outcome reporting bias

Outcome reporting bias arises from the selective reporting of some outcomes but not others, depending on the nature and direction of the results; it is also known as *selective reporting bias*. In many studies, a range of PROs are assessed but frequently not all are reported. If it is intended to present information about only a subset of PROs, that should be clearly stated in the study protocol prior to commencing the study. Once a study has started, the subsequent choice of outcomes that are reported can be influenced by the results. This can potentially make the published results misleading.

Compliance and attrition bias

Poor compliance and missing data (as well as other forms of *attrition*, including patient withdrawal and death) are a major problem in QoL studies. This particularly applies to chronic diseases and cancer, where some clinical trials report that 50% or fewer of the anticipated questionnaires (i.e. from living patients) were received.

The concern is that there may be systematic differences between the comparison groups in the loss of patients from the study. Many investigators have found that poor compliance, leading to incomplete outcome data, is frequently associated with less well patients who have a poorer QoL, and so trials with high levels of missing data are susceptible to bias and are of low validity; they should be assigned a low quality rating.

The approach to handling losses also has great potential for biasing the results, as we have seen in Chapter 15. The problem is further clouded in that some studies fail to publish the extent of the missing data, or do not report the methods of handling missing values. Increasingly, *imputation* is used when analysing trials with missing data. If published reports of trials are used for the meta-analysis there may be little control over whether or not imputed results are used – one is at the mercy of the publications – but if individual patient data are available there is more flexibility over the decision about whether to impute or not.

In Section 10.3 we discussed the *five-and-twenty rule* that was mentioned by Schulz and Grimes (2002). This suggests that "less than 5% loss is thought probably to lead to little bias, while greater than 20% loss potentially poses serious threats to validity." Perhaps this is a starting point for assessing attrition bias, although it might be found that these levels are too harsh for QoL outcomes and result in loss of too many trials. Although there is no consensus as to what is an acceptable level of compliance, consideration should be given to excluding from the meta-analysis all trials that fall below some pre-specified minimum threshold (although they may be retained in the systematic review).

Fortunately, in many cases the QoL meta-analyses may be carried out for diseases in which improvement of QoL is the principal objective of treatment, for example relief of back pain or treatment of depression. Then compliance with assessment is likely to be high. One such example is palliative care, where QoL is by definition the aim of management and therapy. However, two particular problems arise in this setting. Firstly, when patients deteriorate, it may be regarded as unethical to risk further stress by asking them to complete questionnaires, and many patients also refuse during their final months. Secondly, a substantial proportion of patients may die before the target time point for assessment. This *attrition* can raise additional problems of interpretation. At the very least, it is essential that the meta-analysis reports the levels of attrition observed in the various trials.

Validated instruments

Another indicator of quality could be the use of a validated instrument with established high sensitivity. However, this and similar criteria are less likely to be important factors unless they might cause bias in the trial's results. More often, the use of an inferior instrument results in lower precision or sensitivity, but not bias. Despite this, it may be useful to include such criteria in a scoring scheme. Then, trials that use the most sensitive instruments will receive the greatest weight when generating the across-study summary statistics.

20.6 Summarising results

Meta-analyses are relatively straightforward if all included studies use the same outcome measure. Then the treatment difference observed in each study can be shown with its corresponding confidence interval (*CI*). We shall describe how the studies can then be combined to obtain an overall evaluation of treatment effect. Figure 20.1 shows an example of a meta-analysis summary, taken from the Cochrane Library. This example will be followed throughout this chapter.

Example from the literature

Linde *et al.* (2005) reviewed the use of St John's wort for treating depression and identified 26 placebo-controlled trials as suitable for inclusion. Of these, 14 trials reported depression at six to eight weeks using the Hamilton Rating Scale for Depression (HRSD), which is a 17-item interviewer-administered scale. Figure 20.1 shows the results for 10 studies that treated major depression, and a further four studies that were not restricted to major depression. Each study is listed, with its sample size and mean scale score in the two treatment groups. The mean treatment differences are plotted as blocks, with horizontal lines indicating the 95% *CI* values. The interpretation of these results is discussed later in this chapter.

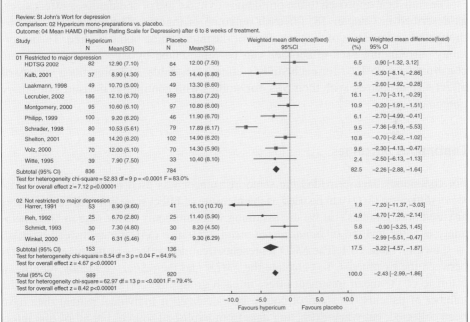

Figure 20.1 Forest plot of St John's Wort for depression. The solid squares denote individual mean effects and the horizontal lines represent 95% *CI*s. The diamonds denote pooled weighted mean differences. Note: See Linde *et al.*, 2005 for detailed references of studies cited. *Source:* Linde *et al.*, 2005, comparison 02, outcome 04. Reproduced with permission of John Wiley & Sons, Ltd.

20.7   Measures of treatment effect

In practice, it is more likely that a variety of instruments will have been used. Clearly, it would not make sense to combine and average the raw mean scores from, say, a four-point numerical scale and a 100-point visual analogue scale (VAS). Thus the main challenge in QoL meta-analyses is to place all studies on a common metric. The outcomes may have been reported on completely different scales, such as perhaps numerical rating scales with ten or more response options, VAS ranging from 0 to 100, short ordered-categorical scales with four- or five-point response levels, and so on. Symptoms and dimensions of QoL may also be presented as dichotomous (binary) outcomes. Thus, for example, pain may be reported as absent/present; it might be graded on a short categorical response scale (e.g. 'no pain', 'a little', 'quite a bit', 'very much', 'unbearable'); it might be rated on a 10-cm VAS; or it might be assessed using a multi-item severity scale.

For the discussion that follows, we shall assume that a decision has been made to include studies that report any of these forms of assessment, and we consider ways to combine dichotomous, ordered categorical and continuous outcome measures. In practice, however, some investigators planning meta-analyses might specify that dichotomous responses are too imprecise and that only studies reporting multilevel categories or continuous outcomes will be included.

The statistical approach to the problem is to make use of standardised effect sizes, as described in Chapter 18, for each outcome of interest. The effect sizes can be thought of as estimates of the true effect of the intervention being studied. The uncertainty surrounding each effect size can be represented by calculating its *SE*, and constructing a 95% *CI* for each study's effect size. Table 20.1 presents a variety of effect-size measures, with their *SE*s, for studies with continuous measures or binary outcomes.

Continuous outcomes

For continuous data, provided the same instrument was used in all studies, the *raw mean difference (MD)* can be used as the measure of effect size. When different scales are used in the studies – as we are assuming will commonly be the case in QoL meta-analyses – the method of *standardised mean difference (SMD)* may instead be used, as shown in Table 20.1. The *SMD* represents treatment effects as the number of *SD*s between the treatments. To calculate the *SMD*s and their *SE*s, we ideally require an estimate of the mean treatment effect in each group, the corresponding *SD* and the number of patients. This can of course be calculated if individual patient data have been collected, but when extracting data from published sources not all of this information may be available explicitly. The Cochrane Handbook for Systematic Reviews (Higgins and Green, 2011) explains methods for imputing the necessary values from other information – for example if *t*-statistics, exact *p*-values or *CI*s are presented, the *SE* and *SD* can usually be estimated.

Table 20.1 Equations for effect sizes and their *SEs*. For continuous outcomes, the means, standard deviations and sample sizes of the control group are $\bar{x}_C$, SD_C^2, n_C, and for the experimental therapy they are $\bar{x}_E$, SD_E^2, n_E. For binary outcomes, a and b are the numbers in the experimental group responding negatively and positively; c and d are the corresponding numbers in the control group

	Effect size	Standard error of effect size
Continuous outcomes, independent groups		
Standardized mean difference (*SMD*) (also called Cohen's *d*)	$$SMD = \frac{\bar{x}_C - \bar{x}_E}{SD_{Pooled}} = t\sqrt{\frac{n_C + n_E}{n_C \times n_E}}$$ where $$SD_{Pooled} = \sqrt{\frac{(n_C - 1)SD_C^2 + (n_E - 1)SD_E^2}{(n_C - 1) + (n_E - 1)}}$$	$$SE_{EMD} = \sqrt{\frac{n_C + n_E}{n_C \times n_E} + \frac{SMD^2}{2(n_C + n_E - 2)}}$$
Glass's Δ	$$\Delta = \frac{\bar{x}_C - \bar{x}_E}{SD_C}$$	$$SE_\Delta = \sqrt{\frac{n_C + n_E}{n_C \times n_E} + \frac{\Delta^2}{2(n_C - 1)}}$$
Hedge's adjusted *g*	$$g = SMD \times \left(1 - \frac{3}{4(n_C + n_E) - 9}\right)$$	$$SE_E = \sqrt{\frac{n_C + n_E}{n_C \times n_E} + \frac{g^2}{2(n_C + n_E - 3.94)}}$$
Continuous outcomes, paired data		
Standardized response mean (*SRM*$_{Paired}$)	$$SRM_{Paired} = \frac{\bar{x}_{Time2} - \bar{x}_{Time1}}{SD_{Difference}} = t\sqrt{\frac{1}{n}}$$ where $$SD_{Difference} = SD\,of\,differences$$	$$SE(SRM_{Paired}) = \sqrt{\frac{1}{n} + \frac{SRM_{Paired}^2}{2(n-1)}}$$
Effect size (*ES*$_{Paired}$) (not recommended)	$$ES_{Paired} = \frac{\bar{x}_{Time2} - \bar{x}_{Time1}}{SD_{Time1}}$$	$$SE(ES_{Paired}) = \sqrt{\frac{2(1-\rho)}{n} + \frac{ES_{Paired}^2}{2(n-1)}},$$ where ρ is the correlation of X_{Time1} with X_{Time2}
Binary outcomes		
Log(Odds-Ratio)	$$\log(OR) = \log\left(\frac{a \times d}{b \times c}\right)$$ $$ES = \sqrt{3}/\pi \times \log(OR) = 0.5513 \times \log(OR)$$	$$SE\{\log(OR)\} = \sqrt{\frac{1}{a} + \frac{1}{b} + \frac{1}{c} + \frac{1}{d}}$$
Log(Relative Risk)	$$\log(RR) = \log\left(\frac{a/(a+b)}{c/(c+d)}\right)$$	$$SE\{\log(RR)\} = \sqrt{\frac{1}{a} - \frac{1}{a+b} + \frac{1}{c} - \frac{1}{c+d}}$$

In line with the policy of the Cochrane Reviews, we recommend the use of Hedges' adjusted g, which is a version of the *SMD* that includes an adjustment for small sample bias. But we shall write '*SMD*' as the generic label for this class of measures that also includes Glass's Δ.

In principle, change scores (i.e. change in a PRO from baseline) can be treated exactly the same way as other continuous variables. The *standardised response mean (SRM)* is the paired-data equivalent of the *SMD*. In practice, however, many published reports fail to supply the *SD* or *SE* of the change scores, and these can be difficult to estimate from the more commonly cited *SD* of the baseline or final score because the *SE* of the change depends on the correlation between the two measurements. In such cases it may be preferable to use the after-treatment time point rather than the change score, because in randomised clinical trials the baseline scores should on average be equal in the two groups.

Example from the literature

Plants from the family Zingiberaceae, which includes ginger, turmeric and galangal, have for centuries been used in traditional medicine and have been claimed to possess anti-inflammatory and analgesic properties. Lakhan *et al.* (2015) carried out a literature search and identified eight randomized, double-blinded, placebo-controlled trials that measured pain using visual analogue scales (VAS) and were eligible for a meta-analysis. The authors present *SMD* values, noting that "The *SMD* is a useful statistical tool when studies all assess the same outcome but measure it in a variety of ways."

Figure 20.2 shows their published forest plot. Lakhan *et al.* conclude from their meta-analysis that Zingiberaceae extracts are clinically effective hypoalgesic agents with a better safety profile than non-steroidal anti-inflammatory drugs.

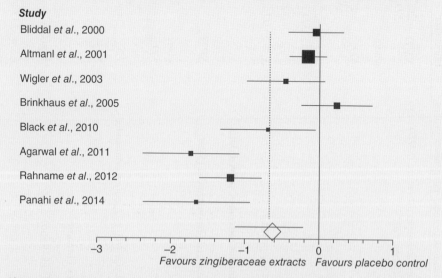

Figure 20.2 Forest plot comparing placebo control against extracts from the Zingiberaceae family of plants for treatment of chronic pain. Standardised mean differences (*SMDs*) are shown for each study, sorted by date of publication. (Based on Lakhan *et al.*, 2015).

Binary outcomes

Several effect-size measures are commonly used for binary data, including the odds ratio (*OR*) or its logarithm, log(*OR*); relative risk (*RR*) or its logarithm log(*RR*); and risk difference. Each possesses certain advantages and disadvantages. Table 20.1 shows log(*OR*) and log(*RR*). The *RR* represents the ratio of the risks of having the event of interest. The *OR* does not have such simple clinical interpretation, although it does approximate the relative risk when the event rate is low. However, a major advantage of OR is its good statistical properties. We shall not consider the risk difference because, although it is probably the easiest effect-size measure to interpret, it has the least desirable statistical properties and tends to give the least consistent results when the event rate is varied. When using the *OR* or *RR*, a value of one represents no difference between the study groups. However, it is common to take a logarithmic transformation of these values before conducting meta-analysis, because the log-transformed effect size is symmetrical about zero and therefore has better statistical properties. Log(*OR*) has the additional advantage that if it is multiplied by $\frac{\sqrt{3}}{\pi} = 0.5513$ it is then commensurate with *SMD* (Chinn, 2000), which provides one approach to combining binary and continuous outcomes (see Section 20.8).

Ordinal outcomes

For ordinal variables, the choice is between assuming they can be treated as if they were continuous variables, converting to binary data by introducing a cut-point, or using more complex analytical methods (see later).

20.8 Combining studies

The previous section discussed how to summarise each study by calculating an effect size and corresponding *SE* of the effect size. The next stage is to combine these estimated treatment effects to provide an overall average treatment effect.

Example from the literature

In a meta-analysis of open mesh versus non-mesh for groin hernia repair, one of the outcome measures was pain (Scott *et al.*, 2001). The open mesh studies were separated into three groups: flat mesh (six studies), plug-and-mesh (two studies) and pre-peritoneal mesh (one study). 'Persisting pain' was defined as groin, thigh or testicular pain at one year after the operation, or at the closest time point to one year provided it was more than three months post-surgery. In Figure 20.3, the disparate ratings of pain have been presented as odds ratios (*OR*s) for the presence of persisting pain lasting longer than three months.

(Continued)

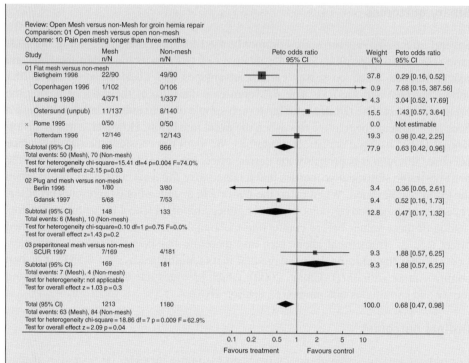

Review: Open Mesh versus non-Mesh for groin hernia repair
Comparison: 01 Open mesh versus open non-mesh
Outcome: 10 Pain persisting longer than three months

Study	Mesh n/N	Non-mesh n/N	Peto odds ratio 95% CI	Weight (%)	Peto odds ratio 95% CI
01 Flat mesh versus non-mesh					
Bietigheim 1998	22/90	49/90		37.8	0.29 [0.16, 0.52]
Copenhagen 1996	1/102	0/106		0.9	7.68 [0.15, 387.56]
Lansing 1998	4/371	1/337		4.3	3.04 [0.52, 17.69]
Ostersund (unpub)	11/137	8/140		15.5	1.43 [0.57, 3.64]
x Rome 1995	0/50	0/50		0.0	Not estimable
Rotterdam 1996	12/146	12/143		19.3	0.98 [0.42, 2.25]
Subtotal (95% CI)	896	866		77.9	0.63 [0.42, 0.96]
Total events: 50 (Mesh), 70 (Non-mesh)					
Test for heterogeneity chi-square=15.41 df=4 p=0.004 I²=74.0%					
Test for overall effect z=2.15 p=0.03					
02 Plug and mesh versus non-mesh					
Berlin 1996	1/80	3/80		3.4	0.36 [0.05, 2.61]
Gdansk 1997	5/68	7/53		9.4	0.52 [0.16, 1.73]
Subtotal (95% CI)	148	133		12.8	0.47 [0.17, 1.32]
Total events: 6 (Mesh), 10 (Non-mesh)					
Test for heterogeneity chi-square=0.10 df=1 p=0.75 I²=0.0%					
Test for overall effect z=1.43 p=0.2					
03 preperitoneal mesh versus non-mesh					
SCUR 1997	7/169	4/181		9.3	1.88 [0.57, 6.25]
Subtotal (95% CI)	169	181		9.3	1.88 [0.57, 6.25]
Total events: 7 (Mesh), 4 (Non-mesh)					
Test for heterogeneity: not applicable					
Test for overall effect z = 1.03 p = 0.3					
Total (95% CI)	1213	1180		100.0	0.68 [0.47, 0.98]
Total events: 63 (Mesh), 84 (Non-mesh)					
Test for heterogeneity chi-square = 18.86 df = 7 p = 0.009 I² = 62.9%					
Test for overall effect z = 2.09 p = 0.04					

0.1 0.2 0.5 1 2 5 10
Favours treatment   Favours control

Figure 20.3 Forest plot of pain severity following open mesh or non-mesh groin hernia repairs. *Source:* Scott *et al.*, 2001. Reproduced with permission of John Wiley & Sons, Ltd.

For simplicity, in this chapter we shall only present the *fixed-effects* approach. This assumes there is no heterogeneity between the study results; that is, we assume all studies are estimating a single true underlying effect. This is in contrast to the *random-effects model*, which incorporates an estimate of between-study variation (heterogeneity) into the calculation of the common effect. This is explained in greater detail in Section 20.10.

Continuous outcomes

For continuous variables, or when continuous, binary and ordinal outcomes have been converted to a common metric that is assumed to be continuous, the simplest method of meta-analysis is known as the *inverse variance weighted* or *weighted mean difference* (*WMD*) method. For this, the average of effect sizes is calculated, giving more 'weight' to estimates from larger studies. The weights are the inverse variances of the means from each study, that is $1/(SE)^2$. This means that studies with the least variability, usually the largest studies, will receive the highest weighting in determining the overall combined result. A 95% *CI* for the combined effect size can then be calculated. This is usually much narrower than those for the individual study estimates.

If there are k studies to be combined, we can use the estimates of treatment effect ($SMDs$ etc.) calculated as in Table 20.1. We represent the treatment effect of the jth study as Y_j, where j varies from 1 to k. The standard errors of the Y_j are SE_j, calculated from the final column of Table 20.1. Then the *inverse variance weights*, W_j, are

$$W_j = \frac{1}{SE_j^2}.$$ (20.1)

The weighted mean effect for, in this case, the *maximum likelihood estimate, fixed-effects model*, is

$$\theta_{\mathrm{MLE}} = \frac{\sum_j W_j Y_j}{\sum_j W_j},$$ (20.2)

with standard error

$$SE(\theta_{\mathrm{MLE}}) = \frac{1}{\sqrt{\sum_j W_j}}.$$ (20.3)

Example from the literature

In Figure 20.1, all studies used the same outcome and so raw *MDs* were used, and combined as weighted mean differences. Linde *et al.* (2005) formed two subgroups, major depression and other studies, and summarise the studies using *WMDs*. They also show the overall effect across all studies. These *WMD* summaries are shown as diamonds. The weights that were applied to each study are listed.

Using a fixed-effects model, Linde *et al.* show that the two subtotals and the overall effect are all statistically highly significant in favour of extracts from St John's wort. The authors concluded that extracts of St John's wort seem more effective than placebo and similarly effective as standard antidepressants for treating mild to moderate depressive symptoms, although they also note that several recent placebo-controlled trials suggest that the tested *Hypericum* extracts have minimal beneficial effects, and that as the preparations available on the market might vary considerably in their pharmaceutical quality, the results of their review apply only to the products tested in the included studies.

Binary outcomes

Although the inverse variance method may also be applied when combining binary data, it is more common to use one of two similar methods instead. The first of these is the Mantel–Haenszel method. Research has shown that this approach is especially beneficial when trials are small or when there are only a small number of trials in the review. The other method, known as *Peto's odds ratio*, involves using $(O - E)/V$ as an estimate of the *OR*, where O and E are the observed and expected events in the treatment group and V is the variance of $O - E$. This estimate has excellent statistical properties and is combined using the inverse variance weighted method. Peto's method is particularly useful when some trials have no events or when events are rare, but does not perform so well when treatment effects are large. Full details are given in Egger *et al.* (2001).

Most QoL meta-analyses include some studies with continuous outcomes, as described under *mixed outcomes*. When all outcomes are binary, the Mantel–Haenszel or Peto methods may be used, as described in more detail in the references under Further Reading.

Example from the literature

In Figure 20.3, Scott *et al.* (2001) used Peto's estimates of the *OR*s to combine the results from different studies. The overall treatment comparison, indicated by the bottom diamond in Figure 20.3, suggests that persisting pain was less frequent after mesh repair than after non-mesh repair. However, the authors note that this result was dependent on one trial, and that data were not available for an additional 11 trials.

Ordinal outcomes

For ordinal variables, which are commonly encountered in QoL assessments, there are two possible approaches. If the ordinal scale data appear to be approximately Normally distributed, or if the analyses reported by the investigators suggest that parametric methods and a Normal approximation are appropriate, the outcome measures can be treated as continuous variables. The second approach is to concatenate the data into two categories that best represent the contrasting states of interest, and to treat the resultant outcome measure as binary.

Mixed outcomes

Often in QoL meta-analyses there will be a combination of dichotomous and continuous data (and also possibly ordinal scales). It may be useful to present separate tables for the continuous data and dichotomous data, while also combining all data for a statistical analysis. There are statistical approaches available that will re-express *OR*s as *SMD*s.

This allows the dichotomous and continuous data to be pooled together, subject to the assumption that the underlying distribution of the dichotomous measurements follows a logistic distribution (roughly similar in shape to the normal distribution). Then, as noted earlier, the *OR*s can be re-expressed as an *SMD* according to the simple formula $SMD = 0.5513 \times \log(OR)$. Alternatively, *SMD*s can be converted to $\log(OR)$. Similarly, the *SE* of the $\log(OR)$ can be converted to the SE of an *SMD* by multiplying by 0.5513. After this, an inverse variance weighted analysis can be carried out as usual.

The simplest approach, as in the example of Figure 20.3, is to convert the continuous outcomes to dichotomous ones – in the given example, these are presence or absence of persisting pain.

Individual patient data

Traditional methods for meta-analysis synthesise aggregate study level data obtained from study publications. An alternative but increasingly popular approach is meta-analysis of individual patient data (IPD), in which the raw individual level data for each study are obtained and used for synthesis. Obtaining IPD is inevitably labour intensive, and usually involves contacting the principal investigator of each study, converting the separate datasets into a common format and merging them to provide a uniform database. Various approaches to analysis are possible, including allowance for baseline characteristics and other prognostic factors (Riley *et al.*, 2010; Simmonds *et al.*, 2005). Frequently the results will differ from those based on published aggregate data, in which case IPD meta-analysis is more convincing and to be preferred.

Example from the literature

McCormack *et al.* (2004) reported that there have been over 40 randomised trials exploring the relative merits and potential risks of laparoscopic surgery for the repair of inguinal hernia. The outcomes were hernia recurrence and persisting pain. The authors carried out a meta-analysis using IPD, and compared this with an earlier analysis based on aggregate published data to determine whether there were statistically significant changes in estimates of either of the two outcomes.

The results for hernia recurrence changed little. However, the IPD update led to divergent conclusions for persisting pain. The published data implied a statistically significant benefit in favour of open repair, whereas the revised result implied a statistically significant benefit in favour of laparoscopic repair ($p < 0.001$). Methodological quality did not account for this difference. Although the IPD study was resource intensive and costly, it greatly increased the amount of data available for meta-analysis by recovering data that was not reported in the trial publications. This led to greater precision in some estimates of effectiveness for one primary outcome, hernia recurrence, and yielded great benefits for persisting pain, an outcome that was rarely included in published reports.

Longitudinal data

QoL and PROs are frequently reported as longitudinal data. Most meta-analyses adopt a simple cross-sectional approach, and frequently this is the only feasible way when using aggregate data from published clinical trials. Cross-sectional analyses at multiple time points, however, fail to take into account the correlations between successive observations, and where IPD is available alternative analyses are possible (Jones *et al.*, 2009).

20.9   Forest plot

The standard way to display the results of a meta-analysis is a *forest plot*, as has been shown in the figures. The confidence limits of the estimates of effect size can be calculated in the usual way, using their SEs, both for individual study effect sizes (Y_j) and the weighted mean effect size (θ). For example, the 95% CI of θ is

$$\theta - 1.96 \times SE(\theta) \text{ to } \theta + 1.96 \times SE(\theta). \tag{20.4}$$

The results from a meta-analysis are then displayed as point estimates for the separate studies and also for the overall effect, together with their associated *CI*s. Figure 20.1 and Figure 20.3 show forest plots produced using the Cochrane Collaboration's Review Manager software, commonly known as 'RevMan' (Review Manager, 2011). While this provides the most comprehensive information in a standardised format, one commonly sees slightly simpler styles of representation in journal publications, such as that of Figure 20.2.

As we have seen, each of the included studies is shown on a separate line, together with the mean treatment effect, the corresponding *CI* and the inverse-variance weight applied to the trial. These results are also shown graphically as a block whose area indicates the weight assigned to that study in the meta-analysis, with a horizontal line depicting the *CI* (usually with a 95% level of confidence). The area of the block and the *CI* convey similar information, but both make different contributions to the graphic. The *CI* depicts the range of treatment effects compatible with the study's result and indicates whether each was individually statistically significant. The size of the block draws the eye towards the studies with larger weight (narrower *CI*s), which dominate the calculation of the pooled result. The pooled result is also shown, with a diamond indicating the overall estimate and with the overall *CI*.

20.10   Heterogeneity

A further complication in meta-analysis is the issue of heterogeneity. All the methods mentioned so far have been *fixed-effect methods* and make the assumption that the true effect sizes for each study are the same (homogeneity); in other words, it is assumed that if all studies enrolled huge numbers of patients they would all have the same effect size. In terms of forest plots, homogeneity implies that the *CI*s of the studies should be largely overlapping. Frequently, a visual inspection of the forest plots will suffice to confirm homogeneity or reveal heterogeneity.

Homogeneity may not be a reasonable assumption, especially when studies have varying entry criteria, for example in age or severity of disease. Another frequent cause of heterogeneity is that if studies apply treatments using varying dosage levels there may be corresponding variations in the response rates. In such cases, the association between the presumed factors (age, disease severity or dosage) and the reported individual-study effect sizes can be explored. However, a more insidious cause of heterogeneity may be publication bias, as discussed in Section 20.11.

In addition to visual checks, homogeneity between studies should also be assessed with a statistical test, although this may lack power if there are few studies. When significant heterogeneity is identified, there are a number of options available. One is to use the fixed-effect method possibly with exploration of the reasons for the heterogeneity; an alternative is to carry out a systematic review without a meta-analysis; another option is to consider a *random-effects model* instead. However, if the cause of heterogeneity is thought to be publication bias, the results of the meta-analysis may be difficult to interpret.

Random-effects methods do not assume the same underlying effect size for each study, but do allow random study-to-study variability. Although often the results from both random- and fixed-effects models may be similar, in practice the random-effects method will tend to give more weight to smaller studies and result in wider *CI*s than the fixed-effect method. There is no consensus as to which is the best approach to use when heterogeneity is present.

Heterogeneity may be explored by calculating the statistic

$$Q = \sum_j W_j \times \left(Y_j - \theta_{MLE}\right)^2.$$ (20.5)

There is statistically significant heterogeneity if Q exceeds the value from a χ^2 distribution with $k - 1$ degrees of freedom (Higgins and Thompson, 2002).

The level of inconsistency may be measured using the following statistic, which represents the percentage of total variation that is due to heterogeneity as opposed to sampling error; a value greater than 50% indicates substantial heterogeneity:

$$I^2 = \frac{Q - (k-1)}{Q} \times 100\%.$$ (20.6)

Examples from the literature

The forest plot in Figure 20.1 also provides the Q-statistics *test for heterogeneity chi-square*. There was strong evidence of heterogeneity in both the analysis of the 10 studies 'restricted to major depression' and the overall comparison of all studies. The figure also reports the I^2 statistics of 83.0% and 79.4% which both indicate substantial heterogeneity.

Linde *et al.* (2005) comment that their previous reviews had found that smaller trials tended to report larger treatment effects, which could be due to publication bias or bias introduced by lower methodological quality of smaller trials. As a consequence, they had chosen to use a fixed-effects model, as this gives more weight to larger trials. They also explored the use of a random-effects regression models.

Lakhan *et al.* (2015), when assessing the role of Zingiberaceae extracts for chronic pain as illustrated in, found that heterogeneity between studies was very high ($I^2 = 87.5\%$). They also speculate that "Earlier studies tended to use lower doses, which may explain the tendency for more recent studies to have larger effect sizes." Thus they used the more conservative random-effects model as "This was necessary because of the heterogeneity of effects in the included studies."

The hernia meta-analysis of Scott *et al.* (2001) shown in Figure 20.3 also displays significant heterogeneity, and as a consequence those authors decided to use a random-effects model.

20.11   Publication bias and funnel plots

Publication bias is a well-known problem in the reporting of clinical trials. Journals are more likely to publish studies that obtain 'interesting' positive results. This is especially the case if the studies are small, when those without such positive findings may fail to be published. In contrast, large and well-conducted randomised clinical trials are more likely to be published, irrespective of their conclusions. Thus one way to explore whether the review might have been prejudiced through publication bias is to draw a *funnel plot*, in which the treatment effect observed in each study (*x*-axis) is plotted against a measure of the study's sample size (*y*-axis). Since the estimates from smaller studies are less precise (larger *SE* and hence wider *CI*), we expect greater scatter at the bottom of the plot. In the absence of any bias, the plot should resemble a symmetrical inverted funnel.

Example from the literature

Linde *et al.* (2005) show a funnel plot of the 23 placebo-controlled trials that reported information on the number of responders according to the HRSD (Figure 20.4). The larger studies have a responder rate close to 1, indicating zero effect, while there is evident asymmetry for the smaller studies, which tend to lie to the right of the larger studies. This substantial asymmetry was reflected by a highly significant *p*-value (< 0.0001).

Despite this, after carrying out many additional analyses, the authors circumspectly conclude: "In summary, we believe that the heterogeneous findings of placebo-controlled trials of *Hypericum* extracts and the clear funnel plot asymmetry found in our analyses are partly due to an overestimation of effects in smaller, older studies, and partly due to variable efficacy of *Hypericum* extracts in different patient populations, while non-publication of negative studies (publication bias) does not seem to play a major role."

Hence they tempered the conclusions of their meta-analysis with the reservation: "Current evidence regarding Hypericum extracts is inconsistent and confusing."

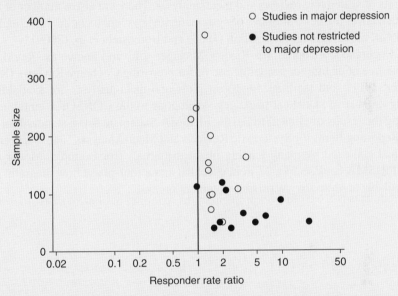

Figure 20.4 Funnel plot of 23 placebo-controlled trials that reported information on the number of responders according to the Hamilton Rating Scale for Depression. *Source:* Linde *et al.,* 2005, Figure 1. Reproduced with permission of John Wiley & Sons, Ltd.

20.12 Conclusions

Now that an increasing number of clinical trials include QoL endpoints, we can expect to see a corresponding increase in the number of meta-analyses of such outcomes that are carried out and published. Although meta-analysis for QoL may seem to be, and in some ways is, more complicated than analyses of other endpoints, there are no fundamental reasons why it cannot be carried out in exactly the same way.

This chapter has discussed and illustrated the particular issues involved in carrying out meta-analyses of QoL endpoints, illustrating some specific problems that arise in this setting and showing how they may be resolved. However, it is also important to emphasise that carrying out a systematic review is a major exercise that calls for appreciable investment of time and resources.

20.13   Further reading

The first port of call for further information should be the Cochrane Collaboration (Website: <http://www.cochrane.org/>). In particular, the *Cochrane Handbook for Systematic Reviews* (Higgins and Green, 2011) is available for electronic access (<http://www.cochrane-handbook.org/>). This provides extensive information about all aspects of systematic reviews and meta-analyses. There are also a number of useful books that cover the general issues of systematic reviews and meta-analysis, including Egger *et al.* (2001), Hedges and Olkin (1985) and Borenstein *et al.* (2009).

The Cochrane Collaboration's Review Manager software, known as 'RevMan', is available free of charge for academic use or for preparing Cochrane Reviews (Review Manager, 2011), and facilities for forest plots and meta-analysis are available in a growing number of statistical packages. Analogous to the CONSORT guidelines for reporting the results of clinical trials, the PRISMA Statement sets a standard for "Preferred Reporting Items for Systematic Reviews and Meta-Analyses" and has been published and endorsed by many leading medical journals (for example, Moher *et al.*, 2009). PRISMA consists of a 27-item checklist and a four-phase flow diagram, and is also available at <http://www.prisma-statement.org/>.

Appendix 1
Examples of Instruments

Generic instruments

PLEASE RESPOND TO (CHECK) <u>ONLY</u> THOSE STATEMENTS THAT YOU ARE <u>SURE</u> DESCRIBE YOU TODAY AND ARE RELATED TO YOUR STATE OF HEALTH.

1. I am confused and start several actions at a time   —

2. I have more minor accidents, for example, drop things, trip and fall, bump into things   —

3. I react slowly to things that are said or done   —

4. I do not finish things I start   —

5. I have difficulty reasoning and solving problems, for example, making plans, making decisions, learning new things   —

6. I sometimes behave as if I were confused or disorientated in place or time, for example, where I am, who is around, directions, what day it is   —

7. I forget a lot, for example, things that happened recently, where I put things, appointments   —

8. I do not keep my attention on any activity for long   —

9. I make more mistakes than usual   —

10. I have difficulty doing activities involving concentration and thinking   —

CHECK HERE WHEN YOU HAVE READ ALL STATEMENTS ON THIS PAGE   ☐

© Johns Hopkins University

For permission to use contact: Mapi Research Trust, 27, Rue de la Villette, 69003 Lyon, FRANCE (www.mapi-trust.org)

Appendix E1 Continued

Page 2 of 2

Sickness Impact Profile (SIP) [Extract only]

PLEASE RESPOND TO (CHECK) <u>ONLY</u> THOSE STATEMENTS THAT YOU ARE <u>SURE</u> DESCRIBE YOU TODAY AND ARE RELATED TO YOUR STATE OF HEALTH.

1. I am having trouble writing or typing —

2. I communicate mostly by gestures, for example, moving head, pointing, sign language —

3. My speech is understood only by a few people who know me well —

4. I often lose control of my voice when I talk, for example, my voice gets louder or softer, trembles, changes unexpectedly —

5. I don't write except to sign my name —

6. I carry on a conversation only when very close to the other person or looking at him —

7. I have difficulty speaking, for example, get stuck, stutter, stammer, slur my words —

8. I am understood with difficulty —

9. I do not speak clearly when I am under stress —

CHECK HERE WHEN YOU HAVE READ ALL STATEMENTS ON THIS PAGE ☐

At the end of the SIP, a reminder:

NOW, PLEASE REVIEW THE QUESTIONNAIRE TO BE CERTAIN YOU HAVE FILLED OUT ALL THE INFORMATION. LOOK OVER THE BOXES ON EACH PAGE TO MAKE SURE EACH ONE IS CHECKED SHOWING THAT YOU HAVE READ ALL OF THE STATEMENTS. IF YOU FIND A BOX WITHOUT A CHECK, THEN READ THE STATEMENTS ON THAT PAGE.

For permission to use contact: Mapi Research Trust, 27, Rue de la Villette, 69003 Lyon, FRANCE (www.mapi-trust.org)

Appendix E2 Nottingham Health Profile (NHP) [Extract only]   *Page 1 of 1*

Nottingham Health Profile

Please do
not write in
this margin

LISTED BELOW ARE SOME PROBLEMS PEOPLE MIGHT HAVE IN THEIR
DAILY LIVES.
READ THE LIST CAREFULLY AND PUT A TICK IN THE BOX □ UNDER
YES FOR ANY PROBLEM THAT APPLIES TO YOU AT THE MOMENT. TICK
THE BOX □ UNDER NO FOR ANY PROBLEM THAT DOES NOT APPLY
TO YOU. PLEASE ANSWER EVERY QUESTION. IF YOU ARE NOT SURE
WHETHER TO ANSWER YES OR NO, TICK WHICHEVER ANSWER YOU THINK
IS MOST TRUE AT THE MOMENT.

	YES	NO
I'm tired all the time	□	□
I have pain at night	□	□
Things are getting me down	□	□

	YES	NO
I have unbearable pain	□	□
I take tablets to help me sleep	□	□
I've forgotten what it's like to enjoy myself	□	□

	YES	NO
I'm feeling on edge	□	□
I find it painful to change position	□	□
I feel lonely	□	□

Please turn over the page

For permission to use contact: Galen Research Ltd, Enterprise House, Manchester Science Park,
Manchester M15 6SE, UK (www.galen-research.com)

Appendix E3 SF36v2™ Health Survey Standard Version *Page 1 of 3*

SF-36v2

QM QualityMetric

SF-36v2™ Health Survey Standard Version

This survey asks for your views about your health. This information will help you keep track of how you feel and how well you are able to do your usual activities.

Please answer every question. Some questions may look like others, but each one is different. Please take the time to read and answer each question carefully, and click on the circle that best describes your answer. *Thank you for completing this survey!*

1) In general, would you say your health is:

Excellent	Very good	Good	Fair	Poor
○	○	○	○	○

2) Compared to one year ago, how would you rate your health in general now?

Much better now than one year ago	Somewhat better now than one year ago	About the same as one year ago	Somewhat worse now than one year ago	Much worse now than one year ago
○	○	○	○	○

3) The following questions are about activities you might do during a typical day. Does your health now limit you in these activities? If so, how much?

	Yes, limited a lot	Yes, limited a little	No, not limited at all
a. Vigorous Activities, such as running, lifting heavy objects, participating in strenuous sports	○	○	○
b. Moderate Activities, such as moving a table, pushing a vacuum cleaner, bowling, or playing golf	○	○	○
c. Lifting or carrying groceries	○	○	○
d. Climbing several flights of stairs	○	○	○
e. Climbing one flight of stairs	○	○	○
f. Bending, kneeling, or stooping	○	○	○
g. Walking more than a mile	○	○	○
h. Walking several hundred yards	○	○	○
i. Walking one hundred yards	○	○	○
j. Bathing or dressing yourself	○	○	○

For permission to use contact: Quality Metric, 24 Albion Road, Building 400, Lincoln, RI 02865 USA (www.qualitymetric.com)

Appendix E3 Continued   *Page 2 of 3*

SF36v2™ Health Survey Standard Version

SF-36v2

QualityMetric

SF-36v2™ Health Survey Standard Version

---

4) During the <u>past 4 weeks,</u> how much of the time have you had any of the following problems with your work or other regular daily activities <u>as a result of your physical health?</u>

	All of the time	Most of the time	Some of the time	A little of the time	None of the time
a. Cut down on the <u>amount of time</u> you spent on work or other activities	○	○	○	○	○
b. <u>Accomplished less</u> than you would like	○	○	○	○	○
c. Were limited in the <u>kind</u> of work or other activities	○	○	○	○	○
d. Had <u>difficulty</u> performing the work or other activities (for example, it took extra effort)	○	○	○	○	○

5) During the <u>past 4 weeks,</u> how much of the time have you had any of the following problems with your work or other regular daily activities <u>as a result of any emotional problems</u> (such as feeling depressed or anxious)?

	All of the time	Most of the time	Some of the time	A little of the time	None of the time
a. Cut down on the <u>amount of time</u> you spent on work or other activities	○	○	○	○	○
b. <u>Accomplished less</u> than you would like	○	○	○	○	○
c. Did work or activities <u>less carefully</u> than usual	○	○	○	○	○

6) During the <u>past 4 weeks,</u> to what extent has your physical health or emotional problems interfered with your normal social activities with family, friends, neighbors, or groups?

Not at all	Slightly	Moderately	Quite a bit	Extremely
○	○	○	○	○

7) How much <u>bodily</u> pain have you had during the <u>past 4 weeks?</u>

None	Very Mild	Mild	Moderate	Severe	Very Severe
○	○	○	○	○	○

For permission to use contact: Quality Metric, 24 Albion Road, Building 400, Lincoln, RI 02865 USA (www.qualitymetric.com)

Appendix E3 Continued   *Page 3 of 3*

SF36v2™ Health Survey Standard Version

SF-36v2

QM
QUALITYMETRIC
HEALTH OUTCOMES SOLUTIONS

SF-36v2™ Health Survey Standard Version

8) During the <u>past 4 weeks</u>, how much did <u>pain</u> interfere with your normal work (including both work outside the home and housework)?

Not at all	A little bit	Moderately	Quite a bit	Extremely
O	O	O	O	O

9) These questions are about how you feel and how things have been with you <u>during the past 4 weeks</u>. For each question, please give the one answer that comes closest to the way you have been feeling. How much of the time during the <u>past 4 weeks</u>...

	All of the time	Most of the time	Some of the time	A little of the time	None of the time
a. Did you feel full of life?	O	O	O	O	O
b. Have you been very nervous?	O	O	O	O	O
c. Have you felt so down in the dumps that nothing could cheer you up?	O	O	O	O	O
d. Have you felt calm and peaceful?	O	O	O	O	O
e. Did you have a lot of energy?	O	O	O	O	O
f. Have you felt downhearted and depressed?	O	O	O	O	O
g. Did you feel worn out?	O	O	O	O	O
h. Have you been happy?	O	O	O	O	O
i. Did you feel tired?	O	O	O	O	O

10) During the <u>past 4 weeks</u>, how much of the time has your <u>physical health or emotional problems</u> interfered with your social activities (like visiting friends, relatives, etc.)?

All of the time	Most of the time	Some of the time	A little of the time	None of the time
O	O	O	O	O

11) How TRUE or FALSE is <u>each</u> of the following statements for you?

	Definitely true	Mostly true	Don't know	Mostly false	Definitely false
a. I seem to get sick a little easier than other people	O	O	O	O	O
b. I am as healthy as anybody I know	O	O	O	O	O
c. I expect my health to get worse	O	O	O	O	O
d. My health is excellent	O	O	O	O	O

For permission to use contact: Quality Metric, 24 Albion Road, Building 400, Lincoln, RI 02865 USA (www.qualitymetric.com)

Appendix E4 EuroQoL EQ-5D-5L

Under each heading, please tick the ONE box that best describes your health TODAY

MOBILITY

I have no problems in walking about ☐

I have slight problems in walking about ☐

I have moderate problems in walking about ☐

I have severe problems in walking about ☐

I am unable to walk about ☐

SELF-CARE

I have no problems washing or dressing myself ☐

I have slight problems washing or dressing myself ☐

I have moderate problems washing or dressing myself ☐

I have severe problems washing or dressing myself ☐

I am unable to wash or dress myself ☐

USUAL ACTIVITIES *(e.g. work, study, housework, family or leisure activities)*

I have no problems doing my usual activities ☐

I have slight problems doing my usual activities ☐

I have moderate problems doing my usual activities ☐

I have severe problems doing my usual activities ☐

I am unable to do my usual activities ☐

PAIN / DISCOMFORT

I have no pain or discomfort ☐

I have slight pain or discomfort ☐

I have moderate pain or discomfort ☐

I have severe pain or discomfort ☐

I have extreme pain or discomfort ☐

ANXIETY / DEPRESSION

I am not anxious or depressed ☐

I am slightly anxious or depressed ☐

I am moderately anxious or depressed ☐

I am severely anxious or depressed ☐

I am extremely anxious or depressed ☐

For permission to use contact: EuroQol Group Executive Office, Marten Meesweg 107, 3068 AV Rotterdam, The Netherlands (www.euroqol.org)

Appendix E4 Continued
(EuroQoL EQ-5D-5L)

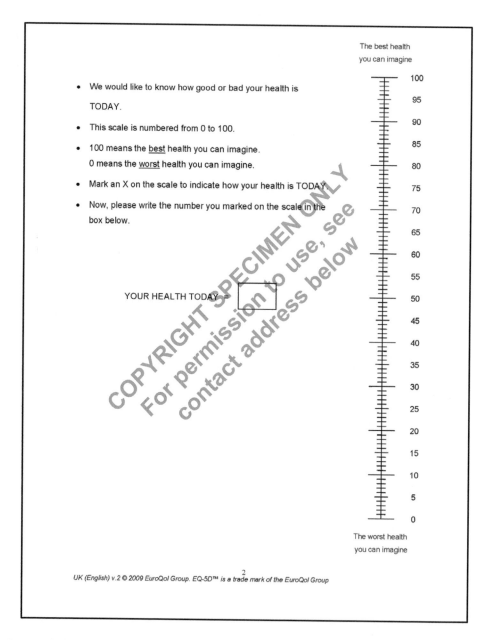

- We would like to know how good or bad your health is TODAY.
- This scale is numbered from 0 to 100.
- 100 means the <u>best</u> health you can imagine.
  0 means the <u>worst</u> health you can imagine.
- Mark an X on the scale to indicate how your health is TODAY.
- Now, please write the number you marked on the scale in the box below.

YOUR HEALTH TODAY =

The best health you can imagine

100
95
90
85
80
75
70
65
60
55
50
45
40
35
30
25
20
15
10
5
0

The worst health you can imagine

UK (English) v.2 © 2009 EuroQol Group. EQ-5D™ is a trade mark of the EuroQol Group

For permission to use contact: EuroQol Group Executive Office, Marten Meesweg 107, 3068 AV Rotterdam, The Netherlands (www.euroqol.org)

Appendix E5 Patient Generated Index of quality of life (PGI)

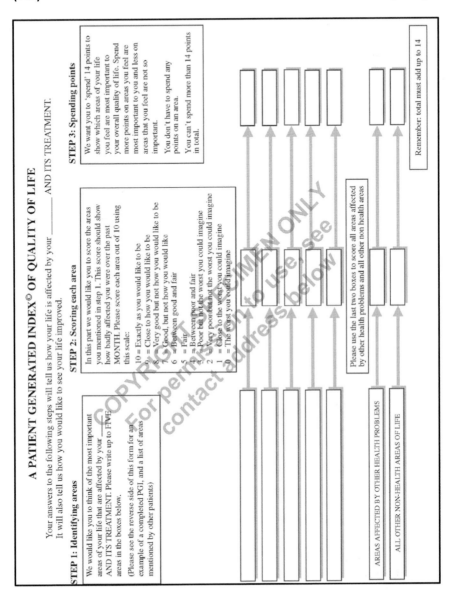

A PATIENT GENERATED INDEX© OF QUALITY OF LIFE

Your answers to the following steps will tell us how your life is affected by your _____ AND ITS TREATMENT.
It will also tell us how you would like to see your life improved.

STEP 1: Identifying areas

We would like you to think of the most important areas of your life that are affected by your _____ AND ITS TREATMENT. Please write up to FIVE areas in the boxes below.

(Please see the reverse side of this form for an example of a completed PGI, and a list of areas mentioned by other patients)

STEP 2: Scoring each area

In this part we would like you to score the areas you mentioned in step 1. This score should show how badly affected you were over the past MONTH. Please score each area out of 10 using this scale:

10 = Exactly as you would like to be
9 = Close to how you would like to be
8 = Very good but not how you would like to be
7 = Good, but not how you would like
6 = Between good and fair
5 = Fair
4 = Between poor and fair
3 = Poor but not the worst you could imagine
2 = Very poor but not the worst you could imagine
1 = Close to the worst you could imagine
0 = The worst you could imagine

STEP 3: Spending points

We want you to 'spend' 14 points to show which areas of your life you feel are most important to your overall quality of life. Spend more points on areas you feel are most important to you and less on areas that you feel are not so important.

You don't have to spend any points on an area.

You can't spend more than 14 points in total.

Please use the last two boxes to score all areas affected by other health problems and all other non health areas

AREAS AFFECTED BY OTHER HEALTH PROBLEMS

ALL OTHER NON-HEALTH AREAS OF LIFE

Remember: total must add up to 14

For permission to use contact: Danny Ruta, Public Health Office, Division of Health and Social Care Research, School of Medicine, King's College London, SE1 3QD (danny.2.ruta@kcl.ac.uk, danny.ruta@nhs.net)

Disease-Specific Instruments

Appendix E6 European Organisation for Research and Treatment of Cancer QLQ-C30 (EORTC QLQ-C30)

EORTC QLQ-C30 (version 3)

We are interested in some things about you and your health. Please answer all of the questions yourself by circling the number that best applies to you. There are no "right" or "wrong" answers. The information that you provide will remain strictly confidential.

Please fill in your inititals: ⬜⬜⬜⬜

Your birthdate (Day, Month, Year): ⬜⬜⬜⬜⬜⬜⬜⬜

Today's date (Day, Month, Year): ⬜⬜⬜⬜⬜⬜⬜⬜

	Not at All	A Little	Quite a Bit	Very Much
1. Do you have any trouble doing strenuous activities, like carrying a heavy shopping bag or a suitcase?	1	2	3	4
2. Do you have any trouble taking a <u>long</u> walk?	1	2	3	4
3. Do you have any trouble taking a <u>short</u> walk outside of the house?	1	2	3	4
4. Do you need to stay in bed or a chair during the day?	1	2	3	4
5. Do you need help with eating, dressing, washing yourself or using the toilet?	1	2	3	4

During the past week:	Not at All	A Little	Quite a Bit	Very Much
6. Were you limited in doing either your work or other daily activities?	1	2	3	4
7. Were you limited in pursuing your hobbies or other leisure time activities?	1	2	3	4
8. Were you short of breath?	1	2	3	4
9. Have you had pain?	1	2	3	4
10. Did you need to rest?	1	2	3	4
11. Have you had trouble sleeping?	1	2	3	4
12. Have you felt weak?	1	2	3	4
13. Have you lacked appetite?	1	2	3	4
14. Have you felt nauseated?	1	2	3	4
15. Have you vomited?	1	2	3	4

Please go on to the next page

For permission to use contact: EORTC Quality of Life Department, Ave. E. Mounier 83, B.11, 1200 Brussels, BELGIUM (http://groups.eortc.be/qol)

Appendix E6 Continued
(EORTC QLQ-C30)

During the past week:	Not at All	A Little	Quite a Bit	Very Much
16. Have you been constipated?	1	2	3	4
17. Have you had diarrhea?	1	2	3	4
18. Were you tired?	1	2	3	4
19. Did pain interfere with your daily activities?	1	2	3	4
20. Have you had difficulty in concentrating on things, like reading a newspaper or watching television?	1	2	3	4
21. Did you feel tense?	1	2	3	4
22. Did you worry?	1	2	3	4
23. Did you feel irritable?	1	2	3	4
24. Did you feel depressed?	1	2	3	4
25. Have you had difficulty remembering things?	1	2	3	4
26. Has your physical condition or medical treatment interfered with your <u>family</u> life?	1	2	3	4
27. Has your physical condition or medical treatment interfered with your <u>social</u> activities?	1	2	3	4
28. Has your physical condition or medical treatment caused you financial difficulties?	1	2	3	4

For the following questions please circle the number between 1 and 7 that best applies to you

29. How would you rate your overall <u>health</u> during the past week?

1	2	3	4	5	6	7
Very poor						Excellent

30. How would you rate your overall <u>quality of life</u> during the past week?

1	2	3	4	5	6	7
Very poor						Excellent

For permission to use contact: EORTC Quality of Life Department, Ave. E. Mounier 83, B.11, 1200 Brussels, BELGIUM (http://groups.eortc.be/qol)

Appendix E7 Elderly cancer patients module
(EORTC QLQ-ELD14)

Page 1 of 1

EORTC QLQ-ELD14

Patients sometimes report that they have the following symptoms or problems. Please indicate the extent to which you have experienced these symptoms or problems <u>during the past week</u>. Please answer by circling the number that best applies to you.

During the past week:	Not at All	A Little	Quite a Bit	Very Much
31. Have you had difficulty with steps or stairs?	1	2	3	4
32. Have you had trouble with your joints (e.g.-stiffness, pain)?	1	2	3	4
33. Did you feel unsteady on your feet?	1	2	3	4
34. Did you need help with household chores such as cleaning or shopping?	1	2	3	4
35. Have you felt able to talk to your family about your illness?	1	2	3	4
36. Have you worried about your family coping with your illness and treatment?	1	2	3	4
37. Have you worried about the future of people who are important to you?	1	2	3	4
38. Were you worried about your future health?	1	2	3	4
39. Did you feel uncertain about the future?	1	2	3	4
40. Have you worried about what might happen towards the end of your life?	1	2	3	4
41. Have you had a positive outlook on life in the last week?	1	2	3	4
42. Have you felt motivated to continue with your normal hobbies and activities?	1	2	3	4
43. How much has your illness been a burden to you?	1	2	3	4
44. How much has your treatment been a burden to you?	1	2	3	4

For permission to use contact: EORTC Quality of Life Department, Ave. E. Mounier 83, B.11, 1200 Brussels, BELGIUM (http://groups.eortc.be/qol)

Appendix E8 Functional Assessment of Cancer Therapy - General (FACT-G)

FACT-G (Version 4)

Below is a list of statements that other people with your illness have said are important. **Please circle or mark one number per line to indicate your response as it applies to the past 7 days.**

PHYSICAL WELL-BEING

		Not at all	A little bit	Some-what	Quite a bit	Very much
GP1	I have a lack of energy	0	1	2	3	4
GP2	I have nausea	0	1	2	3	4
GP3	Because of my physical condition, I have trouble meeting the needs of my family	0	1	2	3	4
GP4	I have pain	0	1	2	3	4
GP5	I am bothered by side effects of treatment	0	1	2	3	4
GP6	I feel ill	0	1	2	3	4
GP7	I am forced to spend time in bed	0	1	2	3	4

SOCIAL/FAMILY WELL-BEING

		Not at all	A little bit	Some-what	Quite a bit	Very much
GS1	I feel close to my friends	0	1	2	3	4
GS2	I get emotional support from my family	0	1	2	3	4
GS3	I get support from my friends	0	1	2	3	4
GS4	My family has accepted my illness	0	1	2	3	4
GS5	I am satisfied with family communication about my illness	0	1	2	3	4
GS6	I feel close to my partner (or the person who is my main support)	0	1	2	3	4
Q1	*Regardless of your current level of sexual activity, please answer the following question. If you prefer not to answer it, please mark this box* ☐ *and go to the next section.*					
GS7	I am satisfied with my sex life	0	1	2	3	4

For permission to use contact: FACIT.org, 381 South Cottage Hill Ave, Elmhurst, IL 60126, USA (www.facit.org)

Appendix E8 Continued

Functional Assessment of Cancer Therapy - General (FACT-G)

FACT-G (Version 4)

Please circle or mark one number per line to indicate your response as it applies to the <u>past 7 days</u>.

EMOTIONAL WELL-BEING		Not at all	A little bit	Some- what	Quite a bit	Very much
GE1	I feel sad	0	1	2	3	4
GE2	I am satisfied with how I am coping with my illness	0	1	2	3	4
GE3	I am losing hope in the fight against my illness	0	1	2	3	4
GE4	I feel nervous	0	1	2	3	4
GE5	I worry about dying	0	1	2	3	4
GE6	I worry that my condition will get worse	0	1	2	3	4

FUNCTIONAL WELL-BEING		Not at all	A little bit	Some- what	Quite a bit	Very much
GF1	I am able to work (include work at home)	0	1	2	3	4
GF2	My work (include work at home) is fulfilling	0	1	2	3	4
GF3	I am able to enjoy life	0	1	2	3	4
GF4	I have accepted my illness	0	1	2	3	4
GF5	I am sleeping well	0	1	2	3	4
GF6	I am enjoying the things I usually do for fun	0	1	2	3	4
GF7	I am content with the quality of my life right now	0	1	2	3	4

For permission to use contact: FACIT.org, 381 South Cottage Hill Ave, Elmhurst, IL 60126, USA (www.facit.org)

Appendix E9 Rotterdam Symptom Checklist (RSCL)

Rotterdam Symptom Checklist　　　　　　　　　　　　　　　　　　**Confidential**

date of completion _____19___

In this questionnaire you will be asked about your symptoms. Would you please, for all symptoms mentioned, indicate to what extent you have been bothered by it, by circling the answer most applicable to you. The questions are related to the past week.

Example: Have you been bothered, during the past week, by

headaches	not at all	a little	quite a bit	very much

Have you, during the past week, been bothered by

lack of appetite	not at all	a little	quite a bit	very much
irritability	not at all	a little	quite a bit	very much
tiredness	not at all	a little	quite a bit	very much
worrying	not at all	a little	quite a bit	very much
sore muscles	not at all	a little	quite a bit	very much
depressed mood	not at all	a little	quite a bit	very much
lack of energy	not at all	a little	quite a bit	very much
low back pain	not at all	a little	quite a bit	very much
nervousness	not at all	a little	quite a bit	very much
nausea	not at all	a little	quite a bit	very much
despairing about the future	not at all	a little	quite a bit	very much
difficulty sleeping	not at all	a little	quite a bit	very much
headaches	not at all	a little	quite a bit	very much
vomiting	not at all	a little	quite a bit	very much
dizziness	not at all	a little	quite a bit	very much
decreased sexual interest	not at all	a little	quite a bit	very much
tension	not at all	a little	quite a bit	very much
abdominal (stomach) aches	not at all	a little	quite a bit	very much
anxiety	not at all	a little	quite a bit	very much
constipation	not at all	a little	quite a bit	very much

For permission to use,

see: http://www.rug.nl/research/share/research/tools/handleiding_rscl2edruk.pdf (page 33)

Appendix E9 Continued

Rotterdam Symptom Checklist (RSCL)

diarrhoea	not at all	a little	quite a bit	very much
acid indigestion	not at all	a little	quite a bit	very much
shivering	not at all	a little	quite a bit	very much
tingling hands or feet	not at all	a little	quite a bit	very much
difficulty concentrating	not at all	a little	quite a bit	very much
sore mouth/pain when swallowing	not at all	a little	quite a bit	very much
loss of hair	not at all	a little	quite a bit	very much
burning/sore eyes	not at all	a little	quite a bit	very much
shortness of breath	not at all	a little	quite a bit	very much
dry mouth	not at all	a little	quite a bit	very much

A number of activities is listed below. *We do not want to know whether you actually do these, but only whether you are able to perform them presently. Would you please mark the answer that applies most to your condition of the past week.*

	unable	only with help	without help, with difficulty	without help
care for myself (wash etc)	O	O	O	O
walk about the house	O	O	O	O
light housework/household jobs	O	O	O	O
climb stairs	O	O	O	O
heavy housework/household jobs	O	O	O	O
walk out of doors	O	O	O	O
go shopping	O	O	O	O
go to work	O	O	O	O

All things considered, how would you describe your quality of life during the past week?	O excellent
	O good
	O moderately good
	O neither good nor bad
	O rather poor
	O poor
	O extremely poor

Would you please check whether you answered all questions?

Thank you for your help.

patient number_____

For permission to use,

see: http://www.rug.nl/research/share/research/tools/handleiding_rscl2edruk.pdf (Page 33)

Appendix E10 Quality of Life in Epilepsy Inventory (QOLIE-89) [Extract only]

QUALITY OF LIFE IN EPILEPSY
QOLIE-31 *(Version 1.0)*

Patient Inventory

Today's Date____/____/____

Patient's Name_____

Patient's ID#_____

Gender: ☐ Male ☐ Female   Birthdate____/____/____

INSTRUCTIONS

This survey asks about your health and daily activities. **Answer every question** by circling the appropriate number (1, 2, 3 . . .).

If you are unsure about how to answer a question, please give the best answer you can and write a comment or explanation in the margin.

Please feel free to ask someone to assist you if you need help reading or marking the form.

1.   Overall, how would you rate your quality of life?

(Circle one number on the scale below)

```
  ☺        ☺        ☺        ☹        ☹        ☹
  |_|___|___|___|___|___|___|___|___|___|___|_|
  10   9   8   7   6   5   4   3   2   1   0
```

Best Possible   Worst Possible
Quality of Life   Quality of Life

                                                     (as bad as or
                                                     worse than
                                                     being dead)

Permissions information: "All of the surveys from RAND Health are public documents, available without charge." (http://www.rand.org/health/surveys_tools/qolie.html)

Appendix E10 Continued

Quality of Life in Epilepsy Inventory (QOLIE-89) [Extract only]

3. **Compared to 1 year ago**, how would you rate your health in general **now**?

Do Not Write in This Space

(Circle one number)

Much better now than 1 year ago	1
Somewhat better now than 1 year ago	2
About the same as 1 year ago	3
Somewhat worse now than 1 year ago	4
Much worse now than 1 year ago	5

4–13: The following questions are about activities you might do during a typical day. Does **your health** limit you in these activities? If so, **how much**?

(Circle 1, 2, or 3 on each line)

	Yes, limited a lot	Yes, limited a little	No, not limited at all
4. *Vigorous activities*, such as running, lifting heavy objects, participating in strenuous sports	1	2	3
5. *Moderate activities*, such as moving a table, pushing a vacuum cleaner, bowling, or playing golf	1	2	3
6. Lifting or carrying groceries	1	2	3
7. Climbing *several* flights of stairs	1	2	3
8. Climbing *one* flight of stairs	1	2	3
9. Bending, kneeling, or stooping	1	2	3
10. Walking *more than one mile*	1	2	3
11. Walking *several* blocks	1	2	3
12. Walking *one block*	1	2	3
13. Bathing or dressing yourself	1	2	3

Permissions information: "All of the surveys from RAND Health are public documents, available without charge." (http://www.rand.org/health/surveys_tools/qolie.html)

Appendix E10 Continued

Quality of Life in Epilepsy Inventory (QOLIE-89) [Extract only]

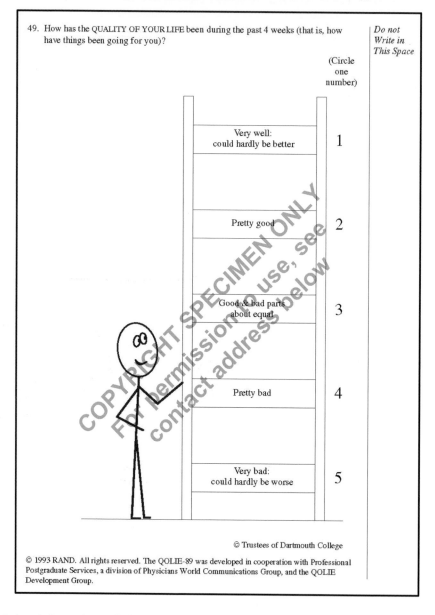

49. How has the QUALITY OF YOUR LIFE been during the past 4 weeks (that is, how have things been going for you)?

Do not Write in This Space

(Circle one number)

Very well: could hardly be better	1
Pretty good	2
Good & bad parts about equal	3
Pretty bad	4
Very bad: could hardly be worse	5

© Trustees of Dartmouth College

Permissions information: "All of the surveys from RAND Health are public documents, available without charge." (http://www.rand.org/health/surveys_tools/qolie.html)

Appendix E10 Continued

Quality of Life in Epilepsy Inventory (QOLIE-89) [Extract only]

89. How good or bad do you think your health is? On the thermometer scale below, the best imaginable state of health is 100 and the worst imaginable state is 0. Please indicate how you feel about your health by circling one number on the scale. **Please consider your epilepsy as part of your health when you answer this question.**

Do Not Write in This Space

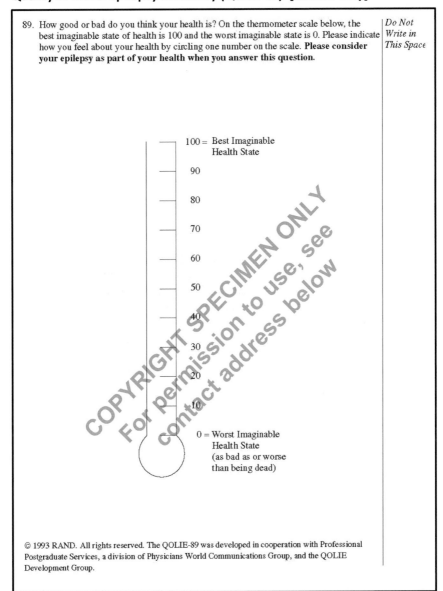

100 = Best Imaginable Health State

90

80

70

60

50

40

30

20

10

0 = Worst Imaginable Health State (as bad as or worse than being dead)

Permissions information: "All of the surveys from RAND Health are public documents, available without charge." (http://www.rand.org/health/surveys_tools/qolie.html)

Appendix E11 Paediatric Asthma Quality of Life Questionnaire (PAQLQ) [Extract only]

Page 1 of 2

PAEDIATRIC ASTHMA QUALITY OF LIFE QUESTIONNAIRE

PATIENT ID _____

SELF-ADMINISTERED   DATE _____

Page 1 of 5

ACTIVITIES

Because you have asthma, you may have found some of the things you like doing difficult or not much fun.

We want you to think about all the things that you do in which you have been bothered by your asthma.

Some people are bothered by asthma when doing some of the following activities. Please read through the list. Think about how your asthma has bothered you during the last week.

On the next page, write down the **three** (3) things in which you have been bothered **most** by your asthma during the last week. These things must be activities that you will be doing regularly during the study. The three activities you choose can be from this list or you can think of other activities as long as you do them regularly.

1. BALL HOCKEY	19. WALKING UPSTAIRS
2. BASEBALL	20. LAUGHING
3. BASKETBALL	21. STUDYING
4. DANCING (BALLET/JAZZ)	22. DOING HOUSEHOLD CHORES
5. FOOTBALL	23. SINGING
6. PLAYING AT RECESS	24. DOING CRAFTS OR HOBBIES
7. PLAYING WITH PETS	25. SHOUTING
8. PLAYING WITH FRIENDS	26. GYMNASTICS
9. RIDING A BICYCLE	27. ROLLERBLADING/ROLLERSKATING
10. RUNNING	28. SKATEBOARDING
11. SKIPPING ROPE	29. TRACK AND FIELD
12. SHOPPING	30. TOBOGGANING
13. SLEEPING	31. SKIING
14. SOCCER	32. ICE SKATING
15. SWIMMING	33. CLIMBING
16. VOLLEYBALL	34. GETTING UP IN THE MORNING
17. WALKING	35. TALKING
18. WALKING UPHILL	

Write your 3 activities on the next page.

For permission to use contact: Professor Elizabeth Juniper, 20 Marcuse Fields, Bosham, West Sussex, PO18 8NA, UK

Appendix E11 Continued

Paediatric Asthma Quality of Life Questionnaire (PAQLQ) [Extract only]

On the lines below, please write down the 3 activities in which you have been bothered **most** by your asthma. We then want you to tell us how much you have been bothered doing these things **during the last week because of your asthma.**

Put an x in the box that best describes how bothered you have been.

HOW **BOTHERED** HAVE YOU BEEN DURING THE LAST WEEK?

	Extremely bothered	Very bothered	Quite bothered	Somewhat bothered	Bothered a bit	Hardly bothered at all	Not bothered	Activity not done
	1	2	3	4	5	6	7	
1. _____	☐	☐	☐	☐	☐	☐	☐	☐
2. _____	☐	☐	☐	☐	☐	☐	☐	☐
3. _____	☐	☐	☐	☐	☐	☐	☐	☐
4. COUGHING	☐	☐	☐	☐	☐	☐	☐	☐

IN GENERAL, **HOW OFTEN** DURING THE LAST WEEK DID YOU

	All of the time	Most of the time	Quite often	Some of the time	Once in a while	Hardly any of the time	None of the time
	1	2	3	4	5	6	7
5. Feel FRUSTRATED because of your asthma?	☐	☐	☐	☐	☐	☐	☐
6. Feel TIRED because of your asthma?	☐	☐	☐	☐	☐	☐	☐
7. Feel WORRIED, CONCERNED OR TROUBLED because of your asthma?	☐	☐	☐	☐	☐	☐	☐

– – – – – – – – – – – – – – – **Example of a later question** – – – – – – – – – – – – – – – –

THINK ABOUT ALL THE ACTIVITIES THAT YOU DID IN THE PAST WEEK:

	Extremely bothered	Very bothered	Quite bothered	Somewhat bothered	Bothered a bit	Hardly bothered at all	Not bothered
	1	2	3	4	5	6	7
22. How much were you bothered by your asthma during these activities?	☐	☐	☐	☐	☐	☐	☐

For permission to use contact: Professor Elizabeth Juniper, 20 Marcuse Fields, Bosham, West Sussex, P018 8NA, UK

Domain-Specific Instruments

Appendix E12 Hospital Anxiety and Depression Scale (HADS) [Extract only]

Hospital Anxiety and Depression (HAD) Scale

Name: _____   Trial No: ☐☐☐

Hospital: _____   Date of Completion: ☐☐ ☐☐ ☐☐
                                                                                              d   m   y

Doctors are aware that emotions play an important part in most illnesses. If your doctor knows about these feelings he will be able to help you more.

This questionnaire is designed to help your doctor to know how you feel. Read each item and place a firm tick in the box opposite the reply which comes closest to how you have been feeling in the past week.

Don't take too long over your replies: your immediate reaction to each item will probably be more accurate than a long thought-out response.

Tick only one box in each section

I feel tense or 'wound up':

Most of the time . . . .

A lot of the time . . . .

Time to time, occasionally . . . .

Not at all . . . .

I still enjoy the things I used to enjoy:

Definitely as much . . . .

Not quite as much . . . .

Only a little . . . .

Hardly at all . . . .

I feel as if I am slowed down:

Nearly all the time . . . .

Very often . . . .

Sometimes . . . .

Not at all . . . .

I get a sort of frightened feeling like 'butterflies' in the stomach:

Not at all . . . .

Occasionally . . . .

Quite often . . . .

Very often . . . .

For permission to use contact: Mapi Research Trust, 27, rue de la Villette, 69003 Lyon, FRANCE (www.mapi-trust.org)

Appendix E13 Short-Form McGill Pain Questionnaire (SF-MPQ)

SHORT-FORM McGILL PAIN QUESTIONNAIRE
RONALD MELZACK

PATIENT'S NAME: _____   DATE: _____

	NONE	MILD	MODERATE	SEVERE
THROBBING	0) ____	1) ____	2) ____	3) ____
SHOOTING	0) ____	1) ____	2) ____	3) ____
STABBING	0) ____	1) ____	2) ____	3) ____
SHARP	0) ____	1) ____	2) ____	3) ____
CRAMPING	0) ____	1) ____	2) ____	3) ____
GNAWING	0) ____	1) ____	2) ____	3) ____
HOT-BURNING	0) ____	1) ____	2) ____	3) ____
ACHING	0) ____	1) ____	2) ____	3) ____
HEAVY	0) ____	1) ____	2) ____	3) ____
TENDER	0) ____	1) ____	2) ____	3) ____
SPLITTING	0) ____	1) ____	2) ____	3) ____
TIRING-EXHAUSTING	0) ____	1) ____	2) ____	3) ____
SICKENING	0) ____	1) ____	2) ____	3) ____
FEARFUL	0) ____	1) ____	2) ____	3) ____
PUNISHING-CRUEL	0) ____	1) ____	2) ____	3) ____

NO PAIN ⊢————————————————————————————⊣ WORST POSSIBLE PAIN

P P I

0 NO PAIN	_____
1 MILD	_____
2 DISCOMFORTING	_____
3 DISTRESSING	_____
4 HORRIBLE	_____
5 EXCRUCIATING	_____

© Ronald Melzack, 1984

For permission to use contact: Dr Ronald Melzack, Department of Psychology, McGill University, 1205 Dr Penfield Avenue, Montreal, Quebec, Canada H3A 1B1

Appendix E14 Multidimensional Fatigue Inventory (MFI-20)

Page 1 of 2

MULTIDIMENSIONAL FATIGUE INVENTORY
MFI-20

Instructions:

By means of the following statements we would like to get an idea of how you have been feeling lately. There is, for example, the statement:

"I FEEL RELAXED"

If you think that this is entirely true, that indeed you have been feeling relaxed lately, please place an X in the extreme left box; like this:

yes, that is true [X][ ][ ][ ] no, that is not true

The more you disagree with the statement, the more you can place an X in the direction of "no, that is not true". Please, do not miss out a statement, and place one X next to each statement.

1. I feel fit   yes, that is true [ ][ ][ ][ ][ ] no, that is not true

2. Physically I feel only able to do a little   yes, that is true [ ][ ][ ][ ][ ] no, that is not true

3. I feel very active   yes, that is true [ ][ ][ ][ ][ ] no, that is not true

4. I feel like doing all sorts of nice things   yes, that is true [ ][ ][ ][ ][ ] no, that is not true

5. I feel tired   yes, that is true [ ][ ][ ][ ][ ] no, that is not true

6. I think I do a lot in a day   yes, that is true [ ][ ][ ][ ][ ] no, that is not true

7. When I am doing something, I can keep my thoughts on it   yes, that is true [ ][ ][ ][ ][ ] no, that is not true

8. Physically I can take on a lot   yes, that is true [ ][ ][ ][ ][ ] no, that is not true

9. I dread having to do things   yes, that is true [ ][ ][ ][ ][ ] no, that is not true

© E. Smets, B. Garssen, B. Bonke

For permission to use contact: Dr Ellen Smets, Academisch Medisch Centrum, Universiteit van Amsterdam, Meibergdreef 9, Postbus 22660, 1100 DD Amsterdam, The Netherlands

Appendix E14 Continued

Multidimensional Fatigue Inventory (MFI-20)

		yes, that is true						no, that is not true
10.	I think I do very little in a day							
11.	I can concentrate well							
12.	I am rested							
13.	It takes a lot of effort to concentrate on things							
14.	Physically I feel I am in a bad condition							
15.	I have a lot of plans							
16.	I tire easily							
17.	I get little done							
18.	I don't feel like doing anything							
19.	My thoughts easily wander							
20.	Physically I feel I am in an excellent condition							

Thank you very much for your cooperation

For permission to use contact: Dr Ellen Smets, Academisch Medisch Centrum, Universiteit van Amsterdam, Meibergdreef 9, Postbus 22660, 1100 DD Amsterdam, The Netherlands.

ADL and Disability

Appendix 15 (Modified) Barthel Index of Disability (MBI)

Activities of Daily Living–Modified Barthel Index

	Unable to perform task	Substantial help required	Moderate help required		Fully independent	Score
Personal hygiene	0	1	3	4	5	
Bathing self	0	1	3	4	5	
Feeding	0	2	5	8	10	
Toilet	0	2	5	8	10	
Stair climbing	0	2	5	8	10	
Dressing	0	2	5	8	10	
Bowel control	0	2	5	8	10	
Bladder control	0	2	5	8	10	
Ambulation	0	3	8	12	15	
or Wheelchair*	0	1	3	4	5	
Chair/Bed transfers	0	3	8	12	15	

Total (0–100)

*Score only if patient is unable to ambulate and is trained in wheelchair management.

For permission to use contact: Dr Surya Shah, School of Health Sciences, University of Teeside, Middlesborough TS1 3BA, UK

APPENDIX 2
Statistical tables

Table T1: Normal distribution

The value tabulated is the probability, α, that a random variable, Normally distributed with mean zero and standard deviation one will be greater than z or less than $-z$. The tabulated values are also known as two-tailed or two-sided p-values.

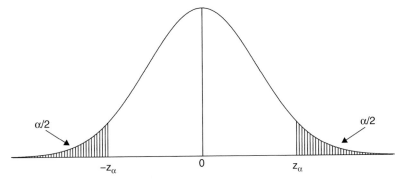

Example: The two-tailed p-value corresponding to $z = 1.96$ is 0.05.

z	α	z	α	z	α	z	α
0.00	1.0000	0.30	0.7642	0.60	0.5485	0.90	0.3681
0.01	0.9920	0.31	0.7566	0.61	0.5419	0.91	0.3628
0.02	0.9840	0.32	0.7490	0.62	0.5353	0.92	0.3576
0.03	0.9761	0.33	0.7414	0.63	0.5287	0.93	0.3524
0.04	0.9681	0.34	0.7339	0.64	0.5222	0.94	0.3472
0.05	0.9601	0.35	0.7263	0.65	0.5157	0.95	0.3421
0.06	0.9522	0.36	0.7188	0.66	0.5093	0.96	0.3371
0.07	0.9442	0.37	0.7114	0.67	0.5029	0.97	0.3320
0.08	0.9362	0.38	0.7039	0.68	0.4965	0.98	0.3271
0.09	0.9283	0.39	0.6965	0.69	0.4902	0.99	0.3222
0.10	0.9203	0.40	0.6892	0.70	0.4839	1.00	0.3173
0.11	0.9124	0.41	0.6818	0.71	0.4777	1.01	0.3125
0.12	0.9045	0.42	0.6745	0.72	0.4715	1.02	0.3077
0.13	0.8966	0.43	0.6672	0.73	0.4654	1.03	0.3030
0.14	0.8887	0.44	0.6599	0.74	0.4593	1.04	0.2983
0.15	0.8808	0.45	0.6527	0.75	0.4533	1.05	0.2937
0.16	0.8729	0.46	0.6455	0.76	0.4473	1.06	0.2891
0.17	0.8650	0.47	0.6384	0.77	0.4413	1.07	0.2846
0.18	0.8572	0.48	0.6312	0.78	0.4354	1.08	0.2801
0.19	0.8493	0.49	0.6241	0.79	0.4295	1.09	0.2757

Normal distribution: Continued

z	α	z	α	z	α	z	α
0.20	0.8415	0.50	0.6171	0.80	0.4237	1.10	0.2713
0.21	0.8337	0.51	0.6101	0.81	0.4179	1.11	0.2670
0.22	0.8259	0.52	0.6031	0.82	0.4122	1.12	0.2627
0.23	0.8181	0.53	0.5961	0.83	0.4065	1.13	0.2585
0.24	0.8103	0.54	0.5892	0.84	0.4009	1.14	0.2543
0.25	0.8026	0.55	0.5823	0.85	0.3953	1.15	0.2501
0.26	0.7949	0.56	0.5755	0.86	0.3898	1.16	0.2460
0.27	0.7872	0.57	0.5687	0.87	0.3843	1.17	0.2420
0.28	0.7795	0.58	0.5619	0.88	0.3789	1.18	0.2380
0.29	0.7718	0.59	0.5552	0.89	0.3735	1.19	0.2340
1.20	0.2301	1.70	0.0891	2.20	0.0278	2.70	0.0069
1.21	0.2263	1.71	0.0873	2.21	0.0271	2.71	0.0067
1.22	0.2225	1.72	0.0854	2.22	0.0264	2.72	0.0065
1.23	0.2187	1.73	0.0836	2.23	0.0257	2.73	0.0063
1.24	0.2150	1.74	0.0819	2.24	0.0251	2.74	0.0061
1.25	0.2113	1.75	0.0801	2.25	0.0244	2.75	0.0060
1.26	0.2077	1.76	0.0784	2.26	0.0238	2.76	0.0058
1.27	0.2041	1.77	0.0767	2.27	0.0232	2.77	0.0056
1.28	0.2005	1.78	0.0751	2.28	0.0226	2.78	0.0054
1.29	0.1971	1.79	0.0735	2.29	0.0220	2.79	0.0053
1.30	0.1936	1.80	0.0719	2.30	0.0214	2.80	0.0051
1.31	0.1902	1.81	0.0703	2.31	0.0209	2.81	0.0050
1.32	0.1868	1.82	0.0688	2.32	0.0203	2.82	0.0048
1.33	0.1835	1.83	0.0672	2.33	0.0198	2.83	0.0047
1.34	0.1802	1.84	0.0658	2.34	0.0193	2.84	0.0045
1.35	0.1770	1.85	0.0643	2.35	0.0188	2.85	0.0044
1.36	0.1738	1.86	0.0629	2.36	0.0183	2.86	0.0042
1.37	0.1707	1.87	0.0615	2.37	0.0178	2.87	0.0041
1.38	0.1676	1.88	0.0601	2.38	0.0173	2.88	0.0040
1.39	0.1645	1.89	0.0588	2.39	0.0168	2.89	0.0039
1.40	0.1615	1.90	0.0574	2.40	0.0164	2.90	0.0037
1.41	0.1585	1.91	0.0561	2.41	0.0160	2.91	0.0036
1.42	0.1556	1.92	0.0549	2.42	0.0155	2.92	0.0035
1.43	0.1527	1.93	0.0536	2.43	0.0151	2.93	0.0034
1.44	0.1499	1.94	0.0524	2.44	0.0147	2.94	0.0033
1.45	0.1471	1.95	0.0512	2.45	0.0143	2.95	0.0032
1.46	0.1443	1.96	0.0500	2.46	0.0139	2.96	0.0031
1.47	0.1416	1.97	0.0488	2.47	0.0135	2.97	0.0030
1.48	0.1389	1.98	0.0477	2.48	0.0131	2.98	0.0029
1.49	0.1362	1.99	0.0466	2.49	0.0128	2.99	0.0028
1.50	0.1336	2.00	0.0455	2.50	0.0124	3.00	0.00270
1.51	0.1310	2.01	0.0444	2.51	0.0121	3.10	0.00194
1.52	0.1285	2.02	0.0434	2.52	0.0117	3.20	0.00137
1.53	0.1260	2.03	0.0424	2.53	0.0114	3.30	0.00097
1.54	0.1236	2.04	0.0414	2.54	0.0111	3.40	0.00067
1.55	0.1211	2.05	0.0404	2.55	0.0108	3.50	0.00047
1.56	0.1188	2.06	0.0394	2.56	0.0105	3.60	0.00032
1.57	0.1164	2.07	0.0385	2.57	0.0102	3.70	0.00022
1.58	0.1141	2.08	0.0375	2.58	0.0099	3.80	0.00014
1.59	0.1118	2.09	0.0366	2.59	0.0096	3.90	0.00010
1.60	0.1096	2.10	0.0357	2.60	0.0093	4.00	0.00006
1.61	0.1074	2.11	0.0349	2.61	0.0091		
1.62	0.1052	2.12	0.0340	2.62	0.0088		
1.63	0.1031	2.13	0.0332	2.63	0.0085		
1.64	0.1010	2.14	0.0324	2.64	0.0083		
1.65	0.0989	2.15	0.0316	2.65	0.0080		
1.66	0.0969	2.16	0.0308	2.66	0.0078		
1.67	0.0949	2.17	0.0300	2.67	0.0076		
1.68	0.0930	2.18	0.0293	2.68	0.0074		
1.69	0.0910	2.19	0.0285	2.69	0.0071		

Table T2: Probability points of the Normal distribution

The value z in Table T1 is called the standard Normal deviate. This table tabulates the value of z corresponding to the probabilities, α, for one- and two-sided p-values.

Example: For an observed test statistic of $z=2.4$, the two-sided p-value is <0.02.

1-sided		2-sided
α	z	α
0.0001	3.891	0.0002
0.0005	3.291	0.0010
0.0025	2.807	0.0050
0.0050	2.576	0.0100
0.0100	2.326	0.0200
0.0125	2.241	0.0250
0.0250	1.960	0.0500
0.0500	1.645	0.1000
0.1000	1.282	0.2000
0.1500	1.036	0.3000
0.2000	0.842	0.4000
0.2500	0.674	0.5000
0.3000	0.524	0.6000
0.3500	0.385	0.7000
0.4000	0.253	0.8000

Table T3: Student's *t*-distribution

The value tabulated is t_α, such that if X is distributed as Student's t-distribution with df degrees of freedom, then α is the probability that $X \le -t_\alpha$ or $X \ge t_\alpha$.

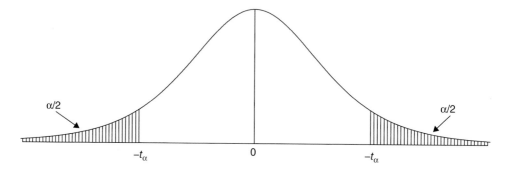

Example: The value of t_α corresponding to a two-tailed p-value of 0.05 is 1.960 if there are infinite degrees of freedom, but this increases to 2.228 if there are only 10 degrees of freedom.

Degrees of freedom	α							
	0.2	0.1	0.05	0.04	0.03	0.02	0.01	0.001
df=1	3.078	6.314	12.706	15.894	21.205	31.821	63.656	636.578
2	1.886	2.920	4.303	4.849	5.643	6.965	9.925	31.600
3	1.638	2.353	3.182	3.482	3.896	4.541	5.841	12.924
4	1.533	2.132	2.776	2.999	3.298	3.747	4.604	8.610
5	1.476	2.015	2.571	2.757	3.003	3.365	4.032	6.869
6	1.440	1.943	2.447	2.612	2.829	3.143	3.707	5.959
7	1.415	1.895	2.365	2.517	2.715	2.998	3.499	5.408
8	1.397	1.860	2.306	2.449	2.634	2.896	3.355	5.041
9	1.383	1.833	2.262	2.398	2.574	2.821	3.250	4.781
10	1.372	1.812	2.228	2.359	2.527	2.764	3.169	4.587
11	1.363	1.796	2.201	2.328	2.491	2.718	3.106	4.437
12	1.356	1.782	2.179	2.303	2.461	2.681	3.055	4.318
13	1.350	1.771	2.160	2.282	2.436	2.650	3.012	4.221
14	1.345	1.761	2.145	2.264	2.415	2.624	2.977	4.140
15	1.341	1.753	2.131	2.249	2.397	2.602	2.947	4.073
16	1.337	1.746	2.120	2.235	2.382	2.583	2.921	4.015
17	1.333	1.740	2.110	2.224	2.368	2.567	2.898	3.965
18	1.330	1.734	2.101	2.214	2.356	2.552	2.878	3.922
19	1.328	1.729	2.093	2.205	2.346	2.539	2.861	3.883
20	1.325	1.725	2.086	2.197	2.336	2.528	2.845	3.850
21	1.323	1.721	2.080	2.189	2.328	2.518	2.831	3.819
22	1.321	1.717	2.074	2.183	2.320	2.508	2.819	3.792
23	1.319	1.714	2.069	2.177	2.313	2.500	2.807	3.768
24	1.318	1.711	2.064	2.172	2.307	2.492	2.797	3.745
25	1.316	1.708	2.060	2.167	2.301	2.485	2.787	3.725
30	1.310	1.697	2.042	2.147	2.278	2.457	2.750	3.646
40	1.303	1.684	2.021	2.123	2.250	2.423	2.704	3.551
50	1.299	1.676	2.009	2.109	2.234	2.403	2.678	3.496
60	1.296	1.671	2.000	2.099	2.223	2.390	2.660	3.460
∞	1.282	1.645	1.960	2.054	2.170	2.327	2.576	3.291

Table T4: The χ^2 distribution

The value tabulated is $\chi^2(\alpha)$, such that if X is distributed as χ^2 with df degrees of freedom, then α is the probability that $X \geq \chi^2$.

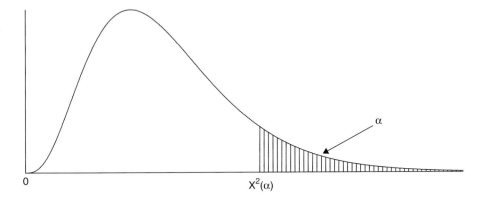

Example: If the observed test statistic, X, has a value of 7.1 with 1 degree of freedom, the p-value lies between 0.01 and 0.001.

Degrees of freedom	α							
	0.2	0.1	0.05	0.04	0.03	0.02	0.01	0.001
df=1	1.64	2.71	3.84	4.22	4.71	5.41	6.63	10.83
2	3.22	4.61	5.99	6.44	7.01	7.82	9.21	13.82
3	4.64	6.25	7.81	8.31	8.95	9.84	11.34	16.27
4	5.99	7.78	9.49	10.03	10.71	11.67	13.28	18.47
5	7.29	9.24	11.07	11.64	12.37	13.39	15.09	20.51
6	8.56	10.64	12.59	13.20	13.97	15.03	16.81	22.46
7	9.80	12.02	14.07	14.70	15.51	16.62	18.48	24.32
8	11.03	13.36	15.51	16.17	17.01	18.17	20.09	26.12
9	12.24	14.68	16.92	17.61	18.48	19.68	21.67	27.88
10	13.44	15.99	18.31	19.02	19.92	21.16	23.21	29.59
11	14.63	17.28	19.68	20.41	21.34	22.62	24.73	31.26
12	15.81	18.55	21.03	21.79	22.74	24.05	26.22	32.91
13	16.98	19.81	22.36	23.14	24.12	25.47	27.69	34.53
14	18.15	21.06	23.68	24.49	25.49	26.87	29.14	36.12
15	19.31	22.31	25.00	25.82	26.85	28.26	30.58	37.70
16	20.47	23.54	26.30	27.14	28.19	29.63	32.00	39.25
17	21.61	24.77	27.59	28.44	29.52	31.00	33.41	40.79
18	22.76	25.99	28.87	29.75	30.84	32.35	34.81	42.31
19	23.90	27.20	30.14	31.04	32.16	33.69	36.19	43.82
20	25.04	28.41	31.41	32.32	33.46	35.02	37.57	45.31
21	26.17	29.62	32.67	33.60	34.76	36.34	38.93	46.80
22	27.30	30.81	33.92	34.87	36.05	37.66	40.29	48.27
23	28.43	32.01	35.17	36.13	37.33	38.97	41.64	49.73
24	29.55	33.20	36.42	37.39	38.61	40.27	42.98	51.18
25	30.68	34.38	37.65	38.64	39.88	41.57	44.31	52.62
26	31.79	35.56	38.89	39.89	41.15	42.86	45.64	54.05
27	32.91	36.74	40.11	41.13	42.41	44.14	46.96	55.48
28	34.03	37.92	41.34	42.37	43.66	45.42	48.28	56.89
29	35.14	39.09	42.56	43.60	44.91	46.69	49.59	58.30
30	36.25	40.26	43.77	44.83	46.16	47.96	50.89	59.70

Table T5: The F-distribution

The value tabulated is $F(\alpha, v_1, v_2)$, such that if X has an F-distribution with v_1 and v_2 degrees of freedom, then α is the probability that $X \geq F(\alpha, v_1, v_2)$.

Example: For an observed test statistic of $X = 5.1$ with 3 and 4 degrees of freedom, $0.10 > \alpha > 0.05$.

v_2	α	1	2	3	4	5	6	7	8	9	10	20	∞
1	0.10	39.86	49.50	53.59	55.83	57.24	58.20	58.91	59.44	59.86	60.19	61.74	63.30
1	0.05	161.45	199.50	215.71	224.58	230.16	233.99	236.77	238.88	240.54	241.88	248.02	254.19
1	0.01	4052.18	4999.34	5403.53	5624.26	5763.96	5858.95	5928.33	5980.95	6022.40	6055.93	6208.66	6362.80
2	0.10	8.53	9.00	9.16	9.24	9.29	9.33	9.35	9.37	9.38	9.39	9.44	9.49
2	0.05	18.51	19.00	19.16	19.25	19.30	19.33	19.35	19.37	19.38	19.40	19.45	19.49
2	0.01	98.50	99.00	99.16	99.25	99.30	99.33	99.36	99.38	99.39	99.40	99.45	99.50
3	0.10	5.54	5.46	5.39	5.34	5.31	5.28	5.27	5.25	5.24	5.23	5.18	5.13
3	0.05	10.13	9.55	9.28	9.12	9.01	8.94	8.89	8.85	8.81	8.79	8.66	8.53
3	0.01	34.12	30.82	29.46	28.71	28.24	27.91	27.67	27.49	27.34	27.23	26.69	26.14
4	0.10	4.54	4.32	4.19	4.11	4.05	4.01	3.98	3.95	3.94	3.92	3.84	3.76
4	0.05	7.71	6.94	6.59	6.39	6.26	6.16	6.09	6.04	6.00	5.96	5.80	5.63
4	0.01	21.20	18.00	16.69	15.98	15.52	15.21	14.98	14.80	14.66	14.55	14.02	13.47
5	0.10	4.06	3.78	3.62	3.52	3.45	3.40	3.37	3.34	3.32	3.30	3.21	3.11
5	0.05	6.61	5.79	5.41	5.19	5.05	4.95	4.88	4.82	4.77	4.74	4.56	4.37
5	0.01	16.26	13.27	12.06	11.39	10.97	10.67	10.46	10.29	10.16	10.05	9.55	9.03
6	0.10	3.78	3.46	3.29	3.18	3.11	3.05	3.01	2.98	2.96	2.94	2.84	2.72
6	0.05	5.99	5.14	4.76	4.53	4.39	4.28	4.21	4.15	4.10	4.06	3.87	3.67
6	0.01	13.75	10.92	9.78	9.15	8.75	8.47	8.26	8.10	7.98	7.87	7.40	6.89
7	0.10	3.59	3.26	3.07	2.96	2.88	2.83	2.78	2.75	2.72	2.70	2.59	2.47
7	0.05	5.59	4.74	4.35	4.12	3.97	3.87	3.79	3.73	3.68	3.64	3.44	3.23
7	0.01	12.25	9.55	8.45	7.85	7.46	7.19	6.99	6.84	6.72	6.62	6.16	5.66
8	0.10	3.46	3.11	2.92	2.81	2.73	2.67	2.62	2.59	2.56	2.54	2.42	2.30
8	0.05	5.32	4.46	4.07	3.84	3.69	3.58	3.50	3.44	3.39	3.35	3.15	2.93
8	0.01	11.26	8.65	7.59	7.01	6.63	6.37	6.18	6.03	5.91	5.81	5.36	4.87
9	0.10	3.36	3.01	2.81	2.69	2.61	2.55	2.51	2.47	2.44	2.42	2.30	2.16
9	0.05	5.12	4.26	3.86	3.63	3.48	3.37	3.29	3.23	3.18	3.14	2.94	2.71
9	0.01	10.56	8.02	6.99	6.42	6.06	5.80	5.61	5.47	5.35	5.26	4.81	4.32
10	0.10	3.29	2.92	2.73	2.61	2.52	2.46	2.41	2.38	2.35	2.32	2.20	2.06
10	0.05	4.96	4.10	3.71	3.48	3.33	3.22	3.14	3.07	3.02	2.98	2.77	2.54
10	0.01	10.04	7.56	6.55	5.99	5.64	5.39	5.20	5.06	4.94	4.85	4.41	3.92
20	0.10	2.97	2.59	2.38	2.25	2.16	2.09	2.04	2.00	1.96	1.94	1.79	1.61
20	0.05	4.35	3.49	3.10	2.87	2.71	2.60	2.51	2.45	2.39	2.35	2.12	1.85
20	0.01	8.10	5.85	4.94	4.43	4.10	3.87	3.70	3.56	3.46	3.37	2.94	2.43
30	0.10	2.88	2.49	2.28	2.14	2.05	1.98	1.93	1.88	1.85	1.82	1.67	1.46
30	0.05	4.17	3.32	2.92	2.69	2.53	2.42	2.33	2.27	2.21	2.16	1.93	1.63
30	0.01	7.56	5.39	4.51	4.02	3.70	3.47	3.30	3.17	3.07	2.98	2.55	2.02
40	0.10	2.84	2.44	2.23	2.09	2.00	1.93	1.87	1.83	1.79	1.76	1.61	1.38
40	0.05	4.08	3.23	2.84	2.61	2.45	2.34	2.25	2.18	2.12	2.08	1.84	1.52
40	0.01	7.31	5.18	4.31	3.83	3.51	3.29	3.12	2.99	2.89	2.80	2.37	1.82
50	0.10	2.81	2.41	2.20	2.06	1.97	1.90	1.84	1.80	1.76	1.73	1.57	1.33
50	0.05	4.03	3.18	2.79	2.56	2.40	2.29	2.20	2.13	2.07	2.03	1.78	1.45
50	0.01	7.17	5.06	4.20	3.72	3.41	3.19	3.02	2.89	2.78	2.70	2.27	1.70
100	0.10	2.76	2.36	2.14	2.00	1.91	1.83	1.78	1.73	1.69	1.66	1.49	1.22
100	0.05	3.94	3.09	2.70	2.46	2.31	2.19	2.10	2.03	1.97	1.93	1.68	1.30
100	0.01	6.90	4.82	3.98	3.51	3.21	2.99	2.82	2.69	2.59	2.50	2.07	1.45
∞	0.10	2.71	2.31	2.09	1.95	1.85	1.78	1.72	1.68	1.64	1.61	1.43	1.08
∞	0.05	3.85	3.00	2.61	2.38	2.22	2.11	2.02	1.95	1.89	1.84	1.58	1.11
∞	0.01	6.66	4.63	3.80	3.34	3.04	2.82	2.66	2.53	2.43	2.34	1.90	1.16

References

Aaronson NK, Ahmedzai S, Bergman B, Bullinger M *et al.* (1993) The European Organisation for Research and Treatment of Cancer QLQ-C30: A quality-of-life instrument for use in international clinical trials in oncology. *Journal of the National Cancer Institute* **85**: 365–376.

Al-Ruthia YS, Hong SH and Solomon D (2015) Do depressed patients on adjunctive atypical antipsychotics demonstrate a better quality of life compared to those on antidepressants only? *Research in Social and Administrative Pharmacy* **11**: 228–240.

Albrecht GL and Devlieger PJ (1999) The disability paradox: high quality of life against all odds. *Social Science & Medicine* **48**: 977–988.

Altman DG (1991) *Practical Statistics for Medical Research.* London, Chapman & Hall.

Altman DG, Machin D, Bryant TN and Gardner M (2000) *Statistics with Confidence.* Chichester, British Medical Association.

Andrich D, Sheridan B and Luo G (2010) *Rasch models for measurement: RUMM2030.* Perth, RUMM Laboratory.

Ang E, Lee ST, Gan CSG, Chan YH *et al.* (2003) Pain control in a randomized, controlled, clinical trial comparing moist exposed burn ointment and conventional methods in patients with partial-thickness burns. *Journal of Burn Care & Rehabilitation* **24**: 289–296.

Apajasalo M, Sintonen H, Holmberg C, Sinkkonen J *et al.* (1996) Quality of life in early adolescence: A sixteen-dimensional health-related measure (16D). *Quality of Life Research* **5**: 205–211.

Apgar V (1953) A proposal for a new method of evaluation of the newborn infant. *Current Researches in Anesthetics and Analgesics* **32**: 260–267.

Arbuckle JL (2009) *Amos 18 User's Guide.* Crawfordville, FL, Amos Development Corporation.

Aristotle 384–322BCE (1926) *Nichomachean Ethics, Book 1 (iv).* Translated by H.Rackham. London, Heinemann.

Baker F and Intagliata J (1982) Quality of life in the evaluation of community support systems. *Evaluation and Program Planning* **5**: 69–79.

Baron-Epel O and Kaplan G (2001) General subjective health status or age-related subjective health status: does it make a difference? *Social Science & Medicine* **53**: 1373–1381.

Barrett P (2007) Structural equation modelling: adjudging model fit. *Personality and Individual Differences* **42**: 815–824.

Bartholomew DJ, Knott M and Moustaki I (2011) *Latent Variable Models and Factor Analysis.* Chichester, Wiley-Blackwell.

Quality of Life: The Assessment, Analysis and Reporting of Patient-Reported Outcomes, Third Edition.
Peter M. Fayers and David Machin.
© 2016 John Wiley & Sons, Ltd. Published 2016 by John Wiley & Sons, Ltd.

Basch E, Abernethy A, Mullins CD, Spencer M *et al.* (2011) Recommendations for incorporating patient-reported outcomes into the design of clinical trials in adult oncology. Center for Medical Technology Policy (CMTP) Effectiveness Guidance Document: 1–19 (Download from <http://www.cmtpnet.org/effectiveness-guidance-documents/oncology-pro/>).

Baxter J, Fayers PM and McKinlay AW (2010) The clinical and psychometric validation of a questionnaire to assess the quality of life of adult patients treated with long-term parenteral nutrition. *Journal of Parenteral and Enteral Nutrition* **34**: 131–142.

Beck AT, Ward CH, Mendelson M, Mock J and Erbaugh J (1961) An inventory for measuring depression. *Archives of General Psychiatry* **4**: 561–571.

Beller E, Tattersall M, Lumley T, Levi J *et al.* (1997) Improved quality of life with megestrol acetate in patients with endocrine-insensitive advanced cancer: A randomised placebo-controlled trial. *Annals of Oncology* **8**: 277–283.

Benjamini Y and Hochberg Y (1995) Controlling the false discovery rate: a practical and powerful approach to multiple testing. *Journal of the Royal Statistical Society, Series B* **57**: 289–300.

Bentler PM (1995) *EQS Structural Equations Program Manual.* Encino, CA, Multivariate Software, Inc.

Bergner M, Bobbit RA, Carter WB and Gilson BS (1981) The Sickness Impact Profile: development and final revision of a health status measure. *Medical Care* **19**: 787–805.

Berkson J (1938) Some difficulties of interpretation encountered in the application of the chi-square test. *Journal of the American Statistical Association* **33**: 526–536.

Bernhard J and Gelber RD (1998) Workshop on missing data in quality of life research in cancer clinical trials. *Statistics in Medicine* **17**: 511–796.

Bernhard J, Zahrieh D, Coates AS, Gelber RD *et al.* (2004) Quantifying trade-offs: Quality of life and quality-adjusted survival in a randomised trial of chemotherapy in postmenopausal patients with lymph node-negative breast cancer. *British Journal of Cancer* **91**: 1893–1901.

Bjordal K and Kaasa S (1995) Psychological distress in head and neck cancer patients 7–11 years after curative treatment. *British Journal of Cancer* **71**: 592–597.

Bjordal K, Kaasa S and Mastekaasa A (1994) Quality of life in patients treated for head and neck cancer: A follow-up study 7 to 11 years after radiotherapy. *International Journal of Radiation Oncology Biology Physics* **28**: 847–856.

Bjorner JB, Kosinski M and Ware JE Jr. (2003) Calibration of an item pool for assessing the burden of headaches: An application of item response theory to the Headache Impact Test (HIT). *Quality of Life Research* **12**: 913–933.

Blalock HM (1982) *Conceptualization and Measurement in the Social Sciences.* Beverly Hills, CA, SAGE Publications.

Bland JM and Altman DG (1986) Statistical methods for assessing agreement between two methods of clinical measurement. *Lancet* **1**: 307–310.

Bland JM and Altman DG (1996) *Logarithms. British Medical Journal* **312**: 700.

Blazeby JM, Fayers PM, Conroy T, Sezer O *et al.* (2009) Validation of a questionnaire, the EORTC QLQ-LMC21, to assess health-related quality of life after liver resection or palliative treatment of hepatic metastases from colorectal cancer. *British Journal of Surgery* **96**: 291–298.

Bollen KA (1989) *Structural Equations with Latent Variables.* New York, John Wiley & Sons.

Bollen KA and Bauldry S (2011) Three Cs in measurement models: Causal indicators, composite indicators, and covariates. *Psychological Methods* **16**: 265–284.

Borenstein M, Hedges LV, Higgins JPT and Rothstein HR (2009) *Introduction to Meta-Analysis*. Chichester, John Wiley & Sons.

Bowling A (2001) *Measuring Disease: A Review of Disease-specific Quality of Life Measurement Scales* (2nd edn). Buckingham, Open University Press.

Bowling A (2004) *Measuring Health: A Review of Quality of Life Measurement Scales* (3rd edn). Buckingham, Open University Press.

Bradburn NM, Sudman S and Wansink B (2004) *Asking Questions: The Definitive Guide to Questionnaire Design*. San Francisco, Jossey-Bass.

Branski RC, Cukier-Blaj S, Pusic A, Cano SJ *et al.* (2010) measuring quality of life in dysphonic patients: A systematic review of content development in patient-reported outcomes measures. *Journal of Voice* **24**: 193–198.

Brazier JE and Roberts J (2004) the estimation of a preference-based measure of health from the SF-12. *Medical Care* **42**: 851–859.

Brazier JE, Deverill A, Green C, Harper R and Booth A (1999) A review of the use of health status measures in economic evaluation. *Health Technology Assessment* **3**: i–iv, 1–164.

Brazier JE, Ratcliffe J, Salomon JA and Tsuchiya A (2007) *Measuring and Valuing Health Benefits for Economic Evaluation*. Oxford, Oxford University Press.

Brazier JE, Roberts J and Deverill M (2002) The estimation of a preference-based measure of health from the SF-36. *Journal of Health Economics* **21**: 271–292.

Brazier JE, Yang Y, Tsuchiya A, Rowen DL (2010) A review of studies mapping (or cross walking) non-preference based measures of health to generic preference-based measures. *European Journal of Health Economics* **11**: 215–225.

Bridges JFP, Hauber AB, Marshall D, Lloyd A *et al.* (2011) Conjoint analysis applications in health – a checklist: A report of the ISPOR Good Research Practices for Conjoint Analysis Task Force. *Value in Health* **14**: 403–413.

Brod, M, Tesler LE and Christensen TL (2009) Qualitative research and content validity: Developing best practices based on science and experience. *Quality of Life Research* **18**: 1263–1278.

Brooks R with the EuroQol group (1996) EuroQol: The current state of play. *Health Policy* **37**: 53–72.

Browne JP, O'Boyle CA, McGee HM, McDonald NJ and Joyce CRB (1997) Development of a direct weighting procedure for quality of life domains. *Quality of Life Research* **6**: 301–309.

Browne MW and Cudeck R (1992) Alternative ways of assessing model fit. *Sociological Methods & Research* **21**: 230–258.

Bruera E, Kuehn N, Miller MJ, Selmser P and Macmillan K (1991) The Edmonton Symptom Assessment System (ESAS): a simple method for the assessment of palliative care patients. *Journal of Palliative Care* **7**: 6–9.

Brundage M, Bass B, Davidson J, Queenan J *et al.* (2011) Patterns of reporting health-related quality of life outcomes in randomized clinical trials: Implications for clinicians and quality of life researchers. *Quality of Life Research* **20**: 653–664.

Buccheri GF, Ferrigno D, Curcio A, Vola F and Rosso A (1989) Continuation of chemotherapy versus supportive care alone in patients with inoperable non-small-cell lung cancer and stable disease after two or three cycles of MACC: Results of a randomized prospective study. *Cancer* **63**: 428–432.

Burnham KP and Anderson DR (2004) Multimodel inference: Understanding AIC and BIC in Model Selection. *Sociological Methods & Research* **33**: 261–304.

Burton P, Gurrin L and Sly P (1998) Extending the simple linear regression model to account for correlated responses: An introduction to generalized estimating equations and multi-level modeling. *Statistics in Medicine* **17**: 1261–1291.

Byrne BM (1998) *Structural Equation Modeling with Lisrel, Prelis, and Simplis: Basic Concepts, Applications, and Programming*. Mahwah, NJ, Lawrence Erlbaum.

Byrne BM (2006) *Structural Equation Modeling with EQS and EQS/WINDOWS: Basic Concepts, Applications, and Programming* (2nd edn). Mahwah, NJ, Lawrence Erlbaum.

Byrne BM (2009) *Structural Equation Modeling with AMOS: Basic Concepts, Applications and Programming* (2nd edn). New York, NY, Routledge Academic.

Byrne BM (2011) *Structural Equation Modeling with Mplus: Basic Concepts, Applications, and Programming*. New York, NY, Routledge Academic.

Cai L, Thissen D and du Toit SHC (2011) *IRTPRO for Windows* [Computer software]. Lincolnwood, IL, Scientific Software International.

Calman KC (1984) Quality of life in cancer patients: An hypothesis. *Journal of Medical Ethics* **10**: 124–127.

Calvert M, Blazeby JM, Altman DG, Revicki DA *et al.* (2013) Patient reported outcomes in randomized trials. The CONSORT PRO Extension. *Journal of the American Medical Association* **309**: 814–822.

Campbell DT and Fiske DW (1959) Convergent and discriminant validation by the multitrait-multimethod matrix. *Psychological Bulletin* **56**: 81–105.

Campbell MJ, Julious SA and Altman DG (1995) Estimating sample sizes for binary, ordered categorical, and continuous outcomes in two group comparisons. *British Medical Journal* **311**: 1145–1147.

Campbell MJ, Machin D and Walters S (2007) *Medical Statistics: A Textbook for the Health Sciences* (4th edn). Chichester, John Wiley & Sons.

Carod-Artal FJ, Coral LF, Trizotto DS and Moreira CM (2009) Self- and proxy-report agreement on the Stroke Impact Scale. *Stroke* **40**: 3308–3314.

Cattell RB (1966) Scree test for number of factors. *Multivariate Behavioral Research* **1**: 245–276.

Cella D, Hahn EA and Dineen K (2002) Meaningful change in cancer-specific quality of life scores: Differences between improvement and worsening. *Quality of Life Research* **11**: 207–221.

Cella D, Riley W, Stone A, Rothrock N *et al.* (2010) The Patient-Reported Outcomes Measurement Information System (PROMIS) developed and tested its first wave of adult self-reported health outcome item banks: 2005–2008. *Journal of Clinical Epidemiology* **63**: 1179–1194.

Cella DF, Tulsky DS, Gray G, Sarafian B *et al.* (1993) The Functional Assessment of Cancer Therapy scale: Development and validation of the general measure. *Journal of Clinical Oncology* **11**: 570–579.

Chen FF, West SG and Sousa KH (2006) A comparison of bifactor and second-order models of quality of life. *Multivariate Behavioral Research* **41**: 189–225.

Chen W-H, Lenderking W, Jin Y, Wyrwich KW, Gelhorn H and Revicki DA (2014) Is Rasch model analysis applicable in small sample size pilot studies for assessing item characteristics? An example using PROMIS pain behavior item bank data. *Quality of Life Research* **23**: 485–493.

Cherepanov D, Palta M and Fryback DG (2010) Underlying of the five health-related quality of life measures used in utility assessment. *Medical Care* **48**: 718–725.

Cheung G and Rensvold R (2002) Evaluating goodness-of-fit indexes for testing measurement invariance. *Structural Equation Modeling* **9**: 233–255.

Child D (2006) *The Essentials of Factor Analysis* (3rd edn). London, Bloomsbury Publishing.

Chinn S (2000) A simple method for converting an odds ratio to effect size for use in meta-analysis. *Statistics in Medicine* **19**: 3127–3131.

Cicardi M, Banerji A, Bracho F, Malbran A *et al.* (2010) Icatibant, a new bradykinin-receptor antagonist, in hereditary angioedema. *New England Journal of Medicine* **363**: 532–541.

Cleeland CS (1991) Pain assessment in cancer. In: OsobaD (ed.) *Effect of Cancer on Quality of Life*. Boca Raton, FL, CRC Press: 293–304.

Cleeland CS and Ryan KM (1994) Pain assessment: Global use of the Brief Pain Inventory. *Annals of the Academy of Medicine* **23**: 129–138.

Cnaan A, Laird NM and Slasor P (1997) Using the general linear mixed model to analyze unbalanced repeated measures and longitudinal data. *Statistics in Medicine* **16**: 2349–2380.

Coates A, Gebski V, Bishop JF, Jeal PN *et al.* (1987) Improving the quality of life during chemotherapy for advanced breast cancer: A comparison of intermittent and continuous treatment strategies. *New England Journal of Medicine* **317**: 1490–1495.

Coates A, Porzsolt F and Osoba D (1997) Quality of life in oncology practice: Prognostic value of EORTC QLQ-C30 scores in patients with advanced malignancy. *European Journal of Cancer* **33**: 1025–1030.

Coates A, Thomson D, McLeod GR, Hersey P *et al.* (1993) Prognostic value of quality of life scores in a trial of chemotherapy with or without interferon in patients with metastatic malignant melanoma. *European Journal of Cancer* **29A**: 1731–1734.

Cocks K, King MT, Velikova G, de Castro G *et al.* (2012) Evidence-based guidelines for interpreting change scores for the European Organisation for the Research and Treatment of Cancer quality of life questionnaire core 30 (EORTC QLQ-C30). *European Journal of Cancer* **48**: 1713–1721.

Cocks K, King MT, Velikova G, St-James MM, Fayers PM and Brown JM. (2011) Evidence-based guidelines for determination of sample size and interpretation of the European Organisation for the Research and Treatment of Cancer quality of life questionnaire core 30 (EORTC QLQ-C30). *Journal of Clinical Oncology* **29**: 89–96.

Cohen J (1988) *Statistical Power Analysis for the Behavioral Sciences* (2nd edn). Hillsdale, NJ, Lawrence Erlbaum.

Cole BF, Gelber RD and Anderson KM for the IBCSG (1994) Parametric approaches to quality-adjusted survival analysis. *Biometrics* **50**: 621–631.

Coltman T, Devinney TM, Midgley DF and Venaik S (2008) Formative versus reflective measurement models: Two applications of formative measurement. *Journal of Business Research* **61**: 1250–1262.

Consolidated Standards of Reporting Trials (CONSORT) statement and QoL Extension (2011, 2012) (Download from <http://www.consort-statement.org>).

Cook DJ, Guyatt GH, Juniper EF, Griffith L *et al.* (1993) Interviewer versus self-administered questionnaires in developing a disease-specific, health-related quality of life instrument for asthma. *Journal of Clinical Epidemiology* **46**: 529–534.

Cook L and Eignor D (1989) Using item response theory in test score equating. *International Journal of Educational Research* **13**: 161–173.

Cox DR, Fitzpatrick R, Fletcher AE, Gore SM *et al.* (1992) Quality-of-life assessment: Can we keep it simple? *Journal of the Royal Statistical Society, Series A* **155**: 353–393.

CPMP (1995) Working Party on Efficacy of Medicinal Products: Biostatistical methodology in clinical trials in applications for marketing authorizations for medicinal products. *Statistics in Medicine* **14**: 1659–1682.

Crane PK, Gibbons LE, Jolley L and van Belle G (2006) Differential item functioning analysis with ordinal logistic regression techniques: DIFdetect and difwithpar. *Medical Care* **44** (Suppl 3): S115–S123.

Cronbach LJ (1951) Coefficient alpha and the internal structure of tests. *Psychometrika* **16**: 297–334.

Cronbach LJ (2004) My current thoughts on coefficient alpha and successor procedures. *Educational and Psychological Measurement* **64**: 391–418.

Croog SH, Levine S, Testa MA, Brown B *et al.* (1986) The effects of antihypertensive therapy on the quality of life. *New England Journal of Medicine* **314**: 1657–1664.

Crott R and Briggs A (2010) Mapping the QLQ-C30 quality of life cancer questionnaire to EQ-5D patient preferences. *European Journal of Health Economics* **11**: 427–434.

Curran D, Fayers PM, Molenberghs G and Machin D (1998a) Analysis of incomplete quality of life data in clinical trials. In: StaquetM, HaysRD and FayersPM (eds), *Quality of Life Assessment in Clinical Trials*. Oxford, Oxford University Press.

Curran D, Molenberghs G, Fayers PM and Machin D (1998b) Incomplete quality of life data in randomized trials: Missing forms. *Statistics in Medicine* **17**: 697–709.

Curran D, Pozzo C, Zaluski J, Dank M *et al.* (2009) Quality of life of palliative chemotherapy naïve patients with advanced adenocarcinoma of the stomach or esophagogastric junction treated with irinotecan combined with 5-fluorouracil and folinic acid: Results of a randomised phase III trial. *Quality of Life Research* **18**: 853–861.

de Haes JCJM and Stiggelbout AM (1996) Assessment of values, utilities and preferences in cancer patients. *Cancer Treatment Reviews* **22**(suppl A): 13–26.

de Haes JCJM, Olschewski M, Fayers PM, Visser MRM *et al.* (1996) *The Rotterdam Symptom Checklist (RSCL): A Manual. Second revised edition.* UMCG/University of Groningen, Research Institute SHARE, The Netherlands. (Download from <http://www.rug.nl/research/share/research/tools/handleiding_rscl2edruk.pdf>).

de Vet HCW, Adèr HJ, Terwee CB and Pouwer F (2005) Are factor analytical techniques used appropriately in the validation of health status questionnaires? A systematic review on the quality of factor analysis of the SF-36. *Quality of Life Research* **14**: 1225–1237.

de Vet HCW, Terluin B, Knol DL, Roorda LD *et al.* (2010) Three ways to quantify uncertainty in individually applied "minimally important change" values. *Journal of Clinical Epidemiology* **63**: 37–45.

de Vet HCW, Terwee CB, Knol DL and Bouter LM (2006) When to use agreement versus reliability measures. *Journal of Clinical Epidemiology* **59**: 1033–1039.

Deng N, Allison JJ, Fang HJ, Ash AS and Ware JE (2013) Using the bootstrap to establish statistical significance for relative validity comparisons among patient-reported outcome measures. *Health and Quality of Life Outcomes* **11**: 89.

Devinsky O, Vickrey BG, Cramer J, Perrine K *et al.* (1995) Development of the quality of life in epilepsy inventory. *Epilepsia* **36**: 1089–1104.

Dewolf L, Koller M, Velikova G, Johnson CD, Scott N and Bottomley A (2009) *EORTC Quality of Life Group Translation Procedure* (3rd edn). EORTC, Brussels. (Download from <http://groups.eortc.be/qol/manuals>).

Diamantopoulos A (2008) Formative indicators: Introduction to the special issue. *Journal of Business Research* **61**: 1201–1202.

Diamantopoulos A and Siguaw JA (2006) Formative versus reflective indicators in organizational measure development: A comparison and empirical illustration. *British Journal of Management* **17**: 263–282.

Diggle PJ, Heagarty P, Liang K-Y and Zeger SL (2002) *Analysis of Longitudinal Data* (2nd edn). Oxford, Oxford University Press.

DiStefano C, Zhu M and Mindrila D (2009) Understanding and using factor scores: Considerations for the applied researcher. *Practical Assessment, Research and Evaluation* **14**: 1–11.

Dmitrienko A, D'Agostino RB and Huque MF (2013) Key multiplicity issues in clinical drug development. *Statistics in Medicine* **32**: 1079–1111.

Dobrez D, Cella D, Pickard AS, Lai J-S and Nickolov A (2007) Estimation of patient preference-based utility-weights from the Functional Assessment of Cancer Therapy-General. *Value in Health* **10**: 266–272.

Dolan P, Shaw R, Tsuchiya A and Williams A (2005) QALY maximisation and people's preferences: A methodological review of the literature. *Health Economics* **14**:197–208.

Donner A and Zou G (2002) Testing the equality of dependent intraclass correlation coefficients. *The Statistician* **51**: 367–379.

Drummond MF, Sculpher MJ, Torrance GW, O'Brien BJ and Stoddart GL (2005) *Methods for the Economic Evaluation of Health Care Programmes* (3rd edn). Oxford, Oxford University Press.

Dworkin RH, Turk DC, Wyrwich KW, Beaton D *et al.* (2008) Interpreting the clinical importance of treatment outcomes in chronic pain clinical trials: IMMPACT recommendations. *Journal of Pain* **9**: 105–121.

Edwards AL (1957) *The Social Desirability Variable in Personality Assessments and Research*. New York, Dryden.

Edwards JR (2011) The fallacy of formative measurement. *Organizational Research Methods* **14**: 370–388.

Edwards JR and Bagozzi RP (2000) On the nature and direction of relationships between constructs and measures. *Psychological Methods* **5**: 155–174.

Egger M, Davey-Smith G and Altman DG (eds) (2001) *Systematic Reviews in Health Care: Meta-analysis in Context*. London, BMJ Books.

Embretson SE and Reise SP (2000) *Item Response Theory for Psychologists*. Mahwah, NJ, Lawrence Erlbaum.

Ettema TP, Droes RM, de Lange J, Mellenbergh GJ and Ribbe MW (2005) A review of quality of life instruments used in dementia. *Quality of Life Research* **14**: 675–686.

European Medicines Agency (EMA) (2000) Points to consider on switching between superiority and non-inferiority. CPMP/EWP/482/99. (Download from <www.ema.europa.eu>).

European Medicines Agency (EMA) (2002) Points to consider on multiplicity issues in clinical trials. CPMP/EWP/908/99. (Download from <www.ema.europa.eu>).

European Medicines Agency (EMA) (2003) Points to consider on adjustment for baseline covariates. CPMP/EWP/2863/99. (Download from <www.ema.europa.eu>).

European Medicines Agency (EMA) (2005a) Guideline on the choice of the non-inferiority margin. EMEA/CPMP/EWP/2158/99 Rev. 1. (Download from <www.ema.europa.eu>).

European Medicines Agency (EMA) (2005b) Reflection paper on the regulatory guidance for the use of health-related quality of life (HRQL) measures in the evaluation of medicinal products. (Download from <www.ema.europa.eu/docs/en_GB/document_library/Scientific_guideline/2009/09/WC500003637.pdf>).

European Medicines Agency (EMA) (2010) Guideline on missing data in confirmatory clinical trials. EMA/CPMP/EWP/1776/99 Rev. 1. (Download from <www.ema.europa.eu>).

Fairclough DL (2010) *Design and Analysis of Quality of Life Studies in Clinical Trials* (2nd edn). Boca Raton, FL, Chapman & Hall/CRC.

Fallowfield L, Gagnon D, Zagari M, Cella D *et al.* (2002) Multivariate regression analyses of data from a randomised, double-blind, placebo-controlled study confirm quality of life benefit of epoetin alfa in patients receiving non-platinum chemotherapy. *British Journal of Cancer* **87**: 1341–1353.

Fayers PM (2004) Quality of life measurement in clinical trials: The impact of causal variables. *Journal of Biopharmaceutical Statistics* **14**: 155–176.

Fayers PM (2011) Alphas, betas and skewy distributions: Two ways of getting the wrong answer *Advances in Health Sciences Education* **16**: 291–296.

Fayers PM and Aaronson NK (2012) "It ain't over till the fat lady sings": A response to Cameron N. McIntosh, Improving the evaluation of model fit in confirmatory factor analysis. *Quality of Life Research* **21**: 1623–1624.

Fayers PM and Hand DJ (1997a) Factor analysis, causal indicators, and quality of life. *Quality of Life Research* **6**: 139–150.

Fayers PM and Hand DJ (1997b) Generalisation from phase III clinical trials: Survival, quality of life, and health economics. *Lancet* **350**: 1025–1027.

Fayers PM and Hand DJ (2002) Causal variables, indicator variables and measurement scales: An example from quality of life. *Journal of the Royal Statistical Society Series A* **165**: 233–261.

Fayers PM and Hays RD (2014a) Don't middle your MIDs: Regression to the mean shrinks estimates of minimally important differences. *Quality of Life Research* **23**: 1–4.

Fayers PM and Hays RD (2014b) Should linking replace regression when mapping from profile-based measures to preference-based measures? *Value in Health* **17**: 261–265.

Fayers PM, Aaronson NK, Bjordal K, Groenvold M *et al.* on behalf of the EORTC Quality of Life Study Group (2001) *EORTC QLQ-C30 Scoring Manual* (3rd edn). Brussels, EORTC. (Download from <http://groups.eortc.be/qol/manuals>).

Fayers PM, Bleehen NM, Girling DJ and Stephens RJ (1991) Assessment of quality of life in small-cell lung cancer using a Daily Diary Card developed by the Medical Research Council Lung Cancer Working Party. *British Journal of Cancer* **64**: 299–306.

Fayers PM, Groenvold M, Hand DJ and Bjordal K (1998b) Clinical impact versus factor analysis for quality of life questionnaire construction. *Journal of Clinical Epidemiology* **51**: 285–286.

Fayers PM, Hand DJ, Bjordal K and Groenvold M (1997a) Causal indicators in quality of life research. *Quality of Life Research* **6**: 393–406.

Fayers PM, Hjermstad MJ, Klepstad P, Loge J-H *et al.* (2011) The dimensionality of pain: Palliative care and chronic pain patients differ in their reports of pain intensity and pain interference. *Pain* **152**: 1608–1620.

Fayers PM, Hjermstad MJ, Ranhoff AH, Kaasa S *et al.* (2005) Which Mini-Mental State Exam (MMSE) items can be used to screen for delirium and cognitive impairment? *Journal of Pain and Symptom Management* **30**: 41–50.

Fayers PM, Hopwood P, Harvey A, Girling DJ *et al.* (1997b) Quality of life assessment in clinical trials: Guidelines and a checklist for protocol writers: The UK Medical Research Council experience. *European Journal of Cancer Part A* **33**: 20–28.

Fayers PM, King M (2008a) The baseline characteristics did not differ significantly. *Quality of Life Research* **17**: 1047–1048.

Fayers PM, King M (2008b) A highly significant difference in baseline characteristics: The play of chance or evidence of a more selective game? *Quality of Life Research* **17**: 1121–1123.

Fayers PM, Langston AL and Robertson C (2007) Implicit self-comparisons against others could bias quality of life assessments. *Journal of Clinical Epidemiology* **60**: 1034–1039.

Feeny D, Furlong W, Boyle M and Torrance GW (1995) Multi-attribute health-status classification systems: Health Utilities Index. *Pharmaco Economics* **7**: 490–502.

Feeny DH, Furlong WJ, Torrance GW, *et al.* (2002) Multiattribute and single-attribute utility function: The Health Utility Index Mark 3 system. *Medical Care* **40**: 113–128.

Feinstein AR (1987) *Clinimetrics*. New Haven, CT, Yale University Press.

Ferguson GA (1941) The factorial interpretation of test difficulty. *Psychometrika* **6**: 323–329.

Fielding S, Fayers PM and Ramsay CR (2009) Investigating the missing data mechanism in quality of life outcomes: A comparison of approaches. *Health and Quality of Life Outcomes* **7**: 57.

Fielding S, Fayers PM, Loge JH, Jordhøy MS and Kaasa S (2006) Methods for handling missing data in palliative care research. *Palliative Medicine* **20**: 791–798.

Fielding S, Maclennan G, Cook JA and Ramsay CR (2008) A review of RCTs in four medical journals to assess the use of imputation to overcome missing data in quality of life outcomes. *Trials* **9**: 51.

Fieller EC, Hartley HO and Pearson ES (1957) Tests for Rank Correlation Coefficients. *I. Biometrika* **44**: 470–481.

Fisher RA (1925) *Statistical Methods for Research Workers*. Edinburgh, Oliver and Boyd.

Fleiss JL and Cohen J (1973) The equivalence of weighted kappa and the intraclass correlation coefficient as measures of reliability. *Educational and Psychological Measurement* **33**: 613–619.

Fliege H, Becker J, Walter OB, Bjorner JB, Klapp BF and Rose M (2005) Development of a computer-adaptive test for depression (D-CAT). *Quality of Life Research* **14**: 2277–2291.

Fornell C and Bookstein FL (1982) Two structural equation models: LISREL and PLS applied to consumer exit-voice theory. *Journal of Marketing Research* **19**: 440–452.

Fortune-Greeley AK, Flynn KE, Jeffery DD, Williams MS *et al.* (2009) Using cognitive interviews to evaluate items for measuring sexual functioning across cancer populations: Improvements and remaining challenges. *Quality of Life Research* **18**: 1085–1093.

Fox-Rushby JA and Hanson K (2001) Calculating and presenting disability adjusted life years (DALYs) in cost-effectiveness analysis. *Health Policy and Planning* **16**: 326–331.

Francis JJ, Johnston M, Robertson C, Glidewell L *et al.* (2010) What is an adequate sample size? Operationalising data saturation for theory-based interview studies. *Psychology and Health* **25**: 1229–1245.

Gafni A, Birch S, Mehrez A (1993) Economics, health and health economics – HYEs versus QALYs. *Journal of Health Economics* **2**: 325–339.

Ganz PA, Haskell CM, Figlin RA, La SN and Siau J (1988) Estimating the quality of life in a clinical trial of patients with metastatic lung cancer using the Karnofsky performance status and the Functional Living Index–Cancer. *Cancer* **61**: 849–856.

Geddes DM, Dones L, Hill E, Law K *et al.* (1990) Quality of life during chemotherapy for small-cell lung cancer: Assessment and use of a daily diary card in a randomized trial. *European Journal of Cancer* **26**: 484–492.

Gelber RD, Cole BF, Gelber S and Goldhirsch A (1995) Comparing treatments using quality-adjusted survival: The Q-TWiST method. *American Statistician* **49**: 161–169.

Gibson WA (1960) Nonlinear factors in two dimensions. *Psychometrika* **25**: 381–392.

Giesinger JM, Petersen MAa, Groenvold M, Aaronson NK *et al.* (2011) Cross-cultural development of an item list for computer-adaptive testing of fatigue in oncological patients. *Health and Quality of Life Outcomes* **9**: 19.

Gill TM (1995) Quality of life assessment: Values and pitfalls. *Journal of Royal Society of Medicine* **88**: 680–682.

Gill TM and Feinstein AR (1994) A critical appraisal of the quality of quality-of-life measurements. *Journal of American Medical Association* **272**: 619–626.

Glaser AW, Nik Abdul Rashid NF, U CL and Walker DA (1997) School behaviour and health status after central nervous system tumours in childhood. *British Journal of Cancer* **76**: 643–650.

Glick HA, Doshi JA, Sonnad SS, Polsky D (2007) *Economic Evaluation in Clinical Trials.* Oxford, Oxford University Press.

Gorecki C, Brown JM, Cano S, Lamping DL *et al.* (2013) Development and validation of a new patient-reported outcome measure for patients with pressure ulcers: The PU-QOL instrument. *Health and Quality of Life Outcomes* **11**: 95.

Gorsuch RL (1983) *Factor Analysis* (2nd edn). Hillsdale, NJ, Lawrence Erlbaum.

Gotay CC and Moore TD (1992) Assessing quality of life in head and neck cancer. *Quality of Life Research* **1**: 5–17.

Gotay CC, Kawamoto CT, Bottomley A and Efficace F (2008) The prognostic significance of patient-reported outcomes in cancer clinical trials. *Journal of Clinical Oncology* **26**: 1355–1363.

Gough IR, Furnival CM, Schilder L and Grove W (1983) Assessment of the quality of life of patients with advanced cancer. *European Journal of Cancer Clinical Oncology* **19**: 1161–1165.

Grant A, Wileman S, Ramsay C, Bojke L *et al.* (2008) The effectiveness and cost-effectiveness of minimal access surgery amongst people with gastro-oesophageal reflux disease – a UK collaborative study. The REFLUX trial. *Health Technology Assessment* **12**(31).

Greimel ER, Padilla GV and Grant MM (1997) Physical and psychosocial outcomes in cancer patients: A comparison of different age groups. *British Journal of Cancer* **76**: 251–255.

Greiner W, Weijnen T, Nieuwenhuizen M, Oppe S *et al.* (2003) A single European currency for EQ-5D health states. Results from a six country study. *European Journal of Health Economics* **4**: 222–231.

Grice JW (2001) Computing and evaluating factor scores. *Psychological Methods* **6**: 430–450.

Groenvold M, Bjørner JB, Klee MC and Kreiner S (1995) Test for item bias in a quality of life questionnaire. *Journal of Clinical Epidemiology* **48**: 805–816.

Groenvold M, Fayers PM, Sprangers MAG, Bjørner JB *et al.* (1999) Anxiety and depression in breast cancer patients at low risk of recurrence compared with the general population: A valid comparison? *Journal of Clinical Epidemiology* **52**: 523–530.

Gundy C and Aaronson NK (2008) The influence of proxy perspective on patient-proxy agreement in the evaluation of health-related quality of life: An empirical study. *Medical Care* **46**: 209–216.

Gundy C and Aaronson NK (2010) Effects of mode of administration (MOA) on the measurement properties of the EORTC QLQ-C30: a randomized study. *Health and Quality of Life Outcomes* **8**: 35.

Gundy CM, Fayers PM, Groenvold M, Petersen MA *et al.* (2012) Comparing Higher Order Models for the EORTC QLQ-C30. *Quality of Life Research* **21**: 1623–1624.

Guyatt G and Schunemann H (2007) How can quality of life researchers make their work more useful to health workers and their patients? *Quality of Life Research* **16**: 1097–1105.

Guyatt GH, Feeny DH and Patrick DL (1993) Measuring health-related quality of life. *Annals of Internal Medicine* **118**: 622–629.

Guyatt GH, Juniper EF, Walter SD, Griffith LE and Goldstein RS (1998) Interpreting treatment effects in randomised trials. *British Medical Journal* **316**: 690–693.

Hahn EA, Cella D, Chassany O, Fairclough DL, Wong GY and Hays RD (2007) Precision of health-related quality-of-life data compared with other clinical measures. *Mayo Clinic Procedings* **82**: 1244–1254.

Haley SM, McHorney CA and Ware JE (1994) Evaluation of the MOS SF-36 physical functioning scale (PF-10): (1) unidimensionality and reproducibility of the Rasch item scale. *Journal of Clinical Epidemiology* **47**: 671–684.

Hambleton RK and Swaminathan (1991) *Fundamentals of Item Response Theory*. Thousand Oaks, CA, SAGE Publications.

Han KR and Kim C (2010) The long-term outcome of mandibular nerve block with alcohol for the treatment of trigeminal neuralgia. *Anesthesia and Analgesia* **111**: 550–553.

Hand DJ (2004) *Measurement: Theory and practice*. Chichester, John Wiley & Sons.

Hart O, Mullee MA, Lewith G and Miller J (1997) Double-blind, placebo-controlled, randomized trial of homeopathic arnica C30 for pain and infection after total abdominal hysterectomy. *Journal of Royal Society of Medicine* **90**: 73–78.

Hays RD, Farivar SS and Liu H (2005) Approaches and recommendations for estimating minimally important differences for health-related quality of life measures. *Journal of Chronic Obstructive Pulmonary Disease* **2**: 63–67.

Hays RD, Kim W, Spritzer KL, Kaplan RM *et al.* (2009) Effects of mode and order of administration on generic health-related quality of life scores. *Value in Health* **12**: 1035–1039.

Hedges LV and Olkin I (1985) *Statistical Methods in Meta-analysis*. Orlando, Academic Press.

Helbostad JL, Oldervoll LM, Fayers PM, Jordhøy MS *et al.* (2011) Development of a computer-administered mobility questionnaire. *Supportive Care in Cancer* **19**: 745–755.

Herdman M, Gudex C, Lloyd A, Janssen M *et al.* (2011) Development and preliminary testing of the new five-level version of EQ-5D (EQ-5D-5L). *Quality of Life Research* **20**: 1727–1736.

Hickey AM, Bury G, O'Boyle CA, Bradley F *et al*. (1996) A new short form individual quality of life measure (SEIQoL-DW): Application in a cohort of individuals with HIV/ AIDS. *British Medical Journal* **313**: 29–33.

Higgins JPT and Green S (eds) (2011) *Cochrane Handbook for Systematic Reviews of Interventions 5.1.0* [updated March 2011]. The Cochrane Collaboration, 2011. (Download from <www.cochrane-handbook.org>).

Higgins JPT and Thompson SG (2002) Quantifying heterogeneity in meta-analysis. *Statistics in Medicine* **21**: 1539–1558.

Hjermstad MJ, Fayers PM, Bjordal K and Kaasa S (1998a) Health-related quality of life in the general Norwegian population assessed by the European Organisation for Research and Treatment of Cancer Core Quality-of-Life Questionnaire: The QLQ-C30 (+3). *Journal of Clinical Oncology* **16**: 1188–1196.

Hjermstad MJ, Fayers PM, Bjordal K and Kaasa S (1998b) Using reference data on quality of life: The importance of adjusting for age and gender, exemplified by the EORTC QLQ-C30 (+3). *European Journal of Cancer* **34**: 1381–1389.

Hjermstad MJ, Fayers PM, Haugen DF, Caraceni A *et al*. (2011) Studies comparing numerical rating scales, verbal rating scales, and visual analogue scales for assessment of pain intensity in adults: A systematic literature review. *Journal of Pain and Symptom Management* **41**: 1073–1093.

Hocaoglu MB, Gaffan EA and Ho AK (2012) Health-related quality of life in Huntington's disease patients: A comparison of proxy assessment and patient self-rating using the disease-specific Huntington's disease health-related quality of life questionnaire (HDQoL). *Journal of Neurology* **259**: 1793–1800.

Holland PW and Wainer H (eds) (1993) *Differential Item Functioning*. Hillsdale, NJ, Lawrence Erlbaum.

Holm S (1979) A simple sequentially rejective multiple test procedure. *Scandinavian Journal of Statistics* **6**: 65–70.

Holmes TH and Rahe RH (1967) *The Social Readjustment Rating Scale. Journal of Psychosomatic Research* **11**: 213–218.

Holzner B, Efficace F, Basso U, Johnson CD *et al*. (2013) Cross-cultural development of an EORTC questionnaire to assess health-related quality of life in patients with testicular cancer: The EORTC QLQ-TC26. *Quality of Life Research* **22**: 369–378.

Holzner B, Kemmler G, Sperner-Unterweger B, Kopp M *et al*. (2001) Quality of life measurement in oncology: A matter of the assessment instrument? *European Journal of Cancer* **37**: 2349–2356.

Homma Y, Kakizaki H, Ymaguchi O, Yamanishi T *et al*. (2011) Assessment of overactive bladder symptoms: Comparison of 3-day bladder diary and the overactive bladder symptoms score. *Urology* **77**: 60–64.

Homs MYV, Steyerberg EW, Eijkenboom WMH, Tilanus HW *et al*. (2004) Single-dose brachytherapy versus metal stent placement for the palliation of dysphagia from oesophageal cancer: Multicentre randomised trial. *Lancet* **364**: 1497–1504.

Hopwood P, Stephens RJ and Machin D for the Medical Research Council Lung Cancer Working Party (1994) Approaches to the analysis of quality of life data: Experiences gained from a Medical Research Council Lung Cancer Working Party palliative chemotherapy trial. *Quality of Life Research* **3**: 339–352.

Hsieh C-M (2012) Should we give up domain importance weighting in QoL measures? *Social Indicators Research* **108**: 99–109.

Hu LT and Bentler PM (1999) Cutoff criteria for fit indexes in covariance structure analysis: Conventional criteria versus new alternatives. *Structural Equation Modeling* **6**: 1–55.

Hunt SM and McKenna SP (1992) The QLDS: A scale for the measurement of quality of life in depression. *Health Policy* **22**: 307–319.

Hunt SM, McKenna SP, McEwen J, Williams J and Papp E (1981) The Nottingham Health Profile: Subjective health status and medical consultations. *Social Science & Medicine* **15A**: 221–229.

Hürny C, Bernhard J, Bacchi M, Vanwegberg B *et al.* (1993) The perceived adjustment to chronic illness scale (PACIS): a global indicator of coping for operable breast-cancer patients in clinical-trials. *Supportive Care in Cancer* **1**: 200–208.

Hürny C, Bernhard J, Joss R, Willems Y *et al.* (1992) Feasibility of quality of life assessment in a randomized phase III trial of small-cell lung cancer: A lesson from the real world: The Swiss Group for Clinical Cancer Research SAKK. *Annals of Oncology* **3**: 825–831.

Husted JB, Cook RJ, Farewell VT and Gladmand DD (2000) Methods for assessing responsiveness: A critical review and recommendations. *Journal of Clinical Epidemiology* **5**: 459–468.

Islam S, Ahmed M, Walton GM, Dinan TG and Hoffman GR (2010) The association between depression and anxiety disorders following facial trauma—A comparative study. *Injury* **41**: 92–96.

Jachuk SJ, Brierly H, Jachuk S and Willcox PM (1982) The effect of hypotensive drugs on quality of life. *Journal of the Royal College of General Practitioners* **32**: 103–105.

Jaeschke R, Singer J and Guyatt GH (1989) Measurement of health status: Ascertaining the minimally clinically important difference. *Controlled Clinical Trials* **10**: 407–415.

Jarvis C, MacKenzie S and Podsakoff P (2003) A critical review of construct indicators and measurement model misspecification in marketing and consumer research. *Journal of Consumer Research* **30**: 199–218.

Jenkins CD (1992) Quality-of-life assessment in heart surgery. *Theoretical Surgery* **7**: 14–17.

Johnson C, Aaronson N, Blazeby JM, Bottomley A *et al.* (2011) *EORTC Quality of Life Group Guidelines for Developing Questionnaire Modules* (4th edn). Brussels, EORTC. (Download from <http://groups.eortc.be/qol/manuals>).

Johnson C, Fitzsimmons D, Gilbert J, Arrarras J-I *et al.* (2010) Development of the European Organisation for Research and Treatment of Cancer quality of life questionnaire module for older people with cancer: The EORTC QLQ-ELD15. *European Journal of Cancer* **46**: 2242–2252.

Johnson T, Kulesa P, Cho YI and Shavitt S (2005) The relation between culture and response styles evidence from 19 countries. *Journal of Cross-Cultural Psychology* **36**: 264–277.

Jones AP, Riley RD, Williamson PR and Whitehead A (2009) Meta-analysis of individual patient data versus aggregate data from longitudinal clinical trials. *Clinical Trials* **6**: 16–27.

Jones DA and West RR (1996) Psychological rehabilitation after myocardial infarction: Multicentre randomised controlled trial. *British Medical Journal* **313**: 1517–1521.

Jordhøy MS, Fayers PM, Loge JH, Ahlner-Elmqvist M and Kaasa S (2001) Quality of life in palliative cancer care. Results from a cluster randomized trial. *Journal of Clinical Oncology* **19**: 3884–3894.

Jordhøy MS, Saltvedt I, Fayers PM, Loge JH, Ahlner-Elmqvist M and Kaasa S (2003) Which cancer patients die in nursing homes? Quality of life, medical and sociodemographic characteristics. *Palliative Medicine* **17**: 433–444.

Jöreskog KG and Sörbom D (2006) *LISREL 8.8 for Windows [Computer software]*. Lincolnwood, IL, Scientific Software International, Inc.

Joyce CRB, Hickey A, McGee HM and O'Boyle CA (2003) A theory-based method for the evaluation of individual quality of life: The SEIQoL. *Quality of Life Research* **12**: 275–280.

Julious SA and Campbell MJ (1996) Sample sizes calculations for ordered categorical data. *Statistics in Medicine* **15**: 1065–1066.

Julious SA, George S, Machin D and Stephens RJ (1997) Sample sizes for randomized trials measuring quality of life in cancer patients. *Quality of Life Research* **6**: 109–117.

Juniper EF, Guyatt GH, Feeny DH, Ferrie PJ et al. (1996) Measuring quality of life in children with asthma. *Quality of Life Research* **5**: 35–46.

Juniper EF, Guyatt GH, Ferrie PJ and Griffith LE (1993) Measuring quality of life in asthma. *American Review of Respiratory Disease* **147**: 832–838.

Juniper EF, Guyatt GH, Streiner DL and King DR (1997) Clinical impact versus factor analysis for quality of life questionnaire construction. *Journal of Clinical Epidemiology* **50**: 233–238.

Junker BW and Sijtsma K (2000) Latent and manifest monotonicity in item response models. *Applied Psychological Measurement* **24**: 65–81.

Kahan BC and Morris TP (2012) Improper analysis of trials randomised using stratified blocks or minimisation. *Statistics in Medicine* **31**: 328–340.

Kahan BC and Morris TP (2013) Analysis of multicentre trials with continuous outcomes: When and how should we account for treatment effects? *Statistics in Medicine* **32**: 1136–1149.

Kahneman D and Tversky A (1984) Choices, values and frames. *American Psychologist* **39**: 341–350.

Kaiser HF (1960) The application of electronic computers to factor analysis. *Educational and Psychological Measurement* **20**: 141–151.

Kaplan RM, Bush JW and Berry CC (1979) Health status index category rating versus magnitude estimation for measuring levels of well-being. *Medical Care* **17**: 501–525.

Karnofsky DA and Burchenal JH (1947) The clinical evaluation of chemotherapeutic agents in cancer. In: MacleadCM (ed) *Evaluation of Chemotherapeutic Agents*. New York, Columbia University Press.

Katz LA, Ford AB, Moskowitz RW, Jackson BA and Jaffe MW (1963) Studies of illness in the aged: The index of ADL: A standardized measure of biological and psychosocial function. *Journal of American Medical Association* **185**: 914–919.

Kenward MG and Carpenter J (2007) Multiple imputation: Current perspectives. *Statistical Methods in Medical Research* **16**: 199–218.

Kerr, C, Nixon A and Wild D (2010) Assessing and demonstrating data saturation in qualitative inquiry supporting patient reported outcomes research. *Expert Review of Pharmacoeconomics & Outcomes Research* **10**: 269–281.

Khanna D, Maranian P, Rothrock N, Cella D et al. (2012) Feasibility and Construct Validity of PROMIS and Legacy Instruments in an Academic Scleroderma Clinic—Analysis from the UCLA Scleroderma Quality of Life Study. *Value in Health* **15**: 128–134.

Kharroubi SA, Brazier JE, Roberts J and O´Hagan A (2007) Modelling SF-6D health state preference data using a nonparametric Bayesian method. *Journal of Health Economics* **26**: 597–612.

King MT (2011) A point of minimal important difference (MID): a critique of terminology and methods. *Expert Review of Pharmacoeconomics and Outcomes Research* **11**: 171–184.

King MT and Dobson A (2000) Estimating the responsiveness of an instrument using more than two repeated measures. *Biometrics* **56**: 1197–1203.

King MT, Stockler MR, Cella DF, Osoba D *et al.* (2010) Meta-analysis provides evidence-based effect sizes for a cancer-specific quality of life questionnaire, the FACT-G. *Journal of Clinical Epidemiology* **63**: 270–281.

Kline RB (2010) *Principles and Practice of Structural Equation Modeling* (3rd edn). New York, Guilford Press.

Klinkhammer-Schalke M, Koller M, Steinger B, Ehret C *et al.* (2012) Direct improvement of quality of life using a tailored quality of life diagnosis and therapy pathway: Randomised trial in 200 women with breast cancer. *British Journal of Cancer* **106**: 826–838.

Knols RH, de Bruin ED, Uebelhart D, Aufdemkampe G *et al.* (2011) Effects of an outpatient physical exercise program on hematopoietic stem-cell transplantation recipients: A randomized clinical trial. *Bone Marrow Transplantation* **46**: 1245–1255.

Kolen MJ and Brennan RL (2010) *Test Equating, Scaling, and Linking: Methods and Practices* (2nd edn). New York, Springer.

Koller M, Aaronson NK, Blazeby JM, Bottomley A *et al.* (2007) Translation procedures for standardised quality of life questionnaires: The European Organisation for Research and Treatment of Cancer (EORTC) approach. *European Journal of Cancer* **43**: 1810–1820.

Kottner J, Audig L, Brorsonc S, Donner A *et al.* (2011) Guidelines for reporting reliability and agreement studies (GRRAS) were proposed. *Journal of Clinical Epidemiology* **64**: 96–106.

Kottschade LA, Sloan JA, Mazurczak MA, Johnson DB *et al.* (2011) The use of vitamin E for the prevention of chemotherapy-induced peripheral neuropathy: Results of a randomized phase III clinical trial. *Support Care Cancer* **19**: 1769–1777.

Kraemer HC, Periyakoil VS and Nodal A (2002) Kappa coefficients in medical research. *Statistics in Medicine* **21**: 2109–2129.

Krueger RA and Casey MA (2000) *Focus Groups A practical guide for applied research* (3rd edn). Thousand Oaks, Sage Publications, Inc.

Kvam AK, Fayers PM and Wisløff F (2010) What changes in health-related quality of life matter to multiple myeloma patients? A prospective study. *European Journal of Haematology* **84**: 345–353.

Lai J-S, Cella D, Chang C-H, Bode RK and Heinemann AW (2003) Item banking to improve, shorten and computerize self-reported fatigue: An illustration of steps to create a core item bank from the FACIT-Fatigue Scale. *Quality of Life Research* **12**: 485–501.

Lai J-S, Cella D, Dineen K, Bode RK *et al.* (2005) An item bank was created to improve the measurement of cancer-related fatigue. *Journal of Clinical Epidemiology* **16**: 1188–1196.

Landgraf JM (2005) Practical considerations in the measurement of HRQoL in child/adolescent clinical trials. In: FayersPM and HaysRD (eds), *Assessing Quality of Life in Clinical Trials: Methods and Practice* (2nd edn). Oxford, Oxford University Press.

Landis JR and Koch GG (1977) The measurement of observer agreement for categorical data. *Biometrics* **33**: 159–74.

Lee N and Cadogan JW (2013) Problems with formative and higher-order reflective variables. *Journal of Business Research* **66**: 242–247.

Lee N, Coxeter P, Beckmann M, Webster J *et al.* (2011) A randomised non-inferiority controlled trial of a single versus a four intradermal sterile water injection technique for relief of continuous lower back pain during labour. *BMC Pregnancy and Childbirth* **11**: 21.

Lee SY, Poon WY and Bentler PM (1995) A 2-stage estimation of structural equation models with continuous and polytomous variables. *British Journal of Mathematical and Statistical Psychology* **48**: 339–358.

Lehoux P, Poland B and Daudel G (2006) Focus group research and 'the patient's view'. *Social Science & Medicine* **63**: 2091–2104.

Lemmens J, Bours GJ, Limburg M and Beurskens AJ (2013) The feasibility and test–retest reliability of the Dutch Swal-Qol adapted interview version for dysphagic patients with communicative and/or cognitive problems. *Quality of Life Research* **22**: 891–895.

Likert RA (1932) A technique for the measurement of attitudes. *Archives of Psychology* **140**: 1–55.

Likert RA (1952) A technique for the development of attitude scales. *Educational and Psychological Measurement* **12**: 313–315.

Linacre JM (2011) *WINSTEPS: Rasch Measurement Computer Program*. Beaverton, OR, Winsteps.com.

Linde K, Mulrow CD, Berner M and Egger M (2005) St John's Wort for depression. *The Cochrane Database of Systematic Reviews: Issue 3*. Chichester, John Wiley & Sons.

Linder JA and Singer DE (2003) Health-related quality of life of adults with upper respiratory tract infections. *Journal of General Internal Medicine* **18**: 802–807.

Lindley C, Vasa S, Sawyer WT and Winer EP (1998) Quality of life and preferences for treatment following systemic therapy for early-stage breast cancer. *Journal of Clinical Oncology* **16**: 1380–1387.

Little RJA and Rubin DB (2002) *Statistical Analysis with Missing Data* (2nd edn.) New York, John Wiley & Sons.

Lohr KN for the Scientific Advisory Committee of the Medical Outcomes Trust (2002) Assessing health status and quality of life instruments: Attributes and review criteria. *Quality of Life Research* **11**: 193–205.

Lord FM and Novick MR (1968) *Statistical Theories of Mental Test Scores*. Reading, MA, Addison-Wesley.

Luckett T, King MT, Butow PN, Oguchi M *et al.* (2011) Choosing between the EORTC QLQ-C30 and FACT-G for measuring health-related quality of life in cancer clinical research: Issues, evidence and recommendations. *Annals of Oncology* **22**: 2179–2190.

Lunn D, Spiegelhalter DJ, Thomas A, Best NG (2009) The BUGS project: Evolution, critique and future directions (with discussion). *Statistics in Medicine* **28**: 3049–3082.

Lydick E, Epstein RS, Himmelberger DU and White CJ (1995) Area under the curve: A metric for patient subjective responses in episodic diseases. *Quality of Life Research* **4**: 41–45.

Machin D and Weeden S (1998) Suggestions for the presentation of quality of life data from clinical trials. *Statistics in Medicine* **17**: 711–724.

Machin D, Campbell MJ, Tan S-B and Tan S-H (2008) *Sample Size Tables for Clinical Studies* (3rd edn). Chichester, Wiley Blackwell.

Machin D, Cheung YB and Parmar MKB (2006) *Survival Analysis: A Practical Approach* (2nd edn). Chichester, John Wiley & Sons.

Magasi S, Ryan G, Revicki D, Lenderking W *et al.* (2012) Content validity of patient-reported outcome measures: Perspectives from a PROMIS meeting. *Quality of Life Research* **21**: 739–746.

Mahoney FI and Barthel DW (1965) Functional evaluation: The Barthel Index. *Maryland State Medical Journal* **14**: 61–65.

Marino BS, Tomlinson RS, Wernovsky G, Drotar D *et al.* (2010) Validation of the Pediatric Cardiac Quality of Life Inventory. *Pediatrics* **126**: 498–508.

Marquise P, Keininger D, Acquadro C and de la Loge C (2005) Translating and evaluating questionnaires: Cultural issues for international research. In: FayersPM and HaysRD (eds), *Assessing Quality of Life in Clinical Trials: Methods and Practice* (2nd edn). Oxford, Oxford University Press.

Martin F, Camfield L, Rodham K, Kliempt P and Ruta D (2007) Twelve years' experience with the Patient Generated Index (PGI) of quality of life: A graded structured review. *Quality of Life Research* **16**: 705–715.

Martin M, Blaisdell B, Kwong JW and Bjorner JB (2004) The Short-Form Headache Impact Test (HIT-6) was psychometrically equivalent in nine languages. *Journal of Clinical Epidemiology* **57**: 1271–1278.

Marx RG, Bombardier C, Hogg-Johnson S and Wright JG (1999) Clinimetric and psychometric strategies for development of a health measurement scale. *Journal of Clinical Epidemiology* **52**: 105–111.

Matthews JNS, Altman DG, Campbell MJ and Royston P (1990) Analysis of serial measurements in medical research. *British Medical Journal* **300**: 230–235.

McBride JR (1997) Research antecedents of applied adaptive testing. In: SandsWA, WatersBK and McBrideJR (eds), *Computerized Adaptive Testing: From Inquiry to Operation*. Washington, American Psychological Association.

McColl E and Fayers PM (2005) Context effects and proxy assessments. In: FayersPM and HaysRD (eds), *Assessing Quality of Life in Clinical Trials: Methods and Practice* (2nd edn). Oxford, Oxford University Press.

McCormack HM, Horne DJ and Sheather S (1988) Clinical applications of visual analogue scales: A critical review. *Psychological Medicine* **18**: 1007–1019.

McCormack K, Grant A and Scott N (2004) Value of updating a systematic review in surgery using individual patient data. *British Journal of Surgery* **91**: 495–499.

McDonald RP (1999) *Test Theory: A Unified Treatment*. Mahwah, NJ, Lawrence Erlbaum.

McDowell I and Newell C (2006) *Measuring Health: A Guide to Rating Scales and Questionnaires* (3rd edn). New York, Oxford University Press.

McEwan MJ, Espie CA, Metcalfe J, Brodie MJ and Wilson MT (2004) Quality of life and psychosocial development in adolescents with epilepsy: A qualitative investigation using focus group methods. *Seizure* **13**: 15–31.

McGraw KO and Wong SP (1996) Forming inferences about some intraclass correlation coefficients. *Psychological Methods* **1**: 30–46.

McHorney CA and Cohen AS (2000) Equating health status measures with item response theory: Illustrations with functional status items. *Medical Care* **38** (suppl II): 43–59.

McIntosh CM (2012) Improving the evaluation of model fit in confirmatory factor analysis: A commentary on Gundy CM, Fayers, PM, Groenvold, M, Petersen MAa *et al. Quality of Life Research* **21**: 1619–1621.

McKenzie L and van der Pol M (2009) Mapping the EORTC QLQ C-30 onto the EQ-5D instrument: The potential to estimate QALY's without generic preference data. *Value in Health* **12**: 167–17.

Medical Research Council Lung Cancer Working Party (1992) A Medical Research Council (MRC) randomized trial of palliative radiotherapy with 2 fractions or a single fraction in patients with inoperable non-small-cell lung cancer (NSCLC) and poor performance status. *British Journal of Cancer* **65**: 934–941.

Medical Research Council Lung Cancer Working Party (1996) Randomised trial of four-drug vs. less intensive two-drug chemotherapy in the palliative treatment of patients with small-cell lung cancer (SCLC) and poor prognosis. *British Journal of Cancer* **73**: 406–413.

Melzack R (1975) The McGill Pain Questionnaire: Major properties and scoring methods. *Pain* **1**: 277–299.

Melzack R (1987) The short-form McGill Pain Questionnaire. *Pain* **30**: 191–197.

Moher D, Hopewell S, Schulz KF, Montori V *et al.*, for the CONSORT Group (2010) CONSORT 2010 Explanation and Elaboration: Updated guidelines for reporting parallel group randomised trial. *British Medical Journal* **340**: c869.

Moher D, Liberati A, Tetzlaff J, Altman DG, The PRISMA Group (2009) Preferred Reporting Items for Systematic Reviews and Meta-Analyses: The PRISMA Statement. *British Medical Journal* **339**: b2535.

Mokkink LB, Terwee CB, Patrick DL, Alonso J *et al.* (2010) The COSMIN checklist for assessing the methodological quality of studies on measurement properties of health status measurement instruments: An international Delphi study. *Quality of Life Research* **19**:539–549.

Morton AP and Dobson AJ (1990) Analyzing ordered categorical data from 2 independent samples. *British Medical Journal* **301**: 971–973.

Moum T (1988) Yea-saying and mood-of-the-day effects in self-reported quality of life. *Social Indicators Research* **20**: 117–139.

Muraki E and Bock RD (2003) *PARSCALE-4: IRT item analysis and test scoring for rating-scale data [Computer software]*. Chicago, Scientific Software International.

Murray C (1997) *Understanding DALYs*. *Journal of Health Economics* **16**: 703–730.

Muthén BO and Kaplan D (1992) A comparison of some methodologies for the factor-analysis of non-normal Likert variables: A note on the size of the model. *British Journal of Mathematical and Statistical Psychology* **45**: 19–30.

Muthén LK and Muthén BO (2002) How to use a Monte Carlo study to decide on sample size and determine power. *Structural Equation Modeling* **4**: 559–620.

Muthén LK and Muthén BO (2010) *Mplus User's Guide* (6th edn). Los Angeles, CA, Muthén & Muthén.

Nager CW, Brubaker L, Daneshgari F, Litman HJ *et al.* (2009) Design of the Value of Urodynamic Evaluation (ValUE) trial: A non-inferiority randomized trial of preoperative urodynamic investigations. *Contemporary Clinical Trials* **30**: 531–539.

Nelson EC, Landgraf JM, Hays RD, Wasson JH and Kirk JW (1990) The functional status of patients: How can it be measured in physicians' offices? *Medical Care* **28**: 1111–1126.

NICE: National Institute for Health and Care Excellence (2013) Guide to the methods of technology appraisal 2013. (Download from <http://publications.nice.org.uk/pmg9>).

Nordic Myeloma Study Group (1996) Interferon-alpha2b added to melphalan-prednisone for initial and maintenance therapy in multiple myeloma. *Annals of Internal Medicine* **124**: 212–222.

Norman GR (2003) Hi! How are you? Response shift, implicit theories and differing epistemologies. *Quality of Life Research* **12**: 239–249.

Norman GR (2010) Likert scales, levels of measurement and the 'laws' of statistics. *Advances in Health Sciences Education* **15**: 625–632.

Norman GR (2012) Sample size calculations: Should the emperor's clothes be off the peg or made to measure? *British Medical Journal* **345**: e5278.

Norman GR, Sloan JA and Wyrwich KW (2003) Interpretation of changes in health-related quality of life: The remarkable universality of a half a standard deviation. *Medical Care* **41**: 582–592.

Norquist JM, Fitzpatrick R, Dawson J and Jenkinson C (2004) Comparing alternative Rasch-based methods vs. raw scores in measuring change in health. *Medical Care* **42**: I25–I36.

Nunnally J and Bernstein I (1994) *Psychometric Theory* (3rd edn). New York, McGraw-Hill.

O'Connell KA and Skevington SM (2012) An international quality of life instrument to assess wellbeing in adults who are HIV-positive: A short form of the WHOQOL-HIV (31 items). *AIDS and Behavior* **16**: 452–460.

Osoba D, Aaronson NK, Zee B, Sprangers MAG and te Velde A (1997) Modification of the EORTC QLQ-C30 (version 2.0) based upon content validity and reliability testing in large samples of patients with cancer. *Quality of Life Research* **6**: 103–108.

Osoba D, Rodrigues G, Myles J, Zee B and Pater J (1998) Interpreting the significance of changes in health-related quality-of-life scores. *Journal of Clinical Oncology* **16**: 139–144.

Osterlind SJ and Everson HT (2009) *Differential Item Functioning* (2nd edn). Thousand Oaks, CA, SAGE Publications.

Pallant JF and Tennant A (2007) An introduction to the Rasch measurement model: An example using the Hospital Anxiety and Depression Scale (HADS). *British Journal of Clinical Psychology* **46**: 1–18.

Patrick DL and Erickson P (1993) *Health Status and Health Policy: Quality of Life in Healthcare Evaluation and Resource Allocation.* New York, Oxford University press.

Pauler DK, McCoy S and Moinpour C (2003) Pattern mixture models for longitudinal quality of life studies in advanced stage disease. *Statistics in Medicine* **22**: 795–809.

Perneger TV (1998) What's wrong with Bonferroni adjustments. *British Medical Journal* **316**: 1236–1238.

Petersen MAa, Giesinger JM, Holzner B, Arraras JI *et al.* (2013) Psychometric evaluation of the EORTC computerized adaptive test (CAT) fatigue item pool. *Quality of Life Research* **22**: 2443–2454.

Petersen MAa, Groenvold M, Aaronson N, Brenne E *et al.* for the EORTC Quality of Life Group (2005) Scoring based on item response theory did not alter the measurement ability of the EORTC QLQ-C30 scales. *Journal of Clinical Epidemiology* **58**: 902–908.

Petersen MAa, Groenvold M, Aaronson N, Fayers PM *et al.* (2006) Multidimensional computerized adaptive testing of the EORTC QLQ-C30: basic developments and evaluations. *Quality of Life Research* **15**: 315–329.

Petersen MAa, Groenvold M, Aaronson NK, Chie W-C *et al.* (2010) Development of computerised adaptive testing (CAT) for the EORTC QLQ-C30 dimensions—General approach and initial results for physical functioning. *European Journal of Cancer* **46**: 1352–1358.

Petersen MAa, Groenvold M, Aaronson NK, Chie W-C *et al.* (2011) Development of computerized adaptive testing (CAT) for the EORTC QLQ-C30 physical functioning dimension. *Quality of Life Research* **20**: 479–490.

Petersen MAa, Groenvold M, Bjorner J, Aaronson N *et al.* (2003) Use of differential item functioning analysis to assess the equivalence of translations of a questionnaire. *Quality of Life Research* **12**: 373–385.

Pfeffer RI, Kurosaki TT, Harrah CH Jr., Chance JM and Filos S (1982) Measurement of functional activities in older adults in the community. *Journal of Gerontology* **37**: 323–329.

Post WJ, Buijs C, Stolk R, de Vries EGE and le Cessie S (2010) The analysis of longitudinal quality of life measures with informative drop-out: A pattern mixture approach. *Quality of Life Research* **19**: 137–148.

Priestman TJ and Baum M (1976) Evaluation of quality of life in patients receiving treatment for advanced breast cancer. *Lancet* **1**: 899–901.

Quinten C, Coens C, Mauer M, Comte S *et al.* (2009) Baseline quality of life as a prognostic indicator of survival: A meta-analysis of individual patient data from EORTC clinical trials. *Lancet Oncology* **10**: 865–71.

Ramsey S, Willke R, Briggs A, Brown R *et al.* (2005) Good research practice for cost-effectiveness analysis alongside clinical trials: The ISPOR RCT-CEA Task Force report. *Value in Health* **8**: 521–533.

Rapkin BD and Schwartz CE (2004) Toward a theoretical model of quality-of-life appraisal: Implications of findings from studies of response shift. *Health and Quality of Life Outcomes* **2**: 14.

Rasbash J, Steele F, Browne WJ and Goldstein H. (2015) *A User's Guide to MLwiN v2.33*. Centre for Multilevel Modelling, University of Bristol.

Rasch G (1960) *Probabilistic Models for Some Intelligence and Attainment Tests*. Copenhagen, Danish Institute for Educational Research.

Raudenbush SW, Bryk AS and Congdon R (2004) *HLM 6 for Windows*. Lincolnwood IL, Scientific Software International Inc.

Ravens-Sieberer U, Wille N, Badia X, Bonsel G *et al.* (2010) Feasibility, reliability, and validity of the EQ-5D-Y: Results from a multinational study. *Quality of Life Research* **19**: 887–897.

Redelmeier DA, Guyatt GH and Goldstein RS (1996) Assessing the minimal important difference in symptoms: A comparison of two techniques. *Journal of Clinical Epidemiology* **49**: 1215–1219.

Reeve BB, Hays RD, Bjorner JB, Cook KF *et al.* (2007) Psychometric evaluation and calibration of health-related quality of life item banks: Plans for the Patient-Reported Outcomes Measurement Information System (PROMIS). *Medical Care* **45**(Suppl. 1): S22–S31.

Reeve BB, Wyrwich KW, Wu AW, Velikova G *et al.* (2013) ISOQOL recommends minimum standards for patient-reported outcome measures used in patient-centered outcomes and comparative effectiveness research. *Quality of Life Research* **22**: 1889–1905.

Regidor E, Barrio G, de la Fuente L, Domingo A *et al.* (1999) Association between educational level and health related quality of life in Spanish adults. *Journal of Epidemiology & Community Health* **53**: 75–82.

Reise SP and Waller NG (2009) Item response theory and clinical measurement. *Annual Review of Clinical Psychology* **5**: 27–48.

Reise SP, Morizot J and Hays RD (2007) The role of the bifactor model in resolving dimensionality issues in health outcomes measures. *Quality of Life Research* **16**(suppl 1): 19–31.

Revicki D, Hays RD, Cella D and Sloan J (2008) Recommended methods for determining responsiveness and minimally important differences for patient-reported outcomes. *Journal of Clinical Epidemiology* **61**: 102–109.

Revicki DA (2005) Reporting analyses from clinical trials. In: FayersPM and HaysRD (eds), *Assessing Quality of Life in Clinical Trials: Methods and Practice* (2nd edn). Oxford, Oxford University Press.

Revicki DA, Feeny D, Hunt TL and Cole BF (2006) Analyzing oncology clinical trial data using the Q-TWiST method: Clinical importance and sources for health state preference data. *Quality of Life Research* **15**: 411–423.

Review Manager (RevMan) [Computer program] (2011) Version 5.1. Copenhagen, The Nordic Cochrane Centre, The Cochrane Collaboration. (Download from <www.ims.cochrane.org/revman/>).

Riley RD, Lambert PC, Abo-Zaid G (2010) Meta-analysis of individual participant data: Conduct, rationale and reporting. *British Medical Journal* **340**: c221.

Ring L, Höfer S, Heuston F, Harris D and O'Boyle CA (2005) Response shift masks the treatment impact on patient reported outcomes (PROs): the example of individual quality of life in edentulous patients. *Health and Quality of Life Outcomes* **3**: 55.

Rose M, Bjorner JB, Becker J, Fries JF and Ware JE (2008) Evaluation of a preliminary physical function item bank supported the expected advantages of the Patient-Reported Outcomes Measurement Information System (PROMIS). *Journal of Clinical Epidemiology* **61**: 17–33.

Rosenberg M (1965) *Society and the Adolescent Self Image*. Princeton, NJ, Princeton University Press.

Rothman KJ (1976) *Causes*. American Journal of Epidemiology **104**: 587–592.

Rothman M, Burke L, Erickson P, Leidy NK, Patrick DL and Petrie CD (2009) Use of existing patient-reported outcome (PRO) instruments and their modification: The ISPOR Good Research Practices for Evaluating and Documenting Content Validity for the Use of Existing Instruments and Their Modification PRO Task Force Report. *Value in Health* **12**: 1075–1083.

Rowen D, Brazier JE, Young TA, Gaugris S *et al.* (2011) Deriving a preference-based measure for cancer using the EORTC QLQ-C30. *Value in Health* **14**: 721–731.

Rubin DB (1987) *Multiple Imputation for Nonresponse in Surveys*. New York, John Wiley & Sons.

Russell LB, Hubley AM, Palepu A and Zumbo BD (2006) Does weighting capture what's important? Revisiting subjective importance weighting with a quality of life measure. *Social Indicators Research* **75**: 141–167.

Ruta DA, Garratt AM, Leng M, Russell IT and Macdonald LM (1994) A new approach to the measurement of quality-of-life: The Patient Generated Index. *Medical Care* **32**: 1109–1126.

Ryan M (1999) Using conjoint analysis to take account of patient preferences and go beyond health outcomes: An application to in vitro fertilisation. *Social Science & Medicine* **48**: 535–546.

Ryan M and Gerard K (2005) Discrete choice experiments. In: FayersPM and HaysRD (eds), *Assessing Quality of Life in Clinical Trials: Methods and Practice* (2nd edn). Oxford, Oxford University Press.

Ryan M, Netten A, Skåtun D and Smith P (2006) Using discrete choice experiments to estimate a preference-based measure of outcome – An application to social care for older people. *Journal of Health Economics* **25**: 927–944.

Saban KL, Bryant FB, Reda DJ, Stroupe KT and Hynes DM (2010) Measurement invariance of the kidney disease and quality of life instrument (KDQOL-SF) across Veterans and non-Veterans. *Health and Quality of Life Outcomes* **8**: 120.

Sadura A, Pater J, Osoba D, Levine M *et al.* (1992) Quality-of-life assessment: Patient compliance with questionnaire completion. *Journal of the National Cancer Institute* **84**: 1023–1026.

Salek S (2004) *Compendium of Quality of Life Instruments: Volume 6.* Haslemere, Euromed Communications Ltd.

Salmon P, Manzi F and Valori RM (1996) Measuring the meaning of life for patients with incurable cancer: The Life Evaluation Questionnaire (LEQ). *European Journal of Cancer* **32A**: 755–760.

SAS Institute Inc. (2008) *SAS/STAT® 9.2 User's Guide.* Cary, NC, SAS Institute Inc.

Sassi F (2006) Calculating QALYs, comparing QALY and DALY calculations. *Health Policy and Planning* **21**: 402–408.

Schag CA, Ganz PA, Kahn B and Petersen L (1992) Assessing the needs and quality of life of patients with HIV infection: Development of the HIV Overview of Problems – Evaluation System (HOPES). *Quality of Life Research* **1**: 397–413.

Schulz KF and Grimes DA (2002) Sample size slippage in randomised trials: Exclusions and the lost and wayward. *Lancet* **359**: 781–785.

Schulz KF, Altman DG and Moher D for the CONSORT Group (2010) The CONSORT 2010 statement: Updated guidelines for reporting parallel group randomised trials. *British Medical Journal* **340**: c332.

Schulz KF, Chalmers I, Hayes RJ and Altman D (1995) Empirical evidence of bias: Dimensions of methodological quality associated with estimates of treatment effects in controlled trials. *Journal of the American Medical Association* **273**: 408–412.

Schwartz CE and Sprangers MAG (1999) Methodological approaches for assessing response shift in longitudinal health-related quality-of-life research. *Social Science & Medicine* **48**: 1531–1548.

Schwartz CE and Sprangers MAG (2010) Guidelines for improving the stringency of response shift research using the then-test. *Quality of Life Research* **19**: 455–464.

Schwartz CE, Ahmed S, Sawatzky R, Sajobi T *et al.* (2013) Guidelines for secondary analysis in search of response shift. *Quality of Life Research* **22**: 2663–2673.

Schwartz CE, Bode R, Repucci N, Becker J, Sprangers MAG and Fayers PM (2006) The clinical significance of adaptation to changing health: A meta-analysis of response shift. *Quality of Life Research* **15**: 1533–1550.

Schwartz N and Sudman S (1994) *Autobiographical Memory and the Validity of Retrospective Reports.* New York, Springer-Verlag.

Scott N, Go PMNYH, Graham P, McCormack K *et al.* (2001) Open mesh versus non-mesh for groin hernia repair. *The Cochrane Database of Systematic Reviews Issue 3.*

Scott NW, Fayers PM, Aaronson NK, Bottomley A *et al.* (2007) The use of differential item functioning analyses to identify cultural differences in responses to the EORTC QLQ-C30. *Quality of Life Research* **16**: 115–129.

Scott NW, Fayers PM, Aaronson NK, Bottomley A *et al*. (2009a) Differential item functioning (DIF) in the EORTC QLQ-C30: a comparison of baseline, on-treatment and off-treatment data. *Quality of Life Research* **18**: 381–388.

Scott NW, Fayers PM, Aaronson NK, Bottomley A *et al*. (2009b) The practical impact of differential item functioning (DIF) analyses in a health-related quality of life instrument. *Quality of Life Research* **18**: 1125–1130.

Scott NW, Fayers PM, Aaronson NK, Bottomley A *et al*. (2010) Differential item functioning (DIF) analyses of health-related quality of life instruments using logistic regression. *Health and Quality of Life Outcomes* **8**: 81.

Scott NW, Fayers PM, Aaronson NK, Bottomley A, de Graeff A, Groenvold M, Gundy C, Koller M, Petersen MA, Sprangers MAG on behalf of the EORTC Quality of Life Group (2008) *EORTC QLQ-C30 Reference Values* (2nd edn). Brussels, EORTC. (Download from <http://groups.eortc.be/qol/manuals>).

Scott NW, Fayers PM, Bottomley A, Aaronson NK *et al*. on behalf of the EORTC and the Quality of Life Cross-Cultural Meta-Analysis Group (2006) Comparing translations of the EORTC QLQ-C30 using differential item functioning analyses. *Quality of Life Research* **15**: 1103–1115.

Selby PJ, Chapman JA, Etazadi-Amoli J, Dalley D and Boyd NF (1984) The development of a method for assessing the quality of life in cancer patients. *British Journal of Cancer* **50**: 13–22.

Senn S (2003) *Cross-over Trials in Clinical Research* (2nd edn). Hoboken, NJ, J Wiley & Sons.

Shah S, Vanclay F and Cooper B (1989) Improving the sensitivity of the Barthel Index for stroke rehabilitation. *Journal of Clinical Epidemiology* **42**: 703–709.

Sharp DM, Walker MB, Chaturvedi, Upadhyay S *et al*. (2010) A randomised, controlled trial of the psychological effects of reflexology in early breast cancer. *European Journal of Cancer* **46**: 312–322.

Shaw GB ([1900] 1972) *Collected Letters Vol. 2: (1898–1910)*. Dan Laurence (ed.), page 203; London, Max Reinhart.

Shrout PE and Fleiss JL (1979) Intraclass correlations: Uses in assessing rater reliability. *Psychological Bulletin* **86**: 420–428.

Silveira AP, Gonçalves J, Sequeira T, Ribeiro C *et al*. (2010) Patient reported outcomes in head and neck cancer: Selecting instruments for quality of life integration in clinical protocols. *Head & Neck Oncology* **2**: 32.

Simmonds MC, Higgins JPT, Stewart LA, Tierney JF, Clarke MJ, Thompson SG (2005) Meta-analysis of individual patient data from randomized trials: A review of methods used in practice. *Clinical Trials* **2**: 209–217.

Slevin ML, Stubbs L, Plant HJ, Wilson P *et al*. (1990) Attitudes to chemotherapy: Comparing views of patients with cancer with those of doctors, nurses, and general public. *British Medical Journal* **300**: 1458–1460.

Sloan JA, Frost MH, Berzon R, Dueck A *et al*. (2006) The clinical significance of quality of life assessments in oncology: A summary for clinicians. *Supportive Care in Cancer* **14**: 988–998.

Smets EMA, Garssen B, Bonke B and de Haes JCJM (1995) The Multidimensional Fatigue Inventory (MFI) psychometric qualities of an instrument to assess fatigue. *Journal of Psychosomatic Research* **39**: 315–325.

Smets EMA, Visser MR, Willems-Groot AF, Garssen B *et al*. (1998) Fatigue and radiotherapy: (B) experience in patients 9 months following treatment. *British Journal of Cancer* **78**: 907–912.

Snyder CF, Aaronson NK, Choucair AK, Elliott TE *et al.* (2012) Implementing patient-reported outcomes assessment in clinical practice: A review of the options and considerations. *Quality of Life Research* **21**: 1305–1314.

Solans M, Pane S, Estrada M-D, Serra-Sutton V *et al.* (2008) Health-related quality of life measurement in children and adolescents: A systematic review of generic and disease-specific instruments. *Value in Health* **11**: 742–764.

Spearman C (1904) General intelligence objectively determined and measured. *American Journal of Psychology* **15**: 201–293.

Spector PE (1992) *Summated Rating Scale Construction: An Introduction.* London, Sage Publications.

Spitzer RL (2003) Can some gay men and lesbians change their sexual orientation? *Archive of Sexual Behavior* **32**: 402–417.

Spitzer RL (2012) Spitzer reassesses his 2003 study of reparative therapy of homosexuality (Letter to the Editor). *Archive of Sexual Behavior* **41**: 757.

Spitzer RL, Kroenke K, Williams JBW (1999) Validation and utility of a self-report version of PRIME-MD: The PHQ primary care study. Primary Care Evaluation of Mental Disorders. *Patient Health Questionnaire. Journal of the American Medical Association* **282**: 1737–1744.

Sprangers MAG and Schwartz CE (1999) Integrating response shift into health-related quality of life research: A theoretical model. *Social Science & Medicine* **48**: 1507–1515.

Sprangers MAG, van Dam FSAM, Broerson J, Lodder L *et al.* (1999) Revealing response shift in longitudinal research on fatigue: Use of the then-test approach. *Acta Oncologica* **38**: 709–718.

Sprent P and Smeeton NC (2007) *Applied Nonparametric Statistical Methods* (4th edn). Boca Raton, FL, Chapman and Hall/CRC.

Stansbury JP, Ried LD, Velozo CA (2006) Unidimensionality and bandwidth in the Center for Epidemiologic Studies Depression (CES-D) Scale. *Journal of Personality Assessment* **86**: 10–22.

Stanton AL, Danoff-Burg S, Cameron CL, Snider PR and Kirk SB (1999) Social comparison and adjustment to breast cancer: An experimental examination of upward affiliation and downward evaluation. *Health Psychology* **18**: 151–158.

StataCorp (2013) *STATA Statistical Software: Release 13.* College Station, TX, StataCorp LP.

Sterne JA, White IR, Carlin JB, Spratt M *et al.* (2009) Multiple imputation for missing data in epidemiological and clinical research: Potential and pitfalls. *British Medical Journal* **338**: b2393.

Stone AA, Broderick JE, Schiffman SS and Schwartz JE (2004) Understanding recall of weekly pain from a momentary assessment perspective: Absolute agreement, between- and within-person consistency, and judged change in weekly pain. *Pain* **107**: 61–69.

Stout W and Roussos L (1996) *SIBTEST Manual.* Statistical Laboratory for Educational and Psychological Measurement, University of Illinois at Urbana-Champaign.

Strack F, Martin LI and Schwarz N (1988) Priming and communication: Social determinants of information use in judgements of life satisfaction. *European Journal of Social Psychology* **18**: 429–442.

Streiner DL and Norman GR (2008) *Health Measurement Scales: A Practical Guide to their Development and Use* (4th edn). Oxford, Oxford Medical Publications.

Suñer IJ, Kokame GT, Yu E, Ward J *et al.* (2009) Responsiveness of NEI VFQ-25 to changes in visual acuity in neovascular AMD: Validation studies from two phase 3 clinical trials. *Investigative Ophthalmology & Visual Science* **50**: 3629–3635.

Svensson E (2012) Different ranking approaches defining association and agreement measures of paired ordinal data. *Statistics in Medicine* **31**: 3104–3117.

Tai B-C and Machin D (2014) *Regression Methods for Medical Research*. Chichester, Wiley Blackwell

Temel JS, Greer JA, Muzikansky A, Gallagher ER *et al.* (2010) Early palliative care for patients with metastatic non-small-cell lung cancer. *New England Journal of Medicine* **363**: 733–742.

Teresi JA (2006) Overview of quantitative measurement methods: Equivalence, invariance, and differential item functioning in health applications. *Medical Care* **44** (Suppl 3): S39–S49.

Terwee CB, Bot SDM, de Boer MR, van der Windt DAWM *et al.* (2007) Quality criteria were proposed for measurement properties of health status questionnaires. *Journal of Clinical Epidemiology* **60:** 34–42.

Terwee CB, Dekker FW, Wiersing WM, Prummel MF and Bossuyt PMM (2003) On assessing responsiveness of health-related quality of life instruments: Guidelines for instrument evaluation. *Quality of Life Research* **12**: 349–362.

Terwee CB, Roorda LD, DFekker J, Bierma-Zeinstra SM *et al.* (2010) Mind the MIC: Large variation among populations and methods. *Journal of Clinical Epidemiology* **63**: 524–534.

Testa MA, Anderson RB, Nackley JF and Hollenberg NK (1993) Quality of life and antihypertensive therapy in men: A comparison of captopril with enalapril: The Quality-of-Life Hypertension Study Group. *New England Journal of Medicine* **328**: 907–913.

Thissen D (2003) *MULTILOG 7: Multiple categorical item analysis and test scoring using item response theory [Computer software]*. Chicago, IL, Scientific Software International.

Thissen D, Reeve BB, Bjorner JB and Chang C-H (2007) Methodological issues for building item banks and computerized adaptive scales. *Quality of Life Research* **16**: 109–119.

Tong A, Sainsbury P and Craig J (2007) Consolidated criteria for reporting qualitative research (COREQ): a 32-item checklist for interviews and focus groups. *International Journal for Quality in Health Care* **19**: 349–357.

Torrance GW, Feeny DH, Furlong WJ, Barr RD *et al.* (1996) Multi-attribute utility function for a comprehensive health status classification system. Health Utilities Index Mark 2. *Medical Care* **34**: 702–722.

Tourangeau R (1984) *Cognitive Science and Survey Methods* (Vol. 73). Washington, DC, National Academy Press.

Tourangeau R, Rips LJ and Rasinski K (2000) *The Psychology of Survey Response*. Cambridge, Cambridge University Press.

Traa MJ, Orsini RG, Den Oudsten BL, De Vries J *et al.* (2014) Measuring the health-related quality of life and sexual functioning of patients with rectal cancer: Does type of treatment matter? *International Journal of Cancer* **134**: 979–987.

Tsuchiya A, Brazier J and Roberts J (2006) Comparison of valuation methods used to generate the EQ-5D and the SF-6D value sets. *Journal of Health Economics* **25**: 334–346.

Turner D, Griffiths AM, Steinhart AH, Otley AR and Beaton DE (2009a) Mathematical weighting of a clinimetric index (Pediatric Ulcerative Colitis Activity Index) was superior to the judgmental approach. *Journal of Clinical Epidemiology* **62**: 738–744.

Turner D, Schünemann HJ, Griffith LE, Beaton DE *et al.* (2009b) Using the entire cohort in the receiver operating characteristic analysis maximizes precision of the minimal important difference. *Journal of Clinical Epidemiology* **62**: 374–379.

Turner D, Schünemann HJ, Griffith LE, Beaton DE *et al.* (2010) The minimal detectable change cannot reliably replace the minimal important difference. *Journal of Clinical Epidemiology* **63**: 28–36.

United States Department of Health and Human Services Food and Drug Administration (FDA) (2009) Guidance for Industry: Patient-reported outcome measures: Use in medical product development to support labelling claims. (Download from <www.fda.gov/downloads/Drugs/GuidanceComplianceRegulatoryInformation/Guidances/UCM193282.pdf>).

United States Department of Health and Human Services Food and Drug Administration (FDA) (2010) Guidance for Industry: Non-Inferiority Clinical Trials (Download from <http://www.fda.gov/downloads/Drugs/GuidanceComplianceRegulatoryInformation/Guidances/UCM202140.pdf>).

Valderas JM, Ferrer M, Mendivil J, Garin O *et al.* (2008) Development of EMPRO: A tool for the standardized assessment of patient-reported outcome measures. *Value in Health* **11**: 700–708.

van de Poll-Franse LV, Mols F, Gundy CM, Creutzberg CL *et al.* (2011) Normative data for the EORTC QLQ-C30 and EORTC-sexuality items in the general Dutch population. *European Journal of Cancer* **47**: 667–675.

Veenhof C, Bijlsma JW, Van den Ende CH, Van Dijk GM, Pisters MF and Dekker J (2006) Psychometric evaluation of osteoarthritis questionnaires: A systematic review of the literature. *Arthritis and Rheumatism* **55**: 480–492.

Visser MRM, Oort FJ, van Lanschott JB, van der Velden J *et al.* (2013) The role of recalibration response shift in explaining bodily pain in cancer patients undergoing invasive surgery: An empirical investigation of the Sprangers and Schwartz model. *Psycho-Oncology* **22**: 515–522.

Von Winterfeld D and Edwards W (1982) Costs and payoffs in perceptual research. *Psychological Bulletin* **91**: 131–138.

Wainer H (2000) *Computerized Adaptive Testing: A Primer* (2nd edn). Mahwah, NJ, Lawrence Erlbaum.

Walter SD, Eliasziw M and Donner A (1998) Sample size and optimal designs for reliability studies. *Statistics in Medicine* **17**: 101–110.

Walters SJ and Campbell MJ (2005) The use of bootstrap methods for estimating sample size and analysing health-related quality of life outcomes. *Statistics in Medicine* **24**: 1075–1102.

Wang J, Zhao Z, Barber B, Sherrill B, Peeters M and Wiezorek J (2011) A Q-TWiST analysis comparing panitumumab plus best supportive care (BSC) with BSC alone in patients with wild-type KRAS metastatic colorectal cancer. *British Journal of Cancer* **10**: 1848–1853.

Ware JE Jr., Harris WJ, Gandek B, Rogers BW and Reese PR (1998) *MAP-R Multitrait/Multi-Item Analysis Program – Revised, for Windows: User's Guide*. Boston, Health Assessment Lab.

Ware JE Jr, Kosinski M, Bjorner JB, Bayliss MS *et al.* (2003) Applications of computerized adaptive testing (CAT) to the assessment of headache impact. *Quality of Life Research* **12**: 935–952.

Ware JE Jr, Snow KK, Kosinski M and Gandek B (1993) *SF-36 Health Survey Manual and Interpretation Guide.* Boston, New England Medical Centre.

Watt T, Rasmussen ⊠K, Groenvold M, Bjorner JB *et al.* (2008) Improving a newly developed patient-reported outcome for thyroid patients, using cognitive interviewing. *Quality of Life Research* **17**: 1009–1017.

Weir JP (2005) Quantifying test-retest reliability using the intraclass correlation coefficient and the SEM. *Journal of Strength and Conditioning Research* **19**: 231–240.

Wettergren L, Kettis-Lindblad A, Sprangers MAG and Ring L (2009) The use, feasibility and psychometric properties of an individualised quality-of-life instrument: A systematic review of the SEIQoL-DW. *Quality of Life Research* **18**: 737–746.

Wheelwright S, Darlington A-S, Fitzsimmons D, Fayers PM *et al.* (2013) International validation of the European Organisation for Research and Treatment of Cancer QLQ-ELD14 questionnaire for assessment of health related quality of life in elderly patients with cancer. *British Journal of Cancer* **109**: 852–858.

Whistance RN, Conroy T, Chie W, Costantini A *et al.* (2009) Clinical and psychometric validation of the EORTC QLQ-CR29 questionnaire module to assess health related quality of life in patients with colorectal cancer. *European Journal of Cancer* **45**: 3017–3026.

Whitehead J (1993) Sample-size calculations for ordered categorical-data. *Statistics in Medicine* **12**: 2257–2271.

Wild D, Eremco S, Mear I, Martin M *et al.* (2009) Multinational trials – recommendations on the translations required, approaches to using the same language in different countries, and the approaches to support pooling the data: The ISPOR Patient-Reported Outcomes Translation and Linguistic Validation Good Research Practices Task Force report. *Value in Health* **12**: 430–440.

Wild D, Grove A, Martin M, Eremco S *et al.* (2005) Principles of good practice for the translation and cultural adaptation process for patient-reported outcomes (PRO) measures: Report of the ISPOR Task Force for Translation and Cultural Adaptation. *Value in Health* **8**: 94–104.

Willis GB (2005) *Cognitive Interviewing: A Tool for Improving Questionnaire Design.* Thousand Oaks, CA, SAGE Publications.

Wills TA (1981) Downward comparison principles in social psychology. *Psychological Bulletin* **90**: 245–271.

Wisløff F, Hjorth M, Kaasa S and Westin J (1996) Effect of interferon on the health-related quality of life of multiple myeloma patients: Results of a Nordic randomized trial comparing melphalan-prednisone to melphalan-prednisone + alpha-interferon: The Nordic Myeloma Study Group. *British Journal of Haematology* **94**: 324–332.

Wood JV, Taylor SE and Lichtman RR (1985) Social comparison in adjustment to breast cancer. *Journal of Personality and Social Psychology* **49**: 1169–1183.

World Health Organization (1948) *Constitution of the World Health Organization.* Geneva, WHO Basic Documents.

Wright JG and Young NL (1997) A comparison of different indices of responsiveness. *Journal of Clinical Epidemiology* **50**: 239–246.

Wu CH (2008) Can we weight satisfaction score with importance ranks across life domains? *Social Indicators Research* **86**: 468–480.

Wyrwich KW, Bullinger M, Aaronson NK, Hays RD *et al.* (2005) Estimating clinically significant differences in quality of life outcomes. *Quality of Life Research* **14**: 285–295.

Wyrwich KW, Norquist JM, Lenderking and Acaster S for the Industry Advisory Committee of ISOQOL (2013) Methods for interpreting change over time in patient-reported outcome measures. *Quality of Life Research* **22**: 475–483.

Young T, de Haes JCJM, Curran D, Fayers PM *et al.* on behalf of the EORTC Quality of Life Study Group (2002) *Guidelines for Assessing Quality of Life in EORTC Clinical Trials*. Brussels, EORTC. (Download from <http://groups.eortc.be/qol/manuals>).

Youngblut JM and Casper GR (1993) Focus on psychometrics: Single-item indicators in nursing research. *Research in Nursing & Health* **16**: 459–465.

Zigmond AS and Snaith RP (1983) The Hospital Anxiety and Depression Scale. *Acta Psychiatrica Scandinavica* **67**: 361–370.

Zou GY (2012) Sample size formulas for estimating intraclass correlation coefficients with precision and assurance. *Statistics in Medicine* **31**: 3972–3981.

Zumbo BD (1999) *A Handbook on the Theory and Methods of Differential Item Functioning (DIF): Logistic Regression Modeling as a Unitary Framework for Binary and Likert-type (Ordinal) Item Scores*. Ottawa, ON, Directorate of Human Resources Research and Evaluation, National Defense Headquarters.

Zung WWK (1983) A self-rating Pain and Distress Scale. *Psychosomatics* **24**: 887–894.

Index